K. Kayser

Analytical Lung Pathology

With 40 Figures

Springer-Verlag
Berlin Heidelberg New York
London Paris Tokyo
Hong Kong Barcelona
Budapest

Professor Klaus Kayser, M.D., Ph.D.
Head, Department of Pathology
Thoraxklinik, W-6900 Heidelberg
Federal Republik of Germany

ISBN 3-540-54263-9 Springer-Verlag Berlin Heidelberg New York
ISBN 0-387-54263-9 Springer-Verlag New York Berlin Heidelberg

Printed in Hong Kong

Typesetting: Data conversion by comed, Heidelberg
Printing and binding: South Sea International Press Ltd., Hong Kong
19/3130/5 4 3 2 1 0 - Printed on acid-free paper

To Maria Consuelo

Preface

> So eine Arbeit wird eigentlich nie fertig, man muß sie für fertig erklären, wenn man nach Zeit und Umständen das möglichste getan hat.
>
> Johann Wolfgang von Goethe, Italienische Reise, 16. März 1787

The daily work of a pathologist is no longer limited to analyzing macroscopic and microscopic images, but has been extended to include other aspects relating to diagnosis and prognosis. Our understanding of the morphological features of a disease has now expanded to dynamic subcellular, cellular, and intercellular processes. Their recognition and analysis often require sophisticated and highly specific biochemical and biophysical techniques which can only be performed if the "general direction" of the search is known. Is the analysis of abnormal light-microscopic textures a useful and effective procedure allowing conclusions to be made about the severity of malfunctions? What is the set of the limited pattern of structures seen in various diseases? What are the corresponding radiological and clinical findings, and what are the patient's symptoms?
To answer these questions, information that is usually spread over a wide variety of specific books and articles must be collected and summarized. This book is meant to give the reader fast access to essential information about lung diseases. We thought it would be helpful to provide the reader with separate descriptions of each disease which may involve the lung, each description being divided into sections covering the major aspects of the disease. These aspects include definition, etiology/pathophysiology, clinical and radiological findings, and prognosis. The emphasis is on the microscopic findings. We have tried to divide these findings into consistent subdivisions which we have named "descriptors". These descriptors correspond to the same specific alterations of the lung parenchyma that are seen in various different diseases. They reflect the limited number of reaction patterns of the lung tissue, which are associated with a large number of possible underlying causes. Some of these descriptors are illustrated in the accompanying micrographs. Readers may use these components according to their needs or may neglect them if they are more used to evaluating diseases by retaining more general impressions.

The practical realization of the book would not have been possible without the assistance of Dr. Bernard Fox, Hans-Ulrich Burkhardt, John Moyers, Corinna Kayser and Gian Kayser, to whom I want to express my deep gratitude. Dr. B. Fox performed the corrections of the English manuscript. H.-U. Burkhardt was responsible for the layout and the final corrections and J. Moyers for the preparation of the microphotographs. C. Kayser and G. Kayser assisted in various technical matters such as proof correction and typing. I am also greatly endebted to my publishers for their cooperation and their assistance throughout the production of this book. In particular, I must thank my family for their patience and tolerance.

I hope that this book will not only be useful beside the microscope but will also offer new perspectives in the understanding and judging of morphological findings and, thus, be of benefit to patients.

Heidelberg, October 1991 Klaus Kayser, M.D., Ph.D.

Foreword

It is now clear that it is not respirology or respiratory medicine but pulmonary medicine that has evolved as one of the most exciting subspecialties within medicine. It has its roots in phthisiology, the art of dealing with consumption, and in physiology, i.e., the art of measuring airflow, lung volumes, and, finally, diffusion capacity. With these measurements now firmly established in everyday practice by the use of flexible fiberoptic bronchoscopy and lung lavage, which provides a window to the cellular components of the alveolar spaces, and with the widespread availability of open lung biopsy, we are most certainly in the Golden Age of lung biology.

For some, the bewildering architecture of the lung with its fractal branching patterns, and the yet to be discovered metabolic functions have always had a special attraction. After all, this is the organ that accommodates the entire blood flow during its passage between the ventricles of the heart, and also receives blood flow from both sides of the heart. It is also an organ with a bewildering number of cell types, an enormous number of different types of tumors, and two circulations – one of which (even today) we know very little about – and at the same time an organ which takes in air but most certainly is much more than just a pump.

The lungs are the environmental organ par excellence. They are vulnerable to attack from the blood side and from the air side. High blood flow and high airway pressure can also cause damages to these filter organs, which funtion in series with the large capillary bed of the liver. Yet at the same time, being open to the blood and to the air, they have an enormous concentration of antioxidants in the alveolar lining fluid and thus also a great potential for recovery and repair. We are truly at a watershed in pulmonary medicine. At this time we think we understand how lung volume changes affect the blood flow through Starling resistors and create waterfalls. We now learn that shear stress and stretch receptors affect ion channels and that distension activates metabolism of lung cells, perhaps even gene expression.

Cardiac catheterization, spirometry, exercise testing, sleep monitoring, and pharmacological tools like the metacholine and allergen provocation tests and the assessment of the degree of pulmonary vasodilation after infusion of prostacyclin that have expanded the armamentarium of the pulmonologist. The specialist has to be knowledgeable and manage diseases like the adult respiratory distress syndrome (ARDS), and he has to be constantly watchful for the appearance of new forms of occupational diseases like the "sick building syndrome" and "air conditioner lung", or "baker's asthma".

Modern transplant medicine provides a different group of clinical and investigational challanges. Clinical observation led to the description of once exotic fungal diseases in the immune compromised, and the acquired immune deficiency syndrome (AIDS) continues to impact on the field of pulmonary medicine not only because of the pulmonary infections, but also because of its association with severe pulmonary vascular disease. There are also familial pulmonary diseases to consider. Familial clusters of pulmonary hypertension have been described, and there is the genetic susceptibility to lung disease has been recognized; passive smoking is likely to affect the immune response in small children and may even determine their future handling of environmental stresses.

We are just beginning to recognize that the lung participates as an immunological organ in lymphocyte trafficking, that collapse of lung areas and microatelectasis may be important as pathogenetic factors in the development of interstitial lung disorders. It is against this background of challanges and new frontiers that the field of modern pulmonary medicine defines itself. The discovery of inflammatory mechanisms and the in-depth exploration of mediator and cytokine networks have changed our understanding of classic lung diseases like asthma. A reassessment, reinvestigation, and redefinition of old concepts regarding the structure and the function of the lung is under way. There incidence of lung cancer is increasing worldwide and international air travel is facilitating the spread of exotic lung diseases. It is thus perhaps time for pulmonary medicine to leave its exile in the sanatorium, where it has been sidelined for decades — at least in some countries. Professor Kayser's book, entitled Analytical Lung Pathology, certainly pays tribute to such an understanding of the field of lung medicine. This text, in alphabetical order from "abscess" to "zirkonium", does not shy away from listing commonly used drugs and drug toxicities, and it is comprehensive and suitable for storage in a data bank – ready for continual expansion and updating. The book goes far beyond describing tissue sections, tumor cell types, and special staining techniques. Emphasis is also placed on a discussion of epidemiological information and on the clinical presentation of the illness under discussion as well as on the differential diagnoses. Access to the key issues and the pertinent facts is easy; modern techniques like DNA hybridization and immunofluorescence are discussed. This text, with its emphasis on the analytical approach, has also absorbed recent developments in cell physiology, electron microscopy, biochemistry, and immunology. Thus, it goes beyond the examination of "dead tissues" and the reiteration of "dead issues". It broadens the scientific basis of modern pulmonary medicine. The appreciation of the lung as an enormously complex organ, which began with Julius Comroe's question, "Do the lungs have any function?", is most certainly going to grow during the next decade.

Norbert. F. Voelkel, M.D.
Health Sciences Center,
University of Colorado,
Denver, USA

Denver, October 1991

Foreword

Many misunderstandings in diagnosis and treatment with their possible disadvantages for the sick, are caused by the uneven and sometimes incorrect application of terms in medical diagnosis, especially when they are not well defined or not generally accepted. It is the great merit of the author to present here an encyclopedic collection of special terms dealing with diseases and pathological conditions of the respiratory organs, especially the lung. He has not only included clinical terms and pathological entities, but also many definitions of terms dealing with etiologic factors such as environmental, chemotoxic, infectious, and many other noxae. The book is not limited to diseases and pathological conditions of the lung in a narrow sense, but includes many disease entities in which the lung may be involved, even if rarely.

The author has been very successful in presenting the carefully collected data in a uniform and clearly arranged system. This makes the book easy to survey, and the reader can find a specific term without difficulties and within a short time. The size of a publication like this is usually subject to technical and financial limitations, and so concentrating on the main criteria has been necessary. Despite this, the value of the information in the volume in extremely high, and numerous carefully selected criteria and definitions have been included.. The definitions include epidemiological, etiological, pathophysiological, clinical, and prognostic factors, as well as further morphological details including radiological information, but concentrating on gross pathological and histological criteria. In the latter, many differential diagnostic questions have been taken into consideration.

This book can thus be regarded as an encyclopedic source of great informative worth not only for pathologists, but also for clinicians and practitioners interested in lung pathology. They will be able to use it as a valuable aid for solving diagnostic problems and questions in daily practical work.

J. H. Holzner, M.D.,Ph.D.
Department of Clinical Pathology,
University of Vienna,
Vienna, Austria

Vienna, November 1991

Contents

General Aspects

Clinical Techniques

Diagnostic pulmonary pathology is usually the last step in a series of various diagnostic procedures. Except in an emergency the clinical diagnostic procedure begins with a detailed history of the disease, a thorough physical examination and chest radiographs. Computed tomography (CT) follows in the majority of cases, especially where there are solid, circumscribed masses, subpleural densities, or mediastinal lymphomas. Sonography confirms or rules out pleural effusions. Detailed lung function analyses are necessary for calculating the preoperative risk and may contribute to the diagnostic and therapeutic process. Perfusion and ventilation scintigraphy gives information about topographic disturbances of lung function and is normally performed prior to invasive diagnostic procedures. Magnetic resonance imaging (MRI) is especially useful for distinguishing mediastinal lymphomas from major blood vessels. Filtered tomography of the hilar region or of the whole chest may detect additional lesions as small as 2 mm in diameter.

Analysis of peripheral blood including blood counts, immuno-electrophoresis, and measurements of pO_2, pCO_2, and enzymes are usually performed within the first hours of hospitalization. Of special importance and easy to measure are the levels of tumor markers in the peripheral blood and – if present – in pleural effusions. Increased levels of neuron specific enolase (NSE), carcinoembryonic antigen (CEA), and squamous cell tumor markers (SCC) are highly suggestive of malignancy.

The pathologist, in general, is not involved in determining the diagnostic invasive procedures performed by the clinicians. On the other hand, he has to examine the morphological changes of the tissue taken by invasive techniques, provide the clinician with a proper description of the morphological changes and, if possible, define the disease of the patient, i.e., give a representative diagnosis which automatically includes therapeutic strategies. He has no access to the complete clinical information under normal circumstances, but this is not necessary in the majority of cases.

What is the minimum information needed for a proper diagnosis? Sex and age of the patient are absolutely necessary. A clearcut clinical question indicating the diagnostic problem is another conditio sine qua non. Three simple words (carcinoma? tuberculosis? sarcoidosis?) accompanying a bronchus biopsy from the upper lobe indicate that the clinician is dealing with a solid circumscribed mass in the upper lobe and probably mediastinal lymphomas. The morphologic changes of the tissue specimen can confirm one of the differential diagnoses. On the other hand, an additional biopsy or a different biopsy technique may be indicated if the tissue specimen shows only nonspecific inflammatory infiltrations. It is very unlikely that these infiltrations are caused by a chronic bronchitis which may be the correct histopathological diagnosis, if there is no knowledge of the responses to the clinical questionnaire.

Bronchial and transbronchial biopsies are usually performed in anesthetized patients, i.e., when the condition of the patient is strong enough to withstand anesthesia lasting 15–20 min. The same holds true for mediastinoscopy and for pleural biopsies. Intrabronchial tumors can be seen very clearly during bronchoscopy in most cases. Biopsies taken from these lesions are usually sufficient for an adequate histopathological diagnosis. Submucosal growth of tumors or lymphangiosis carcinomatosa, frequently found with small cell anaplastic carcinoma and adenocarcinoma, can also be seen clearly by bronchoscopy. However, biopsy specimens taken from these suspicious areas quite frequently fail to confirm the endoscopic impression. Significant endoscopic findings are, therefore, necessary information to be sent to the pathologist.

The submission of specimens taken from bronchial or transbronchial biopsies indicates to the pathologist that the patient may be selected for surgical treatment if not otherwise noted. This is of importance with borderline lesions or diagnostic problems due to sampling errors or insufficient material. A second bronchoscopy performed because of these reasons requires that the patient undergoes anesthesia again including its – even if limited – risk. Appropriate histopathological information given to the clinician (for example, "probably epidermoid carcinoma; however, large cell anaplastic carcinoma or poorly differentiated adenocarcinoma cannot be ruled out") may obviate the need for a second bronchoscopy and lead directly to surgical treatment. A mediastinoscopy may be the next diagnostic step if a small cell anaplastic carcinoma cannot be confirmed or ruled out definitively.

Transcutaneous fine needle biopsies do not require the concurrent use of anesthesia. Thus, they can be performed with patients who cannot tolerate general anesthesia. The adequate treatment of peripheral circumscribed lesions is excision. Intraoperative sections are appropriate to confirm the diagnosis if the clinician cannot rule out a malignancy by macroscopic analysis of the excised tissue. Therefore, surgery is not the adequate treatment planned in the majority of patients undergoing transcutaneous fine needle aspiration. They may be selected for radiotherapy or chemotherapy if the pathologist is able to confirm a malignancy. Inflammatory diseases and benign lesions have to be ruled out very carefully by the pathologist in these cases.

Bronchial biopsies are usually representative samples of the main lesion. The pathologist does not need detailed information about the radiographic findings in these cases except in special clinical diagnoses (amyloidosis, granulomatous diseases, etc.). However, reports of unusual endoscopic findings such as submucosal tumor growth can strongly support the histopathological diagnosis.

Transbronchial biopsies are accompanied by sampling errors quite frequently. They tend to contain only necrotic material if taken from the center of the lesion or unrepresentative inflammatory infiltrations if taken from the boundary. Information from the gross findings of the chest radiographs is necessary to inform the pathologist about the nature of the lesion. The transbronchial biopsy may be representative if the chest radiograph shows a diffuse granular infiltrate and the morphologic changes seen on the biopsy are interstitial inflammation and fibrosis. The same transbronchial biopsy has presumably missed the lesion of concern if a peripheral circumscribed mass can be noted on the chest radiographs.

Pleural biopsies are taken either blind, with the transcutaneous fine needle procedure, or in combination with a thoracoscopy. In both cases they are beset with the hazard of sampling errors. The pathologist should avoid designating diseases of the pleura as benign even in cases with clearly demonstrable mesothelial cells as long as the clinical history and the condition of the patient favor malignant disease. The same holds true for pleuritis tuberculosa. In contrast, even the demonstration of atypical mesothelial cells including a considerable number of mitotic figures is not representative of a malignant tumor as long as the clinical findings support a nonspecific inflammatory event and as long as an invasive tumor growth cannot be confirmed.

Mediastinoscopy is a reliable technique for confirming or ruling out benign diseases accompanied by mediastinal lymphomas, especially sarcoidosis. Sampling errors are more frequent in the case of metastasis into the mediastinum, especially with malignant tumors of the left lung.

Lung function is of minor importance for the histopathological diagnosis as long as the major clinical problem is a circumscribed solid lesion. With diffuse interstitial infiltrates data on lung function will be necessary. The same holds true of sonographic findings.

Cytology specimens are usually sent to the pathologist together with biopsy specimens. Fluids obtained by bronchoscopy are especially useful in peripherally located lesions and may confirm a tumor not reachable by rigid or flexible bronchoscopy. Sputum cytology is usually performed in mass screening programs or in patients not strong enough to submit to anesthesia. Due to the low redundance of information, cytologic diagnoses are handicapped by a higher error rate than histopathological ones. On the other hand, sampling errors are fewer. Cytologic diagnosis of pleural effusions requires special experience and additional clinical information in order to avoid major errors. Unlike with biopsy findings, the pathologist tends to be tempted to diagnose malignancies in cases of nonspecific inflammation due to marked cellular atypia including mitotic figures.

Wedge biopsies taken in combination with diagnostic thoracotomy necessitate special handling in general. The clinician suspects a rare disease if he decides to perform a diagnostic thoracotomy in order to obtain larger biopsy specimens. He takes into account the higher intraoperative risk compared with transbronchial biopsy or fine needle aspiration. He would prefer a simple thoracotomy and lobectomy, which for a common malignant disease would perform both a diagnostic and possible curative therapeutic procedure at the same time. The pathologist should, therefore, be aware of unusual, normally benign diseases in the case of wedge biopsies. Additional specific clinical information should be demanded.

Radiological Techniques

Modern radiological equipment includes the classic instrumentation for chest radiographs as well as computerized imaging techniques. The latter allow nearly error-free computation of the exact localization of circumscribed masses, including measurements of volume, maximum diameter, etc.. A precise definition of the topography of the surgical specimens is only possible by use of in vivo images. Cutting the gross surgical specimens and sampling the tissue for histopathological analysis is very much to be recommended if the chest radiographs or corresponding images are available. The information given by these images should be included in the histopathological statement. The pathologist should be aware of the following:

1) Small circumscribed masses present in radiological images can easily be overlooked during tissue preparation. In rare events, no corresponding morphological result is obtained. In these cases, it is very helpful to analyze the time between the date of taking the chest radiographs and the date of pathological examination. Additional information may be hidden in the radiographic history of the lesion.

2) In the majority of cases diffuse radiological infiltrates have a strong histopathological equivalent. The pathologist tends to overinterpret the histopathological findings. Even the demonstration of a moderate diffuse interstitial fibrosis may give no radiological or functional evidence. Intraalveolar cellular infiltrates or an interstitial edema exhibit a radiological sign only if the lesion is several centimeters in diameter. Lung functions are normally not altered.

3) Calcified bodies or fibrotic areas have a distinct radiologic appearance and can be detected down to a few millimeters in diameter by filtered tomographic examinations. The pathological demonstration of these lesions is sometimes very difficult and requires serial sectioning of the specimen over a distance of a few millimeters. Palpation of the specimen and the marking of the topography prior to fixation is sometimes helpful.

4) Angiography of the surgical specimens is indicated for arteriovenous shunts, angiomas, etc. It should be performed with fresh unfixed material. The images obtained can be compared with the in vivo images in order to assure correct surgical treatment. The histopathological examination of arteriovenous fistulas or tumors is very difficult without corresponding angiological images.

5) Bronchographic images give detailed information about abnormalities of the bronchial tree and are necessary for correct pathoanatomical examination in these cases. They provide the pathologist with in vivo data about the size of the major bronchi and the proper coordination of minor bronchi. Occluded bronchi can easily be found by comparison of bronchographic X-radiographs with the corresponding surgical specimen without requiring serial sectioning.

6) With lymphadenectomy due to bronchogenic carcinoma CT and MR images allow a comparison between the size of the excised extrapulmonary lymph nodes and that on the in vivo images. In instances of great differences of size between the excised lymph nodes and the in vivo images, lymphatic material probably invaded by tumorous masses may have been left by the surgeon. The pathologist can then make a correct residual grading (R stage) of the TNM classification. A potentially curative resection is correctly considered as a noncurative resection in these cases, and the patient has to be treated by adjuvant chemotherapy or radiation.

Tissue Handling

Biopsies

Bronchial and transbronchial biopsies are comparable in size to fine needle biopsies and seldom exceed $3 \times 2 \times 2$ mm. They are usually too small for frozen sections. They should be placed directly into the fixative with minimum exposure to air, a process best performed by the endoscopist. Lung biopsies are very sensitive to crushing and squeezing artefacts. Several fixatives may be used. The use of buffered formalin ($6.8<pH<7.8$) is necessary when immunostaining is being contemplated. Bronchial and transbronchial biopsies should be cut in serial sections. It is important to cut the maximum area of the specimen due to its limited size and the crushing artefacts existing at its boundary. The thickness of the cut influences the diagnosis and should be less than 4 µm. The clinician must be provided with a special form indicating the kind of biopsy and the location from which it was taken. If it takes less time to transmit necessary information from the endoscopist to the pathologist, more of such information can be conveyed.

Cultures of bacteria, mycobacteria, fungi, and viruses are normally made from the bronchial secretions. The material should be directly sent to the corresponding laboratory by the endoscopist.

Cytological Specimens

Analysis of cytological specimens is mostly performed while searching for cancer cells. Approaches to quantification of inflammatory subpopulations in chronic inflammatory diseases (sarcoidosis) based upon cytological fluids (lavage) are a second goal. They can be performed easily on conventional stained cytological smears and provide the clinician with stage-related data about the disease. A third aim is the search for and quantification of inorganic deposits (asbestos fibers) in bronchial fluids. These cytological smears require concentrating the material by centrifugation of the fluids. In addition, an iron stain is helpful for recognition of ferruginous bodies.

Preparation of cytological fluids can either be performed by a process similar to preparation of bronchial biopsies, i.e., fixation of cells, embedding in paraffin, and cutting the blocks, or cytological smears can be made and treated with special stains, for example, Papanicolaou stain.

When searching for cancer cells the general problem that precancerous and inflammatory cells by far exceed the number of cancer cells has to be addressed. Some authors see an advantage in cytocentrifugation and paraffin embedding of fixed cells, but others prefer cytocentrifugation and preparation of conventional smears to overcome this problem.

Preparation of smears is only useful if fresh material is available. Cancer cells and precancerous lesions (dysplastic cells) are easier to discriminate in smears than in blocks due to the better preserved nuclear chromatin. The nuclear/cytoplasm ratio (NC ratio) can be estimated in greater detail. However, preparation of good, i.e., homogeneous, smears demands lengthy experience from the technician. The pathologist has to screen and examine quite a number of slides (four or more) in order to exclude malignancy.

Analysis of inorganic deposits (asbestos fibers) in bronchial fluids can be performed with techniques similar to those used in lung tissue, i.e., by digestion with alkali or by burning the organic material at high temperature (700–800° C) and then counting the asbestos fibers under conventional light microscopy. The minerals contained in the fluid can be assayed by X-ray diffraction or by chemical analysis of silicates, phosphates, oxalates, etc. The major problem in quantification of the minerals is the reference volume, i.e., the number of alveoli washed out by the lavage procedure. Quantification of distinct enzymes has been described as a useful reference system for estimation of the washed-out alveoli. However, none of these enzyme activities has been found to be independent of the underlying disease.

Flow cytometry for automated analysis of bronchial fluids is only practicable for differentiating inflammatory subpopulations due to its low sensitivity for cancer cells. Only hyperploid cells can be distinguished from inflammatory and normal epithelial cells. An additional handicap is that its high background level prohibits exact proof of rare events such as cancer cells in bronchial fluids. This may change when monoclonal tumor markers for distinguishing cancer cells with a high sensitivity are available.

High resolution image analysis applied to Feulgen-stained smears is a very useful method to assist in the diagnostic procedure. However, it is troubled by major sampling problems. Its greatest application is to tumor imprints, allowing correct DNA quantitation and an estimation of the percentage of proliferating tumor cells (S/GM1 phase).

Immunocytology for detecting cancerous cells in cytological smears is beset by major technical problems. These are mainly artifacts due to the air drying of slides. Air drying of smears or related techniques lead to a concentration of fluid proteins at the cell boundaries with subsequent nonspecific absorption of applied monoclonal antibodies or of similar probes. Paraffin embedding of fluids avoids these artifacts. Judgement concerning immunohistochemical results is, however, more difficult in the case of formalin-fixed cells because of shrinking artifacts.

In making a diagnosis based upon cytological specimens it is necessary to keep in mind that cytological classification of tumors is not necessarily identical with their histopathological counterpart which is mainly based upon texture analysis. The cytological diagnosis should specify the existence/nonexistence of cancer cells, the grading of dysplastic cells (I: dysplasia; II: moderate dysplasia; III: severe dysplasia; IV: carcinoma in situ), the demonstration of hyperplastic cells (basal cells, goblet cells), the predominant inflammatory cell type (neutrophilic, eosinophilic leukocytes, lymphocytes, plasma cells, macrophages), and the existence of metaplastic squamous cells. The semiquantitative grading of inflammatory cells is fairly reproducible and is of special interest to the clinician in the case of chronic inflammatory lesions. The existence of epithelioid cells and multinucleated giant cells should, of course, be noted. In the case of clearly demonstrable cancer cells the cytological classification of the tumor cell population has to be marked as "cytological diagnosis" in order to avoid a misunderstanding if the textural pattern of the tumor in the histological specimen leads to a different "histological" tumor classification.

Surgical Specimens

Macroscopic and histopathological examination of surgical specimens (lobes and lungs) should be performed with a standardized technique. Prior to fixation, fresh tissue should be preserved for special examinations, especially if the malignancies were not classifiable by biopsies taken before the operation. Cancer cells live on in surgical specimens for about 3–4 h. They can be used for tissue cultures if taken from the surgical specimens no later than 2 h after operation and if carefully handled and placed in the appropriate medium. Preservation of tumor tissue for preparation of DNA (for example, amplification of oncogenes) can be performed by freezing the unfixed tissue even 2–3 h after operation. Preparation of RNA, however, is very sensitive to postoperative tissue handling and demands deep freezing of tissue specimens 10–20 min after surgical excision at the latest.

The fixation of the surgical specimens should be performed with buffered formalin instilled via the major bronchi with or without additional insufflation of air at moderate pressure (40 mmH_2O). Injection of buffered formalin into the peripheral lung parenchyma using conventional needles is an appropriate technique if the fixation fluid cannot be insufflated into the major bronchi, for example, in the case of occlusion of the bronchus due to intrabronchial tumor growth. Naturally, lungs can also be fixed by injection of buffered formalin into the pulmonary arteries under moderate pressure. After insufflation, the surgical specimens should be placed completely within the fixation fluid and covered with a wet towel. Complete fixation of lobes or lungs takes at least 24 h if the specimens are insufflated carefully. Fixation may be enhanced by the use of microwave ovens at moderate temperature (50–60°C). The microwave-assisted technique usually leads to complete fixation of the specimens within 4–6 h.

The resection boundaries of the major bronchi and of pulmonary arteries and veins should be excised and separately examined prior to fixation. Fixation leads to tissue shrinkage of about 30%. Gross examination of the resection boundaries of the pulmonary arteries and especially veins is very difficult after fixation.

Nonstandardized examination of fixed lung specimens in the search for representative samples has the disadvantage that the major lesions are usually not seen from the outside. The same holds true for the examination of unfixed specimens. We prefer, therefore, to cut the specimens in serial slices 6 mm thick starting, from the hilar side, in the sagittal direction. This method has the advantage of including the complete lung slice by slice without losing topographic information about the major lesion. The slides can be compared with the radiological images, and even small lesions can be analyzed. An electrical slicing machine (electrical butcher's knife) is very useful in order to obtain homogeneous sections. The major lesion can be examined quantitatively, including detailed measurement of its maximum diameter and, if wanted, its volume. Geometrical reconstruction of the lesion is easily possible without major technical aids by consecutive drawing of the circumferences of the sliced lesions on transparent foils. The intrapulmonary lymph nodes are simple to locate and can be studied separately. The slides can be recorded on image-analyzing machines and subsequently processed. The representative images can be stored for further assessment or documentation.

The following parameters are of importance and should be noted, especially in the case of tumor growth:

1) Distance of tumor boundary to resection boundary of the major bronchus (pulmonary artery, vein)

2) Distance of tumor boundary to pleura including area of tumorous infiltration into the pleura, if present

3) Tumorous infiltration into the lung tissue, if present

4) Tumorous infiltration into the intrapulmonary vessels and lymph nodes

5) Presence and area of intrapulmonary lesions caused by obstructive tumor growth

6) Size of additional (inflammatory) lesions and their relation to the tumor

7) Major changes of lung parenchyma (emphysema, pneumonia, anthracotic scars, etc.).

One complete tumor cross-section should be taken out and examined under light microscopy. In addition, representative samples of peripheral lung tissue should be studied. The complete weight of the surgical specimens prior to fixation should be measured. In my experience this is more representative than the geometrical properties of the specimen.

It is very useful to provide the laboratory with special standardized forms for the documentation of the gross findings. Under these circumstances the cutting of the specimens is carried out by well-trained technicians, and standard information can be judged by the pathologist afterwards. Naturally, the lung slices can be analyzed for inorganic deposits by digestion with alkali. They can be stained as a whole, for example, prior to resin embedding, and plastinated (for example, according to the method of von Hagens); they can be analyzed by X-rays (X-ray diffraction), etc..

Autopsy Specimens

Gross examination of autopsy specimens does not differ from the examination of surgical specimens in general. However, the lungs and the heart form one physiological entity, and the findings in both organs are related to each other in many diseases. I prefer, therefore, to excise the lungs and the heart from the body in a block including the aorta thoracica. Depending upon the cause of death the heart can later be examined separately from the lungs, for example, in the case of heart infarction. Both lungs are normally fixed with buffered formalin without being separated. This technique is also indicated for safety reasons, for example, to avoid contact with unexpected infections such as tuberculosis. Both lungs are separated from each other after complete fixation and cut into serial sections as described.

Staining Techniques

Conventional Techniques

Standardization of staining techniques is a prerequisite for obtaining reproducible slides, a necessity for reliable diagnoses. Only a limited number of slides can be obtained from transbronchial and bronchial biopsies due to their small size. Bronchial biopsies being a little bit larger than transbronchial biopsies, they are mostly employed for confirmation or exclusion of malignancies. PAS stain is the most useful one in bronchial biopsies in addition to the classic hematoxylin eosin, especially for separating small cell anaplastic carcinoma from undifferentiated non-small cell carcinoma such as adenocarcinoma or epidermoid carcinoma. It is employed for delineating basement membranes, for demonstrating the presence of organisms, especially fungus, and for assessing extracellular fluids. To demonstrate the nature of inflammatory cells and to separate them from malignant ones, the Romanowsky-Giemsa stain is the most useful.

Transbronchial or lung biopsies require an elastic collagen stain in addition to the hematoxylin eosin stain and to the PAS stain. A modified Sirius stain (combined with hematoxylin) allows the differentiation between fresh, reversible collagen (type III) and adult, irreversible collagen (type I). Reticulin fibers become visible if one uses a common silver stain such as Gomori's. Collagen staining (Sirius) is a prerequisite for defining the reversible or irreversible nature of granulomatous diseases, especially in sarcoidosis.

Depending on the special nature of the disease or on the histo-morphological image, the following stains are applied:

1) Congo red for amyloidosis, colloidal iron for hemorrhages or asbestos fibers, auramine for tuberculosis, argentophil and argyrophil for some rare neoplasms (reticulosis), Grocott for pneumocystis *carinii* and for some fungi (*Candida*, histoplasmosis), metallous for *Legionella* bacteria.

2) Feulgen, being proportional to the DNA content of nuclei, is necessary for image analysis of bronchus carcinoma. It may be combined with a protein stain for demonstrating the chromatin distribution of the nuclei. The nuclear organizing regions can be visualized by use of a modified silver stain.

3) Histochemistry for demonstration of intracytoplasmic enzymes or deposits is of limited practical use in bronchial and transbronchial biopsies. The classic techniques are the PAS stain with and without diastase digestion and the muciamin stain with subsequent digestion for differentiating mesothelioma of the pleura from metastatic adenocarcinoma. Similar results can be obtained with colloidal iron or alcian blue stain performed at pH<4 with and without subsequent hyaluronidase digestion. However, these techniques are not very sensitive and have now been replaced by more appropriate immunoperoxidase methods.

Immunohistochemistry

Immunohistochemistry using monoclonal or polyclonal antibodies is a very useful technique for detecting biological entities not distinguishable by conventional staining methods. Some of the antibodies can only be applied to fresh, unfixed tissue (frozen sections); some detect antigens not destroyed or altered by the fixatives. A positive reaction to a monoclonal antibody can be demonstrated by different techniques like direct immunofluorescence, the peroxidase-antiperoxidase method, the biotin-avidin method, and the immunogold method. Their sensitivity is similar. The peroxidase-antiperoxidase technique is used in the majority of histopathological laboratories, although it exhibits no outstanding advantages when compared with the avidin-biotin technique. The immunogold technique is based upon a photoreaction and is, therefore, somewhat sensitive to overstaining. The immunofluorescence techniques are easier to apply. Slides stained with immunofluorescent dyes have to be analyzed immediately and cannot be stored over a long period of time.

The following antisera or antibodies are useful for the characterization and classification of the diseases noted:

1) Chronic inflammatory diseases

- Probes for detecting immunoglobulins such as IgA, IgE, IgG, IgM, and for detecting complement, fibrin, and albumin, interleukin, human leukocyte antigen (HLA-DR)
- Probes for distinguishing subsets of lymphocytes, i.e., T, B, T4, T8, T6, monocytes,

granulocytes, macrophages, transferrin receptor of monocytes (for exclusion of partial immunodeficiency)

- Probes for detecting endogenous sugar receptors (normal lung parenchyma without previous history of severe inflammation expresses no endogenous lectins detectable by glycohistochemical techniques.)

2) Chronic systemic diseases, including vasculitis, lupus erythematosus, rheumatoid arthritis, etc.

- Probes for detection of antiglomerulus basement membranes, fibronectin, immunoglobulins, complement subsets, lymphocytic subpopulations, granulocytes, monocytes, macrophages, autoantibodies, DNA and RNA fractions

3) Detection of bacteria, fungi, etc.

- Probes against *Legionella*, *Pneumocystis carinii*, tuberculosis, *Candida*, histoplasmosis, *Aspergillus*, etc.

4) Amyloidosis

- Probes against immunoglobulins (IgA, IgE, IgG, IgM) and their fragments for separating primary from secondary amyloidosis

5) Neoplasms

- Probes against cytoskeleton proteins for separating tumors with epithelial differentiation from those with leukocytic or sarcomatous differentiation (demonstration of actin, cytokeratin, vimentin, neurofilaments, desmin, desmoplakin)
- Probes for the classification of lymphomas (common lymphocytic antigen, B-lymphocytic antigens, T-lymphocytic antigens, HLA-related probes, immunoglobulins (IgM, IgD, IgE, IgG, IgA, kappa and lambda light chains), granulocyte-associated probes (Hodgkin's disease)
- Probes for distinguishing small cell anaplastic carcinoma from malignant lymphoma and from undifferentiated non-small cell carcinoma such as adenocarcinoma or undifferentiated epidermoid carcinoma (neuroendocrine markers: neuron-specific enolase (NSE), synaptophysin (sy38), chromogranin A, bombesin, secretogranin; lymphocytic markers (common lymphocytic antigen); epithelial markers: carcinoembryonic antigen (CEA), squamous cell antigen (SCC), epithelial membrane antigen (EMA); histiocytic markers (lysozyme); and endogenous lectins (specific for fucose or mannose))
- Probes for detecting hormones, especially in small cell anaplastic carcinoma and metastatic carcinoma in the lung (calcitonin, gastrin-releasing peptide (bombesin), adrenocorticotropic hormone (ACTH), estrogen and progesterone receptors, etc.)
- Probes related to tumor markers in serum or body fluids (NSE, CEA, SCC, etc.)
- Probes for separating metastatic tumors in the lung from primary tumors of the lung (epithelial membrane antigen (EMA), neuroendocrine markers, prostatic phosphatase, prostatic specific antigen, alpha-fetoprotein, gonadotropin, thyroglobulin, endogenous lectins (heparin receptor), etc.)
- Probes related to tumor growth (Ki67 antibody, etc.)
- New techniques that will probably be developed in the near future include in-situ hybridization for the detection of viruses (papilloma-virus, herpes simplex virus, etc.).
- Analysis of endogenous lectins (sugar receptors) is useful for distinguishing mesothelioma of the pleura from metastatic adenocarcinoma of the lung. In addition, it can be used for separating small cell anaplastic carcinoma from the non-small cell form.
- Binding sites of tumor cells to growth hormone may provide the clinician with additional, therapeutically useful information. Data show that particular receptors for epidermal growth factor are expressed in more differentiated tumors such as epidermoid carcinoma and adenocarcinoma.
- Binding sites to cytokines such as tumor necrosis factor or to immunostimulants such as mistletoe lectin.
- The prognostic value of amplification and expression of oncogenes has still to be worked out.

Normal Histopathology

General Remarks

Morphological examination of histopathological specimens is based upon knowledge of normal cellular populations, upon the characteristics of the normal texture of the tissue, and upon certain changes within these "normal" findings. The lung itself has only a limited number of reactions to damage caused by internal or external factors. These affect the substructures of the lung to varying degrees. Consequently, analysis of the morphological changes can be used to reason out the underlying causes a posteriori. Herein I attempt to analyze and summarize the possible morphological changes of lung tissue in respect of the affected substructures. The changes will be classified into certain entities which may depend on each other or not. The changes themselves and the causes which lead to these changes are not discussed in this chapter. They are listed in the detailed description of the diseases involving the lung. If one is familiar with the structural entities of morphological alterations of lung tissue, it is possible to analyze any given image of lung tissue and to draw conclusions about the possible underlying diseases. In addition, functional abnormalities related to the structural changes can be determined. The basic entities of the structural alterations are the descriptive features which are called descriptors in the following. The analysis of their composition is based upon the knowledge of the structures of the healthy lung tissue and is of great importance for the histomorphological judgement and classification of the underlying disorder.

Normal Lung Biopsy and Biopsy Artifacts

The lung consists microscopically of different subunits which have to be described separately if present: bronchus, bronchiolus, alveolus, interstitium, pulmonary artery, bronchial artery, pulmonary vein, lymphatic vessels, nerves, and pleura. Excision of peripherally located tumors may, in addition, involve compartments of the chest wall, i.e., ribs, intercostal muscles, skin. Biopsies taken from the proximal bronchi normally contain parts of the mucosa, the submucosa with mucinous glands, cartilage, and smooth muscles. Transbronchial biopsies tend to contain peribronchially located lung tissue including bronchioles, arterioles, and interalveolar interstitium. If performed by an experienced endoscopist they contain 10–20 peripherally located alveoli, with some arterioles and interalveolar interstitium. Transcutaneous fine needle biopsies are effective in penetrating peripherally located malignant tumors but are less so in penetrating calcified scars and hamartomas. Biopsies of pleural tissue tend to contain samples of the parietal pleura and less often parts of the visceral pleura.

Bronchi and Bronchioles

The bronchi and bronchioles generally bifurcate. In general, 22–25 generations of division of the conductive airways between the trachea and the alveolus exist. Alveolar ducts generally trifurcate. Cartilaginous skeletons, being circumferential in the proximal bronchi and only partially so in the more distantly located bronchi, are found generally up to the twelfth generation. Bronchi tend to be located within >2 cm below the pleura in an adult person, a fact of some radiographic interest. The inner surface of the bronchi is covered by pseudostratified respiratory epithelium connected to the basement membrane; i.e., all epithelial cells reach the basement membrane. Six epithelial cell types can be distinguished morphologically. Of major importance are the following:

1) The basal cell, an undifferentiated regenerative cell located on the basement membrane but not connected to the bronchial lumen. It is a small cell with dark cytoplasm and a "condensed" dark nucleus.

2) The neurosecretory or Kulchitski's cell similar to the basal cell, with a small round nucleus but pale cytoplasm.

3) The ciliated cell, which is covered with small cilia at the intrabronchial lumen.

4) The mucous cell, whose number is approximately equal to that of the ciliated cell and which contains either small mucous granules or a large single mucous vacuole (goblet cell). It is not covered with cilia in general.

The two additional cell types, which are found infrequently, are ones having cilia together with mucous granules, and nonspecific cells with pale cytoplasm reaching the bronchial lumen. They are not provided with cilia or mucous granules.

Epithelial cells are separated from the subepithelial smooth connective tissue by the basal membrane. The mucous glands in the bronchial mucosa are composed of approximately equal numbers of serous and mucinous glands. The connective tissue contains scattered lymphocytes and plasma cells as well as a varied number of blood vessels and lymphatic vessels. The cartilage is surrounded by a thin fibrous layer (perichondrium) containing spindle-shaped nuclei. It lacks its own blood supply. Its cells are evenly spaced in adults and are mostly closely packed near the perichondrium in children. The outer layer of the bronchi consists of a circumferential anastomotic network of smooth muscle cells penetrated by the ducts of the mucous glands. No muscularis mucosa is formed, i.e., the muscular layer is discontinuous. The accompanying lymphatic vessels tend to show poor structural organization in the major bronchi (bronchus associated lymphoid tissue, BALT). Lymph nodes with capsules and sinuses commonly exist in the surrounding tissue of the lobar and segmental bronchi. The capsules of the lymphoid follicles are lost if situated along the subsegmental bronchi. The bronchioles may have lymphoid aggregates which do not show germinal centers. Localized lymphoid hyperplasia is a common finding in adult lungs, causing corresponding radiologic nodules, especially on high resolution filtered tomogram of the complete lung.

Bronchioles occupy the lung tissue up to 5 mm from the pleural surface in adults. They consist of an inner surface of ciliated epithelial cells and do not have bronchial cartilage. They are divided into terminal bronchioli defining a polyconducting airway and respiratory bronchioli with alveoli as part of their wall. The terminal bronchioles divide approximately six times, being followed by one to three generations of respiratory bronchioles. All kinds of epithelial cells are found in the bronchioles, while the ciliated type dominates in the respiratory bronchioles. Mucous glands become smaller in size and less frequent, similar to the declining number of smooth muscle cells with decreasing diameter of the bronchiolus. Direct connections between terminal bronchioles and adjacent alveoli are referred to as channels of Lamberth, forming collateral ventilation pathways. These alveoli often have deposits of various dusts.

The artifacts found in bronchial biopsies may result in the following:

- Crush artifacts frequently found at the edge of rigid bronchoscopic biopsies. Smears of DNA and of nuclear chromatin do not allow identification of single cells or the nature of the underlying cells.
- Squeezing of epithelial cells of mucous glands, causing difficulty in identifying mucous glands and misinterpretation as lymphangiosis carcinomatosa.
- Dislodging of squamous epithelial cells from the pharynx or larynx during the procedure of bronchoscopy. Such dislodging gives the impression of squamous metaplasia of the bronchial epithelium. Squamous epithelial cells of the pharynx or larynx can be identified by the larger amount of glycogen shown by PAS staining.
- Biopsies containing only epithelial cells or, vice versa, biopsies showing only mucous glands and cartilage. Naturally, the content of morphological information is limited; malignant tumors, however, can be excluded in nearly all of these biopsies.

Distant Lung Parenchyma

The distant respiratory lung parenchyma is composed of alveolar ducts, alveolar sacs and alveoli. The alveolar ducts are tubes surrounded by a spiral of smooth muscle cells forming an outline of the duct. The alveolar duct normally leads into three alveolar sacs and is simply the space between the alveoli as they face one another. This alveolar lung parenchyma is lined by two types of epithelial cells, called pneumocytes type I and II. Type I pneumocytes are flat, long, stretched cells with extremely thin and elongated nuclei. They form about 90% of the inner surface of the alveolar parenchyma. The remaining 10% consists of type II pneumocytes, being cuboidal cells with dark nuclei and granular cytoplasm. Ultrastructurally, they show characteristic osmiophilic lamellar bodies and are the morphological counterpart of the surfactant. They tend to be located in the angiolar recesses of the alveoli. They respond rapidly to noxious stimuli, especially obstruction, and may show mitosis and a highly increased number under these circumstances. They are considered to be the regenerative cell type for both types of pneumocytes.

Although the air spaces are empty under normal conditions, some alveoli are found to contain small numbers of cells not connected to the alveolar walls. They are generally dark brown and contain black dust pigment. They are considered to derive from circulating macrophages migrating through the capillary wall and the alveolar epithelium into the air space.

The alveolar walls or the interalveolar septi consist of a central localized system of capillaries surrounded by a capillary basement membrane. The space between the capillary basement membrane and the alveolar epithelial basement membrane is called interstitium. It contains extracellular fluid, some fibers of collagen, and a few lymphocytes, histiocytes, and mast cells. The capillary system and the interstitium are just visible with optimal fixation of tissue. They can be demonstrated clearly by fixation using a microwave oven. The connective tissue of the bronchi, arteries, veins, pleura, and interlobular septula forms a continuous interstitial space including the interstitium of the interalveolar septula.

Artifacts of transbronchial biopsies may consist of the following:

- Obstructive altered, i.e., uninflated lung tissue difficult to interpret, and simulating obstructive lung diseases.
- Compression of lung tissue caused by forceps. This area, usually found on one side of the biopsy, should not be interpreted as increased interstitial fibrous tissue.
- Polypoid appearance of lung tissue circumferentially covered by respiratory epithelium. This is caused by the compression of the specimens at one edge and by histological sectioning of the specimen out of the biopsy plane.
- Contents of a small bronchial and peribronchial lung parenchyma showing some increased fibrosis. Lung parenchyma located near major bronchi should not be considered as representative of interstitial lung diseases.

Pulmonary Artery

Pulmonary arteries accompany the bronchi and may be divided according to their size into five types of vessels:

1) Pulmonary trunk and its main branches, having a thick internal and external elastic lamina.

2) Intrapulmonary elastic arteries having a relatively thick adventitia and a more continuous internal and external elastic lamina with scattered smooth muscle cells.

3) Muscular arteries having a distinct internal and external elastic lamina and an external diameter of approximately 100–500 μm. The diameter of these arteries is smaller than that of the accompanying bronchioles in the peripheral lung zones.

4) Arterioles having an external diameter of approximately 70–100 μm. They gradually lose the complete circumference of smooth muscle cells and the internal elastic lamina.

5) Capillaries forming a dense network in the interstitial lung parenchyma and being 8 μm in diameter on average.

Small elastic or muscular pulmonary arteries are difficult to differentiate from bronchioles. If both are present in a biopsy, the formation with the larger diameter and with the more irregularly oriented inner and outer elastic fibers belongs to the bronchioli.

Bronchial Artery

Bronchial arteries belong to the systemic arteries originating from the aorta adjacent to the right and left main stem bronchi. A distinct internal elastic lamina, a fully developed thick muscular media, and a small, polydeveloped external elastic lamina are their hallmarks. They supply the mucosa of the bronchi and its surrounding connective tissue and are, therefore, found at the inner and outer side of the bronchial cartilage. Pulmonary arteries on the inner side of the cartilage do not exist. Bronchial arteries, bronchial veins of equal size, and nerve fascicles often form a structural system surrounding the major bronchi. They split up into the capillary network emerging with the pulmonary arterial capillary network in the distant airway conducting system. They are easily studied in bronchial ectasia due to their reactive hypertrophy.

Bronchial and Pulmonary Veins

Venous plexuses consisting of small capillaries can be found in the walls of the major bronchi. They have broad anastomoses with their pulmonary veins. The medial pleura and the hilar bronchi are drained by superficial bronchial veins entering into the systemic venous system by way of the vena azygos or hemiazygos. In contrast to the pulmonary veins the bronchial veins have walls and thin valves.

Pulmonary veins drain the blood from the pulmonary arteries, and most of the blood from the bronchial arteries enters into the interlobular fibrous septa at a maximum diameter of approximately 100 µm. They have an internal elastic membrane and a continuous merging of the media and adventitia, i.e., no external elastic membrane. The larger size of their lumen compared with the thickness of their walls may be used for distinguishing the pulmonary veins from pulmonary arteries. Similar in size, the pulmonary arteries exhibit the opposite characteristics.

Lymphatic System

The intrapulmonary lymphatic system starts around the terminal bronchioles to drain the lung towards the central portion of the lung; i.e., these lymphatic vessels follow the bronchi along the mucosa and the adjacent connective tissue as well as along the adventitia of the pulmonary arteries. A second system starts as a superficial network of lymphatic vessels within the pleura visceralis following the pleural and pulmonary veins into the septa of the hilum. The first system is responsible for the central portion of the lung, the second for the peripheral lung tissue. Both systems enter the hilar and tracheobronchial lymph nodes, being connected with the right and left bronchomediastinal lymphatic trunk. Lymphatic vessels are not present within the interalveolar septula, within the alveolar ducts, or along the respiratory bronchioles.

Histomorphologically, the lymphatic vessels within the lung are formed similar to the lymphatic system found in other organs of the body. The smallest vessels consist of purely endothelial cells covering a basement membrane. Smooth muscle cells and collagen are found within the lymphatic walls of larger vessels. Being of larger size, the lymphatic vessels are very variable in caliber due to dilatations followed by constrictions. The larger lymphatic vessels have numerous, usually bicuspid, lymphatic valves.

Pleura

The pleura is divided into two parts, the visceral and the parietal pleura. It should be considered as a distinct organ with special physiological functions and special alterations due to injuries. Five layers form the visceral pleura histologically. A single layer of cuboidal or flattened mesothelial cells without a basement membrane form the first, most superficial, so-called mesothelial layer. Loose connective tissue approximately equal in thickness to the mesothelial layer is found beneath the mesothelial cells. A thick elastic membrane forms the external elastic layer, i.e., the third layer. Occasionally it is molded, sometimes duplicated, and lymphatic vessels can be found there. Loose connective tissue containing arterial and venous blood vessels as well as lymphatic vessels, small nerve fibers and smooth muscle cells form the fourth layer lying beneath the external elastic membrane. The boundary of the pleura against the lung consists of segments of elastic fibers continuously connected with the elastic fibers of the interalveolar septula. In this layer, lymphatic vessels occasionally can be seen. Boundaries between the five layers are not distinct, and sometimes the external and internal elastic membranes seem to merge.

The structure of the parietal pleura is similar to that of the visceral pleura. The layers are less distinct, and often only one elastic layer can be found. Beneath the parietal pleura, fat cells are normally seen belonging to the chest wall. The endothoracic fascia separates these fat cells from the inner periostium of the ribs. In so-called pleuraectomy, the endothoracic fascia is the plane of surgical dissection.

The mesothelial layer of both the visceral and parietal pleura is often absent in biopsies obtained by limited thoracotomy. Severe reactive hyperplasia of pleural cells mimicking a mesothelioma can be found in cases with chronic irritation of the pleural cavity. Artifacts caused by prolonged thoracic surgery consist of fibrin smears at the pleural surface and a moderate number of neutrophilic lymphocytes within the capillaries and within the interstitial external and internal layer. The small capillaries tend to contain eosinophilic leukocytes in these cases. The eosinophilic leukocytes are also seen in the capillaries of the lung under these circumstances and may not be interpreted as abnormal findings.

Biopsies of the pleura are frequently handicapped by sampling problems. Mesotheliomas are often accompanied by severe fibrosis of the pleura which is not invaded by tumor cells. Many biopsies contain only fibrin without any mesothelial cells. Fibrinous plaques can distort the endoscopic appearance of pleura. They are commonly biopsied, and the diagnostically important areas are missed.

Pieces of visceral or parietal pleura are occasionally found in transbronchial fiberoptic bronchoscopy specimens. These biopsies sometimes contain a saclike piece of pleura with some skeletal muscle cells or compact sheets of mesothelial cells together with the adjacent submesothelial layer. The appearance of muscle cells may be confused with that of aspirated material. However, they do not show peptic digestion. Fine-needle biopsies of the pleura sometimes do not reach the mesothelial layer and contain only fat cells and interstitial connective tissue. Others may contain only fibrinous material of the pleural cavity.

Descriptors of Normal Findings

1) Normal major bronchus

Findings: Continuous basal membrane with a connected layer of basal cells, enclosed goblet cells, and ciliary cells. Beneath the basal membrane loose connective tissue with smooth muscle cells, scattered lymphocytes, plasma cells, normal mucinous and serous glands. Compartments of cartilage with surrounding layer of fibrous tissue.

Absent: Necrosis, eosinophilic and neutrophilic lymphocytes, macrophages, hyalin deposits, calcified areas, compartments of lymphatic tissue, ectatic veins, larger arteries.

2) Normal minor bronchus

Findings: Continuous basal membrane with a connected layer of basal cells, ciliated cells, and, less frequently, goblet cells. Beneath the basal membrane loose connective tissue with scattered lymphocytes and plasma cells, infrequently smooth muscle cells, small mucinous and serous glands, little fragments of cartilage with surrounding layer of fibrous tissue. Sometimes peribronchial connective tissue, alveoli of normal size with flat pneumocytes, small deposits of anthracotic pigment.

Absent: Necrotic areas, macrophages, neutrophilic and eosinophilic granulocytes, granulomatous areas, hyalin deposits, calcified areas, compartments of lymphatic tissue, ectatic veins, larger arteries.

3) Normal lung tissue

Findings: Thin interalveolar septula with flat pneumocytes (in case of microwave fixation expanded capillaries), small arteries and veins, peribronchial slight fibrosis with included anthracotic pigment, sometimes macrophages and lymphocytes in the alveoli, sometimes eosinophilic granulocytes in small arteries, hemorrhage.

Absent: Necrotic areas, intraalveolar fluid, dense infiltrates of lymphocytes, plasma cells, neutrophilic granulocytes, granulomatous areas, dense macrophages with connection to cuboidal pneumocytes.

4) Normal pleura

Findings: Lined up mesothelial cells, absent basal membrane, loose connective tissue with scattered fat cells and sometimes skeletal muscle cells, scattered lymphocytes and plasma cells, ectatic veins, in case of visceral pleura, adjacent normal lung tissue and small deposits of anthracotic pigment.

Absent: Necrotic areas, granulomas, macrophages, layer of multiple mesothelial cells, fibrinous or calcified plaques, eosinophilic and neutrophilic infiltrates, fibrin, hemorrhage.

5) Normal pulmonary and bronchial artery

Findings: The pulmonary and bronchial arteries are of the elastic type. Small tunica intima and dense network of elastic fibers within the tunica media. Relatively dense smooth muscle cells.

In large pulmonary arteries missing lamina elastica externa in contrast to bronchial arteries. Between large pulmonary and bronchial arteries connective arterial vessels, so-called blocking arteries with dense and enlarged smooth muscle cells, small adventitia.
Absent: Even in aged patients larger intima plaques and incrustation of lipoproteins, inflammatory infiltrations, disarrangement of elastic fibers, hyalinosis of small arteries in the adventitia.
6) Normal vein
Findings: Relatively thin walls of the veins. Circularly arranged reticular fibers in the lamina elastica. Dense collagenous fibers and smooth muscle cells in the adventitia.
Absent: Inflammatory infiltrations, incrustations of lipoproteins.

Alphabetical Index of Lung Diseases

Abscess – Azathioprine

Abscess

Definition: Accumulation of inflammatory cells causing complete destruction of the lung parenchyma.

Incidence/Epidemiology: The disease is not rare, usually affecting alcoholics with aspiration, persons with traumatic lesions, elderly and immunocompromised patients with bacterial infection, and patients with bronchial obstruction.

Etiology/Pathophysiology: The causes of the lung abscess include (a) aspiration of foreign bodies, infected own-body material such as pus, teeth, tonsils, (b) septic emboli, (c) traumatic lesions, (d) secondary to bacterial pneumonia (synpneumonic lung abscess), (e) secondary to infarctions, (f) secondary to bronchial obstruction, (g) secondary to malignant growth, (h) transpleural spread of infections, (i) secondary to ruptured hydatid cyst. The fulminant growth of bacteria destroys the peripheral lung parenchyma, bronchi, and arteries. The bacteria are often composed of anaerobic and mixed flora that have been described as appearing in the mouth cavity. The anaerobic cultures include *Fusobacterium nucleatum, Bacteroides melaninogenicus* and *fragilis, Haemophilus, Pseudomonas, Klebsiella*. Nonfetid abscesses are related to *Staphylococcus aureus, Pneumococcus, Typhi* and *Paratyphi bacteria, Pseudomonas tularensis* and *pseudomallei*. Diminished host response including alcoholism, diabetes mellitus, renal failure, malnutrition, treatment with immunosuppressive agents, and (inborn) defects of the immune system favor the formation of abscesses.

Clinical Presentation: The characteristic signs are fever, cough, production of pus, and subpleural pain; after some days, hemoptysis arises. Expectoration of pus is present if the abscess has connection to a major bronchus. Fetid breathing in case of aerobic infections.

Prognosis: Usually good, or depending on the underlying disease.

Radiology: Poorly defined lesions with thick-walled, irregular cavities, located most frequently in the upper right lobe, often subpleural.

Pathology:

Gross: Well-defined, circumscribed, necrotic area of yellowish-red color. The central areas often disintegrate, leaving some remnant trabeculae with thin walls. Ruins of larger bronchi or granulation tissue polyps may be present in older lesions. The consistency of the surrounding lung tissue is solid. Older lesions tend to contain a thin and fibrotic capsule, often without any bronchial attachments.

Histology: In the central area an ill-defined zone of acute inflammatory cells often with colonies of bacteria. Complete destruction of the former lung tissue. The outer zone is marked by acutely inflamed granulation tissue with some scattered remains of smaller bronchi and arterial walls. A fibrotic lamina is present in older lesions, sometimes with squamous metaplasia and dysplastic cells. A small zone of "interstitial pneumonitis" with predominant macrophages in the air spaces surrounds the granulation tissue. Additional small necrotic areas of a few millimeters in diameter are frequently seen besides the main lesion. Fusobacteria and spirochetes are best demonstrated with crystal violet stain. Periodic acid Schiff (PAS) stain demonstrates fungus and *Actinomyces*, Gram stain pneumococci. Silver stains and connective tissue stains are useful to demonstrate remains of connective tissue and to identify possible cancer cells.

➤ *Descriptors:* Lung parenchyma with altered structure:

- necrosis and hemorrhage
- mixed inflammatory infiltrates
- bacteria (*Actinomyces*)
- macrophages
- multinucleated giant cells (foreign body)
- fungus
- calcification
- focal interstitial fibrosis

■ *Special stains:* PAS, collagenous stains, Giemsa.

Hallmark of Diagnosis: Homogeneous "mixed" inflammatory cells with predominant neutrophilic granulocytes. The important zones are the central zone for the demonstration of bacteria such as *Actinomyces* or fungus, and the granulomatous outer zone for exclusion of malignant growth. In surgical specimens additional "healthy" lung tissue has to be examined histologically in search of additional alterations such as angiitis, bronchiolitis obliterans, thromboembolism, fibrosis, and abnormal lymphocytic subpopulations (immunoglobulin alterations).

Differential diagnosis: Necrotic lung cancer (epidermoid carcinoma or large cell anaplastic carcinoma), necrotizing granulomatous diseases such as allergic angiitis and granulomatosis (Churg-Strauss syndrome) or necrotizing sarcoid-like granulomatosis.

Absidia

Definition: Agent of mucormycosis (opportunistic infection), see Mucormycosis.

Acanthamebiasis

Definition: Infection of the lung parenchyma with protozoan species of *Acanthamoeba*.
Incidence/Epidemiology: Very rare infections in humans, about 30 patients are recognized who have died due to granulomatous encephalitis caused by *Acanthamoeba*. Infections of the upper respiratory tract are somewhat more common. One case with granulomatous amebic encephalitis and *Acanthamoeba castellani* infection of the lung has been described.
Etiology/Pathophysiology: The protozoans are common in fresh water and soil of the median and southern hemispheres. These nonparasitic, free-living organisms probably enter the lungs and central nervous system when introduced into the nasal cavity. Infections are usually fulminating, especially in immunocompromised patients.
Clinical Presentation: Unknown, rhinitis and infection of the lower respiratory tract may precede manifestation in the brain.
Prognosis: Poor.
Radiology: Unknown, slight pulmonary edema may be present.
Pathology:
Gross: Necrotizing pneumonitis in mice. Probably, edema and small abscesses arise prior to granulomatous encephalitis.
Histology: Probably interstitial edema with an increased number of granulocytes, in mice abscess. The trophocoites can be demonstrated by Giemsa and Masson's trichrome technique. The amebas range from 10–25 µm in diameter. They present a sharply outlined nucleus with a predominant nucleolus. Immunofluorescence and immunoenzymatic tests are available.

➤ *Descriptors:* Lung parenchyma with altered structure:
- caseous epithelioid granulomas
- infectious organisms (intragranulomatous, ameba of H-A group)
- eosinophils;
- Lung parenchyma with preserved structure:
- interstitial edema
- intraalveolar serous fluid
- mononuclear inflammatory infiltrates

■ *Special stains:* PAS, collagenous stains, Giemsa.

Hallmark of Diagnosis: Interstitial edema, microabscess, identification of the infectious organisms, immunofluorescence or immunoenzymatic tests have been described.
Differential diagnosis: Various protozoan infections including suppurative inflammations caused by *Naegleria, Entamoeba histolytica, Toxoplasma gondii*. The trophocoites of *Acanthamoeba* are usually larger and contain a denser nucleolus than their counterparts of *Naegleria, Entamoeba*, or *Toxoplasma*.

Acariasis

Definition: Pulmonary infection caused by inhalation of acarids (mites).
Incidence/Epidemiology: Acarine parasites live in unclean houses and feed from blood, sweat, food crumbs, fungi, and human keratin fragments. Allergic reactions caused by mites are not infrequent, as well as to the demonstration of mites in sputum. The mites, however, have seldom been found in lung tissue.
Etiology/Pathophysiology: Inhalation of acaridia, especially during sleep.
Clinical Presentation: The inhaled mites act as allergens. Allergic rhinitis and asthmatic bronchitis are the common findings. Blood eosinophilia may be present.
Prognosis: Excellent.
Radiology: Signs of asthmatic bronchitis. Bronchiectasis may be associated with infection with mites.
Pathology:
Gross: No specific changes have been described.
Histology: The mites have 6 or 8 legs and an unarmed hypostome. They measure less than 1 mm long, and their eggs are approximately

60 µm in diameter. Both stain well with HE. They may be seen in sputum and bronchial fluids. Rarely, they may cause pulmonary eosinophilia. Specific infectious reactions of lung tissue have not been described.

➤ *Descriptors:* Bronchial mucosa with preserved structure:
- ectatic lumen
- mites (intrabronchial)
- mixed inflammatory infiltrates
- eosinophils

■ *Special stains:* PAS, collagenous stains.

Hallmark of Diagnosis: Clinical history, identification of acarids in sputum, bronchial washings, or bronchial biopsies.

Differential diagnosis: The parasites are characteristic if demonstrable. The eggs have a strongly hematoxyphil shell and may be confused with eggs of trematode flukes (*Paragonimus westermani*).

Accessory Bronchus

Definition: A bronchus that originates from an abnormal location outside the lung, i.e., from the trachea, main bronchi, or structures derived from the embryonic foregut.

Incidence/Epidemiology: Malformations of the lung are rare. About 2.2% of childhood autopsies show pulmonary malformations. Accessory bronchi and lungs participate in about 10% of all lung malformations.

Etiology/Pathophysiology: The ventral surface of the primitive pharynx forms a primitive laryngotracheal bud at 22–26 days, which is the basis for developing the bronchial tree. The tracheo-bronchial tree develops coincidentally with the esophagus, both being separated by growing mesoderm during this stage. A second respiratory bud may arise from the parts later forming the esophagus or even from the stomach. Depending upon the local rate of growth and upon the exact location, the accessory bronchus may communicate with the main bronchial system or may develop its own peripheral lung tissue.

Clinical Presentation: Most of the accessory bronchi supply an accessory lobe of lung separated from the main lung. It is more frequently found on the left side. The development of adjacent lung tissue influences the symptoms.

Prognosis: Excellent.

Radiology: Hilar filtered tomography may give some information about the anatomical situation.

Pathology:

Gross: Additional major bronchus arising from the trachea or main (left) bronchus often accompanied by accessory lung tissue.

Histology: Fully developed bronchial configuration with normal mucosa and submucosa including bronchial cartilage.

➤ *Descriptors:* Bronchial mucosa with preserved structure:
- no morphological abnormalities

■ *Special stains:* None.

Hallmark of Diagnosis: Gross findings.

Differential diagnosis: Broncho-(tracheo)-esophageal fistula, abnormal variation of the bronchus tree.

Accessory Lung

Definition: Organ-like formation of lung tissue separated from the main lung. The term "sequestrated lung" has often been used synonymously.

Incidence/Epidemiology: Similar to the frequency of accessory bronchi.

Etiology/Pathophysiology: Disturbance of development of bronchi and lung from the primitive laryngotracheal bud, either in an early stage or a later stage. The following forms of accessory lung have to be distinguished:

1. Accessory lung with normal or abnormal bronchial supply
2. Accessory lung without bronchial supply (sequestration)
   a. separated from main lung with own pleura
   (extralobular sequestration)
   b. localization within the main lung and common pleura visceralis
   (intralobular sequestration)
   c. Connection of accessory lung with esophagus or stomach
   (broncho-pulmonary-foregut malformation, BPFM)

The blood supply of all sequestrated lungs is mainly transported by systemic arteries arising from the aorta. Besides radiography, angiography is, therefore, of importance.

Clinical Presentation: Depending upon the size and localization of the accessory lung severe disturbances of lung function and burden in the right heart may characterize the clinical findings. Chronic infections are frequent in patients with BPFM. Extralobular sequestration is often combined with additional malformations and is predominant in early childhood. Intralobular sequestration is mainly seen in adults.

Prognosis: Usually good; however, chronic infection can spread to other lung areas and induce honeycombing.

Radiology: Chest radiographs vary to a large extent and may display consolidated peripheral masses with pleural thickening. Angiography usually identifies the abnormal blood supply.

Pathology:

Gross: Extralobular lungs have a solid consistency and often consist of immature lung tissue. Intralobular lungs are mainly recognized by circumscribed, dense lung tissue usually confined to the posterior basal segment, sometimes with cystic alterations due to chronic infections. In both conditions larger abnormal arteries connected to the aorta can frequently be found.

Histology: No characteristic findings, immature lung tissue or altered lung tissue due to chronic infections may be present.

➤ *Descriptors:* Bronchial mucosa with preserved structure:
- ectatic lumen (bronchial and bronchiolar)
- viscous mucus
- mononuclear inflammatory infiltrates;
- Lung parenchyma with altered structure:
- diffuse interstitial fibrosis
- mononuclear inflammatory infiltrates
- immature lung parenchyma

■ *Special stains:* PAS, collagenous stains.

Hallmark of Diagnosis: Clinical history, gross findings.

Differential diagnosis: According to subclassification of accessory lung, congenital bronchiectasis, malformation.

Accessory Trachea

Definition: Complete or partial doubling of the trachea.

Incidence/Epidemiology: Extremely rare.

Etiology/Pathophysiology: Malformation due to disturbance of development of the primitive laryngotracheal bud.

Clinical Presentation: Depends on the degree of malformation.

Prognosis: Usually poor.

Radiology: Abnormalities of the mediastinum may be present.

Pathology:

Gross: Additional (complete) part of the trachea located beside the original trachea. Part of the accessory trachea may be fibrotic, and additional malformations are common.

Histology: No specific findings.

➤ *Descriptors:* Bronchial mucosa with preserved structure:
- mononuclear inflammatory infiltrates

■ *Special stains:* None.

Hallmark of Diagnosis: Gross findings.

Differential diagnosis: Tracheobronchial fistula.

Acetoaminophen

Definition: Alteration of the lung parenchyma associated with intake of acetoaminophen. See Drug Toxicity.

Acid Gastric Aspiration

Definition: Aspiration of gastric acid with immediate respiratory distress (synonym Mendelson's syndrome).

Incidence/Epidemiology: The classic study of Mendelson revealed a frequency of 0.15% in obstetrical patients under ether anesthesia. In childhood it is accompanied by diaphragmatic hernia. Mixed with food or liquid contents of the stomach, massive aspiration is frequently seen in alcoholics.

Etiology/Pathophysiology: Aspiration of sterile acidic gastric contents causes an acute – abacterial – inflammation. The inflammation is characterized by immediate widespread intraalveolar hemorrhage, edema, congestion and degeneration of bronchiolar lining cells and of pneumocytes. Pneumonic consolidation is followed by invasion of neutrophilic leukocytes after approximately 4 h, and hyaline membranes are found after approximately 48 h. Resolution starts after 72 h. The outcome is either complete restoration of lung parenchyma or residual postpneumonic scars.

If the gastric fluid contains food particles, an infection with predominantly anaerobic bacteria is likely, among which may be *Bacteroides melaninogenicus* and *fragiles,* streptococci, *Fusobacterium nucleatum, Clostridii, Borrelia vincenti, Escherichia coli*. These bacteria cause a gangrenous pneumonia with evil-smelling decomposition products.

Clinical Presentation: Acute pain with cyanosis, tachypnea, and tachycardia.

Prognosis: Usually good.

Radiology: Widespread mottled densities mainly located in the axillary branches of the subsegments of the apical and posterior upper lobe bronchi.

Pathology:

Gross: Localized, circumscribed, widespread, brownish-yellowish, necrotic areas.

Histology: Necrotic areas with predominant granulocytes located around the terminal bronchioles. The surrounding lung parenchyma is similarly affected. Large areas of hemorrhage; at a later stage hyaline membranes are present. In the stage of consolidation, mixed inflammatory infiltrates are predominant. Bronchiolitis obliterans can frequently be observed at this stage. Irregularly formed scars or granulomatous areas characterize the "burned out" stage.

➤ *Descriptors:* Lung parenchyma with preserved structure:

- mixed inflammatory infiltrates;
- Lung parenchyma with altered structure:
- necrosis and hemorrhage
- bacteria (anaerobic)
- intrabronchiolar fibrinoid material and histiocytes
- ulceration of bronchiolar mucosa
- focal interstitial fibrosis

■ *Special stains:* PAS, collagenous stains.

Hallmark of Diagnosis: Acute necrotic areas with former terminal bronchioles in the center, hemorrhage, edema, congestion with distinct boundary; in later stages mixed inflammatory infiltrates, focal fibrosis with irregular, fingerlike, fibrotic bundles.

Differential diagnosis: Acute bacterial pneumonia, acute infarction, lung abscess, necrotic lung cancer.

Acid Maltase Deficiency (Pompe's disease)

Definition: Lung involvement in type II glycogenosis (acid maltase deficiency).

Incidence/Epidemiology: Isolated reports of pulmonary involvement.

Etiology/Pathophysiology: The enzymatic deficiency may lead to pulmonary manifestation of glycogenesis, i.e., accumulation of glycogen in pneumocytes and macrophages.

Clinical Presentation: One adult patient is reported to have had dyspnea, restrictive pulmonary function defect, and diaphragmatic paralysis.

Prognosis: Involvement of the lung is usually not severe, and death occurs due to cardiac failure.

Radiology: No specific manifestations are known.

Pathology:

Gross: No specific findings.

Histology: Increased accumulation of glycogen in macrophages. It is unclear whether interstitial glycogen deposits exist.

➤ *Descriptors:* Lung parenchyma with preserved structure:

- macrophages (glycogen deposits)

■ *Special stains:* PAS, endogenous lectins.

Hallmark of Diagnosis: Clinical history, intraalveolar accumulation of glycogen-laden macrophages, biochemical identification of acid maltase deficiency.

Differential diagnosis: Desquamative interstitial pneumonitis, chronic obstructive lung disease, etc. Pulmonary symptoms may be related to dysfunction of the diaphragm or unrelated intrinsic lung diseases.

Acinus Cell Tumor

Definition: Generally benign tumor of the major bronchi arising from acinus cells. Indistinguishable from acinus cell tumor of the salivary glands.

Incidence/Epidemiology: A few cases have been described in the literature.

Etiology/Pathophysiology: Benign tumor originating in the acinus cells of the bronchial glands.

Clinical Presentation: The tumors are manifested by obstructive pneumonia in the lung parenchyma produced by the bronchus with the growing tumor. The polypous tumor growth may cause asthmoid bronchitis.

Prognosis: Usually good.

Radiology: Besides signs of peripheral obstructive pneumonia, hilar thickening and solid mass on hilar tomogram.

Pathology:
Gross: Circumscribed, pale tan tumor with endobronchial polypous growth.

Histology: Sheets of cells with granular cytoplasm and adenoid growth pattern. Small eccentric nuclei. Two cellular populations: one darker with smaller cells scattered among the predominant lighter and larger cells. No or unsuspicious inflammatory reaction of host tissue. Complete destruction of submucosal structures, absent tumor cell necrosis, very rare mitoses. The cytoplasm stains positively with the PAS stain, with small granules resistant to diastase pretreatment.

➤ *Descriptors:* Newly formed textures without metastasis potential:
- epithelial growth pattern
- adenoid textures
- solid textures
- homogeneous nuclear and cellular size
- finely distributed nuclear chromatin
- abundant cytoplasm (granular)
- absent or infrequent mitoses
- preserved bronchial mucosa
- absent inflammatory infiltrates

■ *Special stains:* PAS (digestion with diastase), Giemsa, DNA analysis, immunohistochemistry for cytokeratin, carcinoembryonic antigen (CEA), endogenous lectins.

Hallmark of Diagnosis: Arrangement of tumor cells in acinar groups and elongated columns, tumor cells with small nuclei and abundant PAS-positive cytoplasm, diastase resistance, absent necrosis, only few mitoses, diploid DNA distribution.

Differential diagnosis: Benign sugar tumor, bronchial oncocytoma, bronchial gland adenoma, mucoepidermoid tumor, well-differentiated adenocarcinoma, carcinoid.

Acquired Immunodeficiency Syndrome (AIDS)

Definition: Syndrome caused by a RNA retrovirus (human immunodeficiency virus, HIV).

Incidence/Epidemiology: Increasing incidence has been reported in various risk groups including homosexuals, patients needing repeated blood transfusions, intravenous drug abusers. It is estimated that worldwide more than five million persons are infected by the AIDS virus and that more than 800 000 patients are suffering from the acute disease. About 20% of infected persons develop an AIDS-related symptom complex (ARC) such as unexplained loss of weight or fever, oral thrush, or diffuse lymphadenopathy syndrome (enlarged lymph nodes at two or more extrainguinal sites for more than 3 months). The virus is transmitted by infected body fluids occurring through sexual contact, shared use of intravenous needles, or transfusion of contaminated blood.

Etiology/Pathophysiology: HIV is a retrovirus with special tropism for T lymphocytes, mainly leading to the death of the T helper cells. A decrease in natural killer cells and profound defects in the B cell-mediated immune response are accompanied by a decrease in the production of antigen-specific antibodies and an increase of nonspecific polyclonal production of antibodies. The infection seems to persist lifelong with an unpredictable variable course, ranging from asymptomatic carriers over self-limited development of influenza or mononucleosis-like stages to complete loss of the immune system with resultant AIDS.

Clinical Presentation: Fully developed AIDS is characterized by severe opportunistic infections such as *Pneumocystis carinii*, cytomegalovirus pneumonia, mycobacteria pneumonia, or a fulminant variety of Kaposi's sarcoma. Involvement of the central nervous system is common (*Toxoplasma gondii* infections).

Prognosis: The patients have a poor prognosis with a lethality of 50% and a median survival of less than 1 year.

Radiology: Chest radiographs may be normal or present characteristic signs of the opportunistic infection.

Pathology:

Gross: Macroscopic changes are characterized by the particular opportunistic infection. The lungs are normally heavy, moist, edematous, and bloody. Infiltrates of Kaposi's sarcoma are often multiple and seldom exceed 2 cm in diameter.

Histology: The reaction pattern of lung in immunocompromised patients includes a broad variety of findings, namely diffuse alveolar damage which may be histologically related to chronic organizing pneumonia, interstitial pneumonia with foamy exudate, alveolar proteinosis, necrotizing pneumonias with and without granulomatous reaction or infarction, bronchiolitis, and diffuse pulmonary hemorrhage. The reactive pattern of the alveolar lining cells is often reduced and weak in comparison to the reaction in nonimmunocompromised patients suffering from the same infection. The degree of granulomatous reactive patterns such as typical tuberculous or fungal granulomas is frequently diminished, a pattern which may cause diagnostic difficulties.

➤ *Descriptors:* Lung parenchyma with altered structure:

- necrosis and hemorrhage
- infectious organisms (intraalveolar)
- caseous epithelioid granulomas (ill defined)
- noncaseous epithelioid granulomas (ill defined);
- Lung parenchyma with preserved structure:
- intraalveolar serous fluid
- desquamation, hypertrophy, hyperplasia and dysplasia of pneumocytes
- inclusion bodies (viral, pneumocytes, macrophages)
- intraalveolar fibrinoid material

■ *Special stains:* PAS to exclude fungus, Grocott's to exclude *Pneumocystis carinii*, Ziel-Neelsen for tuberculosis, elastic tissue stains to characterize the degree of fibrosis.

Hallmark of Diagnosis: Clinical history, unusual opportunistic infection of the lung, weak inflammatory response of host tissue.

Differential diagnosis: Pulmonary infiltrates caused by a variety of opportunistic infections, drug toxicity, rheumatoid lung, infarction, alveolar proteinosis.

Actinomycosis

Definition: Pulmonary infection usually caused by *Actinomyces israelii*. Additional causal organisms include *A. naeslundii, A. odontolyticus, A. vicosus, Arachnia propionica, Bifidobacterium adolescentis.*

Incidence/Epidemiology: Frequent in patients with poor dental hygiene, about three times more common in men than in women, two peak periods of incidence are recognized between the ages 11–20 years and between the ages 35–50 years. The organism has a worldwide distribution and is found to be present around carious teeth and in tonsillar crypts.

Etiology/Pathophysiology: Actinomycosis is described as a primary or secondary infection. The primary infection is caused by inhalation of infected material from the oropharyngeal region. The secondary infection is less common and is usually caused by primary liver or cervicofacial infection. It may also grow in necrotic lesions of different origin such as pulmonary tuberculosis or central necrotizing carcinomas.

Clinical Presentation: The disease is characterized by chest pain, chills, light fever, night sweats, mild leukocytosis, and loss of weight. Chronic onset of the disease hinders correct diagnosis in many cases. Manifestations are local pain and swelling with a tendency to form draining fistulae. The bacteria are not characteristic organisms that infect immunosuppressed patients.

Prognosis: Usually good.

Radiology: Chest radiographs show circumscribed, consolidated masses with pleural thickening. Mediastinal structures can be involved as well as their diaphragm. Osteomyelitis of adjacent ribs may simulate a malignant growth.

Pathology:

Gross: Large fibrotic areas of the lung contain cavities with purulent masses and hard yellow granules about 1 mm in diameter. These granules are characteristic of the disease (so-called sulfur granules) and are mainly located in drainage fistulae leading to adjacent bronchi.

Histology: The purulent abscess is encapsulated by broad granulation tissue containing lymphocytes, plasma cells, histiocytes, and infrequently giant cells. The characteristic sulfur granules are rare and may be difficult to find.

Usually they are located in the center of the purulent area and surrounded by neutrophilic granulocytes. The sulfur granules consist of a granular basophilic center composed of the bacterial colony and radiating eosinophilic, hyaline peripheral clubs (Splendore-Hoeppli phenomenon). The bacteria are anaerobic, gram-positive, and nonmotile.

➤ *Descriptors:* Lung parenchyma with altered structure:
- necrosis and hemorrhage
- mixed inflammatory infiltrates
- bacteria (*Actinomyces*)
- sulfur granules
- focal interstitial fibrosis

■ *Special stains:* Methenamine silver stain, PAS-Gridley stain, Cresyl-Echt violet stain.

Hallmark of diagnosis: Sulfur granules embedded in purulent necrosis and encapsulated by granulation tissue.

Differential diagnosis: *Nocardia* infection, botryomycosis, mycetoma, acid gastric aspiration, necrotic lung cancer.

Acute Lupus Pneumonitis

Definition: Dramatic manifestation of systemic lupus erythematosus (SLE) in the lung.

Incidence/Epidemiology: Rare complication in patients with SLE.

Etiology/Pathophysiology: Immune-complex-mediated acute lung injury probably caused by electron-dense deposits within the alveolar capillary basement membranes.

Clinical Presentation: Fever, tachypnea, hypoxemia, infrequently hemorrhage and renal failure.

Prognosis: Fair; focal fibrosis or honeycombing may develop after a few years.

Radiology: Diffuse infiltrates in both lungs.

Pathology:

Gross: Edematous, wet lung whose consistency is solid.

Histology: Diffuse alveolar damage characterized by interstitial edema, lymphoplasmocytic infiltrations, intraalveolar exudation and formation of hyaline membranes. Rarely, additional intraalveolar hemorrhage. Characteristic changes seen in chronic lupus erythematosus are often not detectable.

➤ *Descriptors:* Lung parenchyma with preserved structure:
- mononuclear inflammatory infiltrates
- intraalveolar serous fluid
- hyaline membranes
- hemorrhage

■ *Special stains:* Immunofluorescence techniques for demonstration of IgG and complement, histones, double-stranded DNA.

Hallmark of Diagnosis: Clinical history, usual interstitial pneumonia with hyaline membranes, desquamated pneumocytes, and mononuclear inflammatory infiltrates.

Differential diagnosis: All causes of diffuse alveolar damage, especially Goodpasture's syndrome, idiopathic pulmonary hemosiderosis (both show no basement staining to IgG and complement).

Adenocarcinoma

Definition: Lung cancer of a special histological type that forms an adenoid growth pattern or produces intracellular or extracellular mucosubstances.

Incidence/Epidemiology: It is now the most frequent lung cancer in the USA, and the second most frequent one in Europe. It comprises about 20% of lung carcinomas of men and 50% of those of women. Within the different types of lung carcinomas its frequency is increasing in Europe and in the USA. Its incidence ranges from 20/100 000 to 60/100 000 cases per year.

Etiology/Pathophysiology: Cigarette smoking is the most important risk factor for all types of lung carcinomas. Radiation exposure and asbestos are additional known risk factors, as are exposure to copper, beryllium, arsenic, chromate, chloromethyl ether, vinyl chloride, benzene, and mustard gas. About 50% of adenocarcinomas are located in the peripheral lung, and the other 50% grow adjacent to main or major bronchi.

Clinical Presentation: Often without any symptoms and accidentally detected by X-ray study performed for various reasons. If the lesion is located in central areas, the patients show symptoms of chronic bronchitis, loss of weight, and – in the case of bronchioloalveolar carcinoma – increased mucus production.

Prognosis: Prognosis is closely associated with the TNM stage. The best indicator is the involvement of lymph nodes: Surgically treated patients with pN0 stage have a median survival of 4–5 years. Those with pN3 stage have a median survival of 6–12 months only. Survival of patients with adenocarcinoma and epidermoid carcinoma is similar and not as poor as that of patients with large cell anaplastic carcinoma or small cell anaplastic carcinoma.

Radiology: Peripherally located tumors present a solid circumscribed mass, sometimes with scarred trabeculae, indicating malignant growth. Diffuse infiltrates indicate the bronchioloalveolar carcinoma. Mediastinal circumscribed masses are seen in centrally located adenocarcinomas.

Pathology:

Gross: Solid, white-yellowish mass with boundaries ill-defined from adjacent lung tissue. Central necrosis and hemorrhage may be present. Small metastases about 1 mm in size are frequent near the boundary of the major tumor mass. Peripheral tumors are often ball-like or ellipsoidally shaped.

Histology: According to the WHO classification (1982) the following four categories of adenocarcinoma should be distinguished:

1. acinar adenocarcinoma
2. papillary adenocarcinoma
3. bronchioloalveolar adenocarcinoma
4. solid adenocarcinoma

The subclassification is, however, obscured by the fact that the majority of adenocarcinomas show mixtures of the different categories depending upon their differentiation. The grading of adenocarcinoma is divided as usual into three categories: well differentiated, moderately differentiated, and poorly differentiated adenocarcinoma. The acinar, papillary, and solid adenocarcinomas consist of medium-sized to large tumor cells with prominent nucleoli in the nuclear chromatin. Mitoses are relatively rare, and the cytoplasm is mainly eosinophilic and often shows a sharp boundary. The tumor proliferates mainly within the air spaces. A mild inflammatory infiltration within the tumor mass and at its boundary is present in the majority of cases. An extracellular mucus production is infrequent, in contrast to PAS-positive granules within the cytoplasm of tumor cells. Bronchioloalveolar carcinoma shows two different growth behaviors: The majority of patients suffer from solid, central scarred tumors with "lined up" tumor cells along the interalveolar septula at the tumor boundary. Additional acinar appearance of tumor textures is frequent. The tumor cells are small, and the tumor cell nuclei show mainly a coarse chromatin distribution. Mitoses are rare and no inflammatory cells can be seen at the tumor boundary. The second type of bronchioloalveolar carcinoma grows in small tumor nests not connected with each other. Usually no major tumor mass is found. These tumors usually produce extracellular mucus, but the surrounding lung tissue is completely normal, and inflammatory cellular infiltrates and necroses are missing. Within the air spaces small tumor cell aggregates are present.

The majority of adenocarcinomas are aneuploid. The percentage of S phases (S-GM1) amounts to 8–15%.

➤ *Descriptors:* Newly formed textures with metastasis potential:

- epithelial growth pattern
- adenoid textures (tubuli, papillary)
- mucus production
- inhomogeneous nuclear and cellular size
- prominent nucleoli
- infrequent mitoses
- eosinophilic cytoplasm (focal PAS positive)

■ *Special stains:* PAS, Giemsa, immunohistochemistry including CEA, cytokeratins, endogenous lectins.

Hallmark of Diagnosis: Adenoid tumor textures, presence of mucosubstance in the cytoplasm, prominent nucleoli, absent intercellular bridges.

Differential diagnosis: Undifferentiated large cell carcinoma, adenoid cystic carcinoma, bronchial adenoma, mucoepidermoid carcinoma, carcinoid, small cell anaplastic carcinoma, metastatic adenocarcinoma into the lung, especially hypernephroid carcinoma, adenocarcinoma of the stomach, ovary, pancreas, endometrium, or colon-rectum. In case of bronchioloalveolar carcinoma, severe atypia of pneumocytes could be suspected.

Adenoid Cystic Carcinoma

Definition: Malignant tumor of the lung which is histologically and electron-microscopically indistinguishable from adenoid cystic carcinoma of the salivary gland.

Incidence/Epidemiology: Most common tumor in the group of salivary gland-like tumors of the lower respiratory tract. It comprises 20–35% of all carcinomas arising from the trachea.

Etiology/Pathophysiology: No risk factors are known, in particular, there is no relation to smoking. Lesion arises from the tracheal and bronchial submucosal glands.

Clinical Presentation: Common in men and women with an average age of onset of 45 years. The symptoms result from partial airway obstruction and include wheezing, cough, dyspnea, hemoptysis, fever, and general cachexia. The tumors tend to spread along the submucosa of the affected bronchus or trachea with late ulceration and late invasion of the adjacent lung tissue. The tumor boundaries are often not visible by endoscopy. Metastases are rare in contrast to local recurrence after surgery.

Prognosis: The prognosis of patients is favorable compared with those suffering from bronchial carcinomas, and 85% of patients are still alive after 5 years.

Radiology: The leading symptom is the manifestation of distal obstruction without centrally placed tumor masses. However, the presence of the submucosal tumor growth may be detectable by computerized tomography (CT) and magnetic resonance (MR) scans.

Pathology:

Gross: Firm tumour masses of white, pink, or light tan color with spreading growth along the bronchus or trachea. At a later stage invasion into adjacent structures and polypoid intraluminal growth can occur. The overlying mucosa is usually unsuspicious, but at a later stage ulceration may occur. The boundaries of the tumors in the submucosa are difficult to detect.

Histology: The characteristic texture of the tumor results from the formation of cystic glands built up of monolayers of epithelial tumor cells mixed with "filled-up" glandular structures, both being embedded in broad bundles of hyalinized stroma. The cystic spaces contain mucin. The tumor cells are of medium size with compact, homogeneous nuclei. Uneffected glands and cartilage circumferentially embedded by tumor cells are common findings. Mitoses are infrequent, necrosis is absent. Inflammatory infiltrations are mild and uncommon. Diploid tumor cells.

➤ *Descriptors:* Newly formed textures with metastasis potential:
- epithelial growth pattern
- adenoid textures (tubuli)
- solid textures
- mucus production
- homogeneous nuclear and cellular size
- finely distributed nuclear chromatin
- infrequent mitoses
- absent necrosis
- absent or weak inflammatory infiltrates

■ *Special stains:* PAS or stains for mucin. Absence of neuroendocrine markers.

Hallmark of diagnosis: Typical "adenoid cystic" tumor textures embedded in hyaline stroma, absence of necroses, medium-sized tumor cells with dense nuclear chromatin, only few mitoses.

Differential diagnosis: Adenocarcinoma, adenoma, lymphangitis carcinomatosa, mucoepidermoid carcinoma, carcinoid.

Adenoma

Definition: Benign circumscribed tumors with adenomatoid tumor textures originating either from the submucosal glands (mucous gland adenoma, pleomorphic adenoma) or from the peripheral lung parenchyma (alveolar adenoma).

Incidence/Epidemiology: Very exceptional tumors. They occur with equal frequency in men and women and can be seen at all ages.

Etiology/Pathophysiology: It is believed that the majority of these tumors arise from the bronchial mucus glands.

Clinical Presentation: The symptoms of the tumors are usually related to bronchial obstruction induced by the proximal tumor localization.

Prognosis: Usually good, and more than 80% of patients are still alive 5 years after curative resection. Local recurrence has been reported.

Radiology: Often unsuspicious or related to proximal obstruction of a major bronchus.

Pathology:

Gross: Circumscribed, endobronchial, yellowish-white tumors measuring 1–2 cm in diameter.

Histology: Medium-sized tumor cells with homogeneous nuclear size and eosinophilic cytoplasm. Tubular growth patterns predominate. Some neoplastic glands may show papillary infolding of epithelial tumor cells. Solid growth patterns, mucus production, and hyalinization of the adjacent bronchial tissue may occur. Necroses, inflammatory response of host tissue, and mitotic figures are absent.

➤ *Descriptors:* Newly formed textures without metastasis potential:

- epithelial growth pattern
- adenoid textures (tubuli, papillary infolding, cysts)
- solid textures
- mucus production
- finely distributed nuclear chromatin
- homogeneous nuclear and cellular size
- absent necrosis
- absent inflammatory infiltrates

■ *Special stains:* PAS, Giemsa, collagenous stains, DNA analysis, endogenous lectins, immunohistochemistry for cytokeratins, CEA.

Hallmark of Diagnosis: Well-differentiated adenoid tumor textures, homogeneous cellular and nuclear size, absence of necroses, inflammation, and mitotic figures.

Differential diagnosis: Carcinoid tumor, adenocarcinoma, mucoepidermoid carcinoma, adenoid cystic carcinoma, benign clear cell tumor of the lung, oncocytoma, metastatic adenocarcinoma into the lung, especially thyroid carcinoma.

Adenomatoid Cystic Malformation of the Lung

Definition: Congenital cystic lung lesion characterized by the presence of abnormal bronchiolar structures of hamartous character and of varying size and/or distribution. Three different types are distinguished by their clinical, radiological, and pathological features:

Type I: (cystic lesion) single or multiple larger cysts 3–7 cm in diameter surrounded by smaller collapsed cysts.

Type II: (intermediate type) smaller, more uniform cysts (5–20 mm) resembling numerous ectatic, overlying bronchioles.

Type III: (solid type) curved channels or randomly distributed bronchiole-like cystic structures (1–3 mm) lined with cuboidal epithelium.

Incidence/Epidemiology: Relatively common with slight predominance in men. Type I is the most frequent (approximately 65%), followed by type II (approximately 25%), and by type III (approximately 10%).

Etiology/Pathophysiology: The more mature type I lesion suggests an onset at 7–10 weeks' gestation in contrast to the more immature type II lesion (estimated onset 3–4 weeks' gestation). Typ III is estimated to start at 3–4 weeks' gestation due to an observed combination with renal agenesis. Overgrowth of bronchioles with consequent suppression of alveolar differentiation has been postulated.

Clinical Presentation: The malformation is usually restricted to one lobe and recognized at birth. However, some adult cases with congenital adenomatoid malformation have been reported. Respiratory distress including cyanosis, retraction, grunting as well as fever, cough, repeated infections, or pneumothorax are common symptoms. Fetal anasarca and stillbirth may be present as well as maternal polyhydramnios.

Prognosis: After adequate surgery 85% of patients will survive with nearly 90% of normal lung volume during later life.

Radiology: Depending upon type, multicystic appearance restricted to one lobe or a solid homogeneous lesion may be present. The solid lesions may transform to empty cysts after several days if fluid becomes depleted.

Pathology:

Gross: Thin-walled cysts surrounded by smaller collapsed cysts with adjacent normal lung parenchyma characterize type I. Type II shows more homogeneous smaller cysts surrounded by normal lung tissue together with some dense lung areas distant from the lesion. A capsule between the cysts and the normal lung tissue is not present. Type III is characterized by rubbery condensed lung tissue normally occupying a whole lobe.

Histology: The large cysts of type I are lined by ciliated pseudostratified columnar cells. Due to collapse during tissue preparation several polypoid projections form the cystic wall. Fragments of cartilage and fibromuscular bundles are often seen between two cysts and are characteristic of type I. The structures may resemble a hamartous lesion. Cuboidal-to-columnar epithelium rarely displaying pseudostratification lines type II cysts. Bundles of striate muscular fibers may be located between the cysts and also between the alveolar ducts and around blood vessels. Mucus producing cells or cartilage fragments are absent in type II malformations. Type III lesions are composed of true "adenomatoid" lesions with randomly distributed irregular bronchiole-like structures. The lesion resembles the structures of the immature lung in the pseudoglandular phase. A thin fibromuscular layer may form the base of the epithelium of the bronchiolar cysts.

➤ *Descriptors:* Newly formed textures with altered structure:
- immature lung parenchyma
- cysts (ciliated pseudostratified columnar cells)
- fragments of cartilage
- smooth muscle cells
- mucinous cells (papillary infoldings)

■ *Special stains:* PAS, elastic stains, DNA analysis.

Hallmark of Diagnosis: Combined features of hamartoma, immature lung, and dysplastic growth. Single or multiple cysts occupying parts of one lobe with distinct boundary adjacent to healthy lung tissue (type I and type II). Small cystic "pseudobronchioles" are randomly distributed in one lobe (type III).

Differential diagnosis: Hamartoma, congenital pulmonary lymphangiectasis, infantile lobar emphysema, pulmonary sequestration.

Adenosquamous Carcinoma

Definition: Malignant lung tumor composed of squamous and glandular structures.

Incidence/Epidemiology: It represents 0.4–4% of all lung carcinomas; associated with the common risk factors of bronchial carcinomas, especially smoking and exposure to asbestos.

Etiology/Pathophysiology: Similar to adenocarcinomas.

Clinical Presentation: Peripherally or centrally located tumor with early metastases into the lymph nodes, liver, brain, skeleton. Symptoms are related to tumor localization. Patients may by asymptomatic or present with cough, dyspnea, shortness of breath during exercise, and loss of weight.

Prognosis: Patients with adenosquamous carcinomas have a worse prognosis than those with adenocarcinoma or with epidermoid carcinomas; less than 5% are still alive after 5 years.

Radiology: Mainly a circumscribed, peripherally located mass with thin radial densities.

Pathology:

Gross: Yellowish tumor mass with distinct boundary. Central necrotic areas may be present as well as intrapulmonary lymph node metastases.

Histology: Moderately differentiated glandular differentiation in one area of the tumor is combined with epidermoid structures in another. Keratin production is generally poor, and there are extracellular deposits of mucus. Inflammatory infiltrations are poor, just distinct stroma bundles. Goblet cells may be present. The majority of the tumors are aneuploid.

➤ *Descriptors:* Newly formed textures with metastasis potential:
- epithelial growth pattern
- adenoid textures (tubuli)
- epidermoid textures
- mucus production
- keratin production
- intercellular bridges
- inhomogeneous nuclear and cellular size
- prominent nucleoli
- frequent mitoses
- necrosis
- absent or weak inflammatory infiltrates

■ *Special stains:* PAS, Giemsa, immunohistochemistry for CEA, cytokeratin, epithelial membrane antigen (EMA), endogenous lectins.

Hallmark of Diagnosis: Geometrically, separated, moderately differentiated glandular and epidermoid growth pattern.

Differential diagnosis: Mucoepidermoid carcinoma, poorly differentiated epidermoid carcinoma, mixed adeno-large cell carcinoma.

Adenovirus Infection

Definition: Respiratory infection caused by one of the 41 different types of adenovirus.

Incidence/Epidemiology: This infection comprises about 5% of all acute respiratory diseases in young children. It is also found in immunosuppressed adults and rarely in healthy ones. It is slightly more common in winter and has occurred as epidemics in military camps.

Etiology/Pathophysiology: Infection by droplets and person-to-person spread.

Clinical Presentation: Acute systemic illness including fever, malaise, headache, cough, and wheezing. An exudative pharyngitis and a flu-like syndrome may precede the pulmonary manifestation. Severe bronchiolitis and fatal pneumonia have been described in young children.

Prognosis: Usually good, but in about 20% of patients severe lung damage such as bronchiectasis and bronchiolitis obliterans may follow.

Radiology: Findings vary from "classic interstitial infiltrates" to necrotizing pneumonia. Alveolar filling or a micronodular pattern is often present as well as patchy infiltrates.

Pathology:

Gross: Heavy, edematous, and airless lung, often with small necrotic areas or hemorrhage. Micronodular thickening may be present.

Histology: Manifestation usually in two different patterns of damage: (a) necrotizing inflammation of bronchioles and small to medium-sized bronchi and (b) interstitial pneumonitis. The necrotizing inflammation mainly affects the mucosa and parts of the submucosa with usually preserved muscularis. The lumina are filled with coagula of fibrin, necrotic material, and inflammatory infiltrations including neutrophilic granulocytes, lymphocytes, and plasma cells. The surrounding lung parenchyma is also affected in the manner of interstitial pneumonitis and shows an alveolar exudate, intraalveolar hemorrhage, and edema. Hyaline membranes and focal necrosis of interalveolar septula may be present. Inclusion bodies can be found in the bronchiolar epithelium and in the cells of the alveolar lining. They occur in two types: one showing a homogeneous, basophilic or amphophilic, Feulgen-positive inclusion located in an enlarged so-called smudge cell. The second, less common type of inclusion is smaller, round, eosinophilic, Feulgen-negative, and surrounded by an often incomplete, clear halo. Chronically damaged lungs may proceed to a destructive stage characterized by bronchiectasis, bronchiolitis obliterans, or fibrotic scarring. Inclusion bodies are absent in these stages.

➤ *Descriptors:* Bronchial mucosa with preserved structure:
- ectatic lumen;
- Bronchial mucosa with altered structure:
- necrosis (segmental)
- ulceration
- fibrinoid material
- inclusion bodies (bronchiolar epithelial cells);
- Lung parenchyma with preserved structure:
- mononuclear inflammatory infiltrates
- hemorrhage
- hyaline membranes
- intraalveolar fibrinoid material
- inclusion bodies (pneumocytes);
- Lung parenchyma with altered structure:
- intrabronchiolar fibrinoid material and histiocytes
- ulceration of bronchiolar mucosa
- focal interstitial fibrosis

■ *Special stains:* PAS, collagenous stains, Feulgen stain, immunoperoxidase or immunofluorescence with special antibodies, in situ hybridization (sensitivity approximately 90%).

Hallmark of Diagnosis: No special morphological alterations exist. Necrotizing bronchiolitis combined with interstitial pneumonitis may suggest virus infection. Detection of inclusion bodies is a prerequisite for correct diagnosis. Final proof by immunohistochemical and in situ hybridization techniques, and by virus cultures.

Differential diagnosis: Infections caused by other viruses, aspiration pneumonia, allergic extrinsic alveolitis, necrotizing bronchocentric granulomatosis.

Adiaspiromycosis

Definition: Pulmonary fungus infection caused by the dimorphic *Chrysosporium parvum, Emmonsia parva*, and *crescens*.

Incidence/Epidemiology: Worldwide distribution, living in soil, usually an infection of rodents and other small mammalian animals, very seldom (approximately 10–20 reports) infection of human lung.

Etiology/Pathophysiology: Solely primary infection of human lung. No multiplication in lung tissue.

Clinical Presentation: Often clinically and radiologically inapparent, sometimes slight symptoms, including cough and mild progressive dyspnea.

Prognosis: Good, severe involvement of the lung is only seen in heavy infections.

Radiology: Often unsuspicious, sometimes, in severe cases, detectable, bilateral, solid nodules 1–2 mm in diameter.

Pathology:

Gross: Discrete or confluent, solid, white granulomas (1–2 mm in diameter).

Histology: Typical adiaspores with trilaminar composition of wall which contains an outer eosinophilic and an inner hyaline layer. Size of the adiaconidia 200–500 µm, thickness of the wall 20–70 µm. The adiaconidia are embedded in granulomatous tissue with concentrically arranged fibroblasts, collagen fibers, and scattered giant cells. The adjacent lung tissue is unsuspicious.

➤ *Descriptors:* Lung parenchyma with altered structure:
- noncaseous epithelioid granulomas
- fungus (intragranulomatous, adiaspores)
- multinucleated giant cells
- palisading histiocytes
- focal interstitial fibrosis

■ *Special stains:* PAS, Mayer's mucicarmine technique, Gridley, gallocyanin, toluidine blue.

Hallmark of diagnosis: Demonstration of adiaconidia embedded in granulomatous collagenous tissue with scattered giant cells.

Differential diagnosis: Lentil pneumonia (grain aspiration).

α-Adrenergic Nasal Sprays

Definition: Alteration of the lung parenchyma associated with intake of α-adrenergic nasal sprays, see Drug Toxicity.

Adult Respiratory Distress Syndrom (ARDS)

Definition: Clinical syndrome related to damage of the alveolar capillary membrane representing a heterogeneous group of disorders.

Incidence/Epidemiology: Common, and it affects about 150 000 persons per year in the USA.

Etiology/Pathophysiology: Development of severe pulmonary edema after various injuries, leading to leaking capillaries. The preclinical phase is characterized by lung parenchymal injuries due to invasion of activated polymorphonuclear leukocytes that release their lysosomal enzymes and generate oxygen-free radicals. This process can be activated by infectious agents, inhaled substances, chemotherapeutic agents, shock, trauma, sepsis, radiation, acute pancreatitis, fat or air embolism, uremia, etc.

Clinical Presentation: It often affects persons who are quite healthy prior to onset. Acute onset of dyspnea and diffuse pulmonary infiltrates. Manifestation of severe hypoxemia and decreasing lung compliance.

Prognosis: High mortality (about 50%), or recovery may occur after several days or within weeks. Mild obstructive defects may remain in survivors.

Radiology: Diffuse increase in density of chest radiographs, so-called white-out.

Pathology:

Gross: Heavy, congested, airless lung in the early phase, while after about 7 days lungs appear stiff, firm and gray. Cystic formation as seen in honeycomb lung may be the end-stage.

Histology: The disease is histologically characterized by two different stages, the edematous one (diffuse alveolar damage) and the organizing one. The exudative (edematous) stage forms hyaline membranes within 24 h. Fibrinous exudates and cellular debris are located within the alveoli, arranged in a layer along the interalveolar septula. Erythrocytes, fibrin, and an increased number of neutrophilic granulocytes accompany the hyaline membranes within the alveolar spaces. A marked interstitial edema is usually present. After 3–7 days the proliferation of pneumocytes of type II can be observed. Hyperplasia of cells of the alveolar lining is a sign that the acute stage of ARDS is being transformed to the organizing stage. Proliferating type II cells replace the damaged type I cells and stick to the basement membrane. Atypia and mitotic figures are present and should not be mistaken for bronchioloalveolar carcinoma. The organizing stage starts with deposits of collagenous fibers within the interstitium which are clearly demonstrable by light microscopy after 14 days. The hyperplastic type II pneumocytes remain prominent. The hyaline membranes are phagocytosed by macrophages, but remnants of fibrin and cellular debris can still be seen. Fibrinous thrombi in small pulmonary arteries are detectable. At a later stage (within 2 weeks) severe diffuse fibrosis may lead to death.

➤ *Descriptors:* Lung parenchyma with preserved structure:

- intraalveolar serous fluid
- interstitial edema
- hemorrhage
- intraalveolar fibrinoid material
- hyaline membranes
- neutrophils
- desquamation, hypertrophy, hyperplasia and dysplasia of pneumocytes
- Pulmonary vessels with preserved structure:
- thrombosis (fibrinoid, capillaries, small arteries)
- Lung parenchyma with altered structure:
- mononuclear inflammatory infiltrates
- proliferating fibroblasts
- diffuse interstitial fibrosis
- honeycombing

■ *Special stains:* PAS, elastic tissue stains, Giemsa, endogenous lectins.

Hallmark of Diagnosis: Hyaline membrane formation, increased number of neutrophils, marked interstitial edema, hypertrophy, hyperplasia and dysplasia of cells of the alveolar lining, proliferating fibroblasts, diffuse interstitial fibrosis.

Differential diagnosis: Usual interstitial pneumonia, bronchiolo alveolar carcinoma, viral pneumonia.

Agenesis of Lung

Definition: Absence of lung tissue beyond the trachea or main stem bronchus.

Incidence/Epidemiology: Depending upon the degree of malformation, bilateral pulmonary agenesis is very rare (less than 10 reported cases), unilateral absence of lung is more frequent, with a slight predominance in females. Unilateral agenesis may be compatible with normal life, especially agenesis of the left lung. Additional congenital anomalies are frequent and include the VATER association. Isolated absence of one or more lobes occurs very rarely.

Etiology/Pathophysiology: Disturbance of development of airway formation during the period from 6–16 weeks of gestation.

Clinical Presentation: Patients show severe respiratory distress and mediastinal shift.

Prognosis: Most patients die within a few days after birth. Agenesis of right lung seems to be associated with higher mortality due to more severe cardiovascular abnormalities.

Radiology: Mediastinal shift, findings depend upon the degree of agenesis (in the instance of right lung agenesis dextrocardia may exist).

Pathology:

Gross: Macroscopic findings include absence of one or both lungs with rudimentary, blind-ending bronchus, tracheobronchus, or tracheal agenesis. Absence of one or more lobes should not be confused with "bilateral left lungs" seen in association with cardiac malformations. Existing lung is often enlarged.

Histology: No specific findings. Existing lung has normally mature lung parenchyma and may present an increased number of alveoli and a reduced number of bronchial branches and arterial branches.

➤ *Descriptors:* Lung parenchyma with preserved structure:

- increased number of distant air spaces (in existing lung);
- Bronchial mucosa with preserved structure:
- reduced number of bronchial generations (in existing lung)

Special stainings: None, morphometry of existing lung.

Hallmark of Diagnosis: Gross findings, increased number of alveoli, and reduced number of bronchial generations in the existing lung.

Differential diagnosis: Pulmonary hypoplasia, bronchial isomerism syndrome (bilateral right or left lungs).

Agenesis of Trachea

Definition: Absence or almost complete absence of trachea due to congenital malformation

Incidence/Epidemiology: Very rare, about 40 cases have been described.

Etiology/Pathophysiology: Maldevelopment of trachea from the primitive laryngotracheal bud starting late in the 4th week of gestation.
Clinical Presentation: Most children with tracheal agenesis present with esophageal fistulae and additional anomalies related to the VATER association.
Prognosis: All children reported died before the 6th week of life.
Radiology: Missing trachea in filtered mediastinal tomography.
Pathology:
Gross: Complete or incomplete absence of trachea, in the majority of cases broncho-esophageal fistula. Complete agenesis of lung may be present. Existing lungs are described as being identical with extralobular sequestration.
Histology: No specific findings.

➤ *Descriptors:* Lung parenchyma with preserved structure:
- no morphological abnormalities

■ *Special stains:* None.

Hallmark of Diagnosis: Gross findings.
Differential diagnosis: Esophageal agenesis, congenital tracheal stenosis, congenital tracheomalacia.

Aging Lung

Definition: Morphological and functional changes of lung due to aging with special reference to the environment (air pollution, etc.).
Incidence/Epidemiology: No exact data exist except general morphological changes such as emphysema with increasing age and in smoking and nonsmoking persons. The emphysema score increases in nonsmokers from 1 at age 40–49 to 8 at age 90–99 years, and in smokers from 4 at age 40–49 to 20 at age 90–99 years.
Etiology/Pathophysiology: External damage of lung causes increased proteolytic activity, digesting the lung parenchyma. Elastase derived from polymorphonuclear leukocytes is thought to be one of the most effective agents destroying elastic fibers. Local scars may develop and cause additional damage by physical stretching forces, in addition to deposits of dust and foreign material.
Clinical Presentation: Decrease of lung function with mainly restrictive, partly obstructive components.
Prognosis: It is still debatable whether air pollution affects the life span. Very old persons usually die due to cardio-respiratory failure.
Radiology: Increased transparency of lung, sometimes with focal scarring.
Pathology:
Gross: Increasing anteroposterior diameter, perimeter, area, and height up to the 6th decade with "outrounding" of the surface.
Histology: Increasing size (volume) of respiratory bronchioles, alveolar ducts, and alveolar sacs with relative decrease in the volume fraction of alveolar volume. Decrease of alveolar surface area (surface/volume ratio), loss of alveolar wall tissue resulting in loss of capillary bed. Loss of elastic tissue fibers in the alveolar walls. The changes are hardly visible by light microscopy, and morphometric (stereologic) measurements have to be applied except in cases with clearly demonstrable emphysema.

➤ *Descriptors:* Lung parenchyma with preserved structure:
- enlarged distant air spaces
- atrophic interalveolar septula
- dust (anthracotic pigment);
- Pulmonary vessels with altered structure:
- hyaline material (small arteries and veins);
- Lung parenchyma with altered structure:
- focal interstitial fibrosis

■ *Special stains:* Elastic stains, stains of reticular fibers, application of monoclonal antibodies against the various types of collagen, morphometry.

Hallmark of Diagnosis: Diffuse emphysema with atrophic interalveolar septula, deposits of anthracotic pigment, hyaline scars.
Differential diagnosis: All types of emphysema (especially panacinar), normal lung, anthracosis.

Air Embolism

Definition: Rapid influx of air into the vascular system.
Incidence/Epidemiology: Rare, it may occur during head and neck surgery, traumas, intravenous and intraarterial injections, intrauterine and intravaginal manipulations, gas distension of the peritoneal space for laparoscopy, hyperbaric decompression, forced positive pressure ventilation, and similar circumstances.

Etiology/Pathophysiology: The introduced air blocks the pulmonary blood flow, and, depending on the amount, rapid death may occur due to shock. The increase of intracapillary pressure causes pulmonary edema.

Clinical Presentation: Decrease of cardiac output, acute right-heart strain and acute heart failure.

Prognosis: Depending upon the amount of air embolism, an air volume of 20 cm^3 or more usually causes rapid death.

Radiology: Diffuse pulmonary infiltrations due to pulmonary edema.

Pathology:

Gross: Dilated right heart and vena cava inferior, contracted and empty left ventricle, frothy blood in the pulmonary artery and veins. Wet, heavy, bloody, and partly foamy lungs.

Histology: Acute pulmonary edema with dilated veins, and if the dying process was prolonged, an increased number of eosinophilic and neutrophilic granulocytes in the small arteries, capillaries, and interstitial tissue.

➤ *Descriptors:* Lung parenchyma with preserved structure:

- eosinophils (intravascular, interstitial)
- neutrophils
- intraalveolar serous fluid;
- Pulmonary vessels with preserved structure:
- ectatic lumen (veins and arteries)

■ *Special stains:* PAS, elastic tissue stains, silver stain.

Hallmark of Diagnosis: Clinical history, dilated veins and capillaries, increased number of eosinophilic and neutrophilic granulocytes in the small arteries and capillaries.

Differential diagnosis: *Clostridia* sepsis, pulmonary edema due to acute heart failure.

Alagille's Syndrome

Definition: Congenital anomaly with paucity of intrahepatic bile ducts, cholestasis, characteristic facies, and often stenotic lesions of the peripheral pulmonary arteries.

Incidence/Epidemiology: Rare, reported to be related to α_1-antitrypsin deficiency, chromosomal defects (45/XO, trisomy 17-18, Down's syndrome).

Etiology/Pathophysiology: Inborn error with less than the normal number of bile ducts (less than one per portal triad).

Clinical Presentation: One group of patients with special facies (hypertelorism, deeply set eyes, broad forehead) present with a systolic murmur which is related to stenosis of the pulmonary artery. Additional anomalies may be present.

Prognosis: Prognosis is fair, and progression into liver cirrhosis seldom occurs.

Radiology: Unsuspicious except for stenosis of the pulmonary arteries.

Pathology:

Gross: Gross findings are normal except for moderate stenosis of one or both pulmonary arteries.

Histology: No specific findings.

➤ *Descriptors:* Lung parenchyma with preserved structure:

- no morphological abnormalities

■ *Special stains:* Elastic tissue stains.

Hallmark of Diagnosis: Clinical history, circumcribed stenosis of pulmonary arteries.

Differential diagnosis: Neonatal liver cirrhosis, isolated stenosis of pulmonary arteries.

Alariasis

Definition: Human infection with mesocercaria larvae of species of *Alaria.*

Incidence/Epidemiology: Very rare human infections may occur in North America from species that are common parasites of canids. Frogs or snakes are mentioned as the intermediate hosts.

Etiology/Pathophysiology: Infection may occur by eating raw amphibians or snakes.

Clinical Presentation: The infection may be systemic, or the parasites may settle down in the eyes or skin. In one reported systemic case the lung was involved. The disease started with cough, hemoptysis, and dyspnea.

Prognosis: The outcome of the reported case was fatal.

Radiology: Several dense infiltrations in both lungs were reported.

Pathology:

Gross: The gross findings revealed living worms in both lungs. In addition, liver, heart, kidneys, pancreas, lymph nodes, brain, and skin were involved.

Histology: The parasites are 300-800 μm long. The four penetration glands, the number of rings of spines on the ventral sucker and the arrangement of spines on the back are of diagnostic value.

➤ *Descriptors:* Lung parenchyma with altered structure:

- parasites (larvae, alive)
- necrosis
- mixed inflammatory infiltrates
- eosinophils

■ *Special stains:* PAS, elastic tissue stains.

Hallmark of Diagnosis: Clinical history, identification of the parasites, severe inflammatory response of host tissue.

Differential diagnosis: Infections of various trematodes, especially *Angiostrongylus*, larva migrans.

Albinism Oculocutaneous

Definition: Ceroid-like storage disorder involving skin, lung, large bowel, eyes. Also called Hermansky-Pudlak syndrome.

Incidence/Epidemiology: Very rare, less than 10 patients with lung involvement have been reported. Most patients are reported from Puerto Rico and Holland.

Etiology/Pathophysiology: Autosomal recessive disorder with oculocutaneous (tyrosine-positive) albinism showing a defect in the second stage of platelet aggregation and ceroid storage of histiocytes.

Clinical Presentation: Patients present with albinism and accumulation of ceroid-filled histiocytes in various organs including liver, skin, lung, colon. Albinism is not essential for diagnosis; some patients present only with disturbance of second stage platelet aggregation, granulomatous colitis, and lung involvement similar to that of idiopathic usual interstitial pneumonia. Patients'age ranges from 20–45 years.

Prognosis: The prognosis of patients is fair.

Radiology: Diffuse infiltrations of various intensity in both lungs.

Pathology:

Gross: Heavy, yellowish lungs with interstitial fibrosis.

Histology: Preserved lung tissue with interstitial mononuclear infiltrations, various degrees of interstitial fibrosis, and dense foamy histiocytic infiltrates in the alveoli. Image may be indistinguishable from the usual idiopathic interstitial pneumonia. The intraalveolar histiocytes stain positively with PAS and Fontana's stain, weakly positively with acid-fast stains, negatively with iron and fluorescent orange.

➤ *Descriptors:* Lung parenchyma with preserved structure:

- mononuclear inflammatory infiltrates
- hyaline membranes
- macrophages;
- Lung parenchyma with altered structure:
- diffuse interstitial fibrosis

■ *Special stains:* PAS, acid-fast, Fontana, Prussian blue, fluorescence orange.

Hallmark of Diagnosis: Usual interstitial pneumonia, clinical and family history, PAS-positive histiocytes.

Differential diagnosis: Various storage diseases such as Fabry's disease, infantile GM1-gangliosidosis, Gaucher's disease, adult Niemann-Pick-disease, idiopathic usual interstitial pneumonia.

Algae

Definition: Uncommon infection of lung caused by certain species of genus *Prototheca* (achlorophyllus algae, *Prototheca wickerhamii* and *zopfii*).

Incidence/Epidemiology: Widely distributed organism living in soil, sewage, stream water. About 30 cases are reported, mainly from the USA.

Etiology/Pathophysiology: Progressive papular or eczematous infection of the skin in patients with diminished immunoresponse such as those suffering from diabetes mellitus, malnutrition, alcoholism or olecranon bursitis. In healthy patients, it may proceed to regional lymphadenitis and hematogenous spread, causing repetitive pneumonia.

Clinical Presentation: Cutaneous lesions of one extremity precede pulmonary infections. Olecranon bursitis often associated with local injury may show either little cellular reaction or a mixed granulomatous necrotizing dermatitis which may resemble rheumatoid nodules.

Prognosis: Usually good.

Radiology: Localized, circumscribed, dense infiltrates depending upon the degree of infection.

Pathology:

Gross: Circumscribed, yellowish-white nodules.

Histology: Mixed cellular infiltrates with central necrosis and granulomatous organization including multinucleated giant cells similar to rheumatoid nodules.The organism can be recognized by the yeastlike colonies which consist of endosporulating sporangia. The oval cells contain vacuolated cytoplasm and small, dark nuclei. The hyaline walls of the sporangia stain positively with PAS, Gomori's methenamine silver stain (GMS), Gridley's stains.

➤ *Descriptors:* Lung parenchyma with altered structure:

- necrosis
- mixed inflammatory infiltrates
- caseous epithelioid granulomas
- algae (intragranulomatous, yeastlike colonies)
- multinucleated giant cells

■ *Special stains:* PAS, GMS, Gridley's, direct immunofluorescence.

Hallmark of Diagnosis: Characteristic staining of organism, skin lesions with identical histopathological appearance; ill-defined, epithelioid granulomas with central necrosis.

Differential diagnosis: Rheumatoid nodules, tuberculosis, fungal infections.

Allergic (Extrinsic) Alveolitis

Definition: Predominantly chronic inflammatory disease of the peripheral lung parenchyma caused by sensitization and subsequent exposure to various inhaled agents. It is also referred to as hypersensitivity pneumonitis or microgranulomatous hypersensitivity reaction of the lung.

Incidence/Epidemiology: Patients are usually exposed to the inorganic or organic antigens via their occupation, avocation, or housing conditions. The prevalence varies depending upon the agent and is reported to range between 2.3–8.6% for the farmer's lung disease caused by thermophilic *Actinomyces*.

Etiology/Pathophysiology: Allergic alveolitis is mediated by immune complexes (combination of type III and type IV immune reactions of the lung). Type I includes reagin-mediated or immediate hypersensitivity (IgE) with the histological hallmark of eosinophilic infiltrates (asthma); type II includes cytotoxic antibody-mediated hypersensitivity as seen in Goodpasture's syndrome; type III displays activated complement and intravascular adhesive immune complexes; in type IV cell-mediated or delayed hypersensitivity is mediated by sensitized T lymphocytes forming granulomas as seen in tuberculosis. The agents causing hypersensitivity pneumonitis can be divided into four general categories: (a) thermophilic *Actinomyces* (farmer's lung, mushroom worker's lung, bagassosis, humidifier lung, etc.); (b) molds (maple bark stripper's lung, malt workers lung, sequoiosis, etc.); (c) animal products (bird fanciers' disease, pigeon handler's disease, pituitary snuff-taker's lung, fish meal worker's lung, furrier's lung, bat lung, miller's lung, etc.); (d) unknown (sauna taker's lung, coptic lung, coffee worker's lung, tea grower's lung, thatched roof lung, etc.).

Clinical Presentation: The disease may present in two different stages: an acute or subacute stage consisting of fever, malaise, chills, dyspnea, cough 4–6 h after inhalation of the antigen, and a chronic form resulting from prolonged exposure to small amounts of the antigen with complaints of chronic fatigue, dyspnea on exertion, anorexia, and occasionally progressive respiratory failure. Skin testing is useful in the acute form as well as in the search for precipitating antibodies. Symptoms in the acute form usually resolve after 1–2 days following cessation of exposure.

Prognosis: Usually good if the offending antigen is evaluated. In the contrary case interstitial fibrosis and honeycombing can occur.

Radiology: In the acute form are seen diffuse, soft, interstitial infiltrates, and fine, microgranular densities. Unsuspicious lung or bilateral interstitial linear infiltrates in the chronic form.

Pathology:

Gross: Depending upon the stage, normal lung tissue or consolidated, firm, reddish-gray, and rubbery lung parenchyma with uniform diffuse pattern.

Histology: The characteristics of allergic alveolitis are interstitial, noncaseating granulomas in the acute and chronic forms of the disease. Prominent, patchy interstitial infiltrates not fully developed into granulomas are located near the terminal bronchioles. At a later stage they contain epithelioid histiocytes, plasma cells, lymphocytes, multinucleated giant cells, and foamy histiocytes resembling sarcoidlike granulomas. The peripheral lung tissue is normally altered by hypertrophied and hyperplastic lining cells. The small bronchi are often altered by bronchiolitis obliterans. Additional infrequent findings include desquamative interstitial pneumonitis, organizing pneumonia (often in connection with bronchiolitis obliterans), diffuse interstitial (normally slight or moderate) fibrosis, and focal acute vasculitis involving the small arteries.

➤ *Descriptors:* Lung parenchyma with altered structure:

- noncaseous epithelioid granulomas
- eosinophils
- multinucleated giant cells
- intrabronchiolar fibrinoid material and histiocytes
- ulceration of bronchiolar mucosa;
- Lung parenchyma with preserved structure:
- macrophages
- desquamation, hypertrophy, hyperplasia and dysplasia of pneumocytes
- mononuclear inflammatory infiltrates
- intraalveolar serous fluid

■ *Special stains:* PAS, collagenous stains, silver stains. With immunohistochemistry, predominant lymphocytes positive to OKT8 in allergic alveolitis and to OKT4 in sarcoidosis.

Hallmark of Diagnosis: Noncaseating granulomatous interstitial pneumonia with additional alveolitis (hyperplasia and hypertrophy of cells of the alveolar lining), history of occupation.

Differential diagnosis: Sarcoidosis, granulomatous infections, usual interstitial pneumonia, desquamative interstitial pneumonia, berylliosis, lymphoid interstitial pneumonia, drug toxicity.

Allergic Angiitis and Granulomatosis (Churg-Strauss Syndrome)

Definition: A disease of unknown origin characterized by extensive parenchymal necrosis and vasculitis involving arteries and veins.

Incidence/Epidemiology: About 100 patients suffering from this disease have been described. It occurs almost exclusively in asthmatic patients with peripheral blood eosinophilia.

Etiology/Pathophysiology: It is considered to be a true vasculitis, related to Wegener's granulomatosis and periarteritis nodosa.The underlying immunologic mechanism is still unknown.

Clinical Presentation: It occurs at any age and in both sexes equally. The patients present with a history of chronic asthma or suffer from asthma at the time of presentation. Allergic rhinitis, peripheral blood eosinophilia, and moderate fever are common findings. The skin, nervous system (mononeuritis multiplex), and gastrointestinal tract are commonly involved, rarely the kidneys. Destructive upper respiratory tract lesions are not reported. The clinical course may vary from a fulminant process to an indolent disease; the response of patients to corticosteroids is generally good.

Prognosis: Usually good, although fatal cases have been reported.

Radiology: Findings are similar to eosinophilic pneumonia, consisting of patchy migratory infiltrates. Fine nodular densities or interstitial infiltrates are less common.

Pathology:

Gross: Irregularly shaped, necrotic areas several millimeters in diameter.

Histology: Irregularly shaped infarctlike zones of necrosis with surrounding palisading histiocytes, prominent eosinophilic infiltrates, and multinucleated giant cells. Free eosinophilic granules and Charcot-Leyden crystals are a frequent finding within and around the necrotic areas. The walls of the medium-sized arteries and veins are infiltrated by eosinophilic granulocytes. The arteries may be occluded by thrombotic agglutinations. The bronchioles and small bronchi elsewhere in the lung are not affected by the dense eosinophilic infiltrates; however, morphologic evidence of chronic asthma is a characteristic observation.

➤ *Descriptors:* Lung parenchyma with preserved structure:
- mononuclear inflammatory infiltrates;
- Bronchial mucosa with preserved structure:
- eosinophils
- hyaline basal membrane;
- Pulmonary vessels with preserved structure:
- eosinophils;
- Lung parenchyma with altered structure:
- necrosis and hemorrhage
- palisading histiocytes
- eosinophils
- multinucleated giant cells

■ *Special stains:* PAS, collagenous stains, silver stains.

Hallmark of Diagnosis: Infarctlike necroses with palisading histiocytes, giant cells, and predominant eosinophilic infiltrates. Dense involvement of eosinophilic granulocytes in arteries and veins and chronic asthmatic changes of bronchi elsewhere in the lung. Clinical and radiological presentation.

Differential diagnosis: Abscess, infectious fungal diseases, tuberculosis, Wegener's granulomatosis, necrotizing sarcoid granulomatosis, lymphomatoid granulomatosis.

Allergic Bronchopulmonary Aspergillosis

Definition: Hypersensitivity reaction of lung caused by *Aspergillus* mold.

Incidence/Epidemiology: Frequent in the UK, also well recognized in the USA.

Etiology/Pathophysiology: Patients exposed to mold of *Aspergillus fumigatus* may inhale the organism which can grow in the bronchi especially in preexisting bronchiectases. Mucoid impactions as well as a hypersensitivity reaction including asthma develop.

Clinical Presentation: Patients present with chronic asthma and cough up plugs of mucus containing *Aspergillus* hyphae. Peripheral blood eosinophilia is usually present. The history of asthma usually lasts for several years before one can specify the cause of the allergic reaction.

Prognosis: Good if the diagnosis is established prior to severe subsequent alterations of lung parenchyma.

Radiology: The lungs show fleeting areas with homogeneous consolidation, the bronchial walls present with thicker parallel lines (tram lines) and tubular shadows, including proximal saccular bronchiectases. Some patients present with radiological findings similar to those of chronic eosinophilic pneumonia.

Pathology:

Gross: Thickened walls of the major bronchi with saccular bronchiectases, often filled with yellowish-brown detritus. Additional pneumonic changes of peripheral lung tissue may be present.

Histology: Intensive chronic inflammatory infiltrates in the bronchial mucosa and submucosa, often with ulceration of the epithelial cells. Usually no granulomatous configurations in the larger bronchi; the bronchioles, however, may show foreign body response and abrupt transition to granulomatous changes. In the lumen are found aggregations of eosinophilic granular debris containing fragments of *Aspergillus* hyphae. The ectatic lumen of the larger bronchi usually contains dense hyphae of *Aspergillus.*

➤ *Descriptors:* Bronchial mucosa with preserved structure:
- ectatic lumen (bronchial and bronchiolar)
- atrophy
- ulceration
- viscous mucus
- fungus (intrabronchial, aspergillus)
- mononuclear inflammatory infiltrates
- eosinophils;
- Bronchial mucosa with altered structure:
- caseous epithelioid granulomas (small bronchi)
- fungus (intragranulomatous, *Aspergillus*);
- Lung parenchyma with preserved structure:
- eosinophils
- macrophages (foamy)

■ *Special stains:* PAS, Grocott's silver stain, collagenous stains.

Hallmark of Diagnosis: Chronic eosinophilic bronchitis with fragments of *Aspergillus* hyphae, bronchiectases with dense agglutinations of *Aspergillus*. (Characteristic of *Aspergillus* is the acute angle branching of hyphae). No signs of infiltrative aspergillosis.

Differential diagnosis: Chronic asthmoid bronchitis, mucoid impactions, and bronchiectasis of various origins, invasive aspergillosis.

Allergy

Definition: Alteration of the lung parenchyma associated with sensitization and subsequent exposure to various (inhaled) substances, see Allergic (Extrinsic) Alveolitis.

Allescheria boydii

Definition: Pneumonia caused by *Allescheria boydii*, the usual agent of maduromycosis or pheohyphomycosis.

Incidence/Epidemiology: The fungi including *Madurella mycetomi*, *M. grisea*, *Allescheria boydii*, *Cephalosporium sp.*, *Phialophora jeanselmei*, *Pyrenochaeta romeroi*, *Leptosphaeria senegalensis*, and *Neotestudina rosatii* are widely distributed in the tropical countries. Infections occur mainly in the lower extremities.

Etiology/Pathophysiology: The common infections of the lower extremities (feet) support the theory of local implantation of the organisms. Secondary infection of the lung is generally assumed.

Clinical Presentation: The patients usually present with swelling and many elevated nodules in the lower extremities with purulent exudate. In immunocompromised patients extensive pneumonic infiltrations may occur. Fever and nonproductive cough as well as dyspnea, pleuritic chest pain, and hemoptysis are present.

Prognosis: Good in immunocompetent patients, worse in immunocompromised patients.

Radiology: Circumscribed, dense infiltrations with central necroses and irregular margins.

Pathology:

Gross: Irregularly formed, necrotic areas of yellowish-brown color and occasionally cavitations.

Histology: Necrotic areas containing densely packed masses of microorganisms surrounded by amorphous eosinophilic material and invaded by accumulated neutrophilic granulocytes, lymphocytes, and plasma cells. The broad septate hyphae resemble *Aspergillus* and grow in disorganized, clustered patterns. The boundaries of the granules, which are similar to *Actinomyces*, present with chlamydospores and broad hyphae measuring 2–5 μm in diameter.

➤ *Descriptors:* Lung parenchyma with altered structure:
- necrosis
- fungus (septated hyphae, chlamydospores)
- mixed inflammatory infiltrates
- eosinophils

■ *Special stains:* PAS, silver stains, Gridley's, Gram.

Hallmark of Diagnosis: Demonstration of fungus with characteristic appearance of the mycetoma and of the hyphae. PAS and Gridley's stain will color the fungus but not bacteria (botryomycosis, demonstrable by Brown and Brenn stains).

Differential diagnosis: Other fungal infections, especially aspergillosis, botryomycosis, *actinomyces*.

Althesin

Definition: Alteration of the lung parenchyma associated with intake of Althesin, see Drug Toxicity.

Altitude

Definition: Alteration of the lung parenchyma (acute edema) associated with high altitude, see Mountain Sickness.

Aluminum Dust

Definition: Environmental disease of peripheral lung caused by exposure to aluminum dust, related to bauxite lung (Shaver's disease).

Incidence/Epidemiology: Persons working in mines or factories dedicated to explosives, fireworks, aluminum purification are endangered.

Etiology/Pathophysiology: The granular type has been reported to be less fibrotic in lungs of exposed rats and guinea pigs, as opposed to the flake type which causes severe fibrosis with or without added stearin or oil.

Clinical Presentation: Fatal cases have been reported. Characteristic are shortness of breath, dyspnea, cough, a progressive course.

Prognosis: Aluminum has a fibrogenic potency and progressive fibrosis can occur.

Radiology: Fibrotic lesions may be seen as early as 3 months after exposure. Larger silicotic nodules are absent.

Pathology:

Gross: Identical with the findings in bauxite lung, shrunken lungs with thickened pebbled pleura and subpleural emphysema.

Histology: See Bauxite Lung: Marked interstitial fibrosis with scattered mononuclear infiltrates. Agglutinations of dust-laden macrophages in the distant airways, endarteritis obliterans.

➤ *Descriptors:* Lung parenchyma with altered structure:

- diffuse interstitial fibrosis
- focal interstitial fibrosis
- mononuclear inflammatory infiltrates
- macrophages (dust-laden)
- multinucleated giant cells
- dust (crystal clefts);
- Pulmonary vessels with preserved structure:
- mononuclear inflammatory infiltrates
- thrombosis (small arteries)

■ *Special stains:* Collagenous stains, aurine stain, X-ray diffraction and similar physical techniques for identification of aluminum.

Hallmark of Diagnosis: Severe lung damage with predominant fibrosis, dense deposits of dust and dust-laden macrophages, absence of larger silicotic nodules, clinical history, identification of aluminum by physical techniques.

Differential diagnosis: Pneumoconioses due to other agents, diffuse interstitial fibrosis due to other causes.

Alveolar Calcification

Definition: Deposits of calcium salts in the lung parenchyma usually associated with related altered serum calcium and phosphorus levels (synonyms, calcinosis of lung, interstitial or metastatic calcification of lung).

Incidence/Epidemiology: Most cases remain undetected until death. In chronic uremic and chronic dialyzed patients the prevalence may reach 40–50%.

Etiology/Pathophysiology: Disorders related to metastatic calcification include primary and secondary diseases of the skeleton, chronic renal diseases, hypervitaminosis D, and unclear cases such as pyloric stenosis. Focal tissue alkalosis is thought to be responsible for the calcium deposits.

Clinical Presentation: Most patients are asymptomatic, others develop terminal pulmonary edema or respiratory failure. The heart, the stomach, and kidneys are frequently involved. Rapid progress of the disease has been reported. The age of the patients varies from 8 weeks to 70 years.

Prognosis: Usually good and defined by the underlying disorder.

Radiology: Chest X-radiographs are usually unsuspicious, or may show early increases in lung density detectable by a negative or black pleural shadow.

Pathology:

Gross: The lungs are heavy, gritty, dry, and gray to gray-yellowish. They usually do not collapse during cutting.

Histology: Calcium deposits are usually small in size and located in the elastic tissue of the alveolar septula, arteries, veins, bronchioles, and bronchi. Inflammatory infiltrations are normally absent, in later stages a foreign body reaction including multinucleated giant cells may be present. The tissue texture is generally preserved. The deposits may be granular, diffuse, focal, or nodular. Both lungs are normally involved.

➤ *Descriptors:* Lung parenchyma with preserved structure:

- calcium deposits (interstitial, both lungs)
- multinucleated giant cells (foreign body)

■ *Special stains:* PAS, collagen stains, Kossa's stain.

Hallmark of Diagnosis: Fine deposits of calcified material along the alveolar walls without any inflammatory reaction of lung tissue, preserved lung textures.

Differential diagnosis: Dystrophic calcification, calcification occurring in histoplasmosis, tuberculosis, silicosis, *Pneumocystis carinii* infection.

Alveolar Microlithiasis

Definition: Disease of the peripheral lung tissue characterized by concentrically laminated intraalveolar calcospherites.

Incidence/Epidemiology: Very rare disease, about 150 cases having been published in the literature.

Etiology/Pathophysiology: The cause is unknown. About half of the reported cases have a family history with siblings predominantly involved. Equal sex incidence.

Clinical Presentation: The disease can be detected at any age within the range 6–60 years. Most patients are asymptomatic at the time of diagnosis. The progression of the disease is generally slow, ranging over several years. The patients may present, in addition, with pulmonary fibrosis and chronic mitral stenosis.

Prognosis: Slowly progressive with fatal outcome after several years.

Radiology: Chest radiographs show dense miliary mottling over the middle and lower lung fields, sometimes with confluent shadows. The discrepancy between the degree of radiologic findings and the lung functions or the patient's condition is a characteristic finding.

Pathology:

Gross: The stony hard and heavy lungs with well maintained shape and grayish-pale lower parts are difficult to cut. The microliths measure 0.01–0.5 mm in diameter and easily fall out of the lung tissue.

Histology: After decalcification with 20% nitric acid the microscopic examination shows psammous-like bodies located in the alveoli and bronchioles. Typically they are concentrically laminated and consist chemically of calcium, phosphates, iron, and traces of magnesium. The alveolar walls are chronically damaged and present interstitial inflammatory infiltrates and moderate fibrosis. The lung texture is normally preserved. Normally, one microlith is located within one alveolus. Ossification may be found in the more affected areas.

➤ *Descriptors:* Lung parenchyma with preserved structure:

- calcium deposits (intraalveolar, diffuse)
- mononuclear inflammatory infiltrates;
- Lung parenchyma with altered structure:
- diffuse interstitial fibrosis (mild)

■ *Special stains:* PAS and iron stain for positive demonstration of the microliths, collagenous stains for estimating the degree of fibrosis.

Hallmark of Diagnosis: Typical microliths with the corresponding familial background and discrepancy between radiologic and clinical findings.

Differential diagnosis: Alveolar calcification, corpora amylacea of lung, pulmonary ossification.

Alveolar Proteinosis

Definition: Disease of the peripheral lung tissue characterized by diffuse lipid-proteinaceous material located in the alveoli.

Incidence/Epidemiology: Not a rare disease. Has been reported in patients with exposure to various dusts including fine silica, wood, tobacco, aluminum, kaolin, fiberglass, 100% oxygen, welding fumes, talc, cadmium, etc. Sometimes the disease is related to hematolymphoid malignancies (T-cell lymphoma), opportunistic infections, immunosuppression, congenital thymic alymphoplasia, or hypogammaglobulinemia.

Etiology/Pathophysiology: It is still unknown whether the disease is caused by increased production, decreased clearance, or both of the elsewhere normal components of deposits in the alveoli. The deposits consist of surfactant and some protein material reflecting fibrinogen and serum proteins. Alveolar macrophages have been reported to show a decreased proliferative activity.

Clinical Presentation: The disease is mainly seen in men at any age ranging from newborn to 80 years. It presents with slowly progressive dyspnea and increased temperature, cough, fatigue, chest pain. Infants and children have a higher mortality than the adults, familial occurrence having been reported in a few cases. The serum proteins are slightly altered with decreased albumin, and increased α_1- and α_2-globulin. Lung function reveals an impaired diffusion defect of restrictive type without obstruction. The outcome of the disease has been improved after introduction of bronchopulmonary lavage for treatment. Changes to progressive fibrosis are rare.

Prognosis: Usually fair, as it is a slowly progressive disease.

Radiology: Nodular, bilateral, feathery, centrally located infiltrates not affecting the peripheral zones, as seen in acute pulmonary edema, are normally present in chest radiographs.

Prominent air bronchograms and normal hilar nodes, missing pleural effusions are additional findings.

Pathology:

Gross: The heavy, wet lungs show multiple, firm, yellowish areas measuring up to several centimeters in diameter without cavitation.

Histology: The lung tissue shows a normal structure with intraalveolar filling of a finely granular acellular material. This material is PAS-positive, diastase-resistant, and negative to alcian and mucicarmine stains. The interalveolar septula are preserved and normally not at all or only slightly infiltrated by lymphocytes, granulocytes, and plasma cells. Focal cholesterol crystals may be present. The alveoli filled with the proteinaceous masses do not contain additional inflammatory cells such as macrophages or plasma cells, although at the boundary of the lesions ghosts of foamy macrophages mixed with granulocytes and plasma cells may exist. Pneumocytes in these areas may be hyperplastic as opposed to the acellular areas. Calcification and fibrinous exudation are uncommon.

➤ *Descriptors:* Lung parenchyma with preserved structure:
- intraalveolar serous fluid
- absent inflammatory infiltrates
- unsuspicious pneumocytes

■ *Special stains:* PAS with diastase digestion, alcian stain, mucicarmine stain, Grocott's silver stain (for exclusion of *Pneumocystis carinii*), oil red O or Sudan black stain in frozen sections.

Hallmark of Diagnosis: Typical, eosinophilic, intraalveolar, acellular deposits with unaffected pneumocytes and normal interalveolar septula.

Differential diagnosis: *Pneumocystis carinii* infection, desquamative interstitial pneumonia (at the boundary of the lesion), acute pulmonary edema, chronic peribronchial edema.

Alveolitis

Definition: Nonspecific inflammation of the distant air spaces, see Pneumonitis.

Amebiasis

Definition: Infection of lung caused by *Entamoeba histolytica*.

Incidence/Epidemiology: Mainly tropical disease reported to be epidemic in urban populations in Mexico City, Medellin (Colombia), and Durban (South Africa). Social and economic factors such as inadequate sanitation and poor personal hygiene are considered to predispose to the disease.

Etiology/Pathophysiology: Infection of the protozoan *E. histolytica* begins by invasion of the colonic mucosa, where the cysts or trophozoites may remain localized for many years, being asymptomatic or producing minimal ulcers. The trophozoites reproduce on the surface of the mucosa by binary fission. The parasites may involve the lung either by contiguous liver abscess or by hematogenous spread.

Clinical Presentation: Amebic colitis is characterized by increasing discomfort of the lower abdomen, presenting with loose stools sometimes mixed with mucus and blood, malodorous flatus. Intermittent constipation and increased number of stools may alternate. Acute clinical picture suggesting appendicitis, right sided cramps, high fever may result from liver abscess and pneumonia. Cough with amebic pus is usually seen.

Prognosis: Usually good, but pleural involvement worsens the prognosis.

Radiology: Filling defects of right chest radiographs suggest empyema. Hematogenous abscesses may range up to several centimeters in diameter.

Pathology:

Gross: Various sizes of necrotic, nonmalodorous brownish-red areas with edematous surrounding lung tissue or right-sided abscess with continuous extension into the diaphragm, liver, and lung. Typical "flaskshaped" ulcers in the colon, in about 5% of patients so-called amebic pseudotumor of the colon (ameboma).

Histology: Trophozoites and cysts are found in man. Both stain intensely with PAS stain and measure between 15–25 μm in diameter. The spherical nucleus of the trophozoite is surrounded by a thin membrane and has finely dispersed chromatin. The cytoplasm is vacuolated and amphophylic. Ingested erythrocytes may be seen. The organisms are usually present with mixed inflammatory infiltrates at the outer zones of the abscesses. HE stain is considered to demonstrate the morphology of the trophozoites best.

➤ *Descriptors:* Lung parenchyma with altered structure:
- necrosis and hemorrhage
- mixed inflammatory infiltrates
- eosinophils;
- Lung parenchyma with preserved structure:
- intraalveolar fibrinoid material
- infectious organisms (trophozoites, entameba)

■ *Special stains:* PAS, direct immunofluorescence.

Hallmark of Diagnosis: Lung abscess in combination with colonic ulcer and demonstration of trophozoites.

Differential diagnosis: Miscellaneous protozoan infections (such as *Cryptosporidium, Leishmania donovani, Acanthameba castellanii*).

Aminorex

Definition: Alteration of the lung parenchyma associated with intake of aminorex, see Drug Toxicity.

Aminosalicylic acid

Definition: Alteration of the lung parenchyma associated with intake of aminosalicylic acid, see Drug Toxicity.

Amiodarone

Definition: Alteration of the lung parenchyma associated with intake of amiodarone, see Drug Toxicity.

Amitriptyline

Definition: Alteration of the lung parenchyma associated with intake of amitriptyline (tricyclic antidepressant), see Drug Toxicity.

Amniotic Fluid Embolism

Definition: Embolism of amniotic fluid into the maternal veins and maternal pulmonary arteries during birth.

Incidence/Epidemiology: Fatal amniotic fluid embolism has been calculated to occur once in every 26 000 deliveries during the second and third stages of labor. Minimal amounts of amniotic fluid in pulmonary arteries may be present in almost all deliveries.

Etiology/Pathophysiology: Intravenous infusion of amniotic fluid into the maternal veins is caused by intrauterine pressure during partial detachment of the placenta via the open veins at the placental site or into ruptured or surgically incised veins of the uterine wall.

Clinical Presentation: Acute onset of respiratory distress during delivery, hypoxemia, decreased cardiac output, and cardiac shock may lead to death.

Prognosis: Usually good, but massive embolism causes death in 40–70% of patients.

Radiology: Patchy, diffuse densities in both lungs, signs of atelectasis and focal emphysema.

Pathology:

Gross: Both lungs are heavy and wet and show focal areas of atelectasis, emphysema and diffuse edema.

Histology: Amniotic fluid can be identified in the pulmonary arteries, arterioles, and capillaries by the demonstration of amniotic contents such as lanugo hairs, mucin, fetal meconium, fat. The small arteries may be filled with neutrophilic and eosinophilic granulocytes if the patient survives about 24 h. Additional trophoblast emboli and decidual emboli may be found, especially if hydatidiform moles have developed. Pulmonary infarction due to amniotic embolism is uncommon; bacterial pneumonia may subsequently develop.

➤ *Descriptors:* Lung parenchyma with preserved structure:
- intraalveolar serous fluid;
- Pulmonary vessels with preserved structure:
- amniotic fluid (in small arteries and capillaries, lanugo hairs, squamous epithelial cells, fat, mucinous material, meconium)

■ *Special stains:* Phloxine and alcian green for mucus and epithelial squames, Sudan black for fat.

Hallmark of Diagnosis: Clinical history and demonstration of amniotic material in the pulmonary arteries, arterioles or capillaries.
Differential diagnosis: Acute pulmonary edema due to heart failure, acute pneumonia.

Ampicillin

Definition: Alteration of the lung parenchyma associated with intake of ampicillin, see Drug Toxicity.

Amyloidoma

Definition: Circumscribed deposits of amyloid in the peripheral lung parenchyma, see Amyloidosis.

Amyloidosis

Definition: Deposits of hyalin, waxy-pink material (amyloid) in the proximal lung (tracheobronchial) or in the peripheral lung.
Incidence/Epidemiology: Amyloidosis can be classified into primary, secondary, multiple-myeloma-associated, and senile types. Primary systemic amyloidosis involves the lung in 50–80% of cases, the secondary type likewise. Usually slight deposits of amyloid in the lung can be demonstrated in 10–30% of aged people (80 years of age and older).
Etiology/Pathophysiology: Amyloid consists of agglutinations of β-pleated sheets of fibrils of chemically diverse glycoproteins. Characteristically, the deposits occur along preexisting collagenous layers such as the lamina elastica interna and externa in vessels, basal membranes of bronchial mucosa, and capillary membranes. Amyloidosis may develop in association with chronic inflammatory processes (secondary type), in relation to age (senile type), or for unknown reasons (primary type). The patterns of primary pulmonary amyloidosis can be divided into the tracheobronchial group, the nodular parenchymal group, and the diffuse alveolar septal group.
Clinical Presentation: The clinical picture varies depending upon the site and degree of pulmonary involvement. In tracheobronchial amyloidosis most patients have symptoms of airway obstruction. The disease is often assumed to be a centrally localized bronchial carcinoma with submucosal tumor growth. Peripherally localized amyloidosis may correlate with a slight restriction in a lung function test; the senile form of amyloidosis is often asymptomatic. Serum protein abnormalities are – if present at all – only mild.
Prognosis: Usually good in patients with nodular parenchymal amyloidosis, worse in patients with tracheobronchial amyloidosis, which shows mild progression into honeycombing, the worst in patients with diffuse alveolar septal amyloidosis, who usually die within 2 years after development of clinical symptoms.
Radiology: Chest radiographs show either normal findings or an image corresponding to the size and localization of the deposits of amyloid. The lesions are usually marked with clear-cut boundaries. Diffuse radiologic features are present only in diffuse septal alveolar amyloidosis. Peripherally localized lesions may appear as circumscribed densities (amyloidomas).
Pathology:
Gross: Amyloid lesions are white-yellowish and present as irregularly shaped, homogeneous, firm nodules or plaques without central necrosis. The boundaries are clearly identifiable. The surrounding lung is unsuspicious. Tracheobronchial amyloidosis usually forms stenotic lesions of the bronchus with intact mucosa. Secondary calcification and ossification may occur.
Histology: Amyloid deposits are of extracellular origin, hyalin-homogeneous, and destructive in nature. The boundaries normally contain chronic inflammatory infiltrates, occasionally with multinucleated giant cells. Diffuse alveolar septal amyloidosis contains the original configuration of the interalveolar septula and forms broad homogeneous interstitial bands with unsuspicious alveolar-lining cells. Interstitial capillaries are destroyed by the homogeneous deposits. Intraalveolar deposits are uncommon and exist only in close connection with one of the surrounding alveolar septula. Nodular parenchymal amyloidosis forms irregularly shaped, homogeneous, yellowish-translucent masses measuring several millimeters to a centimeter in diameter with complete replacement of the original lung textures. Inflammatory in-

filtrations are rare and only exist at the boundaries of the lesions, whereas the central areas are often calcified or ossified. The transition to normal lung parenchyma is abrupt.

➤ *Descriptors:* Bronchial mucosa with altered structure:
- hyaline material (amyloid, in submucosa)
- mononuclear inflammatory infiltrates
- destruction of submucosal glands;
- Lung parenchyma with altered structure:
- interstitial hyaline material (amyloid)
- mononuclear inflammatory infiltrates
- multinucleated giant cells (foreign-body)
- ossification

■ *Special stains:* Congo red for amyloidosis, showing characteristic apple-green birefringence with polarization. Immunohistochemistry for heavy and light chains of immunoglobulins (heavy chains are reported to be characteristic of secondary amyloidosis, light chains of primary amyloidosis). Special monoclonal antibodies against various glycoproteins are available.

Hallmark of Diagnosis: Homogeneous acellular hyalin deposits with typical staining for Congo red.

Differential diagnosis: Hyalin plaques and scars of various origins, tracheopathia osteoplastica for tracheobronchial amyloidosis, pulmonary hyalinizing granulomas.

Anaerobic Pneumonia

Definition: Infection of the lung with anaerobic bacteria.

Incidence/Epidemiology: Fairly frequent in association with periodontal infections, aspiration related to alcoholism, anaesthesia, impaired consciousness.

Etiology/Pathophysiology: Anaerobic bacteria are normal inhabitants of the gastrointestinal tract. The predominant infectious strains are *Peptostreptococci, Peptococcus, Fusobacterium nucleatum, Bacteroides melaninogenicus.* Most anaerobic infections are polymicrobial.

Clinical Presentation: Anaerobic infection can manifest itself as pneumonitis, lung abscess, or necrotizing pneumonia. Pneumonitis starts as febrile illness with cough, lung abscess is usually accompanied by fever, anemia, loss of weight, and fetor of sputum, and necrotizing pneumonia can show variations in the clinical picture ranging from minimally symptomatic patients to fulminant pneumonia. The most frequent sites of anaerobic infections are the posterior segments of the upper and lower lobes.

Prognosis: Serious infection in immunocompromised patients, infants, and elderly people.

Radiology: Diffuse infiltrations in the posterior segments of the upper and lower lobes, circumscribed densities with central necrosis, or several marked areas of consolidation combined with small multiple areas of cavitation measuring less than 1 cm in diameter are the radiological evidence associated with the clinical manifestations.

Pathology:

Gross: Grayish and airless lungs with multiple necrotic areas and larger firm nodules involving more than one lobe are the typical findings. Fetid odor, thickened pleura, and fibrotic interlobar septa are usually seen as well as ectatic bronchi with edematous and thickened walls.

Histology: The findings vary from necrotic areas filled with debris and pus, and surrounded by dense inflammatory infiltrations to areas with predominantly lymphocytic-plasmacellular infiltrations combined with macrophages and histiocytes and fibrin deposits. Other areas may show fibrotic interalveolar septula with only mild inflammatory infiltrations. Older necrotic lesions frequently have a thin fibrotic capsula. The bronchial walls show dense mononuclear infiltrations, often with accompanying squamous metaplasia of the epithelial cells.

➤ *Descriptors:* Lung parenchyma with preserved structure:
- mixed inflammatory infiltrates
- intraalveolar fibrinoid material
- bacteria;
- Lung parenchyma with altered structure:
- necrosis and hemorrhage
- mononuclear inflammatory infiltrates
- focal interstitial fibrosis;
- Bronchial mucosa with altered structure:
- mononuclear inflammatory infiltrates
- squamous metaplasia and dysplasia

■ *Special stains:* PAS for demonstration or exclusion of additional mycotic infections, Brown and Brenn's stain for demonstration of anaerobic bacteria, collagenous stains.

Hallmark of Diagnosis: Complete focal destruction of tissue texture combined with corresponding inflammatory infiltrates. Culture of anaerobic bacteria.

Differential diagnosis: Pneumonia caused by different infectious organisms, necrotic tumorous infiltrations.

Aneurysm

Definition: Circumscribed ectasia of the arterial pulmonary trunk or its main branches.

Incidence/Epidemiology: Relatively frequent in patients with pulmonary hypertension or in young children with patent ductus arteriosus. Fairly common as poststenotic dilatation in tetralogy of Fallot. True aneurysms such as are seen in syphilitic infections, Marfan's syndrome, or mycotic infections are extremely rare.

Etiology/Pathophysiology: Increased pulmonary pressure dilates the arterial walls. Inborn errors of the collagenous texture of the arterial wall or inflammatory destruction (mycotic infection) causes ectatic dilatation even if the arterial pressure is normal.

Clinical Presentation: Rupture may occur in Marfan's syndrome. The aneurysm may cause degenerative changes in the supplying bronchial arteries, which are referred to as the Hughes-Stovin syndrome if associated with venous thrombophlebosis and pulmonary emboli. The clinical picture is usually dominated by an extension of pulmonary hypertension or an extension of disturbance of blood perfusion.

Prognosis: Usually determined by the underlying disease.

Radiology: The chest X-radiograph findings include mediastinal abnormalities, cor pulmonale, peripheral thrombotic lesions. Angiography combined with measurement of the intraarterial blood pressure is usually of diagnostic value.

Pathology:

Gross: Circumscribed (mostly saccular) ectatic dilatation of the arterial pulmonary trunk or its main arteries with thrombotic sedimentation.

Histology: Disturbance of the collagenous net within the thin media and prominent fragmentation of the lamina elastica can be seen in Marfan's syndrome or in tetralogy of Fallot. Myxomatoid changes of the media with scattered lymphocytic-plasmacellular infiltrations and degenerative changes in the bronchial arteries suggest syphiliticc infection. Normal texture with thinned media and slight sclerosis of the intima are the usual findings in poststenotic aneurysms.

➤ *Descriptors:* Pulmonary vessels with preserved structure:
- ectatic lumen (arteries)
- atrophy of media
- mononuclear inflammatory infiltrates;
- Pulmonary vessels with altered structure:
- fragmentation of elastic fibers
- myxomatoid changes (media)

■ *Special stains:* Collagenous stains, silver stains.

Hallmark of Diagnosis: Gross findings with associated clinical history.

Differential diagnosis: Related to the underlying cause, i.e., differentiation between true aneurysms and general dilatation of the pulmonary arteries.

Angiitis

Definition: Nonspecific inflammation of pulmonary arteries, see Vasculitis.

Angiitis, Lymphocytic and Granulomatosis, Benign

Definition: Benign lymphocytic vasculitis with formation of granulomas, see Lymphocytic Angiitis and Granulomatosis, Benign.

Angiocentric Large Cell Lymphoma

Definition: Pulmonary involvement of highly malignant non-Hodgkin's lymphoma associated with angiocentric necrosis.

Incidence/Epidemiology: Extremely rare disease occurring in young and middle-aged adults with equal sex distribution.

Etiology/Pathophysiology: Non-Hodgkin's lymphoma with abnormal postthymic T cell proliferation and destructive invasion of all layers of pulmonary vessels (arteries and veins).

Clinical Presentation: Usually adult patients presenting with fever, cough, and hemoptysis. Extrapulmonary involvement (skin) may occur.
Prognosis: Most patients die within 2 years after diagnosis.

Radiology: Indistinguishable from Wegener's granulomatosis or metastatic lesions with either single or multiple dense nodules.

Pathology:
Gross: Firm, central, necrotic, yellowish-red areas.

Histology: Large areas of mononuclear atypical lymphomatoid cells surrounding necrotic lesions with centrally localized pulmonary arteries or veins invaded by the tumor cells. Usually diffuse lymphomas classified as mixed large and small cell lymphoma, large cell lymphoma, or large cell immunoblastic lymphoma.

➤ *Descriptors:* Newly formed textures with metastasis potential:

- mesenchymal growth pattern
- lymphomatoid textures
- vascular and pleural invasion
- large tumor cells (lymphomatoid)
- inhomogeneous nuclear and cellular size
- prominent nucleoli
- moderate number of mitosis
- necrosis

■ *Special stains:* Collagenous stains, PAS, immunohistochemistry for distinguishing the subsets of lymphocytic cells.

Hallmark of Diagnosis: Destructive tumor growth of a malignant non-Hodgkin's lymphoma with angiocentric necrosis.

Differential diagnosis: Opportunistic infections of lung, lymphomatoid granulomatosis, benign lymphocytic angiitis and granulomatosis, Wegener's disease, Churg-Strauss syndrome, necrotizing sarcoid granulomatosis.

Angiocentric Lymphoproliferative Processes

Definition: Spectrum of lesions with angioinvasion of the lung associated with lymphoproliferative processes including benign lymphocytic angiitis and granulomatosis, lymphomatoid granulomatosis, and angiocentric large cell lymphoma.

Incidence/Epidemiology: Rare diseases. Benign lymphocytic angiitis and granulomatosis is less frequent than lymphomatoid granulomatosis.

Etiology/Pathophysiology: Diseases of unknown origin. Defects in the proliferation of postthymic T cells are assumed.

Clinical Presentation: Patients suffering from benign lymphocytic angiitis and granulomatosis are somewhat older (mean age 57 years) than patients suffering from Wegener's granulomatosis. All diseases can occur at any age, with slight male preponderance. Symptoms are related to the major site of manifestation and include fever, cough, chest pain, and shortness of breath.

Prognosis: The prognosis is usually good in patients with Wegener's granulomatosis, allergic angiitis and granulomatosis, necrotizing sarcoid-like granulomatosis, and bronchocentric granulomatosis. It is poor in patients with lymphomatoid granulomatosis and the worst in patients with angiocentric large cell lymphoma.

Radiology: All three diseases present the same picture, identical with that seen in Wegener's granulomatosis, including multiple bilateral nodular densities measuring several centimeters in diameter. Solitary masses or areas of consolidation are less frequent.

Pathology:
Gross: Multiple, yellowish-white lesions measuring 1–4 cm in diameter. Central necrosis is rare, but the unaffected lung areas appear slightly edematous. In larger nodules centrally localized affected arteries can be identified.

Histology: The lesions are characterized by central necroses of small and medium-sized arteries of a coagulative type surrounded by dense lymphocytic infiltrations with various degrees of cellular atypias. Benign lymphocytic angiitis and granulomatosis shows faint granuloma formations inside the infiltrates, consisting mainly of mature lymphocytes including some larger, activated lymphocytes. The infiltrates spread mainly within the interstitial tissue and efface normal tissue textures only in the center of the lesions. Lymphomatoid granulomatosis presents a mixed mononuclear infiltrate of small lymphocytes, histiocytes, plasma cells, immunoblasts, and atypical lymphoreticular cells resembling Reed-Sternberg cells. The degree of necrosis varies, all layers of the walls of the small and medium-sized arteries being invaded by the mononuclear infiltrate. Angiocentric large cell lymphomas are characterized by foci of large mononuclear atypical lymphocytes classified as diffuse, mixed large and small cell lymphoma, diffuse large cell lymphoma, and diffuse large cell immunoblastic lymphoma. Necrotic areas are usually extensive.

➤ *Descriptors:* Lung parenchyma with altered structure:
- necrosis and hemorrhage
- palisading histiocytes
- multinucleated giant cells
- eosinophils
- mononuclear inflammatory infiltrates
- atypical lymphoid cells (resembling immunoblasts);
- Bronchial mucosa with altered structure:
- necrosis
- palisading histiocytes
- multinucleated giant cells
- eosinophils
- mononuclear inflammatory infiltrates;
- Pulmonary vessels with preserved structure:
- mononuclear inflammatory infiltrates

■ *Special stains:* Collagenous stains, PAS, immunohistochemistry for distinguishing different subtypes of lymphocytes.

Hallmark of Diagnosis: Angiocentric necrosis surrounded by dense lymphocytic infiltrations with various degrees of cellular atypias.

Differential diagnosis: Opportunistic infections including mycotic pneumonias, Wegener's granulomatosis, Churg-Strauss syndrome, allergic angiitis, necrotizing sarcoid granulomatosis.

Angioimmunoblastic Lymphadenopathy

Definition: Pulmonary involvement in a disorder of T cell proliferation.

Incidence/Epidemiology: Rare disease with quite frequent pulmonary involvement. About 10–30% of patients with generalized angioimmunoblastic lymphadenopathy present with pulmonary involvement.

Etiology/Pathophysiology: Proliferation of T cells related to lymphoma; originally postulated as a hyperimmune B cell proliferation associated with a defect in immunoregulatory T cells.

Clinical Presentation: Patients present with lymphadenopathy, hepatosplenomegaly, fever, loss of weight, Coombs-positive hemolytic anemia, macropapular pruritic rash, polyclonal hypergammaglobulinemia, lymphopenia, or neutrophilic leucocytosis with eosinophilia, dyspnea, and chronic cough.

Prognosis: Good to fair, about 70% of patients will survive 5 years or longer.

Radiology: Alterations of the mediastinum with enlarged hilar lymph nodes, peripherally localized, circumscribed densities, or diffuse interstitial infiltrates.

Pathology:

Gross: Enlarged, white or grayish-red, proximal lymph nodes suggesting involvement of lymphoma. The lungs show diffuse grayish-white infiltrates.

Histology: Characteristic triad of (a) polymorphous infiltrations of immunoblasts, plasma cells and histiocytes, (b) proliferation of small arborizing vessels, and (c) deposits of amorphous acidophilic, interstitial material. In the peripheral lung proliferation of small vessels and eosinophilic intercellular material are usually not predominant. Polymorphous proliferation of lymphoid cells resembles tumorous infiltrations of Hodgkin's lymphoma with complete obliteration of the original lung texture. Scattered histiocytes are present at the boundary of the lesion.

➤ *Descriptors:* Lung parenchyma with altered structure:
- mononuclear inflammatory infiltrates
- acidophilic intercellular material;
- Newly formed textures without metastasis potential:
- mesenchymal growth pattern
- lymphomatoid textures
- angiomatoid textures (small venous vessels)
- atypical lymphoreticular cells

■ *Special stains:* Collagenous stains, PAS, Giemsa, immunohistochemistry for subpopulations of lymphocytes, immunoglobulins, endothelial cells, DNA analysis, endogenous lectins.

Hallmark of Diagnosis: Polymorphous proliferation of immature immunoblasts, plasma cells, histiocytes following the "routes of lymphatic drainage", occasional additional proliferation of small vessels and amorphous interstitial deposits, and related clinical picture.

Differential diagnosis: Hodgkin's lymphoma, angiocentric lymphoproliferative disorders, lymphocytic interstitial pneumonitis.

Angiokeratoma Corporis Diffusum Universale

Definition: Lung involvement of a hereditary storage disease with deposits of crystalline glycosphingolipid.

Incidence/Epidemiology: Lung involvement is fairly common but not predominant in these patients.

Etiology/Pathophysiology: X-linked deficiency of α-galactosidase leads to deposits of crystalline glycosphingolipid in the vessel walls, along the smooth muscle cells, and in a lesser degree in histiocytes throughout the body.

Clinical Presentation: Symptoms appear in young adults, with rheumatoid pains, hyperkeratotic angiomas of skin, renal insufficiency, cardiac dilatation. Lung symptoms are usually chronic bronchitis and emphysema, which may be enhanced by smoking. Normal to slightly decreased lung function tests.

Prognosis: Usually not determined by pulmonary involvement.

Radiology: Usually normal.

Pathology:

Gross: Slightly increased consistency of lung, slight edema.

Histology: Deposits of pale material with Maltese cross polarization in histiocytes and to a lesser degree along the intima of small arteries. Signs of chronic bronchitis.

➤ *Descriptors:* Lung parenchyma with preserved structure:

- hyaline material (birefringent, in histiocytes)
- mononuclear inflammatory infiltrates

■ *Special stains:* PAS, collagenous stains, endogenous lectins.

Hallmark of Diagnosis: Intracytoplasmatic material (Maltese cross polarization, in histiocytes, foamy deposits), clinical history and clinical findings.

Differential diagnosis: Other storage diseases, chronic bronchitis.

Angioma

Definition: Benign vascular lesion in the lung, see Hemangioma, Lymphangioma.

Angiosarcoma

Definition: Pulmonary manifestation of a malignant angiomatous tumor.

Incidence/Epidemiology: Rare intrapulmonary tumor, most commonly described as metastatic lesions.

Etiology/Pathophysiology: Angiosarcoma may arise in sites in which vascular stasis is present, e.g. postmastectomy, after irradiation, Thorotrast-exposed patients, etc.

Clinical Presentation: Depending upon the degree of tumorous infiltrations, cough, fever, chest pain, malaise, shortness of breath.

Prognosis: Poor, most of the reported patients died within 6–9 months after diagnosis.

Radiology: Firm, sometimes bilateral, nodular, parenchymal infiltrates.

Pathology:

Gross: Brown-red, soft tumors with distinct boundary.

Histology: Irregularly formed, spindle-shaped tumor cells forming an arbitrary network of vascular spaces, usually bound to larger vessels. No or unsuspicious inflammatory infiltrations, frequent mitoses.

➤ *Descriptors:* Newly formed textures with metastasis potential:

- mesenchymal growth patterns
- sarcomatous textures
- angiomatoid textures
- plump spindle cells
- frequent mitoses
- absent or weak inflammatory infiltrates

■ *Special stains:* Collagenous stains, PAS, immunohistochemistry including factor VIII, endothelial marker, endogenous lectins.

Hallmark of Diagnosis: Sarcomatous vascular pattern of the tumor with additional confirmation by immunohistochemistry.

Differential diagnosis: Different types of sarcomas, anaplastic carcinomas, and angioimmunoblastic lesions.

Angiostrongylus cantonensis

Definition: Human infection by the nematode *Angiostrongylus cantonensis* (lungworm of rats).

Incidence/Epidemiology: Many human infections have been reported from the smaller islands of Oceania, Thailand, Philippines, Taiwan, Vietnam, Indonesia, New Caledonia, Tahiti, Hawaii (in rats from Madagascar to Hawaii). Man usually acquires the disease by eating raw or insufficiently cooked intermediate hosts containing third-stage larvae. Infections also occur by eating transport hosts including land planarians, freshwater prawns, land crabs and frogs, or raw fruits, green salad, and vegetables contaminated by intermediate or transport hosts or by their mucus.

Etiology/Pathophysiology: Rats, being the definite host of the parasites, are usually infected by eating the intermediate hosts, snails and slugs. In rats the adult parasites live in branches of the pulmonary arteries. Their eggs are swept into the alveolar capillaries, and the hatched larvae enter the alveoli and migrate to the trachea and through the esophagus. The first-stage larvae are excreted and invade their intermediate hosts, where they molt twice and become infective third-stage larvae. Larvae ingested by rats enter the venules of the gastrointestinal lymphatic system and concentrate in the central nervous system (spinal cord, cerebellum, diencephalon) within 4 days. The third-stage larvae molt twice and become young adult worms, being carried to the pulmonary vessels by entering the cerebral veins. In man only adult worms have been found.

Clinical Presentation: Aberrant numbers of parasites are usually found in man because they cannot complete their life cycle. The symptoms are related to those associated with infection of the nervous system and include fever, headache, stiff neck, photophobia, vertigo, nausea, vomiting, radicular paresthesias of the trunk and limbs, facial paralysis, and tenderness of muscles of the extremities. A slight leucocytosis and a high eosinophilia are present in the peripheral blood. Patients can usually be rid of angiostrongyliasis after several weeks. The worm has also been reported to invade the eyes and the pulmonary arteries in humans.

Prognosis: Recovery from parasitic infection is common and usually without sequelae, but healing may take several weeks, and recurrent infection is not infrequently seen.

Radiology: Signs of pulmonary thrombosis or peripherally localized circumscribed densities suggest pulmonary infections.

Pathology:

Gross: The worms in man usually measure 8–15 mm in length and 100–250 µm in diameter and are surrounded by thrombotic lesions in the pulmonary arteries.

Histology: The worms have a cuticle about 5 µm thick, an attached lateral cord, smooth muscle cells, and a central intestinal tract. Living worms cause little or no inflammatory response, whereas dead worms are usually surrounded by granulomatous inflammation consisting of eosinophils, multinucleated giant cells, histiocytes, and hemosiderin.

➤ *Descriptors:* Lung parenchyma with altered structure:

- parasites (alive, intravascular, pulmonary arteries)
- caseous epithelioid granulomas
- intragranulomatous parasites (degenerated)
- mixed inflammatory infiltrates
- eosinophils
- multinucleated giant cells
- hyaline material (interstitial, eosinophilic)

■ *Special stains:* Collagenous stains, PAS, Movat stain.

Hallmark of Diagnosis: Demonstration of the parasites with typical clinical history, caseous epithelioid granulomas with dead (degenerated) parasites.

Differential diagnosis: Various parasitic infections (encephalitides) such as visceral larva migrans, cysticercosis, coenurosis, trichinosis, schistosomiasis, gnathostomiasis, paragonimiasis.

Anisakiasis

Definition: Human infection of larval nematodes of the family Anisakidae.

Incidence/Epidemiology: Common parasites of sea mammals living in the North Sea, Atlantic, and North Pacific oceans. People from Japan and the Netherlands eating raw, salted, slightly pickled, or undercooked fish have been found to be infected.

Etiology/Pathophysiology: At least three different types of larvae have been described: *Anisakis*, *Phocanema*, and *Contracaecum*. Adult worms live in the lumen of the gastrointestinal tract of marine mammals including whales, dolphins, seals, and sea lions. Second-stage larvae develop in the feces before hatching in sea water. Ingested by small crustaceans, they molt to their third stage. Fish eating the crustaceans serve as transport hosts until the mammalians become infected by eating infected fish.

Clinical Presentation: Patients with anisakiasis suffer from acute or chronic gastric symptoms such as nausea, vomiting, epigastric pain mimicking peptic ulcer, chronic gastritis, or gastric carcinoma. In addition, the small bowel is often infected, and patients present with the clinical picture of appendicitis or regional enteritis. Infection of the lung has been reported in one case.

Prognosis: Usually good in patients with infection of the stomach and tonsils, but lethal infection of the small intestines and the colon has been reported.

Radiology: Roentgenograms of the stomach or intestines may demonstrate the worms.

Pathology:

Gross: Thickened edematous wall of the stomach or intestines, in acute cases ulceration.

Histology: The worms present in a thick multilayered cuticle, adjacent large lateral chords and multiple smooth muscle cells, a centrally localized intestine with numerous tall columnar cells, and an excretory gland cell in the anterior region. The larvae measure 10–50 mm in length and about 1 mm in diameter. Inflammatory response of host tissue consists of eosinophilic and neutrophilic granulocytes, lymphocytes, plasma cells, multinucleated giant cells, and histiocytes and is usually associated with destruction of the worm, reported from the case with pulmonary infection.

➤ *Descriptors:* Lung parenchyma with altered structure:

- caseous epithelioid granulomas
- parasites (intragranulomatous, degenerated)
- mixed inflammatory infiltrates
- multinucleated giant cells
- eosinophils
- necrosis (eosinophilic microabscess)

■ *Special stains:* Collagenous stains, PAS, Movat stain.

Hallmark of Diagnosis: Necrotizing granulomas with degenerated parasites, identification of the worms associated with the clinical history.

Differential diagnosis: Various parasitic infections such as enterobiasis, *Angiostrongylus costaricensis*, visceral larva migrans, strongyloidiasis, ancylostomiasis, trichuriasis.

Anomalies, Pulmonary Vascular

Definition: Congenital disorders of one or both pulmonary arteries or veins.

Incidence/Epidemiology: Rare diseases most frequently including segmental stenoses in the pulmonary arterial system, a so-called absent or occult pulmonary artery, "vascular sling" (origin of the left pulmonary artery from the right pulmonary artery), reduced number of intrapulmonary arteries in cases of pulmonary valvular atresia, arteriovenous fistulae, anomalous return of pulmonary veins.

Etiology/Pathophysiology: The majority of malformations arise during the late embryonic period when the sixth aortic arches give rise to the primitive pulmonary arteries.

Clinical Presentation: Children present most frequently with hypoxemia and related symptoms. Additional alterations of lung parenchyma such as atelectasis, pulmonary hypoplasia, lymphangiectasis, or immature lung parenchyma are frequent.

Prognosis: Depending on degree and type of malformation.

Radiology: Angiography usually identifies the lesion.

Pathology:

Gross: The gross findings show circumscribed stenoses of the pulmonary arteries, anomalous origin of the pulmonary arteries, arteriovenous fistulae, total anomalous venous return (all four main veins converge and drain to the innominate vein, coronary veins, or right atrium), or partial anomalous venous return (the so-called scimitar syndrome with drainage of a large (usually right) pulmonary vein into the inferior vena cava), or stenosis of one or more pulmonary veins.

Histology: Unsuspicious layers of arterial or venous walls except in special cases such as Ehlers-Danlos syndrome.

➤ *Descriptors:* Pulmonary vessels with preserved structure:

- ectatic lumen (arteries, veins)
- tortuous vessels (veins)
- stenosis (arteries);
- Lung parenchyma with preserved structure:
- no morphological abnormalities

■ *Special stains:* Collagenous stains.

Hallmark of Diagnosis: Gross findings in association with the angiographic findings.

Differential diagnosis: Biological variations in the size of the affected vessels, stenosis due to postinflammatory scars, neoplasias (angiomas, etc.).

Antacids

Definition: Alteration of the lung parenchyma associated with intake of antacids, see Drug Toxicity.

Anthracosilicosis

Definition: Alterations of the lung parenchyma associated with exposure to silicotic dust, see Silicosis.

Anthracosis

Definition: Pneumoconiosis caused by inhalation of atmospheric soot particles.

Incidence/Epidemiology: With increasing age most if not all persons show intrapulmonary deposits of dust particles related to air pollution. Increase in traffic density and corresponding increase in car exhaust as well as industrial pollution are associated with increased levels of anthracosis.

Etiology/Pathophysiology: Most of the dust particles are removed from the airways by bronchial mucus and ciliary action or are ingested by macrophages and expectorated. Other particles remain in the peripheral lung and are transported via the lymphatic vessels to the proximal intrapulmonary lymph nodes, visible as immobile black deposits. Smoking causes a similar, more impressive picture.

Clinical Presentation: No major symptoms are known.

Prognosis: Good.

Radiology: Unsuspicious.

Pathology:

Gross: Intrapulmonary proximal lymph nodes show a homogeneous black color. Small black spots are visible in the peripheral lung.

Histology: Agglutinations of black dust particles in the intrapulmonary lymph nodes, partly ingested by histiocytic cells. Similar deposits in the peripheral lung surrounded by small proliferating alveolar cells. Some of them have ingested small black particles, not birefringent. No major inflammatory response of host tissue nor major disturbance of lung texture. Dust-laden macrophages suggest smoking or greater chronic exposure.

➤ *Descriptors:* Lung parenchyma with preserved structure:

- dust (amorphous black particles)
- macrophages (dust particles)

■ *Special stains:* Collagenous stain, PAS, Prussian blue, endogenous lectins (absent or weak sugar binding capacities).

Hallmark of Diagnosis: Deposits of dust without birefringence or asbestos particles, absent inflammatory response.

Differential diagnosis: Coal-miner's pneumoconiosis, smoker's lung.

Anthrax Pneumonia

Definition: Pneumonia caused by *Bacillus anthracis*.

Incidence/Epidemiology: The disease is endemic in goats and sheep and may spread to farmers or exposed persons who inhale contaminated particles or by cutaneous contamination. Cutaneous infection is much more common in humans than primary pulmonary infection. Anthrax pneumonia is a rare disease, the last small outbreak occurring in Manchester, NH, USA, in 1957.

Etiology/Pathophysiology: Spores of the large gram-positive bacillus are infectious. The spores are ingested by macrophages and cells of the alveolar lining and are transported into the regional lymph nodes, where they germinate. Following germination and multiplication of the organisms, generalized septicemia involving the lung and other organs including the spleen and the meninges occurs.

Clinical Presentation: The disease evolves in two phases with an initial phase of about 4 days, characterized by mild fever and discomfort, cough, malaise, and myalgia. The second phase starts with abrupt dyspnea, hypotension, and cyanosis, leading to death within 1–2 days.

Prognosis: Most patients die within 1 week.

Radiology: Diffuse, dense infiltrates resembling acute edema and mediastinal enlargement with tracheal compression.

Pathology:

Gross: Massive mediastinal edema, hemorrhagic necrosis of hilar and mediastinal lymph nodes, and congested edematous lungs are the common findings.

Histology: Hemorrhage, acute edema filling the air spaces, invasive lymphocytic infiltrates, and the absence of neutrophilic granulocytes are the findings in peripheral lung tissue. Dense amounts of large gram-positive organisms are visible in the edematous air spaces. The lymph nodes show large irregular areas of hemorrhagic necrosis.

➤ *Descriptors:* Lung parenchyma with preserved structure:

- bacteria (numerous, gram-positive)
- mononuclear inflammatory infiltrates
- intraalveolar serous fluid;
- Lung parenchyma with altered structure:
- necrosis (lymph nodes)

■ *Special stains:* PAS, Gram, Ziehl Neelsen.

Hallmark of Diagnosis: Dense clusters of large gram-positive organisms with missing neutrophilic granulocytes, intraalveolar edema, necrotic proximal lymph nodes, clinical history.

Differential diagnosis: Acute hemorrhagic pneumonia caused by other infectious organisms.

Antibiotics

Definition: Alteration of the lung parenchyma associated with intake of antibiotics, see Drug Toxicity.

Anticoagulants

Definition: Alteration of the lung parenchyma associated with intake of anticoagulants, see Drug Toxicity.

Antiglomerular Basement Membrane Disease

Definition: Synonym Goodpasture's syndrome. Disease with diffuse pulmonary hemorrhage caused by antiglomerular basement membrane-specific antibody with or without additional nephropathy.

Incidence/Epidemiology: Rare disease most frequently seen in men aged 16–30 years and occasionally in young children.

Etiology/Pathophysiology: The etiology of the disease is unknown. It is the prototype of a type II cytotoxic antibody-mediated reaction following exposure to hydrocarbons or penicillamine. Other authors have reported an increased HLA-DR2 haplotype and an increase of HLA-B7 haplotype. There is evidence that the globular domain region of collagen type IV may act as initiating antigen.

Clinical Presentation: Most patients have decreased hemoglobin concentrations in the peripheral blood, elevated white blood count, proteinuria, hemoptysis, weakness, fatigue, and shortness of breath. Hemoptysis occurs most frequently as the initial symptom. A nonspecific (viral) pulmonary infection may precede the outbreak of the disease. Complement-fixing IgG (IgA) can be detected.

Prognosis: The prognosis of patients with antiglomerular basement membrane disease has improved significantly during the past few years, and patients with minimal renal involvement have the most favorable outcome. Complete remission is usually seen by application of modern therapeutic regimes (immunosuppressive therapy combined with plasmapheresis).

Radiology: Diffuse pulmonary consolidations affecting both lungs, mainly localized in the lower parts of the upper and lower lobes, are seen.

Pathology:

Gross: Brown to brownish-red lungs with increased consistency and irregularly formed areas of intrapulmonary hemorrhage.

Histology: The alveoli are filled with blood associated with macrophages laden with hemosiderin. The alveolar septa are mildly thickened and contain scattered mononuclear inflammatory cells. Alveolar type II cells show reactive hyperplasia. Occasionally mild interstitial fibrosis can be documented. The texture of the lung parenchyma is usually preserved, vasculitis, abnormalities of bronchi, necrotic areas, and increased inflammatory cell infiltrates are not present.

➤ *Descriptors:* Lung parenchyma with preserved structure:
- hemorrhage
- macrophages (hemosiderin-laden)
- hyaline material (intraalveolar deposits of IgG, IgA, IgM, linear staining)

■ *Special stains:* Collagenous stain, PAS, Prussian blue, immunohistochemistry for deposits of IgG (linear staining is the common finding), IgA, and IgM (less frequent).

Hallmark of Diagnosis: Intrapulmonary hemorrhage without vasculitis, necrotic areas, or dense inflammatory infiltrates. Large numbers of hemosiderin-laden macrophages. Positive immunohistochemistry of linear deposits of IgG along the alveolar septa. Demonstration of glomerular basement membrane-specific antibody in the serum or in kidney biopsies.

Differential diagnosis: A variety of other diseases may cause diffuse pulmonary hemorrhage. These include immune-complex glomerulonephritis, uremic pneumonitis, Wegener's granulomatosis, lupus pneumonitis, necrotizing acute pneumonia, idiopathic pulmonary hemosiderosis, and pulmonary venoocclusive disease.

Antimony Exposure

Definition: Environmental lung disease in patients exposed to antimony.

Incidence/Epidemiology: Antimony is used in the production of accumulators and electrodes, and its oxide is used as a pigment in paints, plastics, enamels, and rubber. It is refined from antimony sulfide mined in South Africa, China, Mexico, Bolivia, and Europe.

Etiology/Pathophysiology: Antimony belongs to the so-called inert metals and causes no severe inflammatory reaction of lung parenchyma.

Clinical Presentation: Most patients are asymptomatic, but mild shortness of breath and chronic cough may be present.

Prognosis: No serious complications have been reported.

Radiology: Massive lesions are usually absent; however, mild signs of pneumoconiosis may be present.

Pathology:

Gross: Increased size of hilar and intrapulmonary proximal lymph nodes may exist, in addition to a brown coloration of the lung parenchyma.

Histology: Dust particles are usually accumulated in macrophages clustered in the alveolar ducts or in the alveoli. No major changes of interstitial lung parenchyma are found. Similar particles are seen in the proximal lymph nodes.

➤ *Descriptors:* Lung parenchyma with preserved structure:
- dust (black particles)
- macrophages (dust-laden)

■ *Special stains:* Prussian blue, X-ray spectrophotometry, energy-dispersal X-ray analysis, neutron activation analysis.

Hallmark of Diagnosis: Dust-laden macrophages in patients with a relevant history, and identification of antimony by physical techniques.

Differential diagnosis: Exposure of the lung to other "inert" metallic dusts such as titanium, iron, zirconium, tin, barium, cerium.

Antitetanus Serum

Definition: Alteration of the lung parenchyma associated with injection of antitetanus serum, see Drug Toxicity.

α_1-Antitrypsin Deficiency

Definition: Familial emphysema associated with α_1-antitrypsin deficiency.

Incidence/Epidemiology: α_1-antitrypsin deficiency has been reported to occur in 1/1 000 to 1/5 000 births in Northern Europe, and even less frequently in southern Europe, Japan, Africa.

Etiology/Pathophysiology: α_1-antitrypsin deficiency is determined by genetic factors, one of which is a pair of codominant alleles responsible for protease-antiprotease equivalence. The protease-inhibitor alleles (Pi) amount to 30 distinct units associated with a predisposition to emphysema (PiSZ), to chronic airflow obstruction (PiS), and to panacinar emphysema (PiZ). Smoking and additional socioeconomic or environmental factors aggravate the genetic predisposition.

Clinical Presentation: Patients usually exhibit chronic cough and are usually younger (45 years) than patients with chronic airflow obstruction (57 years).

Prognosis: Slow progression of the disease is usually seen.

Radiology: Chest radiograms usually show enlarged lung volumes and increased symmetric transparency of the basal parts of the lungs.

Pathology:

Gross: Increased volume of the lungs is associated with multiple pseudocystic enlarged alveolar ducts and bronchioles equally distributed over the lower parts of the lungs.

Histology: Increased size of terminal air spaces with flattened shape and missing boundary to adjacent air flow structures are the characteristic finding. The destroyed lung parenchyma is replaced by empty spaces demarcated by membranes with different degrees of fenestration. The lesions are focal, positioned in neighboring lung tissue with normal appearance, and are confluent with large cystic air spaces in advanced stages of the disease. Enlarged fibrotic bundles of interstitial tissue are absent, and the bronchial walls are usually infiltrated by moderate mononuclear inflammatory infiltrates.

➤ *Descriptors:* Lung parenchyma with preserved structure:

- enlarged distant air spaces
- atrophic interalveolar septula;
- Lung parenchyma with altered structure:
- focal interstitial fibrosis;
- Bronchial parenchyma with preserved structure:
- mononuclear inflammatory infiltrates

■ *Special stains:* Collagenous stains.

Hallmark of Diagnosis: Panacinar emphysema in younger adults with family history and α_1-antitrypsin deficiency in the serum.

Differential diagnosis: Localized panacinar emphysema, proximal acinar (centrilobular) emphysema, distal acinar (localized, bullous) emphysema, irregular (perifocal) emphysema associated with various agents such as coal, smoking, scars.

Apatite

Definition: Alteration of the lung parenchyma associated with inhalation of apatite, see Nonasbestos Mineral Fibers, Mineral Pneumoconiosis.

Apresoline

Definition: Alteration of the lung parenchyma associated with intake of apresoline (hydralazine), see Drug Toxicity.

Arc Welders Lung

Definition: Occupation-related disorder ranging from systemic "metal fume fever" to mineral dust pneumoconiosis.

Incidence/Epidemiology: Metallic welding fumes composed of particles ranging from 0.1–1 µm in diameter consist of various amounts of iron, titanium, manganese, aluminum, silicates, and carbonates. Shielding of production units and protection of workers have reduced the levels of toxic concentrations in general. Welders have an increased risk of developing bronchogenic carcinoma, especially when working with stainless steel.

Etiology/Pathophysiology: The metallic dust particles are inhaled and deposited in the terminal air spaces. They are mostly inert, and inflammatory response of host tissue is rare. Aluminum oxides are associated with certain reactive patterns such as pleural fibrosis, whereas titanium and iron oxides are relatively inert.

Clinical Presentation: Slightly progressive restrictive lung function with shortness of breath are common. Acute febrile illness noted as "metal fume fever" develops within hours after exposure to fumes from zinc, copper, magnesium, and nickel and will spontaneously remit after a day or two. Interstitial fibrosis is seen in severe cases.

Prognosis: Usually good, but patients with massive exposure may show slow progression into interstitial fibrosis.

Radiology: Chest radiographs may be unsuspicous or may present with prominent interstitial markings suggesting interstitial fibrosis. Pleural thickening is not an unusual finding.

Pathology:

Gross: Deep pigmentation of the lungs with little or no fibrotic changes is a characteristic finding. Dark-brown to black color suggests exposure to iron fumes, whereas a metallic sheen similar to tarnished aluminum indicates exposure to aluminum.

Histology: Large amounts of dust lying in the interstitial peripheral lung tissue without any major inflammatory response is the characteristic finding. Several polarizing particles may be included in the amorphous material. Granulomas are usually not present, and the texture of the peripheral lung tissue is preserved. Agglutination of dust in the proximal lymph nodes is not predominant, and fibrotic alterations of lymph nodes are rare. Diffuse interstitial fibrosis and pleural fibrosis suggest exposure to aluminum or asbestos.

➤ *Descriptors:* Lung parenchyma with preserved structure:

- dust (amorphous black material, birefringent fibers, crystals)
- absent inflammatory infiltrates

■ *Special stains:* Collagenous stains including Sirius stain, Prussian blue for iron stain, endogenous lectins for changes of sugar receptors in pneumocytes. Identification of dust particles by X-ray diffraction, energy-dispersal X-ray spectra due to electron or proton irradiation, scanning electron microscopy.

Hallmark of Diagnosis: Interstitial deposits of dust without any major inflammatory response.

Differential diagnosis: Idiopathic hemosiderosis of the lung, silico-pneumoconiosis, asbestosis, coal worker's pneumoconiosis.

Arsenic Fumes

Definition: Environmental lung disease in patients exposed to arsenic fumes.

Incidence/Epidemiology: Exposure has been reported for persons working at smelting of arsenic-bearing ores or in companies producing arsenical pesticides.

Etiology/Pathophysiology: Chronic inhalation has been reported to be associated with increased risk of lung cancer (3.3 times the normal risk).

Clinical Presentation: Chronic exposure to fumes is usually asymptomatic, although allergic skin reactions may occur.

Prognosis: Usually good, except for the increased risk of lung cancer.

Radiology: No significant changes have been reported.

Pathology:

Gross: The gross appearance of the lungs is usually unsuspicious.

Histology: One observes dust-laden macrophages clustered in the peripheral lung parenchyma with mild interstitial inflammatory reaction and mild reactive hyperplasia of pneumocytes.

➤ *Descriptors:* Lung parenchyma with preserved structure:

- macrophages (dust-laden)
- mononuclear inflammatory infiltrates
- desquamation, hypertrophy, hyperplasia and dysplasia of pneumocytes

■ *Special stains:* Prussian blue, X-ray spectrophotometry, energy-dispersal X-ray analysis, neutron activation analysis.

Hallmark of Diagnosis: Dust-laden macrophages associated with a relevant occupational history, identification of arsenic by physical techniques.

Differential diagnosis: Exposure of the lung to other environmental agents.

Arteriovenous Fistula

Definition: An intrapulmonary abnormal connection between medium-sized to larger arteries with veins of corresponding size, usually confined to one lobe of the lungs.

Incidence/Epidemiology: Rare disease which has been reported mainly as an inborn malformation.

Etiology/Pathophysiology: It occurs with isolated or multiple lesions associated with familial telangiectasis (Osler-Weber-Rendu syndrome). Acquisition of the disease on the basis of trauma has been documented.

Clinical Presentation: Patients suffer from systemic arterial blood desaturation and may present with hypoxemia, cyanosis, or polycythemia.

Prognosis: Usually good, depending on the degree of the shunt.

Radiology: Arteriovenous fistulae are usually identified by angiography.

Pathology:

Gross: Plexus of intercommunicating vessels of larger size than those usually seen in the relevant part of the lung, with great variations in the diameter of the tortuous vessels.

Histology: The vessels are of different diameters and show structures of arterial walls localized beneath structures of veins. The fistulae are usually embedded in lung parenchyma of normal structure.

➤ *Descriptors:* Pulmonary vessels with preserved structure:

- ectatic lumen
- stenosis
- tortuous vessels
- fistula

■ *Special stains:* Collagenous stains, angiography of the surgical specimen.

Hallmark of Diagnosis: Plexus of tortuous vessels with textures of walls beneath being characteristic of arteries and veins, seen by angiography.

Differential diagnosis: Angiomatous neoplasia (hemangioma, angiosarcoma).

Arteriovenous Malformation

Definition: Morphologic alterations of the pulmonary vessels occurring during the developmental period, see also Anomalies, Pulmonary Vascular.

Incidence/Epidemiology: Minor alterations (anatomic variants) of the pulmonary arteries and veins are quite frequent. Severe malformations are usually rare events and associated with other abnormalities.

Etiology/Pathophysiology: Paired segmental arteries arising from the dorsal aorta are the earliest blood supply to the developing lung. The main pulmonary arteries arise from the sixth aortic arches. The venous blood drainage of the lungs is associated with the splanchnic plexus and enters not into the right heart but into a wide variety of veins during the primordial period. Therefore, a broad variety of arterial and venous malformations has been described including aortopulmonary septal defect (usually not associated with patent ductus arteriosus), crossed pulmonary arteries (the left pulmonary artery crosses the right in front), origin of the (left) pulmonary artery from its (right) counterpart, unilateral absence of one pulmonary artery, congenital stenosis and ectasia, dissociation between parts of the bronchial tree and the pulmonary arteries (sequestration), tortuous arteries; drainage of pulmonary veins into the right atrium or into the portal veins, cor triatriatum (accessory atrial chamber connected with the pulmonary veins), stenosis and ectasia of the pulmonary veins, arteriovenous fistula.

Clinical Presentation: Minor abnormalities are usually asymptomatic. Major abnormalities usually induce pulmonary hypertension or are not compatible with life.

Radiology: Chest radiographs are normal or show abnormal configurations of the major pulmonary vessels.

Pathology:

Gross: The findings depend on the malformation and include arterial (venous) ectasia, stenosis, abnormal connections to the right and left heart, aorta, vena cava, etc.

Histology: The arterial and venous walls may be normal or fibrotic. Additional findings include tortuous vessels, intimal fibrosis, organizing thromboses, muscular arteries.

➤ *Descriptors:* Pulmonary vessels with preserved structure:

- ectatic lumen
- stenosis
- intimal fibrosis
- tortuous vessels;
- Pulmonary vessels with altered structure:
- increased number of smooth muscle cells
- fibrosis

■ *Special stains:* Collagenous stains.

Hallmark of Diagnosis: Clinical history, gross findings.

Differential diagnosis: Hamartoma, biological variations in the size of the affected vessels, vascular neoplasias.

Arthropods

Definition: Infection of the lung or bronchi with arthropods.

Incidence/Epidemiology: Arthropods reported to infect the lower respiratory tract are mites (see Acariasis) and larvae of *Diptera* (see Myiasis). Allergic reaction caused by mites is not infrequently seen. Infection of the lung with the larvae of *Diptera* is a very rare event (less than 10 cases have been reported).

Etiology/Pathophysiology: Acarine parasites live in unclean houses and may be inhaled. They usually stick in the nose, or the larger or medium-sized bronchi and induce allergic rhinitis or asthmatic bronchitis. The larvae dipterans invade the skin after a mosquito bite and involve the skin and the parenchymal organs including the lungs. A severe inflammatory reaction of the involved tissue usually takes place.

Clinical Presentation: The patients may be asymptomatic or present with cough, hemoptysis, chest pain, and dyspnea.

Radiology: Chest radiographs are normal (acariasis) or may show coin lesions in the peripheral lung zones (myiasis).

Prognosis: Usually good; however, myiasis may be fatal.

Pathology:

Gross: Mites in the bronchi or multiple, grayish-white, consolidated nodules (myiasis).

Histology: Mononuclear inflammatory infiltrates and eosinophils in the bronchial walls (mites); dense inflammatory infiltrates surrounding the parasites (larvae of *Diptera*). The details are described under their particular headings.

➤ *Descriptors:* Bronchial mucosa with preserved structure:

- ectatic lumen
- mites (intrabronchial)
- eosinophils;
- Lung parenchyma with altered structure:
- parasites (maggots)
- mixed inflammatory infiltrates (dense)
- necrosis and hemorrhage

■ *Special stains:* PAS, collagenous stains, Giemsa, Movat.

Hallmark of Diagnosis: Clinical history, necrotizing bronchitis, identification of the parasites.

Differential diagnosis: Infection of the lung with other parasites, bacterial bronchopneumonia.

Asbestos-Associated Diseases

Definition: Environmental lung diseases (fibrosis of the lung, pleural effusion, pleural plaque, mesothelioma, lung carcinoma) in patients exposed to asbestos fibers.

Incidence/Epidemiology: Asbestos, a generic name for six different asbestiform minerals, is mined in the Ural Mountains and Siberia in Russia, in the Quebec province of Canada, and in the Cape province and the Transvaal in South Africa. It is mainly used in the cement industry in the manufacture of sheets, corrugated roofing, gutters, tiles, drain pipes, and also in the manufacture of fire-resistant textiles, automobile brakes and clutches, filters for various fluids including beer, wines, and drugs, in asbestos paper for insulation, etc. Important sources of exposure include shipyards, dismantling of buildings with asbestos products, special working conditions (among fitters, electricians, plumbers, welders, carpenters), carding and spinning of fibers in the textile industry, buildings with closed ventilation systems constructed out of asbestos tubes, neighborhood exposure such as housewives cleaning contaminated clothes, etc. The prevalence of asbestosis ranges from 6–25% of exposed workers depending upon the number of years of exposure and the asbestos concentration in the air.

Etiology/Pathophysiology: Asbestos fibers are fibrous silicates of two different structures, the curved type (chrysotile derived from serpentine rock) and the straight type (crocidolite, amosite, anthophillite, tremolite, actinolite derived from amphibole rock). The fibers, which measure less than 100 μm in length and 2 μm in diameter, can enter the bronchioles, alveolar ducts and alveoli. Curved fibers tend to stick more proximally in the airways and split into submicroscopic fibrils. The fibers are ingested by macrophages and activate complement-derived chemotactic activity on alveolar surfaces. They enter interstitial tissue, where they remain inert. In the majority of patients they become coated with ferritin and protein and form the so-called ferruginous (asbestos) bodies. The pathophysiology leading to asbestos-related diseases is still unknown. No correlation has been found between the concentration of histologically demonstrable asbestos fibers and lung fibrosis. Experimental findings emphasize the importance of physical properties such as the length of the fibers for the development of fibrosis. These findings could not be confirmed in the analysis of human diseases. Macrophages are probably involved in the genesis of fibrosis which may become activated by asbestos fibers and can then stimulate the functional activity of fibroblasts. Immunologic components have also been described such as increased complement in bronchial lavages, and rise of secretory IgA, serum IgA, IgG, IgM, and IgE.

Clinical Presentation: Depending upon the underlying disease chronic cough may be present as well as shortness of breath during physical exercise, chest pain in case of mesothelioma, etc.

Prognosis: Prognosis of patients with massive or longer-lasting exposure to asbestos is poor due to serious sequelae. Asbestos is one of the most powerful carcinogenic agents and also induces progressive interstitial fibrosis of the lung and of the pleura.

Radiology: Early changes may not be detectable on chest radiographs, which normally demonstrate diffuse pleural and parenchymal disease. Under the ILO scheme (see under Pneumoconiosis) it should be classified into three categories according to size and profusion of the morphologic changes of lung and pleura.

Pathology:

Gross: Pleural effusions are usually clear and of yellowish color and only seldom bloody. Pleural plaques are white to yellowish of irregular shape, homogeneous surface, frequently bilateral and symmetric and range from a few millimeters to 10 cm or more in size. Conventional adhesions between both pleural surfaces occur only secondary to infections; the parietal pleura is almost exclusively involved. Fibrotic lungs have an increased consistency with grayish streaks along the interlobular septa and diffuse scarring. Honeycombing is only seen in advanced stages. Mesotheliomas are usually yellowish with some intratumorous bleeding or small necrotic areas in advanced stages. In early stages, they are macroscopically of similar appearance to pleural plaques. Asbestos-related lung carcinomas look the same and have the same proportions of cell types as those in patients not exposed to asbestos.

Histology: Pleural effusions usually do not contain asbestos fibers. They may show severe atypias of mesothelial cells including mitotic figures, especially if repetitive drainage has been performed. Pleural plaques consist of hyaline collagen fibers with a basket-weave appearance of the collagen. Connective tissue is nearly acellular. Scattered fibroblasts or mononuclear inflammatory cells are only visible near the abrupt edges of the lesions. Central calcification may occur. Identification of noncoated asbestos fibers are usually not possible by light microscopy. Asbestos-associated fibrosis is of diffuse type with inclusions of focal fibrotic scars. The alveolar walls are thickened and filled with collagenous deposits. A few lymphocytes may be seen. The alveoli contain macrophages, lymphocytes, plasma cells, and various amounts of asbestos fibers; the alveolar lining cells are unsuspicious. Fibrosis is marked near the terminal airways, whereas the smaller and larger bronchi and the surrounding lung parenchyma are spared. Presence of smooth muscle cells is only detectable in advanced stages, if at all. Mesotheliomas are usually of the epithelial or biphasic type. Bronchial carcinomas include the four major cell types (epidermoid carcinoma, adenocarcinoma, large cell anaplastic carcinoma, and small cell anaplastic carcinoma).

➤ *Descriptors:* Lung parenchyma with preserved structure:

- asbestos bodies (intraalveolar)
- dust (birefringent, asbestos fibers)
- macrophages (asbestos fibers);
- Lung parenchyma with altered structure:
- diffuse interstitial fibrosis
- mononuclear inflammatory infiltrates;
- Pleura with altered structure:
- hyaline material

- acellular collagen (basket-weave appearance)

■ *Special stains:* Prussian blue for detection of ferruginous bodies, collagenous stains, transmission electron microscopy for detection of asbestos fragments, energy-dispersal X-ray analysis, infrared spectrometry, quantitative analysis of asbestos fibers by digestion of wet lung tissue using 40% KOH or using low temperature (500°C) ashing and counting the fibers filtered through a membrane. More than 100 asbestos fibers should be present per 1 g (1 cm^3) of lung tissue. Blocks of six specific sites are recommended by the International Union Against Cancer (UICC): (a) apex of right upper lobe, pleural surface; (b) right middle lobe, lateral pleural surface; (c) right lower lobe, middle of basal surface; (d) left upper lobe, central section; (e) lingula, central section; (f) left lower lobe, central basal section.

Hallmark of Diagnosis: Identification and quantification of asbestos fibers (100 fibers or more per cm^3 of lung tissue), mild morphological interstitial changes, presence of lung cancer or mesothelioma, in addition to confirmation of exposure to asbestos by the clinical history.

Differential diagnosis: Nonasbestos-related pleural effusion, fibrosis, mesothelioma, or lung cancer. Pseudoferruginous bodies (black-coated fibers with negative staining to Prussian blue).

Asbestos Bodies

Definition: Deposition of fibers coated with iron-protein mucopolysaccharide substances in the lung, see Ferruginous Bodies.

Ascariasis

Definition: Infection of human lung with *Ascaris lumbricoides.*

Incidence/Epidemiology: Cosmopolitan disease with greatest frequency in moist tropical countries, especially in overcrowded rural communities. Most common among children. Infection occurs from fecal contamination of toys, soil, raw vegetables, or drinking water.

Etiology/Pathophysiology: Adult worms of both sexes live in the small intestines (jejunum) and produce about 200 000 eggs daily which are excreted with the feces. They develop into infective eggs containing larvae in moist, warm soil, resisting freezing, drying, and chemicals, and being viable for years. After being eaten the infective eggs hatch in the small intestines, and the larvae penetrate the intestinal wall, enter the portal vein or intestinal lymphatic vessels, migrate from the liver to the heart, and are swept to the lung. Here they become third stage larvae and migrate to the esophagus via the bronchi and trachea. In the intestines they become mature worms after molting twice.

Clinical Presentation: Symptoms are rare in general due to the good adaption of the worms to man. Complications include partial or complete intestinal obstruction, peritonitis, abdominal discomfort, epigastric pain, cholangitis, liver abscess, fever, eosinophilia, pneumonia, mucoid or bloody sputum, tachycardia, cyanosis.

Prognosis: Usually good, but serious complications can develop when the parasites migrate to the ampulla of Vater, perforate the peritoneum, or induce pneumonia.

Radiology: In severe infections increased prominence of peribronchial markings, diffuse mottled infiltrates resembling miliary tuberculosis.

Pathology:

Gross: Lungs contain small, consolidated grayish areas most frequently in the lower lobes. The worms are of cylindrical shape with white to tan color, measuring 220–350 mm in length and 3–6 mm in diameter. The larvae in the lungs reach 2 mm in length by 75 μm in diameter, the fertilized eggs 60 μm by 40 μm.

Histology: The larvae contain prominent lateral alae, paired excretory columns, and a central localized intestine. The cuticle has attached smooth muscle fibers and is transversely striated. The larvae in the lung cause an inflammatory response of host tissue comprising histiocytes, eosinophilic leukocytes, macrophages. They are most numerous in the bronchial lumen, in the bronchioles, and within the alveolar walls.

➤ *Descriptors:* Lung parenchyma with preserved structure:

- parasites (larvae, intraalveolar)
- mononuclear inflammatory infiltrates (dense)

- eosinophils;
- Bronchial mucosa with preserved structure:
- parasites (larvae, intrabronchial)
- mononuclear inflammatory infiltrates (dense)
- eosinophils;

■ *Special stains:* PAS, Movat.

Hallmark of Diagnosis: Eosinophilic pneumonia, identification of the eggs in the feces, of the worms in the intestines, and of the larvae in the lung tissue. Sometimes they can be detected in the sputum.

Differential diagnosis: Infections with other nematodes.

Askin Tumor

Definition: Malignant small cell tumor of the thoracopulmonary region in childhood.

Incidence/Epidemiology: Rare malignancy with an estimated incidence of 0.1/100 000 children. The tumor is more frequently seen in girls than in boys at an age ranging from 2–20 years.

Etiology/Pathophysiology: The neuroendocrine origin of the tumor suggests its development from the intercostal nerves.

Clinical Presentation: The patient's first symptoms include chest pain, shortness of breath, pleural effusions, dyspnea, malaise, mild fever.

Prognosis: Usually poor, about 60–80% of patients die within 5 years after diagnosis.

Radiology: After fine needle aspiration of the pleural effusion, radiographs usually reveal solid tumor masses adjacent to the chest wall, often with destruction of the corresponding ribs.

Pathology:

Gross: Usually large, soft, yellowish tumor masses with large necrotic areas and diffuse, invasive growth.

Histology: Small tumor cells without distinct boundaries of cytoplasm. Scanty nuclear chromatin with one to two unsuspicious nucleoli, focal myxomatoid changes without any reproducible growth textures. In the central tumorous areas hemorrhages and necroses, at tumor boundary some inflammatory cells. High rate of mitoses.

➤ *Descriptors:* Newly formed textures with metastasis potential:
- mesenchymal growth pattern
- lymphomatoid textures
- solid textures
- small tumor cells
- homogeneous nuclear and cellular size
- finely distributed nuclear chromatin
- frequent mitoses
- necrosis
- absent or weak inflammatory infiltrates

■ *Special stains:* PAS, Giemsa, immunohistochemistry for differentiation from small cell anaplastic carcinoma, lymphoma, rhabdomyosarcoma, Ewing's sarcoma (lymphocytic markers negative, neuroendocrine markers partly positive (10–30%), cytoskeleton markers negative), texture analysis, and DNA analysis.

Hallmark of Diagnosis: Small lymphocytic tumor cells with myxomatoid areas, high proliferation rate, characteristic tumor localization, age of the patient.

Differential diagnosis: Malignant non-Hodgkin's lymphomas, neuroblastoma, Ewing's sarcoma, rhabdomyosarcoma, small cell anaplastic carcinoma of the lung.

Aspergillosis

Definition: Mycotic infection of the lung with *Aspergillus (fumigatus, flavus-oryzae).*

Incidence/Epidemiology: Frequent disease in debilitated or immunosuppressed patients. *Aspergillus* conidia are ubiquitous and constantly present in the human environment. *Aspergillus* can be demonstrated in soil and organic debris and on moist inorganic surfaces, decaying plants.

Etiology/Pathophysiology: The fungi colonize (a) in preexisting cavities of patients with intact immunity; (b) in the trachea/main bronchi causing non-invasive or superficially invasive necrotizing tracheobronchitis; (c) in the smaller airways of mildly compromised patients causing chronic progressive and destructive bronchopneumonia; (d) in the peripheral lung of immunosuppressed patients causing severe, rapidly progressive, necrotizing pneumonia. Mild infections in patients with intact immunity can be responsible for a variety of hypersensitivity reactions.

Clinical Presentation: The symptoms depend upon the immunodefensive mechanism of the patient. Colonization in obstructed or ectatic bronchi such as are seen in patients with cystic fibrosis, bronchial asthma, and neoplasms causes no or only mild symptoms. The fungi may grow in ball-like shapes (aspergilloma) in preexisting cavities such as cystic formations caused by tuberculosis, sarcoidosis, infarction, bullous emphysema, necrotic neoplasms. Hemoptysis, positive serology, and radiographic demonstration of the ball-like configuration are clues to the clinical diagnosis of aspergilloma. Necrotizing tracheobronchitis and chronic progressive bronchopneumonia are associated with cough, recurrent mild fever, dyspnea, wheezing, loss of weight. Patients with invasive rapidly progressive infections develop fever, hemoptysis, chest pain, dyspnea.

Prognosis: Patients with noninvasive aspergillosis have a good prognosis, while those with invasive aspergillosis can develop fungemia and serious complications, causing death.

Radiology: Aspergilloma form large round densities in preexisting cysts partly surrounded by crescents of air. Chronic necrotizing pulmonary aspergillosis is characterized by thick-walled cavities often associated with pleural thickening, usually seen in the upper lobes or superior segments of the lower lobes. Patchy, multifocal, or diffuse densities with areas of consolidation or circumscribed nodules with cavitations suggest invasive pneumonia.

Pathology:

Gross: The aspergilloma or mycotic infiltrated lung areas are yellowish-white and soft in consistency. The intrapulmonary nodules measure a few millimeters to several centimeters in diameter and are surrounded by hemorrhagic rims.

Histology: The fungus consists of septated hyphae with characteristic dichotomous branching measuring 3–6 μm in diameter. Viable hyphae are basophilic, as contrasted with necrotic hyphae, which are hyaline or eosinophilic. The mycotic agglutinations are surrounded by lymphocytes, plasma cells, histiocytes, and vascularized connective tissue in cases of aspergilloma or chronic infective lesions. Occasionally, a Splendore-Hoeppli phenomenon exists. Central nodular infarction of mycotic nodules together with viable masses of *Aspergillus* hyphae forming a peripheral rim are characteristic findings in invasive progressive aspergillosis. The inflammatory response of host tissue usually includes monocytes and eosinophilic lymphocytes. A well-formed granulomatous reaction with palisading histiocytes occurs only occasionally and can be encountered when immunoreactivity is intact.

➤ *Descriptors:* Bronchial mucosa with preserved structure:
- fungus (intrabronchial, *Aspergillus*, hyphae)
- mononuclear inflammatory infiltrates
- eosinophils;
- Lung parenchyma with altered structure:
- caseous epithelioid granulomas
- fungus (intragranulomatous, hyphae)
- mononuclear inflammatory infiltrates
- eosinophils

■ *Special stains:* PAS, GMS, collagenous stains, immunofluorescence.

Hallmark of Diagnosis: Demonstration of the hyphae with the characteristic dichotomous rectangular branching and attached aleuriospores; destructive growth and types of host tissue response for correct classification of invasiveness.

Differential diagnosis: Mucormycosis, angioinvasive opportunistic organisms such as *Fusarium* and *Pseudallescheria boydii*.

Aspiration

Definition: Inhalation of fluids or solid material into the lower respiratory tract.

Incidence/Epidemiology: Frequent disease seen in young children or in adults suffering from alterations of the nervous system (due to loss of consciousness, alcoholic stupor, seizures, drugs, debilitation, anesthesia) and from aspiration of gastric acid (due to vomiting, gastrointestinal reflux, achalasia, esophageal dysmotility, fistula to the respiratory tract, nasogastric intubation, swallowing difficulties).

Etiology/Pathophysiology: Foreign bodies partially occlude a segmental or subsegmental bronchus causing chronic inflammatory reaction of the wall and obstructive inflammation of the corresponding lung parenchyma with subsequent bacterial superinfection, leading to features of atelectasis, bronchiectasis, pneumonia, lung abscess. Aspiration of gastric acid causes diffuse alveolar damage ranging from mild bronchiolitis to necrotizing bronchiolitis and lung abscess. Aspiration of lipid-containing fluids such as milk, mineral oil, liquid paraffin, or aerosols containing lipid such as hairspray propellant, oil mist in steel rolling, or products of burning fat leads to the picture of exogenous lipid pneumonia.

Clinical Presentation: Aspiration in young children (peanuts, seeds, beads, fragments of wooden or plastic toys) causes cough, tachypnea, fever, and chest pain. If the cause of the disease is not recognized, chronic symptoms often misinterpreted as chronic asthma may develop. Similar symptoms are seen in patients who have aspirated gastric acid, sometimes called the Mendelson syndrome. The degree of the symptoms and the corresponding damage to the lungs depends, naturally, upon the amount of the aspirate. Aspiration of lipid material produces, in the initial stage, hemoptysis, fever, cough. The later stages are characterized by dyspnea and shortness of breath.

Prognosis: Usually good; however, secondary bacterial infection can occur, which may induce severe abscessing bronchopneumonia.

Radiology: Chest radiographs usually show larger foreign bodies in the corresponding bronchi, signs of atelectasis or dense diffuse or circumscribed infiltrations, sometimes with cavitation.

Pathology:

Gross: Aspirated solid material (peanuts, seeds, etc.) stick in the corresponding bronchi surrounded by thickened walls of white color. Atelectatic lung parenchyma can be recognized by its firm, nearly homogeneous, compact consistency and red-brown color. Lipid pneumonia shows wet red areas in the beginning and fibrotic strings in the later stages.

Histology: Foreign bodies usually cause marked inflammation of granulomatous appearance associated with granulocytes, lymphocytes, histiocytes, and multinucleated giant cells. Fragments of the aspirated material may show calcification and can be mistaken for parasites. In earlier stages of lipid pneumonia the alveoli are filled with lipid-laden macrophages. The pneumocytes are unsuspicious, and a mild interstitial inflammatory response is present. In later stages, the macrophages decline in number and confluent lipid droplets fill the alveoli, accompanied by multinucleated giant cells and a moderate fibroblastic response of host tissue leading to disturbance of the original lung texture and to diffuse interstitial fibrosis. Aspiration of gastric acid causes hyaline membranes and interstitial edema in the beginning and, at a later stage, necrosis of the bronchioles and of the centroacinar regions. The inflammatory infiltrates consist mainly of granulocytes which are later replaced by lymphocytes, fibroblasts, and histiocytes, leading to irreversible injury.

➤ *Descriptors:* Lung parenchyma with preserved structure:
- mixed inflammatory infiltrates
- multinucleated giant cells (foreign body)
- macrophages (lipid-laden)
- hyaline membranes;
- Lung parenchyma with altered structure:
- mononuclear inflammatory infiltrates
- focal interstitial fibrosis
- calcification;
- Bronchial mucosa with altered structure:
- mixed inflammatory infiltrates
- ulceration
- necrosis
- squamous metaplasia and dysplasia

■ *Special stains:* PAS, GMS, collagenous stains.

Hallmark of Diagnosis: Acute (lipid) pneumonia, identification of foreign bodies, clinical history.

Differential diagnosis: Parasitic infections, endogenous lipid pneumonia, opportunistic pneumonia.

Aspirin

Definition: Alteration of the lung parenchyma associated with intake of aspirin, see Drug Toxicity.

Asteroid Bodies

Definition: Star-shaped intracytoplasmic inclusion bodies of multinucleated giant cells, see Berylliosis, Sarcoidosis.

Asthma

Definition: Acute, spasmodic, diffuse airway narrowing with persistent airway hyperreactivity.

Incidence/Epidemiology: Common disease affecting about 1% of the European population with a more rapid course beginning after the age of 40.

Etiology/Pathophysiology: Obstruction of the bronchioles and small bronchi caused by spasms of the smooth muscle cells, by acute edema of the bronchial mucosa, or by hypersecretion of the mucous glands leads to severe disturbance of ventilation and diffusion of the peripheral lung parenchyma. Episodes of asthma are associated with infections, exercise, antigens, occupational stimuli, environmental stimuli, pharmacologic causes, or emotional stress. Besides an acquired hyperreactivity in a nonspecific fashion, specific IgE binding to mast cells mediated by histamines and triggered by inflammatory reactions such as smoking, viral infections, etc. play an important role.

Clinical Presentation: The disease occurs at any age and is characterized by its "asthmatic dyspnea" which occurs in severe cases with cyanosis, exhaustion and expectoration of gelatinous mucus plugs. Short inspiration and prolonged expiration are combined with chest pain, cardiac arrhythmia, and overexpansion of the peripheral lung tissue.

Prognosis: Chronic asthma usually induces cor pulmonale. Acute asthma such as status asthmaticus can have a lethal outcome.

Radiology: Areas with increased air content and deformation of the thorax with flattened diaphragm and anomalous movement of the diaphragm are characteristic findings.

Pathology:

Gross: The lungs do not collapse and are pale in color showing alternating areas of hyperexpansion and collapse. The small bronchi are filled with thick, yellowish mucus, and the bronchial walls are thickened. Emphysematous changes are usually not present.

Histology: The small bronchi and bronchioles present a thickened basal membrane and an increased number of smooth muscle cells. The number of goblet cells is also increased, the bronchial lumen is filled with mucus, numerous eosinophilic granulocytes, desquamated bronchial epithelial cells, and so-called Charcot-Leyden crystals (bipyramidal, hexagonal eosinophilic crystals composed of lysophos-pholipase). The epithelial cells of the smaller bronchi frequently degenerate and detach from the basement membrane (Creola bodies). In the sputum twisted mucous spirals (Curschmann's spirals) are present. The mucous glands in the bronchial walls usually increase in number and size, and the bronchial cartilage sometimes degenerates. The bronchial walls contain numerous eosinophilic granulocytes, lymphocytes, and plasma cells. The alveoli are either collapsed or expanded and empty.

➤ *Descriptors:* Bronchial mucosa with preserved structure:
- hyaline basal membrane
- increased number of smooth muscle cells
- increased number of goblet cells
- viscous mucus
- eosinophils
- desquamation, hypertrophy, hyperplasia and dysplasia of epithelial cells;
- Bronchial mucosa with altered structure:
- squamous metaplasia and dysplasia

■ *Special stains:* PAS, collagenous stains, Papanicolaou's stain, Giemsa.

Hallmark of Diagnosis: Changes in the walls of small bronchi and bronchioles presenting with gelatinous mucus, eosinophilic granulocytes, Creola bodies in the lumen, increased number of goblet cells, broad hyaline basal membrane, hypertrophic smooth muscle cells, submucous edema, and infiltrations of mast cells, eosinophilic granulocytes, lymphocytes, plasma cells. Clinical history.

Differential diagnosis: Chronic bronchitis, bronchocentric granulomatosis, allergic (extrinsic) alveolitis.

Atelectasis

Definition: Acute or chronic collapse of peripheral lung with resulting loss of volume.

Incidence/Epidemiology: Common disease seen in children with infectious diseases (sinobronchitis, i.e., bronchitis with purulent nasal discharge), asthma, cystic fibrosis (right lung), measles, pertussis (multiple), in adults with proximal localized bronchial carcinoma (recurrent atelectasis).

Etiology/Pathophysiology: Atelectasis is caused by disturbance of lung mechanics, gas exchange, hemodynamics, and host defenses. According to the Laplace's law, the tendency for an alveolus to collapse is inversely related to its diameter and to the air pressure. The capillary blood flow is decreased in atelectatic lung areas caused by shunts of the unaffected lung. Hypoxic lung is less effective in killing bacteria or opportunistic organisms.

Clinical Presentation: Depending on the underlying disease the symptoms may include cough, tachypnea, rhonchi, fever, chest pain, shortness of breath. Asymptomatic patients are not infrequently seen. Special types of atelectasis are: (a) middle lobe syndrome (chronic or recurrent atelectasis of the right middle lobe usually associated with cough, pain, hemoptysis, recurrent pneumonia); (b) rounded atelectasis (special "rounded" type of atelectasis predominantly of the right lower lobe with adjacent pleural thickening, usually solitary, often seen in patients with exposure to asbestos).

Prognosis: Usually good.

Radiology: Chest radiographs show compacted lung areas located close to overinflated lung portions. The vessels show crowding if more than two-thirds of the lung volume is collapsed. Shift of the mediastinum is more commonly present in lower lobe collapse. The diaphragm becomes elevated in case of upper lobe collapse.

Pathology:

Gross: The affected areas of the lung show a firm consistency with a somewhat darker color than the adjacent overinflated portions. The proximal supporting bronchus is usually stenotic or occluded with corresponding poststenotic dilatation of the lumen. The volume of the affected lobes or lung is remarkably decreased.

Histology: The lung texture is completely normal. Even in chronic cases no significant histomorphological changes of the lung parenchyma are detectable, except a raised number of intraalveolar macrophages and a moderate number of interstitial mononuclear inflammatory infiltrates.

➤ *Descriptors:* Lung parenchyma with preserved structure:
- atelectatic distant air spaces
- macrophages
- mononuclear inflammatory infiltrates

■ *Special stains:* None.

Hallmark of Diagnosis: Gross findings, normal histology, intraalveolar agglutinations of macrophages, clinical history.

Differential diagnosis: Normal, nonexpanded lung due to poorly discriminating techniques of fixation.

Atherosclerosis of the Pulmonary Trunk

Definition: Narrowing of the lumen of the proximal pulmonary arteries caused by degenerative changes, with lipoid deposits, calcified incrustations, thrombotic adherences.

Incidence/Epidemiology: Commonly seen in middle-aged patients as a singular entity (not related to pulmonary hypertension). More common in young children suffering from congenital heart diseases or associated pulmonary hypertension.

Etiology/Pathophysiology: The general concomitants of atherosclerosis (deposits of lipoid material, proliferative smooth muscle fibers, incrustations of microthrombotic lesions, immunologic alterations) are probably responsible for the atherosclerotic changes of the pulmonary arteries. In children, a close relation to pulmonary hypertension exists. Aged patients usually show minimal changes of the pulmonary walls.

Clinical Presentation: No symptoms in patients with "idiopathic" changes, i.e., in patients without pulmonary hypertension. Cardiac hypertrophy may occur.

Prognosis: Usually good as long as no cardiac involvement occurs.

Radiology: Chest radiographs may show calcified lesions of the proximal pulmonary arteries.

Pathology:

Gross: The same appearance as that in the systemic circulation, i.e., narrowing of the lumen, rough surface of the intima with yellowish plaques, thrombotic adherences, calcifications etc.

Histology: The same alterations of the vessel walls as seen in systemic atherosclerosis, usually extensive fragmentation and dissolution of the elastic fibers with focal incrustation of lipoid material, calcified areas, plaques of the intima consisting of agglutinations of foamy, lipid-laden macrophages, fibrin deposits, etc.

➤ *Descriptors:* Pulmonary vessels with altered structure:
- fragmentation of the elastic fibers
- hyaline material (intima, plaques)
- lipoid material (incrustated, intima, media)
- mononuclear inflammatory infiltrates (media)

■ *Special stains:* Collagenous stains.

Hallmark of Diagnosis: Narrowing of the lumen with characteristic macroscopic and microscopic appearance similar to that in systemic atherosclerosis.

Differential diagnosis: Various causes of pulmonary atherosclerosis, i.e., pulmonary hypertension, high altitude, chronic thromboembolism.

Atresia, Bronchial

Definition: Absent opening of a major bronchus, see Emphysema, Lobar Infantile, Agenesis of Trachea, Agenesis of Lung.

Atresia, Esophageal

Definition: Absent opening of the esophagus, see Fistula.

Attapulgite Fibers

Definition: Deposits of nonasbestos mineral fibers in the lung, see Nonasbestos Mineral Fibers.

Ayerza's Disease

Definition: Alteration of the lung parenchyma associated with pulmonary hypertension, see Hypertension, Pulmonary.

Azathioprine

Definition: Alteration of the lung parenchyma associated with intake of azathioprine (immunosuppressive agent), see Drug Toxicity.

Bacterial Infections – Byssinosis

Bacterial Infections

Definition: Infection of the lung parenchyma with various species of bacteria (bacterial pneumonia).

Incidence/Epidemiology: Pneumonias play an important role in the health care system and can be classified according to their epidemiologic significance as follows: (a) community-acquired infections (outside of the hospital environment, such as pneumonias caused by *Streptococcus pneumoniae* (*pneumococcus*), *Klebsiella, Legionella, Staphylococcus aureus, Hemophilus influenzae*); (b) gram-negative opportunistic bacterial infections (usually seen in immunocompromised or hospitalized patients caused by *Bacterioides, Escherichia coli, Pseudomonas aerugenosa, Serratia marcescens*, or *Klebsiella, Legionella*); (c) chronic bacterial infections (most frequently seen in patients with constitutional anomalies caused by *Actinomyces israelii, Nocardia asteroides, Pseudomonas pseudomallei*); (d) infections with highly pathogenic bacteria (seen in patients with special exposure to *Yersinia pestis, Bacillus anthracis, Francisella tularensis).*

Etiology/Pathophysiology: Community-acquired infections are usually caused by inhalation of the organisms. Viral pulmonary infections may precede bacterial outbreak of the disease. Gram-negative opportunistic bacterial infections are, in addition, often secondarily caused by bacteremia. Chronic pneumonias occur in areas of the lung being damaged by various causes, such as preexisting scars, tumorous lesions, infarctions. Highly virulent bacteria usually infect healthy persons having close contact with infected animals such as sheep and goats (infections with *Bacillus anthracis*), and rodents (*Yersinia pestis* or *Francisella tularensis*).

Bacterial growth causes activation of the defense mechanisms of the lung tissue usually leading to annihilation of the organisms, resolution of the invaded cellular inflammatory infiltrate and restoration of the pulmonary architecture. Incomplete annihilation of the bacteria or resolution of the exudate proceeds to chronic pneumonia or to focal destruction of the lung tissue (healed scars with perifocal emphysema).

Clinical Presentation: The onset of bacterial infections is usually abrupt. Symptoms include fever, cough, chest pain, dyspnea, tachypnea. Resolution of the infiltrate and recession of symptoms are usually seen between the 5th and 10th day.

Prognosis: Fatal outcome is frequently seen in elderly patients with pneumonia, immunocompromised persons, and premature babies if the course of the disease is abrupt and appropriate therapy is still absent. About 30–50% of autopsy cases show acute pneumonias associated with the cause of death.

Radiology: Lobar or lobular increased densities with precise correspondence to the involved portions of the lung.

Pathology:

Gross: In the first stage wet, hyperemic areas of the lung closely restricted to the infected lobe or segment. Increased red color and consistency in the second stage, followed by changes to grayish color in the third stage. The final stage is characterized by firm lungs of yellow-tan color.

Histology: The usually progress of bacterial infection of the lung can be grouped into four stages according to Rokitansky: (a) congestion and spreading edematous stage, characterized by intraalveolar edema and vascular engorgement; (b) red hepatization, characterized by extravasation of red blood cells, deposits of fibrin, and the beginning of invasion of neutrophilic granulocytes from the capillaries into the air spaces; (c) gray hepatization stage, characterized by fibrinous deposits and an enormous number of neutrophilic granulocytes in the alveoli mixed with macrophages and less frequently with lymphocytes and plasma cells; (d) yellow hepatization or resolution stage, characterized by restoration of the tissue texture, decline in the number of neutrophilic granulocytes, cellular debris, emptying of the air spaces. Signs of lobular pneumonia or bronchopneumonia include histologically less dense inflammatory infiltrates in the peripheral lung parenchyma with clusters near the terminal and respiratory bronchioles, associated with chronic infection of the larger bronchi.

➤ *Descriptors:* Lung parenchyma with preserved structure:

- intraalveolar serous fluid
- hemorrhage
- mixed inflammatory infiltrates
- intraalveolar fibrinoid material;

- Pulmonary vessels with preserved structure:
- ectatic lumen (small arteries, veins, capillaries);
- Lung parenchyma with altered structure:
- proliferating fibroblasts
- focal interstitial fibrosis

■ *Special stains:* PAS, collagenous stains, Gram's, immunofluorescence for identification of the organisms.

Hallmark of Diagnosis: Intraalveolar (hemorrhagic) exudate with different numbers of inflammatory cells, preserved lung texture, clinical history, findings of the chest radiograph.

Differential diagnosis: Pneumonias caused by viruses or by mycoplasms (interstitial pneumonias), infarction, abscess, acid gastric aspiration.

Bagassosis

Definition: Extrinsic allergic alveolitis caused by *Thermoactinomyces vulgaris*.

Incidence/Epidemiology: Infrequently seen in sugarcane workers or mushroom workers.

Etiology/Pathophysiology: Usually immune complex formation (type III immune reaction of the lung) in combination with cell-mediated hypersensitivity (type IV).

Clinical Presentation: Acute and chronic courses have been described. Patients present with dyspnea, cough, fever, chills.

Prognosis: Usually good and without sequelae, but chronic pneumonitis with slow progressive respiratory failure can occur.

Radiology: Diffuse, soft infiltrates or fine micronodular densities.

Pathology:

Gross: Firm, rubbery, reddish-gray lungs in chronic cases, while acute cases may still show normal lungs.

Histology: Prominent, patchy interstitial infiltrate with close relation to the terminal bronchioles. It is composed of histiocytes, lymphocytes, plasma cells, and occasional multinucleated giant cells. Noncaseating granulomatous formation and bronchiolitis obliterans occur. Eosinophilic granulocytes are not predominant.

➤ *Descriptors:* Lung parenchyma with altered structure:

- noncaseous epithelioid granulomas
- eosinophils
- multinucleated giant cells
- intrabronchiolar fibrinoid material and histiocytes
- ulceration of bronchiolar mucosa;
- Lung parenchyma with preserved structure:
- macrophages
- desquamation, hypertrophy, hyperplasia and dysplasia of pneumocytes
- mononuclear inflammatory infiltrates
- intraalveolar serous fluid

■ *Special stains:* PAS, collagenous stains, endogenous lectins.

Hallmark of Diagnosis: Noncaseating granulomas with moderate dysplasia of pneumocytes, focal bronchiolitis obliterans, clinical history, findings of chest radiographs.

Differential diagnosis: Sarcoidosis, tuberculosis, fungal infections, berylliosis.

Baritosis

Definition: Occupational lung disease caused by inhalation of barium sulfate.

Incidence/Epidemiology: Exposure has been reported from persons working in mines or in factories using barium sulfate (paints, vulcanized rubber, glass, radiographic contrast media).

Etiology/Pathophysiology: Barium sulfate consists of birefringent, refractile, relatively inert crystals causing moderate inflammatory response of the host tissue.

Clinical Presentation: Usually mild symptoms in occupationally exposed persons. Progress of the disease is more related to silicotic components than to barium.

Prognosis: Usually good and without sequelae.

Radiology: Usually no characteristic findings, but discrete interstitial densities or "snowstorm" appearance of the lung have been described.

Pathology:

Gross: The lungs present grayish macules a few millimeters in diameter randomly distributed in both lungs. Severe fibrosis has not been described.

Histology: The crystals can be demonstrated by polarization. Granulomatous formation of inflammatory cells, including histiocytes, lymphocytes, plasma cells and multinucleated giant cells seldom occurs and independently of the number of inhaled particles. Macrophages contain many ingested birefringent crystals. Pneumocytes are unsuspicious; fibrotic response is weak.

➤ *Descriptors:* Lung parenchyma with preserved structure:
- dust (birefringent crystals)
- macrophages (birefringent crystals)
- unsuspicious pneumocytes;
- Lung parenchyma with altered structure:
- noncaseous epithelioid granulomas
- mononuclear inflammatory infiltrates
- multinucleated giant cells

■ *Special stains:* Collagenous stains, X-ray diffraction and related techniques.

Hallmark of Diagnosis: Birefringent crystals in the air spaces, in the interstitium, and ingested in macrophages, mild response of host tissue, clinical history, X-ray diffraction findings.

Differential diagnosis: Pneumoconioses caused by other agents.

Bat Lung

Definition: Allergic extrinsic alveolitis caused by bat droppings.

Incidence/Epidemiology: Rare disease seen in humans exposed to bat droppings.

Etiology/Pathophysiology: Combination of type III and type IV reaction of immune system. For details see Allergic (Extrinsic) Alveolitis.

Clinical Presentation: Acute or chronic disease.

Prognosis: Usually good without serious sequelae.

Radiology: Chest radiographs are normal or show diffuse, soft, interstitial infiltrates or fine granular densities.

Pathology:

Gross: The lungs are of normal color and consistency or may display small, firm, reddish-gray nodules.

Histology: The characteristic findings include nonnecrotizing epithelioid granulomas near the terminal bronchioles, desquamation, hypertrophy and hyperplasia of cells of the alveolar lining, marked eosinophilic inflammatory infiltrates, bronchiolitis obliterans, and focal acute vasculitis. For details, see Allergic (Extrinsic) Alveolitis.

➤ *Descriptors:* Lung parenchyma with altered structure:
- noncaseous epithelioid granulomas
- eosinophils
- multinucleated giant cells
- intrabronchiolar fibrinoid material and histiocytes
- ulceration of bronchiolar mucosa;
- Lung parenchyma with preserved structure:
- macrophages
- desquamation, hypertrophy, hyperplasia and dysplasia of pneumocytes
- mononuclear inflammatory infiltrates
- intraalveolar serous fluid

■ *Special stains:* PAS, collagenous stains, Giemsa. For details, see Allergic (Extrinsic) Alveolitis.

Hallmark of Diagnosis: Clinical history, nonnecrotizing epithelioid granulomas, morphologic findings related to desquamative interstitial pneumonia, lymphoid interstitial pneumonia, bronchiolitis obliterans.

Differential diagnosis: Infectious and noninfectious granulomatous diseases such as sarcoidosis, fungal infections, or berylliosis. For details, see Allergic (Extrinsic) Alveolitis.

Bauxite Lung

Definition: Disease caused by fumes generated during the manufacture of aluminum (corundum) (synonym Shaver's lung).

Incidence/Epidemiology: Exposed persons may work in the manufacture of explosives, or fireworks, electrolytic extraction of aluminum from bauxite or adding stearine (oil) to the granular or flake aluminum.

Etiology/Pathophysiology: Lung damage occurs most frequently from exposure to flake aluminum with added stearine or oil. The causes are unknown, since lungs of rats and of guinea pigs were reported to be only weakly fibrotic after exposure to granular aluminum and strongly fibrotic after exposure to flake independent of the amounts of added stearine or oil.

Clinical Presentation: Patients present with shortness of breath, cough, progressive dyspnea; fatal cases are known.

Prognosis: Usually good, depending on amount and composition of inhaled particles and fumes, but progressive fibrosis and acute death can occur.

Radiology: Radiologic changes can appear as early as 3 months after exposure, with signs of diffusely distributed fibrosis, pleural adhesions, and zones of coarse emphysema. Larger fibrous nodules are usually not seen.

Pathology:

Gross: The lungs are often shrunken and present a thickened, pebbled pleura with subpleural emphysematous bullae, dark bands of fibrous tissue in the central areas, and a grayish-red color.

Histology: The normal texture of the peripheral lung parenchyma is replaced by thick, fibrotic, acellular bundles showing some monocytes and dust-laden macrophages. The alveoli and bronchioles are expanded and contain dense agglutinations of dust-laden macrophages, and scattered multinucleated giant cells surrounding crystal clefts. Silicotic nodules are lacking, whereas endarteritis obliterans is a common finding.

➤ *Descriptors:* Lung parenchyma with preserved structure:
- dust (birefringent crystals)
- macrophages (dust-laden)
- mononuclear inflammatory infiltrates
- enlarged distant air spaces;
- Lung parenchyma with altered structure:
- intrabronchiolar fibrinoid material and histiocytes
- ulceration of bronchiolar mucosa
- focal interstitial fibrosis
- dust (birefrigent crystals)
- multinucleated giant cells;
- Pulmonary vessels with preserved structure:
- thrombosis (small arteries)
- mononuclear inflammatory infiltrates (small arteries)

■ *Special stains:* Collagenous stains, Prussian blue, aurine stain for aluminum, X-ray diffraction and related techniques.

Hallmark of Diagnosis: Diffuse fibrosis of peripheral lung parenchyma with dust-laden macrophages and deposits of dust, missing silicotic nodules, clinical history, physical techniques for identification of aluminum.

Differential diagnosis: Pneumoconioses due to exposure to other agents.

Baygon

Definition: Alteration of the lung parenchyma associated with intake of baygon, see Drug Toxicity.

Baylisascariasis

Definition: Human parasitic disease caused by the nematode *Baylisascaris procyonis*.

Incidence/Epidemiology: *B. procyonis* is the ascarid of racoons with corresponding geographical distribution. Two patients have been reported to be infected with this parasite.

Etiology/Pathophysiology: The parasite lives in the small intestines of racoons and has a life-cycle similar to that of human ascaris. The infection of humans probably occurs by eating raw food contaminated with the eggs passed in the feces of racoons.

Clinical Presentation: The patients suffered from symptoms of the infected central nervous system and had a fatal course.

Prognosis: Usually fatal outcome.

Radiology: The findings are related to usual infections with ascarid worms.

Pathology:

Gross: Findings related to ascarid infections.

Histology: The living worms were seen in the arteries of the lungs.

➤ *Descriptors:* Lung parenchyma with preserved structure:
- parasites (alive, pulmonary arteries, worms)
- mononuclear inflammatory infiltrates
- eosinophils

■ *Special stains:* PAS, collagenous stains, GMS, Movat.

Hallmark of Diagnosis: Special appearance of the viable parasites, clinical history.

Differential diagnosis: Parasitic infection with other nematodes, especially with *Ascaris lumbricoides*.

BCG Pneumonia

Definition: Iatrogenic lipid pneumonia caused by aerosols containing BCG (bacille Calmette-Guerin).

Incidence/Epidemiology: Administration of BCG-containing aerosols has been reported to induce pulmonary changes in young children.
Etiology/Pathophysiology: Inhalation of lipid-containing aerosols may cause acute and chronic foci of inflammation. The lipids accumulate and are stored in macrophages or remain within the alveoli and induce a foreign-body reaction with progressive destructive characteristics.

Clinical Presentation: Patients may be asymptomatic or may present with shortness of breath and related symptoms.

Prognosis: Usually good and without sequelae.

Radiology: Chest radiographs usually show basilar infiltrates or an intrapulmonary mass resembling a neoplasm or pulmonary infection.

Pathology:
Gross: The firm lungs show areas of yellow or grayish color.

Histology: Numerous vacuolated macrophages fill the alveoli which, in addition, contain lipid droplets surrounded by foreign-body giant cells. Additional lymphocytes and plasma cells are present. The lipid droplets also lie in the interstitium; granulomatous inflammatory formations may suggest fungal infections.

➤ *Descriptors:* Lung parenchyma with preserved structure:
- lipoid material (droplets)
- macrophages (foamy)
- mononuclear inflammatory infiltrates
- multinucleated giant cells (foreign body);
- Lung parenchyma with altered structure:
- noncaseous epithelioid granulomas
- mononuclear inflammatory infiltrates

■ *Special stains:* Collagenous stains, fat stains, PAS.

Hallmark of Diagnosis: Lipid droplets in the airways and in the interstitium, macrophages containing lipid droplets, foreign-body giant cells, occasional cholesterol crystals, preserved lung texture, clinical history.

Differential diagnosis: Extrinsic lipoid pneumonia of other causes, endogenous lipoid pneumonia, fungal infections, desquamative interstitial pneumonia.

BCG Therapy

Definition: Alteration of the lung parenchyma associated with inhalation of BCG-containing aerosols, see BCG Pneumonia.

BCNU

Definition: Alteration of the lung parenchyma associated with intake of BCNU (carmustine), see Drug Toxicity.

Beclomethasone

Definition: Alteration of the lung parenchyma associated with intake of beclomethasone, see Drug Toxicity.

Behçet's Disease

Definition: Pulmonary involvement in a multisystemic disease characterized by relapsing iritis, genital ulcerations, oral aphthous ulcers, and nodules in the skin of the lower limbs.
Incidence/Epidemiology: A few patients suffering from Behçet's disease with pulmonary involvement have been reported.
Etiology/Pathophysiology: The etiology of Behçet's disease is unknown. It is associated with various symptoms including thrombophlebitis migrans, arthritis, recurrent epididymitis, and recurrent perivascular myelitis and occurs during the 3rd decade of life, more often in men than in women.
Clinical Presentation: Pulmonary symptoms include hemoptysis, pleural effusions, and shortness of breath. The related Hughes-Stovin syndrome is characterized by aneurysms of the pulmonary arteries, recurrent thrombophlebitis, and symptoms related to increased intracranial pressure.
Prognosis: Fair, patients usually present with slow progression of pulmonary symptoms.
Radiology: Chest radiographs show transient infiltrates, nodular densities, ectasis of the pulmonary arteries.
Pathology:
Gross: Several small necrotic areas of the lung parenchyma and obliterative older thromboses

in the pulmonary arteries and veins have been described.

Histology: The basic lesion is a chronic necrotizing vasculitis involving both the smaller arteries and veins. The inflammatory infiltrate is comprised of neutrophilic granulocytes, lymphocytes, plasma cell, and less frequently histiocytes. Surrounding fibrosis and scarred vessels are notable.

➤ *Descriptors:* Lung parenchyma with altered structure:
- focal interstitial fibrosis (perivascular);
- Pulmonary vessels with altered structure:
- thrombosis (arteries and veins)
- mixed inflammatory infiltrates (arteries and veins)
- necrosis (arteries and veins)

■ *Special stains:* PAS, collagenous stains, Giemsa.

Hallmark of Diagnosis: Necrotizing arterial and venous angiitis, clinical history.

Differential diagnosis: Miscellaneous vasculitis including polyarteritis nodosa, hypersensitivity vasculitis, intravenous drug abuse.

Benign Clear Cell Tumor of the Lung

Definition: Benign neoplasm of the peripheral lung with a special histologic appearance.

Incidence/Epidemiology: Rare neoplasm seen equally in both sexes of adults.

Etiology/Pathophysiology: Its cellular origin still remains unclear. Suggestions range from an unusual variant of carcinoid to an aberrant form of smooth muscle tumors.

Clinical Presentation: Tumor-related symptoms are rare, most patients being recognized by chest radiographs taken for other reasons.

Prognosis: Usually good, and no malignant aberration has been reported.

Radiology: Solid, firm tumor mass most frequently localized in the lower lobes, measuring several centimeters in diameter.

Pathology:

Gross: Homogeneous tumor mass of pink to red-brown color without detectable capsula. Necrotic areas have been infrequently reported.

Histology: The tumor consists of large, homogeneous tumor cells with abundant pale cytoplasm and small homogeneous nuclei usually localized at the periphery of the cytoplasm. Spindle-shaped tumor cells or multinucleated giant cells of the Tuton type may be present; mitotic figures are very rare. The tumor texture is characterized by its peculiar vascular supply consisting of thin-walled sinusoidal vessels which are comprised of endothelial cells and attached tumor cells. Infarctlike necrotic areas are – if present – small and unsuspicious. The PAS stain is strictly positive for the cytoplasm of the tumor cells which contain enormous amounts of glycogen which is not diastase-resistant. Inflammatory infiltration in the tumor or at the tumor boundary is scarce.

➤ *Descriptors:* Newly formed textures without metastasis potential:
- epithelial growth pattern
- solid textures
- homogeneous nuclear and cellular size
- abundant cytoplasm (pale, PAS-positive, after diastase PAS-negative)
- small nuclei
- absent or infrequent mitoses
- absent inflammatory infiltrates

■ *Special stains:* PAS, Giemsa, immunohistochemistry for neuroendocrine and soft-tissue tumor markers.

Hallmark of Diagnosis: Vascular pattern, glycogen content of tumor cells, clinical history.

Differential diagnosis: Metastatic renal cell carcinoma, granular cell tumor, large cell anaplastic carcinoma, atypical carcinoid, acinus cell tumor, oncocytoma.

Benzene

Definition: Exposure to benzene is associated with increased risk of lung cancer, see Cancer of the Lung.

Berylliosis

Definition: Pneumoconiosis caused by exposure to beryllium.

Incidence/Epidemiology: The source of the metal is beryllium aluminum silicate, which is mined in South Africa, Australia, southern America, and India. Beryllium is used for fluorescent lighting tubes, in the ceramic, electronic, and aerospace industries, and in atomic reactors. About 1 000 persons with beryllium exposure are known to have suffered from the acute or (more frequently) the chronic form of berylliosis.

Etiology/Pathophysiology: Beryllium particles are easily airborne because of their lightness. They cause an acute edematous reaction of the lung in persons exposed to high levels of soluble salts of beryllium, and a chronic hypersensitivity response (type IV) with elevated IgA serum levels in the chronic stage.

Clinical Presentation: The acute form presents with fever, shortness of breath, dyspnea, and vomiting and will proceed, in about 10% of patients, to the chronic stage. Onset of the chronic stage may occur 15 years after initial exposure or later and is characterized by insidious onset of dyspnea, malaise, or shortness of breath. Known complications are the development of a cor pulmonale, renal failure from nephrolithiasis, and increased risk of lung cancer and other malignant neoplasms, especially osteosarcomas.

Prognosis: Good in the acute stage; the chronic stage is associated with slow progressive respiratory failure which brings about death after several years.

Radiology: The acute stage may show signs of acute edema and of bilateral acute bronchiolitis. The chronic stage shows diffuse bilateral densities with small nodular lesions resembling interstitial fibrosis of various degrees.

Pathology:

Gross: The lungs are heavy, wet, and pink to grayish in the acute stage. In the chronic form the pleura is fibrotic and usually adherent. There is a marked diffuse fibrosis with honeycombing, including small, firm nodules several millimeters in diameter. The hilar and proximal intrapulmonary lymph nodes are enlarged.

Histology: The acute stage presents with an intraalveolar exudate made up of fibrin, lymphocytes, plasma cells, and macrophages, whereas neurophilic and eosinophilic granulocytes are quite rare. The inflammatory reaction is pronounced around the bronchioles and arterioles with signs of endarteritis obliterans. The exudate usually discharges after a couple of days, leaving a distinct diffuse fibrosis. The chronic stage has two characteristics: (a) an interstitial diffuse fibrosis with moderate signs of progression mainly visible by virtue of the accumulation of lymphocytes, plasma cells, and macrophages; and (b) noncaseating epithelioid granulomas comprised of Langhans' giant cells with surrounding lymphocytes and plasma cells. These granulomas may be confluent, are often surrounded by acellular bundles of collagenous material, and resemble sarcoid granulomas. They have also been described to occur in the hilar lymph nodes, spleen, liver, bone marrow, kidneys, muscle, and skin. The giant cells occasionally contain conchoidal (Schaumann) bodies, asteroid bodies, and birefringent platelike crystals. Under light microscopy, chronic berylliosis is indistinguishable from sarcoidosis.

➤ *Descriptors:* Lung parenchyma with preserved structure:

- intraalveolar serous fluid
- mononuclear inflammatory infiltrates;
- Pulmonary vessels with preserved structure:
- thrombosis (small arteries)
- mononuclear inflammatory infiltrates;
- Lung parenchyma with altered structure:
- ulceration of bronchiolar mucosa
- noncaseous epithelioid granulomas
- multinucleated giant cells (Langhans)
- mononuclear inflammatory infiltrates
- diffuse interstitial fibrosis

■ *Special stains:* PAS, collagenous stains, X-ray diffraction and related physical techniques, endogenous lectins.

Hallmark of Diagnosis: Sarcoidlike granulomas and interstitial fibrosis resembling sarcoidosis in the chronic stage; acute fibrinous pneumonitis in the acute stage; clinical history; identification of beryllium by physical techniques.

Differential diagnosis: Sarcoidosis, exogenous allergic alveolitis, tuberculosis.

Birbeck's Granules

Definition: Intracytoplasmatic inclusion bodies of histiocytes, see Histiocytosis X.

Bird Fancier's Lung

Definition: Allergic extrinsic alveolitis caused by avian droppings, feathers, serum, or proteins.

Incidence/Epidemiology: Seen in persons handling or raising parakeets, pigeons, chickens, turkeys, etc.
Etiology/Pathophysiology: Combined hypersensitivity reaction of type III and IV.

Clinical Presentation: Acute and chronic stages have been described.

Prognosis: Usually good, but slow progressive respiratory failure and fibrosis can occur.

Radiology: Chest radiographs are normal or show diffuse, soft, interstitial infiltrates or fine granular densities.

Pathology:
Gross: The lungs are of normal color and consistency or may display small, firm, reddish-gray nodules.

Histology: The characteristic findings include nonnecrotizing epithelioid granulomas near the terminal bronchioles, desquamation, hypertrophy and hyperplasia of cells of the alveolar lining, marked eosinophilic inflammatory infiltrates, bronchiolitis obliterans, and focal acute vasculitis. For details, see Allergic (Extrinsic) Alveolitis.

➤ *Descriptors:* Lung parenchyma with altered structure:
- noncaseous epithelioid granulomas
- eosinophils
- multinucleated giant cells
- intrabronchiolar fibrinoid material and histiocytes
- ulceration of bronchiolar mucosa;
- Lung parenchyma with preserved structure:
- macrophages
- desquamation, hypertrophy, hyperplasia and dysplasia of pneumocytes
- mononuclear inflammatory infiltrates
- intraalveolar serous fluid

■ *Special stains:* PAS, collagenous stains, Giemsa. For details, see Allergic (Extrinsic) Alveolitis.

Hallmark of Diagnosis: Clinical history, nonnecrotizing epithelioid granulomas, morphologic findings related to desquamative interstitial pneumonia, lymphoid interstitial pneumonia, bronchiolitis obliterans.

Differential diagnosis: Infectious and noninfectious granulomatous diseases such as sarcoidosis, fungal infections or berylliosis. For details, see Allergic (Extrinsic) Alveolitis.

Black Lung Disease

Definition: Alteration of the lung parenchyma seen in coal miners, see Coal Worker's Pneumoconiosis.

Blastoma

Definition: Malignant tumor of the lung with histologic appearance of embryonic lung during its pseudoglandular period of development.
Incidence/Epidemiology: Blastomas are rare malignancies and comprise about 0.5% of all primary malignant lung tumors. A male predominance of 2:1 and a biphasic age distribution with two peaks at the 1st and 7th decades have been reported.
Etiology/Pathophysiology: Some authors support the theory that these tumors arise from "dormant" or undeveloped areas of the lung parenchyma; other authors assume an "ordinary" malignancy of the lung with "recapitulation of its own life history".
Clinical Presentation: The tumors are usually of large size and compress large bronchi at the time of clinical significance. The symptoms are those of large centrally localized bronchial carcinomas and include cough, fever, loss of weight, dyspnea, malaise, etc.
Prognosis: Usually poor, only 15–20% of patients are still alive 5 years after clinical diagnosis.
Radiology: Usually centrally localized tumor mass with obstruction of a main bronchus and broad extension into the peripheral lung parenchyma.
Pathology
Gross: The bulky tumors are of soft consistency and show a yellow, tan, grayish, or white color with extensive areas of necrosis. They usually invade the pleura and a main bronchus and measure more than 5 cm in diameter.
Histology: The tumor resembles embryonal lung parenchyma of the pseudoglandular stage and grows in primitive epithelial glandular structures combined with broad stromal mesenchymal elements of embryonic appearance. The epithelial cells present with large variations in nuclear size with coarsely distributed nuclear chromatin and subnuclear vacuolization because of abundant glycogen. The glands usually

contain one to two layers of epithelial cells, often with "polarization" of the nuclei and a textural appearance similar to a morula. The primitive stromal cells are directly attached to the glands and have a spindle shape with pale cytoplasm and large nuclei. Occasionally a variation with islands of primitive cartilage or squamoid epithelium can be seen. The growth of the blastoma completely resolves the original lung textures. An inflammatory response of the host tissue is usually absent. Infarctlike necrotic areas are frequent.

➤ *Descriptors:* Newly formed textures with metastasis potential:
- epithelial growth pattern
- mesenchymal growth pattern
- adenoid textures (differentiated tubular glands)
- solid textures (fiberlike)
- inhomogeneous nuclear and cellular size
- granular cytoplasm (PAS-positive, glycogen)
- prominent nucleoli
- moderate number of mitoses
- plump spindle cells
- fragments of primitive cartilage
- absent or weak inflammatory infiltrates

■ *Special stains:* PAS (with and without digestion), collagenous stains, Giemsa, reticulin stains, immunohistochemistry for keratin, vimentin, CEA, neuroendocrine marker, endogenous lectins, DNA analysis.

Hallmark of Diagnosis: Tumorous textures with primitive glandular pattern and stromal elements of embryonic appearance, demonstration of glycogen in the epithelial tumor cells and of islands containing primitive cartilage or squamoid cell clusters, absence of mucus production, age of the patient.

Differential diagnosis: Combined carcinosarcoma, in small biopsies small cell anaplastic carcinoma or adenocarcinoma.

Blastomycosis

Definition: Infection of the lung with *Blastomyces dermatitides*.

Incidence/Epidemiology: Sporadic, not contagious disease occurring in persons living in North America (Great Lakes areas), South America, Africa, and the Middle East.

Etiology/Pathophysiology: Primary infection of the lung is the main cause, and secondary pneumonia due to primary infection of the skin has been reported in a few immunocompromised patients.

Clinical Presentation: The infection is most frequently seen in men 30–50 years old. They suffer from chronic respiratory symptoms with insidious onset or from an acute pneumonia with high fever, chills, and cough. The patients usually recover within a few weeks.

Prognosis: Usually good and without sequelae.

Radiology: Chest radiographs show patchy infiltrates, mediastinal lymphadenopathy, diffuse linear infiltrates, fibronodular densities, or larger nodules with thin walled cavitation.

Pathology:

Gross: The posterior segments of the lower lobes, which are most often involved, show multiple, yellowish to grayish nodules. Fibrous bundles are present. The larger nodules are necrotic and display a small fibrous wall.

Histology: The formed granulomas contain plump palisading histiocytes with scattered multinucleated giant cells which surround necrotic neutrophilic granulocytes intermingled with the organisms. The organisms consist of uniform, round yeast cells. Their granular internal structure is surrounded by a thick "doubly contoured" cell wall. The organisms measure 8–30 μm in diameter. They stain positively to HE, PAS, GMS, PAS-Gridley. Chronic stages may show focal interstitial fibrosis in addition to the granulomatous reaction of the lung.

➤ *Descriptors:* Lung parenchyma with altered structure:
- caseous epithelioid granulomas
- fungus (intragranulomatous, yeast)
- mixed inflammatory infiltrates
- multinucleated giant cells
- focal interstitial fibrosis

■ *Special stains:* PAS, GMS, collagenous stains, immunofluorescence.

Hallmark of Diagnosis: Granulomatous epithelioid reaction of the lung tissue with centrally localized necrotic neutrophilic granulocytes intermingled with yeast cells, identification of yeast, clinical history, chest radiographs.

Differential diagnosis: Fungal infection with other organisms such as cryptococcosis, paracoccidiomycosis, histoplasmosis, etc, necrotizing sarcoid granulomatosis, atypical tuberculosis.

Bleomycin

Definition: Alteration of the lung parenchyma associated with intake of bleomycin, see Drug Toxicity.

Blue Boater

Definition: Syndrome seen in patients with chronic airflow obstruction and severe hypoxemia (hypercarbia, polycythemia and right heart failure), see Chronic Airflow Obstruction.

Blue Bodies

Definition: Intraalveolar, laminated, calcified deposits (associated with histiocytes and giant cells, birefringent), see Desquamative Interstitial Pneumonitis, Usual Interstitial Pneumonitis, Allergic (Extrinsic) Alveolitis.

Bone Marrow Emboli

Definition: Emboli in (small) pulmonary arteries consisting of bone marrow, and usually associated with severe trauma, see Embolism, Pulmonary.

Bordetella Pertussis Infection

Definition: Infection of the lung with *Bordetella pertussis* bacteria.

Incidence/Epidemiology: The incidence of whooping cough caused by *Bordetella pertussis*, *B. parapertussis*, and less commonly by *B. bronchiseptica* declined rapidly after the introduction of vaccination in Europe. It is, however, after the abolition of obligatory vaccination, increasing again in Germany. It occurs most frequently in children below the age of 6 years.

Etiology/Pathophysiology: The pathogenesis of the disease is associated with the production of toxins by the noninvasive bacteria. Three principal components of the toxin are known, heat labile toxin, lipopolysaccharide toxin, and pertussis toxin. The toxins cause an agglutination of lymphocytes with consequent blocking of the small lymphocytic vessels and submucosal edema. *B. pertussis*, in addition, releases an enzyme, adenyl cyclase, which suppresses the chemotactic, phagocytic, and bactericidal activity of macrophages and neutrophilic granulocytes.

Clinical Presentation: The clinical course can be divided into three stages: (a) an initial stage of 1–3 weeks with mild cough, sneezing, lacrimation and mild fever; (b) the marked stage lasting up to 6 weeks with characteristic paroxysms, sudden violent coughs with inspiratory whoop, apnea, cyanosis; (c) the convalescent stage with gradually subsiding symptoms. Secondary pneumonia has been reported to develop in about 30% of the children.

Prognosis: The disease is seldom fatal, and sequelae are rare.

Radiology: Signs of bronchitis and peribronchitis.

Pathology:

Gross: The lumen of the bronchi contains a yellowish viscous mucus. The peripheral lung parenchyma shows areas of air trapping and collapsed lung tissue.

Histology: The lumen of the bronchi and bronchioles contains viscous mucus and cellular debris. The epithelial cells of the mucosa are hyperplastic or partially denuded. A characteristic inflammatory infiltrate of lymphocytes, plasma cells, and neutrophilic granulocytes can be detected beneath the mucosa. The infiltrate is usually limited to the peribronchial and peribronchiolar regions. The bacteria stain gram-positive and lie attached to the ciliated cells.

➤ *Descriptors:* Bronchial mucosa with preserved structure:

- viscous mucus
- fibrinoid material (intrabronchial)
- mixed inflammatory infiltrates
- bacteria (intrabronchial)

■ *Special stains:* Gram, various stains for bacteria including Goodpasture's, collagenous stains.

Hallmark of Diagnosis: Clinical history, mononuclear infiltrate limited to the bronchial walls.

Differential diagnosis: Acute and chronic bronchitis of various causes.

Botryomycosis

Definition: Pulmonary suppurative infection with different bacteria which become enclosed within a hyaline coating (sulfur granules).

Incidence/Epidemiology: Quite common in horses and other mammals. The skin and the subcutaneous tissues are usually involved in humans. A few cases have been reported of lung involvement in children with cystic fibrosis or in nonimmunocompromised adults with sporadic lung abscess.

Etiology/Pathophysiology: Colonies of coated bacteria include *Staphylococcus aureus*, *Proteus aeruginosa*, and various strains of streptococci. The coating of the bacterial colonies is part of the immunodefense of host tissue. The shell contains hyaline refractile eosinophilic material.

Clinical Presentation: The symptoms are closely related to the underlying disease, and in the case of cystic fibrosis include atypical manifestations such as lobar consolidation or mediastinal infections.

Prognosis: Usually defined by the underlying disease. The pulmonary suppurative infection is usually seen in advanced stages.

Radiology: Signs of scarring or abscess formation in patients with prolonged course.

Pathology:

Gross: Usually large infected areas which can be necrotic, suppurative, or firm with small abscess formations. The sulfur granules are usually too small to be seen macroscopically.

Histology: The densely packed bacteria are covered with a homogeneous hyaline shell which can be smooth, fanlike, or inserted in clubs or spikes. The granules measure 100–300 μm in diameter but may be larger and macroscopically visible. They are localized in the center of the lung abscesses, or in epithelioid granulomas or isolated in fibrotic tissue.

➤ *Descriptors:* Lung parenchyma with preserved structure:

- bacteria (hyaline shells, densely packed foci)
- intraalveolar fibrinoid material;
- Lung parenchyma with altered structure:
- mixed inflammatory infiltrates (dense)
- caseous epithelioid granulomas
- bacteria (intragranulomatous);
- Bronchial mucosa with preserved structure:
- bacteria (intrabronchial, hyaline shell)
- mixed inflammatory infiltrates

■ *Special stains:* PAS, Gram (positive), collagenous stains.

Hallmark of Diagnosis: Colonies of gram-positive bacteria coated with a hyaline, eosinophilic shell, clinical history of prolonged course or atypical manifestation (cystic fibrosis).

Differential diagnosis: Infection with *Actinomyces*, various fungal organisms, *Nocardia* infection.

Breast Cancer Metastasis

Definition: Malignant tumors in the lung and pleura secondary to primary carcinoma of the breast.

Incidence/Epidemiology: Metastatic breast carcinoma to the pleura and lung are frequently seen in female patients and account for as much as 30% of all metastatic lesions.

Etiology/Pathophysiology: The tumors may grow years after resection of the primary breast cancer. Tumor cell spread before resection of the breast carcinoma via the lymphatic vessels is assumed.

Clinical Presentation: The metastatic lesions usually grow slowly and are localized in the peripheral lung tissue, causing no or only minimal symptoms. Subpleural growth with or without pleural effusions may occur. The hormone-receptor status of the metastatic carcinoma is weak compared with that of the primary carcinoma.

Prognosis: Pulmonary metastases of breast carcinoma are usually not curable, and most patients die within 2 years after clinical detection.

Radiology: Circumscribed clear-cut peripheral density.

Pathology:

Gross: Solid, yellowish-white tumor mass with no or only small areas of necrosis.

Histology: Tumor growth has adenoid textures with only a few irregularly formed glands, large areas with solid growth pattern of small cells with only mildly enlarged nuclei. The architecture of the original lung tissue is destroyed. Small metastatic lesions can be seen close to the main metastasis. Inflammatory response of the host tissue is nonexistent or weak. Mitoses, stromal elements, and necrotic areas are rare.

➤ *Descriptors:* Newly formed textures with metastasis potential:
- epithelial growth pattern
- adenoid textures
- solid textures
- small tumor cells
- homogeneous nuclear and cellular size
- finely distributed nuclear chromatin
- infrequent mitoses
- micrometastases
- absent or weak inflammatory infiltrates

■ *Special stains:* PAS, collagenous stains, immunohistochemistry including hormone receptors, EMA, neuroendocrine markers, DNA analysis.

Hallmark of Diagnosis: Clinical history, small tumor cells with adenoid growth pattern and missing inflammatory infiltrations.

Differential diagnosis: Primary adenocarcinoma of the lung, small cell anaplastic carcinoma of the intermediate type.

Bromocarbamide

Definition: Alteration of the lung parenchyma associated with intake of bromocarbamide, see Drug Toxicity.

Bronchial Gland Tumors

Definition: A group of neoplasms growing in the bronchial gland region and comprised of carcinoid tumors, adenoid cystic carcinomas, mucoepidermoid carcinomas, mucous gland adenomas, oncocytomas, acinic cell tumors, pleomorphic mixed tumors, low-grade and high-grade adenocarcinomas.

Incidence/Epidemiology: Bronchial gland tumors are rare in relation to all primary tumors of the lower respiratory tract and comprise about 1–2% of these tumors.

Etiology/Pathophysiology: Heterogeneous group of tumors partly of neuroendocrine origin (carcinoid tumors), partly originating in the epithelium of mucous glands (adenoid cystic carcinoma, mucoepidermoid carcinoma, acinic cell tumor, pleomorphic mixed tumor, adenocarcinoma), partly of unknown origin (oncocytoma).

Clinical Presentation: The tumors arise in younger patients more often than those suffering from ordinary carcinomas of the lung. The symptoms are caused by their proximal localization with obstruction of one or more major bronchi and include cough, fever, signs of asthmoid bronchitis, loss of weight, etc.

Prognosis: Usually good and determined by the extent of lung damage induced by chronic obstruction and secondary infection.

Radiology: Proximal stenosis of a bronchus with consequent atelectasis.

Pathology:

Gross: Yellowish to grayish tumor mass in a proximal bronchus with bronchial stenosis or intraluminal growth. Invasion of adjacent lung tissue is rare.

Histology: The microscopic growth patterns include adenoid structures of various degrees of differentiation and "endocrinoid structures" with solid tumor islands. Dense inflammatory infiltrates, necrotic areas, and erosion of cartilage are usually missing. The detailed microscopic description is given under their particular headings.

➤ *Descriptors:* Newly formed textures with metastasis potential:
- epithelial growth pattern
- adenoid textures (tubuli)
- endocrine textures
- solid textures
- polypoid endobronchial textures
- homogeneous nuclear and cellular size
- finely distributed nuclear chromatin
- infrequent mitoses
- absent or weak inflammatory infiltrates

■ *Special stains:* PAS (especially for acinic cell tumors), collagenous stains, Giemsa, immunohistochemistry for neuroendocrine markers, CEA, cytokeratins, S-100 protein, endogenous lectins, DNA analysis.

Hallmark of Diagnosis: Microscopic growth pattern, adenoid textures, endocrine textures, proximal localization, age of the patient.

Differential diagnosis: Common primary carcinomas of the lower respiratory tract, hyperplasia of the bronchial glands, metastatic carcinomas of various origins.

Bronchiectasis

Definition: Circumscribed or diffuse dilatation of one or several bronchi.

Incidence/Epidemiology: Not infrequently seen in patients of any age. The prevalence is estimated to be 0.1–0.5% of the German population.

Etiology/Pathophysiology: Three major causes of bronchiectases are known: (a) congenital bronchiectasis occurring in hypoplasia or anomalies of the bronchi, vessels, or alveolar tissue; (b) nonobstructive (collapse) bronchiectasis usually occurring in adolescents and including poststenotic dilatation of the bronchi; (c) Postpneumonic infective bronchiectasis occurring adjacent to destructive infection of the lung parenchyma. The major cause is a recurrent infection of the lower respiratory tract leading to inflammatory-destructive processes in the bronchial mucosa, including disturbance of mucus secretion, focal mucosal ulcerations, disturbance of neuromuscular tension, and submucosal fibrosis. The bronchial lumen becomes dilated either by increased intrabronchial pressure (mucoviscidosis, chronic cough with viscous mucus, poststenotic flow disturbance,etc.), by decreased tension of the bronchial wall (inflammation, focal tension due to scarring, congenital instability, etc.), or by decreased (negative) pressure from the adjacent lung tissue (shrinkage of the lung parenchyma due to various causes, decreased intraalveolar pressure, etc.).

Clinical Presentation: Symptoms of bronchiectasis are cough, expectoration, hemoptysis, and clubbing in long-standing disease. Fever and malodor indicate secondary complications. Shortness of breath is usually not a sign of bronchiectasis.

Prognosis: Patients can do well for several years but usually develop recurrent infections, progressive destruction of the lung parenchyma and systemic toxicity after some time.

Radiology: Grossly and radiographically, 3 different types of bronchiectasis can be differentiated: (a) saccular or cystic; (b) cylindrical, tubular, or fusiform; and (c) varicose. Cylindrical bronchiectases show foci of mucus retention, and the saccular type is more frequently seen in the distal portions of the bronchi. Abnormalities include increased bronchial markings, overcrowding of bronchi and focal loss of the lung parenchyma.

Pathology:

Gross: The surface of the dilated bronchi is uneven and may present transverse ridging, longitudinal striations, or larger saccular formations with thin atrophic walls. The color may change from violet to grayish-white, and the lumen is either filled with viscous mucus plugs or completely empty (dry bronchiectasis). The bronchi of the 2nd to the 6th order are usually involved. Bilateral manifestation occurs in about 30% of cases.

Histology: In postpneumonic infective bronchiectasis numerous lymphoid follicles or nodules are present in the thickened bronchial walls. The epithelial cells show severe hyperplasia of goblet cells with increased mucus production. The smooth muscle fibers are replaced by fibrotic tissue. Other patients present with squamous metaplasia of the bronchial epithelial cells, inflammatory erosion and destruction of cartilage, atrophy of the bronchial wall with loss of smooth muscle cells, or dense fibrosis of the adjacent lung parenchyma. The inflammatory infiltrations are usually made up of lymphocytes, plasma cells, histiocytes, and less frequently neutrophilic and eosinophilic granulocytes.

➤ *Descriptors:* Bronchial mucosa with preserved structure:

- ectatic lumen
- viscous mucus
- increased number of goblet cells
- mononuclear inflammatory infiltrates
- atrophy;
- Bronchial mucosa with altered structure:
- fibrosis (submucosa)
- squamous metaplasia and dysplasia

■ *Special stains:* Collagenous stains, PAS.

Hallmark of Diagnosis: Macroscopic findings including those of bronchoscopy, and radiology, microscopic fibrosis, or atrophy of the bronchial wall.

Differential diagnosis: Cysts of the lung parenchyma, accessory lung, malformation.

Bronchiolitis

Definition: Acute or chronic inflammation of the small bronchi and bronchioles.

Incidence/Epidemiology: Acute bronchiolitis is a disease of childhood and is often associated with viral infections including influenza virus, parainfluenza virus, adenovirus, rhinovirus, herpes virus, etc. Chronic bronchiolitis has been reported in patients with emphysema, or smoking habits; the special form of bronchiolitis obliterans is associated with inhalation of toxic gases, allergic alveolitis, eosinophilic pneumonia, emphysema, bronchiectasis, Sjögren's syndrome, heart-lung transplantation, drug response of the lung tissue (penicillamine), etc.

Etiology/Pathophysiology: Acute bronchiolitis is usually seen in infective lung disease involving various viruses or *Staphylococcus aureus, Streptococcus pyogenes* (purulent bronchiolitis). Chronic bronchiolitis is reflected in a mild inflammation associated with chronic airway obstruction. Chronic irritation of the epithelial cells is associated with an increased number of goblet cells, increased mucus production and consequent rise of resistance in the small conductive airways.

Clinical Presentation: Acute bronchiolitis is associated with cough, mucus production, fever, shortness of breath. Patients suffering from chronic bronchiolitis have decreased lung function tests, chronic expectoration, cough.

Prognosis: Usually good, but patients with chronic bronchiolitis can develop slow progression of interstitial lung damage.

Radiology: Chest radiographs may be normal or exhibit signs of emphysematous changes of the lung. Bronchiolitis obliterans characteristically show small nodular densities associated with various degrees of overinflammation.

Pathology:

Gross: The lungs are heavy, overinflated, and of reddish color. The small bronchi contain mucus, and the bronchial walls may be thickened. Chronic bronchiolitis is usually associated with emphysematous changes of peripheral lung tissue and signs of chronic bronchitis.

Histology: Acute bronchiolitis is characterized by dense inflammatory granulocytic infiltrates in the bronchiolar walls associated with desquamation of the epithelial cells and debris in the lumen. The inflammation usually spreads into the adjacent lung tissue, i.e., the alveolar ducts and peribronchiolar tissue are also involved. In chronic bronchiolitis the granulocytic inflammatory infiltrates are replaced by lymphocytes and plasma cells, while the epithelial cells often show squamous metaplasia. The lumen may contain proliferative epithelial cells or densely packed histiocytes. Bronchiolitis obliterans is characterized by fibrinoid plugs in the lumen of the bronchioles, extending into the alveolar ducts and sacs and into the small bronchi. Part of the mucosa is usually destroyed by the granulomatous lesion which includes lymphocytes, plasma cells, histiocytes. and macrophages.

➤ *Descriptors:* Bronchial mucosa with preserved structure:
- mixed inflammatory infiltrates (dense)
- desquamation, hypertrophy, hyperplasia and dysplasia of mucosa cells
- viscous mucus;
- Bronchial mucosa with altered structure:
- histiocytes (intrabronchial, dense)
- fibrinoid material;
- Lung parenchyma with altered structure:
- intrabronchiolar fibrinoid material and histiocytes
- ulceration of bronchiolar mucosa
- focal interstitial fibrosis (peribronchiolar)
- mononuclear inflammatory infiltrates

■ *Special stains:* PAS, collagenous stains, Giemsa.

Hallmark of Diagnosis: In acute bronchiolitis, destruction of the bronchiolar mucosa by granulomatous inflammatory infiltrates. In chronic bronchiolitis, mononuclear infiltrates in the mucosa of the bronchioles and small bronchi, squamous metaplasia and intraluminal proliferation of epithelial cells. In bronchiolitis obliterans, fibrinoid granulomatous tissue in the bronchioles and small bronchi with partial ulceration of the bronchiolar mucosa. The granulomas reach into the alveolar ducts and sacs.

Differential diagnosis: Bronchopneumonia, fungal infections (bronchiolitis obliterans), bronchocentric granulomatosis.

Bronchiolitis Obliterans

Definition: Lesion of the small conducting airways which is repaired by proliferation of granulation tissue.

Incidence/Epidemiology: The lesion is common and not infrequently seen in patients of all ages. It is commonly associated with patchy organizing pneumonia of various etiologies.

Etiology/Pathophysiology: The lesion may be focal or a diffuse bilateral process. A rapidly dynamic lesion, it usually starts as an edematous intrabronchiolar polyp with necrosis and mixed inflammatory infiltrates. Focal ulceration of the mucosa is usually present which is followed by granulation repair. Intraluminal fibrinoid material is intermingled with histiocytes and mononuclear inflammatory infiltrates. Later stages show narrowing or occlusion of the lumen followed by scarring. The alveolar ducts may also be involved. The lesion is associated with various toxic or infectious agents such as metal fumes, aspiration of gastric contents, bacteria, fungus, virus, mycoplasma. It is also seen in allergic reaction, or drug toxicity. Bronchiolitis obliterans with prolonged course and unknown origin is sometimes called idiopathic bronchiolitis obliterans.

Clinical Presentation: Patients complain about dyspnea, cough, fever, but seldom chest pain or hemoptysis. The symptoms usually develop over weeks or months, simulating lower respiratory tract infection.

Prognosis: Fair, about 10% of patients will die, usually within a few months after onset of the disease. The rest will recover, but residues are often seen even after years.

Radiology: Chest radiographs often present with bilateral patchy diffuse infiltrates, often seen in the lower lobes, simulating atypical or nonresolving pneumonia.

Pathology:

Gross: The lungs show multiple, patchy, yellowish-white densities of firm consistency.

Histology: The epithelial cells of the bronchioles are destroyed and replaced by dense mononuclear inflammatory infiltrates. The bronchiolar lumen is (partly) occluded by fibrinoid material intermingled with proliferating histiocytes, plasma cells, lymphocytes, and scattered neutrophils. Scarring may be seen in the later stages. The peribronchiolar region is usually affected. The cells of the alveolar lining are unsuspicious as are the larger bronchi and vascular walls.

➤ *Descriptors:* Lung parenchyma with preserved structure:

- unsuspicious pneumocytes;
- Lung parenchyma with altered structure:
- intrabronchiolar fibrinoid material and histiocytes
- ulceration of bronchiolar mucosa
- focal interstitial fibrosis (scars)

■ *Special stains:* PAS, collagenous stains, endogenous lectins.

Hallmark of Diagnosis: Clinical history, ulceration and fibrinoid polyps in the bronchioles, proliferating histiocytes.

Differential diagnosis: According to the underlying cause, organizing bacterial pneumonia, usual interstitial pneumonia.

Bronchioloalveolar Carcinoma

Definition: Malignant lung neoplasm with characteristic histological appearance, subtype of adenocarcinoma of the lung.

Incidence/Epidemiology: These tumors are relatively more frequent in men than in women (ratio 2:1) and comprise 10–20% of all adenocarcinomas. No specific chemical agents are associated with these tumors. Smoking is related to a portion of patients with bronchioloalveolar carcinoma. However, a significant portion of patients have no discernable risk factors.

Etiology/Pathophysiology: There is a close association with scars in these tumors. Some 25–50% are localized adjacent to scars and grow focally whereas a second type grows in a diffuse multilocular pattern. In sheep with the histomorphologically similar lung carcinoma known as jaagsiekte, maedi, or Montana progressive pneumonia, a transmissible agent suggestive of an oncovirus has been identified which is now suggested to be nuclear inclusions of surfactant apoprotein. The majority of bronchioloalveolar carcinomas contain apical mucous granules resembling the granules of Clara cells. In addition, cells resembling type II pneumocytes and ciliated cells can be identified in bronchioloalveolar carcinoma.

Clinical Presentation: The tumor is often detected in younger asymptomatic patients by uncorrelated chest radiographs. Other patients present with symptoms of chronic bronchitis including cough, increased expectoration, dyspnea, fever, and loss of weight.

Prognosis: Extrapulmonary metastases develop in 10–20% of patients, and diffuse intrapulmonary metastases in more than 60% of patients. The 5 year survival is less than 20%.

Radiology: The tumors present with either solid, circumscribed, peripherally localized nodules with "scarring with peduncules" or diffuse pneumonic infiltrates.

Pathology:

Gross: The tumors appear as a peripherally localized, yellowish-grayish scar without larger necrotic areas or as larger, mucinous, confluent, yellowish masses randomly distributed in a complete lobe or lung. Consolidated areas often resemble pneumonic infiltrates.

Histology: The characteristic pattern of bronchioloalveolar carcinoma is its growth along the preformed lung textures without major destruction of the underlying framework. Inflammatory response of host tissue does not take place, and some papillary intraalveolar tumor strings are formed. The tumor cells are either small with "condensed" nuclei or large with intracytoplasmic mucinous inclusions. Mitoses are rare. The tumor cells are relatively homogeneous, causing difficulties with small biopsies for differentiation from dysplastic pneumocytes. Stromal reaction is scarce. Extracellular mucus production may be present, leading to severe clinical problems. Solid tumors are usually related to scars. They show more undifferentiated textures near fibrotic areas and pass into the characteristic growth pattern at the lung parenchyma boundary. The diffuse type presents with small separate islands of tumor cell agglutinations distributed in a complete lobe or lung. The alveoli are usually empty. Sometimes isolated intraalveolar "grapelike" clusters of tumor cells are present, being the characteristic cytologic findings in sputum or bronchial secretions.

➤ *Descriptors:* Newly formed textures with metastasis potential:

- epithelial growth pattern
- adenoid textures (papillary)
- lining of tumor cells (along interalveolar septula)
- islands of tumor cells (small, separated)
- mucus production
- homogeneous nuclear and cellular size
- finely distributed nuclear chromatin
- infrequent mitoses
- micrometastases
- absent or weak inflammatory infiltrates

■ *Special stains:* PAS, collagenous stains, immunohistochemistry for CEA, surfactant apoprotein, neuroendocrine markers, endogenous lectins.

Hallmark of Diagnosis: Characteristic growth textures with preservation of the underlying lung parenchyma framework.

Differential diagnosis: Desquamative interstitial pneumonia, obstructive pneumonitis with dysplastic pneumocytes, viral pneumonia, acute respiratory distress syndrome, other subtypes of adenocarcinoma of the lung.

Bronchitis

Definition: Acute or chronic infection of the air passages.

Incidence/Epidemiology: Acute tracheobronchitis is a frequent disease in autumn and springtime. The incidence of chronic bronchitis increases with its close association to air pollution of various causes. The mortality of chronic bronchitis with associated emphysema has been rising steadily over the past 20 years and has reached values of 60/100 000 inhabitants per year with a predominance of men (3–4:1). Smoking is a major noxa in addition to air pollution which is of great importance in children.

Etiology/Pathophysiology: Acute bronchitis is usually caused by viral and bacterial infections (*Staphylococcus aureus, Hemophilus influenzae, Pseudomonas aeruginosa*) of the upper respiratory tract with subsequent spread of the organisms to the lower airways, or by irritant gases such as sulfur dioxide, smoke, ammonia, nitrogen dioxide, mustard, agent orange,etc. Chronic bronchitis either develops subsequent to unhealed acute bronchitis or from a combination of various factors including an idiopathic reaction pattern of the airways, chronic exposure to irritant components in the air, additional infections, and living habits.

Clinical Presentation: Acute bronchitis causes cough and increased mucus production. Fever and malaise are usually present. Chronic bronchitis is defined to be a disease with increased expectoration of mucus lasting for at least 3 months and chronic cough. Dyspnea and obstructive findings in a lung function test may exist in addition, thus leading to the term chronic obstructive bronchitis.

Prognosis: Acute bronchitis is a self-healing disease in the majority of patients but can proceed to chronic bronchitis, which usually shows a slow progression.

Radiology: Chest radiographs may be normal or demonstrate increased thickness of bronchial walls, peribronchial infiltrates, and increased peribronchial air volume, indicating emphysematous alterations.

Pathology:

Gross: The surface of the bronchi is covered with mucus and is red in acute bronchitis. Chronic bronchitis usually shows thickened bronchial walls with an endobronchial layer of mucus and deformations of bronchial size and configuration.

Histology: The findings in acute bronchitis include desquamation of epithelial cells, debris and mucus in the bronchial lumen, and dense granulocytic and lymphoplasmocytic infiltrates in the bronchial mucosa. Chronic bronchitis is characterized either by an increased number of goblet cells and hyperplasia of basal cells or by squamous metaplasia of the epithelial cells. The basal layer is thickened under both conditions. The muscular layer is thickened or fibrotically altered and contains a mild to dense inflammatory infiltrate with predominantly lymphocytes and plasma cells. Eosinophilic infiltrates are present in asthmoid-allergic reactions but usually do not exceed the number of mononuclear cellular infiltrates. Pseudopolypous endobronchial obliteration consisting of edematous fibrous tissue mixed with scattered lymphocytes may suggest bronchial carcinoma (inflammatory pseudopolyp of the bronchus).

➤ *Descriptors:* Bronchial mucosa with preserved structure:

- viscous mucus
- increased number of goblet cells
- hyaline basal membrane
- increased number of smooth muscle cells
- mixed inflammatory infiltrates
- ulceration of bronchial mucosa;
- Bronchial mucosa with altered structure:
- fibrinoid material (intrabronchial)
- squamous metaplasia and dysplasia
- mononuclear inflammatory infiltrates

■ *Special stains:* PAS, collagenous stains, Giemsa.

Hallmark of Diagnosis: Dense inflammatory infiltrations of acute or chronic reactive pattern in the mucosa, focal ulceration, hyperplasia or metaplasia of epithelial cells, eosinophilic granulocytes in asthmoid bronchitis, thickened basal membrane.

Differential diagnosis: Subspecification due to various organisms.

Bronchobiliary Fistula

Definition: Abnormal connection between a major bronchus and the biliary ducts, see Fistula.

Bronchocentric Granulomatosis

Definition: Granulomatous and necrotizing replacement of bronchial mucous membrane lining.

Incidence/Epidemiology: Rare disease of equal sex distribution, reported in patients over 20 years old.

Etiology/Pathophysiology: The disease is found in asthmatic and nonasthmatic patients. It is considered to be a specific graft-versus-host reaction at least in the group of patients with a history of chronic asthma, who usually fulfil the diagnostic criteria for hypersensitivity reaction of the lung to fragments of noninvasive *Aspergillus*. A similar cause is assumed for the group of nonasthmatic cases, although these patients usually do not present with blood eosinophilia and fragments of inhaled organisms.

Clinical Presentation: Patients present with fever, cough, and severe wheezing, and in about half of the reported cases there is a history of asthma and blood eosinophilia.

Prognosis: Usually good and without or only with mild sequelae.

Radiology: Chest radiographs display diffuse solitary lung infiltrates as well as areas of atelectasis.

Pathology:

Gross: Smaller and larger bronchi are replaced by necrotic, usually firm, grayish material. The peripheral lung parenchyma is usually atelectatic.

Histology: The walls of the bronchi and bronchioles are completely destroyed. The former lumen is filled with necrotic cellular debris surrounded by a granulomatous infiltrate comprised of palisading histiocytes, lymphocytes, plasma cells, eosinophilic granulocytes and focally multinucleated giant cells. The inflammation is restricted to the bronchi and usually does not affect distant lung parenchyma. The necrotic areas may contain fragments of *Aspergillus*, acid-fast bacilli, or *Histoplasma capsulatum*. The arteries and veins are not involved except by spreading inflammation due to adjacent bronchi. The proximal bronchi may show localized necrotizing granulomas in the submucosa, focal ulceration of the mucosa, or erosion of cartilage by a histiocytic infiltrate.

➤ *Descriptors:* Bronchial mucosa with altered structure:

- caseous epithelioid granulomas
- palisading histiocytes
- multinucleated giant cells
- eosinophils
- mixed inflammatory infiltrates
- fungus (fragments of *Aspergillus*, acid-fast bacilli, *Histoplasma capsulatum*)
- necrosis (complete destruction of bronchial walls)
- erosion of cartilage

■ *Special stains:* Collagenous stains, PAS, silver stain, immunofluorescence for *Aspergillus*, Ziehl-Neelsen.

Hallmark of Diagnosis: Necrotizing granulomas of the bronchioles, small and medium-sized bronchi without affecting the vascular system or the peripheral lung parenchyma, clinical history of asthma.

Differential diagnosis: Wegener's granulomatosis, nodular rheumatoid diseases, granulomatous infections of the lung, Churg-Strauss syndrome, lymphomatoid granulomatosis, adenovirus infection.

Broncholithiasis

Definition: Calcified nodules in the bronchial mucosa or in the bronchial lumen, which may be expectorated.

Incidence/Epidemiology: Rare disease. Broncholiths are occasionally observed in patients suffering from tuberculosis or histoplasmosis. Men and women show the same frequency.

Etiology/Pathophysiology: Calcified deposits originating in chronic inflammatory diseases penetrate the bronchial wall and enter the bronchial lumen. In addition, originally intraluminal deposits occur in bronchiectases.

Clinical Presentation: Expectoration usually occurs in combination with chronic suppurative bronchitis. The bronchioliths may be frequently produced or in a single event.

Prognosis: Usually good and not defined by the broncholiths.

Radiology: Calcifications are usually seen on chest radiographs and are frequently localized near the junctions of the bronchi.

Pathology:

Gross: The calcified masses are whitish-yellow, and seldom exceed 1 cm in diameter.

Histology: Homogeneous hyaline mass after decalcification.

➤ *Descriptors:* Bronchial mucosa with altered structure:

- destruction of submucosal glands
- calcium deposits (calcified material in bronchial walls)
- mononuclear inflammatory infiltrates

■ *Special stains:* PAS.

Hallmark of Diagnosis: Macroscopic appearance, calcified material in the bronchial submucosa penetrating into the bronchial lumen.

Differential diagnosis: Aspiration, calcification occurring in histoplasmosis, silicosis, tuberculosis, *Pneumocystis carinii*.

Bronchomalacia (Tracheobronchomalacia)

Definition: Abnormal development or degeneration of tracheo-bronchial cartilage leading to collapse or stenosis of the lumen.

Incidence/Epidemiology: Congenital tracheobronchomalacia has been described in association with a familial syndrome of cryptorchidism, chest deformity, muscular hypoplasia, dolichocephaly, and retardation. It may arise in patients with a history of tracheotomy, or chronic destructive bronchitis or may be idiopathic.

Etiology/Pathophysiology: The congenital disorder is characterized by small islands of immature cartilage with deteriorated consistency. Postinflammatory malacia shows fragments of the original cartilage replaced by loose fibrotic tissue, i.e., a picture that is in accordance with probable enzymatic dissolution of cartilage.

Clinical Presentation: The clinical picture is characterized by the collapse of the bronchial lumen leading to asthmatic symptoms with difficulties in expiration. Acute collapse with cyanosis may occur.

Prognosis: Patients usually suffer from severe sequelae and progressive recurrent respiratory failure; however, implantation of stands may improve the outcome significantly.

Radiology: Stenosis of the trachea/bronchus with poststenotic increased air volume.

Pathology:

Gross: "Floppy" consistency of the trachea/bronchus with poststenotic dilatation.

Histology: In the congenital disorder the cartilage is replaced by immature islands of cartilage, and there are a decreased number of mucosal glands and mild fibrosis. Acquired bronchomalacia characteristically shows a rough surface and substantial loss of cartilage, replaced by scattered histiocytes and fibroblasts. Acute granulocytic infiltrates are usually not present.

➤ *Descriptors:* Bronchial mucosa with altered tissue structure:

- erosion of cartilage
- fragments of immature cartilage
- fibrosis (submucosa)
- decreased number of submucosal glands

■ *Special stains:* Collagenous stains, PAS, Giemsa.

Hallmark of Diagnosis: Immature islands of cartilage, fragmented cartilage with surrounding loose connective tissue, clinical history, radiologic findings.

Differential diagnosis: Cartilage atrophy, Campbell-Williams syndrome, bronchopathia osteoplastica.

Bronchopathia Osteoplastica (Tracheobronchopathia Osteoplastica)

Definition: Disease with multiple nodules of bone and cartilage in the mucosa of the trachea/bronchus leading to stenosis of the lumen.

Incidence/Epidemiology: Rare disorder in middle-aged to elderly men. An association with pulmonary (proximal) amyloidosis has been reported.

Etiology/Pathophysiology: The pathogenesis is not known. A process of cartilaginous metaplasia has been suggested.

Clinical Presentation: The patients usually show few or no symptoms, but severe cases may show obstruction-related complaints.

Prognosis: Usually good and without severe sequelae.

Radiology: Chest radiographs are usually normal, and tomography may detect additional bony formations in the tracheal/bronchial wall.

Pathology:

Gross: Rough surface of the trachea/bronchus with sandpaperlike appearance including rigid circular tubes. The membranous part of the airways is usually not affected.

Histology: The superficial submucosa shows multiple nodules that are formed by mature cartilage or bone formations with surrounding cartilage. Calcification or actively hematopoietic bone marrow is present. The nodules replace the submucosal glands which are reduced in number and show atrophy in some. Severe inflammation is not a sign of tracheobronchopathia osteoplastica.

➤ *Descriptors:* Bronchial mucosa with altered structure:

- fragments of mature cartilage
- fragments of mature bone and bone marrow
- decreased number of submucosal glands

■ *Special stains:* Collagenous stains, PAS, Giemsa.

Hallmark of Diagnosis: Superficial submucosal nodules of bone and cartilage in the trachea/bronchus in addition to the normal cartilage, atrophy of submucosal glands, macroscopic appearance.

Differential diagnosis: Endobronchial hamartoma, bronchomalacia.

Bronchopneumonia

Definition: Bacterial infection of the lower respiratory tract, see Bacterial Infections.

Bronchopulmonary Dysplasia

Definition: Disease of the newborn during the "transition period" which results in bronchiolar epithelial dysplasia, necrotizing bronchiolitis, and peribronchiolar edema.
Incidence/Epidemiology: Bronchopulmonary dysplasia occurs in 2.5–20% of infants with respiratory distress syndrome who receive intermittent positive pressure ventilation. The percentage increases to 40% in children with a birth weight of 1000 g or less.
Etiology/Pathophysiology: This multifactorial disorder is associated with high oxygen breathing levels, immature lungs, pulmonary edema, vitamin E and A deficiency, family history of asthma, ceruloplasmin deficiency.
Clinical Presentation: The children become oxygen-dependent following rather long lasting positive pressure mechanical ventilation. They usually develop respiratory distress soon after birth and are in a premature stage. The mortality in severe cases is high ranging as much as 50%. Damage to lung tissue in survivors causes increased morbidity in this group of patients.
Prognosis: About 50% of patients die within the 1st week. Survivors develop serious sequelae and progressive respiratory failure.
Radiology: Chest radiographs show persistent increased densities, lung opacity being replaced by increased air volume and atelectatic zones.
Pathology:
Gross: The gross appearance of the lungs depends upon the degree of immaturity of the lung, the duration of the disease, and the therapeutic approaches employed. The early stage, lasting 7–14 days after onset of ventilation, is characterized by acute inflammation of the trachea/bronchi with a red color and ulcerations. The reparative or fibroproliferative stage, lasting 2–4 weeks after onset of ventilation, involves firm, heavy, reddish-gray lungs with atelectatic and overinflated lung portions. The chronic fibroproliferative stage shows signs related to interstitial fibrosis such as honeycombing, scarring, areas with bacterial superinfection, etc.
Histology: In the acute stage the mucosa of the trachea and major bronchi show dysplasia and focal necrosis with intraluminal debris. The bronchioles are occluded by hyaline membranes which line the interalveolar septa. The interlobular septa show interstitial edema. Early fibrotic changes may be present in the interstitial tissue. The subacute proliferative stage is characterized by extensive metaplasia of the tracheal and bronchial mucosa, a muscular hyperplasia, and chronic inflammatory infiltrates in the submucosa. The bronchioles show metaplasia and are usually occluded by fibrinoid deposits or proliferating fibroblasts. The interalveolar septa exhibit prominent proliferation of fibroblasts mixed with mononuclear inflammatory infiltrates. The alveolar lining cells show marked dysplasia of cuboidal cells with cellular atypias. The interlobular septa may, in addition, contain multinucleated giant cells. The chronic fibroproliferative stage displays irreversible changes of the lung texture with restructuring of interalveolar septula, proliferating smooth muscle fibers, interstitial fibroblasts, and a mild inflammatory mononuclear infiltrate. The changes are usually diffuse and result in honeycombing.

➤ *Descriptors:* Bronchial mucosa with altered structure:
- necrosis (bronchial mucosa, focal)
- fibrinoid material (intrabronchial)
- mixed inflammatory infiltrates
- squamous metaplasia and dysplasia
- ectasia and hyperplasia of submucosal glands;
- Lung parenchyma with preserved structure:
- hyaline membranes
- intraalveolar fibrinoid material
- desquamation, hypertrophy, hyperplasia and dysplasia of pneumocytes;
- Lung parenchyma with altered structure:
- proliferating fibroblasts
- necrosis (bronchiolar and ductal)
- mononuclear inflammatory infiltrates
- diffuse interstitial fibrosis

■ *Special stains:* Collagenous stains, PAS, Giemsa, immunohistochemistry for surfactant apoprotein, immunoglobulins including light and heavy chains, endogenous lectins.

Hallmark of Diagnosis: Clinical history, and depending on the stage of bronchopulmonary dysplasia, necrotizing bronchiolitis, peribronchiolar edema, hyaline membranes; bronchiolitis obliterans, dysplasia of alveolar lining cells, beginning interstitial fibrosis; interstitial fibrosis, various degrees of honeycombing.

Differential diagnosis: Hyaline membrane disease (idiopathic respiratory distress syndrome), pulmonary interstitial emphysema.

Bronchostenosis

Definition: Narrowing of the bronchial lumen by congenital, inflammatory, or tumorous lesions.

Incidence/Epidemiology: Stenosis of the proximal bronchi is a frequent lesion seen in patients at any age.

Etiology/Pathophysiology: Congenital fibrosis is associated with inflammatory processes of intrauterine life caused by aspiration of meconium, viral or bacterial infections. Other causes are bronchial adenoma, ectopic thyroid tissue, absence of bronchial cartilage (Williams-Campbell syndrome), compression of the bronchus by abnormally located pulmonary arteries, parabronchial teratoma, or bronchogenic cysts. In adults, bronchial stenosis is most frequently associated with submucosal growth of bronchogenic carcinomas such as small cell anaplastic carcinoma or adenocarcinoma. Submucosal inflammation and granulomatous lesions in the lymphatic tissue or in the airways like tuberculosis or sarcoidosis can be seen in 5–10% of patients.

Clinical Presentation: Symptoms include expiratory wheezing, dyspnea, cough, asthmoid complaints, or minimal alterations such as shortness of breath during exercise.

Prognosis: Varies according to the underlying disease, long-standing bronchostenosis usually induces inflammation and destruction of the poststenotic areas of the lung.

Radiology: Chest radiographs may show progressive atelectasis, peribronchial calcified areas, or tumor masses.

Pathology:

Gross: Narrowing of the bronchial lumen to various extents, usually accompanied by parabronchial, whitish-yellow, tumorous masses. The lumen distal to the stenosis is dilated.

Histology: The epithelial cells often show squamous metaplasia with various degrees of cellular atypias. The mucosa is fibrotic, the number of submucous glands is decreased except in cases of glandular adenomas. Tumor cells usually do not extend to the epithelial layer of the mucosa, and superficial bronchial biopsies are often unsuspicious.

➤ *Descriptors:* Bronchial mucosa with altered structure:

- squamous metaplasia and dysplasia
- stenosis

■ *Special stains:* PAS, Giemsa.

Hallmark of Diagnosis: Macroscopic and endoscopic findings, radiology. Narrowing of the bronchial lumen in surgical specimens.

Differential diagnosis: Chronic asthmatic inflammation.

Brucellosis

Definition: Infection of human lung with *Brucella abortus*, *B. melitensis*, *B. suis*.

Incidence/Epidemiology: Brucellosis is a worldwide disease occurring in ranchers, farmers, veterinarians, or abattoir workers. Infection from unpasteurized dairy products is most frequent; in the arctic region intake of raw bone marrow is associated with infection of *B. suis*.

Etiology/Pathophysiology: Chronic infection of domestic animals serves as a reservoir of the disease. Humans become infected by eating unpasteurized milk products or raw meat. The bacteria invade through the alimentary tract or through the skin and spread to the regional lymph nodes or to organs of the reticuloendothelial system. The organisms multiply in histiocytes and may settle in the spleen, liver, bone marrow, and other organs including the lung.

Clinical Presentation: After an infection period ranging from 5 days to several months the clinical course can be classified into 3 different types: (a) The acute malignant type, usually occurring after a clearcut occupational exposure, has a sudden onset of high fever, chills, headache, prostration, and abdominal complaints. Local or generalized swollen lymph nodes may be present, and death can occur within a few days or after a few weeks, usually caused by infection of the nervous system. (b) The second type is characterized by recurrent "undulant" fever with headache, constipation, insomnia, generalized aching, and signs of chronic bronchitis. The patients usually suffer several weeks until the symptoms disappear. (c) The third type, called the chronic or intermittent type, involves loss of weight, increase in malaise, depression, insomnia, somatic and joint pains. The leading neurotic signs may persist for years.

Prognosis: Poor in the acute malignant type, good in the prolonged and chronic types.

Radiology: Chest radiographs are often normal. Sometimes peribronchial infiltrates or hilar adenopathy are present. Long-lasting brucellosis can end in multiple, calcified, small nodules detectable on chest radiographs.

Pathology:

Gross: The lungs are usually unsuspicious, while the bronchi are reddish and contain viscous mucus. Spherical, grayish-white, necrotic nodules enclosed by a fibrous capsule resembling tuberculoid lesions have been reported from infections with *B. suis*.

Histology: The bacteria cause caseous granulomas consisting of epithelioid cells, histiocytes, scattered surrounding lymphocytes and plasma cells. Multinucleated giant cells may be present. Smaller lesions only show a focal suppurative appearance with enclosed neutrophilic granulocytes, but older lesions tend to calcify. The bacteria can be demonstrated in the histiocytes present at the margins of the granulomas.

➤ *Descriptors:* Lung parenchyma with altered structure:

- caseous epithelioid granulomas
- multinucleated giant cells
- macrophages
- bacteria (histiocytes)
- neutrophils (numerous)
- necrosis
- calcification

■ *Special stains:* PAS, collagenous stains, Goodpasture's stain for the bacteria.

Hallmark of Diagnosis: Clinical history including occupational exposure and agglutination tests, caseous epithelioid granulomas resembling tuberculosis, demonstration of the bacteria in the histiocytes.

Differential diagnosis: Infectious granulomatous diseases including tularemia, melioidosis, tuberculosis, listeriosis; non-infectious granulomatous diseases such as sarcoidosis, Wegener's disease, etc.

Bulla

Definition: Large subpleural emphysematous changes of the lung.

Incidence/Epidemiology: Frequently seen in centrilobular and panlobular emphysema.

Etiology/Pathophysiology: Emphysematous destruction of the lung in centrilobular emphysema is associated with cigarette smoking. An imbalance between the levels of protease and antiprotease is assumed to be of major importance for emphysematous changes of the lung. Congenital bullae are frequently seen and may clinically impress the observer as pneumothorax.

Clinical Presentation: Focal emphysema (bulla) is usually clinically silent. Acute pneumothorax occurs especially in congenital bullae or in bullae associated with obstructive airway disease.

Prognosis: Subpleural emphysematous changes usually show progression and chronic infection if they are connected to the major conducting airways. They usually remain silent in case of encapsulation.

Radiology: Increased transparency of the affected lobe/lung portion.

Pathology:

Gross: Large, subpleural, "empty" air space with pseudocystic appearance.

Histology: Atrophic pleura with focal fibrosis, eradication of the lung texture. The supplying bronchi have thickened walls and show chronic inflammatory infiltrates in the mucosa and submucosa.

➤ *Descriptors:* Lung parenchyma with preserved structure:

- enlarged distant air spaces (empty);
- Lung parenchyma with altered structure:
- focal interstitial fibrosis (at the margins);
- Pleura with preserved structure:
- atrophy

■ *Special stains:* None.

Hallmark of Diagnosis: Macroscopic appearance, pseudocysts in the peripheral lung parenchyma.
Differential diagnosis: Congenital cyst.

Busulfan

Definition: Alteration of the lung parenchyma associated with intake of busulfan, see Drug Toxicity.

Byssinosis

Definition: Environmental lung disease seen in flax and hemp workers (Flax worker's disease).
Incidence/Epidemiology: Retting, crushing, beating, spinning, combing, and carding produce a mixture of dust fibers contaminated with bacteria and fungi. The degree of byssinosis is determined by the dust concentration (10% of workers inhaled air contaminated with dust 0.5 mg/m^3) and by the duration of exposure (40 years or more will cause symptoms). Affected are various types of textile cotton workers.
Etiology/Pathophysiology: Dust contaminated with bacteria and fungi may act in three different ways, (a) Nonallergic histamine release was observed in vitro by surgical specimens exposed to cotton bracts. This model with induced smooth muscle concentration and increased mediators such as prostaglandin, arachidonic acid metabolites, and leukokines can explain the functional changes of first-day responses in cotton workers. (b) Chronic exposure may result in antigen-antibody complexes consistent with a hypersensitivity reaction of the lung and the shift of increased IgE levels from Monday to Sunday. (c) Endotoxins released by gram-positive bacteria present in the air of cotton mills may cause histamine release and subsequent disturbance in lung function (FEV1 decrease).
Clinical Presentation: Characteristic symptoms are recurring tightness in the chest and shortness of breath on the first day of exposure and abatement of the symptoms during the weekend. Chronic manifestation has not been reported from all exposed workers; however, progressive loss of ventilatory capacity and increased prevalence of chronic bronchitis with mucus production have been seen.
Prognosis: Usually good, but sequelae of chronic bronchitis and slow progressive emphysematous changes can occur.
Radiology: No characteristic features are known.
Pathology:
Gross: Emphysematous changes exist with predominantly inflammatory proximal emphysema or panacinar and disclosed emphysema may be seen, especially in workers who smoke. The role of byssinosis in these patients remains, however, unclear.
Histology: The bronchi show an increased number of goblet cells, a thickened basal membrane, and a mononuclear infiltrate in the mucosa and submucosa. Emphysematous changes are associated with intraalveolar and interstitial macrophages, histiocytes, lymphocytes, and plasma cells. The number of plasma cells containing immunoglobulins of IgA type is reduced. Interstitial fibrosis is not a sign of byssinosis.

➤ *Descriptors:* Bronchial mucosa with preserved structure:

- increased number of goblet cells
- viscous mucus
- hyaline basal membrane
- mononuclear inflammatory infiltrates;
- Lung parenchyma with preserved structure:
- enlarged distant air spaces
- macrophages
- mononuclear inflammatory cells

■ *Special stains:* Collagenous stains, immunohistochemistry for immunoglobulins, endogenous lectins.

Hallmark of Diagnosis: Clinical history, signs of chronic mucoid bronchitis and emphysematous changes of the lung, decrease of IgA-containing plasma cells.
Differential diagnosis: Smoking-related changes of the conducting and distant airways.

Cadmium Fumes – Cytosine Arabinoside

Cadmium Fumes

Definition: Damage of the lung parenchyma by cadmium fumes.

Incidence/Epidemiology: Cadmium is used for corrosion protection in various metals built into exhaust systems, atomic reactors, alkaline accumulators, electroplating, alloys, etc.. Cadmium mines are located in North and South America, South Africa, Australia, and the USSR. Heating and welding as well as coal-burning power stations produce cadmium oxide fumes which are hazardous for the lung. Workers exposed to cadmium fumes have higher risks for lung cancer and prostatic cancer.

Etiology/Pathophysiology: Cadmium particles are ingested by macrophages and histiocytes. They act as chronic irritants for cells of the alveolar lining, which become necrotic or dysplastic, probably caused by direct cytotoxity of cadmium fumes.

Clinical Presentation: Acute symptoms include shortness of breath, fever, malaise; they usually develop several hours after exposure to high levels of fumes. Chronic exposure to low levels leads to a decrease of lung function of a restrictive type, progressive shortness of breath followed by dyspnea after years of exposure.

Prognosis: Usually good, but slow progression of respiratory failure can occur.

Radiology: Chest radiographs reveal emphysematous changes of both lungs in chronic stages. Acute poisoning usually results in diffuse interstitial infiltrates in both lungs.

Pathology:

Gross: The acute stage is characterized by heavy, fluid, reddish-yellowish lungs. The chronic stage is evidenced by emphysematous alterations of various degrees with focal fibrotic nodules measuring a few millimeters in diameter.

Histology: Necrosis of the cells of the alveolar lining caused by acute poisoning, fibrinoid exudation into the alveoli mixed with macrophages, neutrophilic granulocytes, lymphocytes, and plasma cells. The bronchioles and alveolar ducts are also involved. The course of the damage leads to a proliferation of pneumocytes of type II, and emphysematous eradication of peribronchiolar tissue. The chronic stages present with empty enlarged air spaces diffusely distributed in both lungs. Bronchitis is not a sign of chronic cadmium damage.

➤ *Descriptors:* Lung parenchyma with preserved structure:

- intraalveolar fibrinoid material
- macrophages
- desquamation, hypertrophy, hyperplasia and dysplasia of pneumocytes
- enlarged distant air spaces;
- Lung parenchyma with altered structure:
- mixed inflammatory infiltrates
- necrosis (pneumocytes)
- diffuse interstitial fibrosis
- focal interstitial fibrosis

■ *Special stains:* PAS, collagenous stains, endogenous lectins, X-ray diffraction methods and related physical techniques.

Hallmark of Diagnosis: Clinical history, diffuse panalveolar emphysema with absent bronchitis, identification of cadmium deposits by physical methods.

Differential diagnosis: Lung damage from fumes composed of other metals, due to smoking, or idiopathic emphysema, usual interstitial pneumonia.

Calcification of the Lung

Definition: Deposits of calcium salts into injured or scarred lung tissue.

Incidence/Epidemiology: Frequent disease seen after traumatic tissue alterations, hemorrhagic infarcts, organizing pneumonia, old infectious or silicotic granulomas, berylliosis.

Etiology/Pathophysiology: Local tissue alkalinity and organization of debris is associated with the formation of calcium salts.

Clinical Presentation: Usually no complaints, severe cases present with shortness of breath, progressive dyspnea, or cyanosis.

Prognosis: Usually good, but progression to respiratory failure can occur.

Radiology: Dense nodules which may be single or multiple usually surrounded by fibrotic tissue.

Pathology:

Gross: Yellowish, circumscribed, hard nodules sometimes with loose adhesion to the lung tissue.

Histology: Amorphous, calcified, extracellular material often surrounded by acellular fibrous tissue.

➤ *Descriptors:* Lung parenchyma with preserved structure:
- desquamation, hypertrophy, hyperplasia and dysplasia of pneumocytes (focal)
- mononuclear inflammatory infiltrates;
- Lung parenchyma with altered structure:
- focal interstitial fibrosis
- calcium deposits (calcified material, fibrosis)

■ *Special stains:* PAS, collagenous stains, Prussian blue, Kossa stain, alizarin red.

Hallmark of Diagnosis: Macroscopic findings, amorphous material.

Differential diagnosis: Metastatic calcification (alveolar microlithiasis).

Calcium Salts

Definition: Alteration of the lung parenchyma associated with intake of calcium salts, see Drug Toxicity.

Cancer of the Lung

Definition: Malignant neoplasms of the lung with varied microscopic appearance.

Incidence/Epidemiology: The incidence of lung cancer amounts to 80–100/100 000 cases per year in men and 15–30/100 000 cases per year in women in the industrialized countries. A dramatic increase in Western Europe was seen after the First World War. Lung cancer rates are still increasing in Western Europe whereas they are decreasing nowadays in North America. The sex ratio is changing to higher levels in women.

Etiology/Pathophysiology: Cigarette smoking is the most important factor associated with lung cancer. About 90% of patients with lung cancer are heavy smokers. A dose-response relationship between the number of cigarettes smoked and lung cancer risk has been proven. Passive smoking increases the risk of lung cancer as well. Exsmokers have close to a nonsmokers' risk of lung cancer 12–15 years after stopping smoking. Additional risk factors positively associated with lung cancer are radiation exposure, (inhalation of radioactive particles or external radiation), exposure to asbestos and various metallic fumes (cadmium, beryllium, nickel, etc.), various organic substances such as chloromethyl ether, flax substances, benzene, mustard gas, etc. Genetic factors associated with the BW-44 allele or chromosomal abnormalities or vitamin A deficiency may also be involved.

Clinical Presentation: The clinical picture of lung cancer shows great variation. Cancer occurring in the proximal bronchi (about 70%) causes cough, recurrent bronchopneumonia, expectoration, hemorrhage, dyspnea, etc. Peripherally localized lung cancer may be silent and is occasionally detected by chest radiographs. Loss of weight, fever, and malaise are additional symptoms, as is pain associated with metastatic growth. About 40–60% of all lung cancer patients cannot be treated by potentially curative operations.

Prognosis: Survival of patients with lung cancer is poor and strongly dependent upon the stage of the disease: In non-small cell carcinomas about 50–60% of patients with stage I survive 5 years or longer, but only 30% of patients with stage II, and less than 20% of patients with stage III. Involvement of lymph nodes (N stage) is considered to be the best prognostic factor. Other prognostic factors are size and location of the tumor (T stage), inflammatory response of host tissue, invasion of bronchial cartilage, chromosomal abnormalities, proliferation index, microscopic growth textures for small cell carcinomas. About 90% of patients with small cell carcinoma die within 2 years after diagnosis.

Pathology:

Gross: Lung cancer appears as white or yellowish, often central, necrotic, circumscribed masses, sometimes with diffuse margins resembling pneumonic infiltrations. The surrounding lung parenchyma may be transformed into atelectatic or bacterially superinfected regions. Tumor invasion into the regional lymph nodes has its macroscopic equivalence in grayish, necrotic, crumb-like alterations. Tumor staging (TNM classification) is performed according to the following rules (UICC):

T0 no evidence of primary tumor

TIS carcinoma in situ

T1 a tumor measuring 3 cm or less in greatest diameter, surrounded by lung tissue or visceral pleura, and without evidence of invasion proximal to a lobar bronchus at bronchoscopy. A superficial tumor of any size (inside the epithelial cells, mucosa, submucosa, and bronchus lumen) and extending proximal to the main bronchus.

T2 a tumor more than 3 cm in greatest dimension, or one of any size that either invades the visceral pleura or has associated atelectasis or obstructive pneumonitis extending to the hilar region. At bronchoscopy, the proximal extent of demonstrable tumor must be within a lobar bronchus or at least 2 cm distal to the carina. Any associated atelectasis or obstructive pneumonitis must involve less than an entire lung.

T3 a tumor of any size with direct extension into the chest wall (including superior sulcus tumors), diaphragm, mediastinal pleura or pericardium without involving the heart, great vessel, trachea, esophagus, or vertebral body, or a tumor in the main bronchus less than 2 cm of the carina without involving it.

T4 a tumor of any size with invasion of the mediastinum or involving the heart, great vessels, trachea, esophagus, vertebral body, or carina or presence of malignant pleural effusion.

TX tumor proven by the presence of malignant cells in bronchopulmonary secretions but not visualized roentgenographically or bronchoscopically, or any tumor that cannot be assessed, as in a retreatment staging.

Lymph node involvement:

N0 no demonstrable metastasis to regional lymph nodes.

N1 metastasis to lymph nodes in the peribronchial or the ipsilateral hilar region, or both, including direct extension.

N2 metastasis to ipsilateral mediastinal lymph nodes and subcarinal lymph nodes.

N3 metastasis to contralateral mediastinal lymph nodes, contralateral hilar lymph nodes, ipsilateral or contralateral scalene or supraclavicular lymph nodes.

Metastasis

M0 no evidence of distant metastasis.

M1 evidence of distant metastasis such as bone, brain, liver, etc.

In practice staging causes the following macroscopic difficulties:

It is often not possible to measure exactly the greatest dimension of the tumor in the surgical specimen. This can be performed only by three-dimensional reconstruction.

Differentiation between the tumor mass and surrounding inflammatory infiltrations is not always possible and may cause major discrepancies between the radiological and pathological size.

The distance to the carina cannot be measured in the majority of surgical specimens and has to be estimated.

Infiltration of the visceral pleura cannot always be proven in larger tumors due to the number of histological slides necessary.

Tumor invasion into lymph nodes can be missed in histological slides if tissue is not cut in serial sections.

Clinical data needed for correct classification (pleural effusions, details of bronchoscopy, etc.) are often incomplete.

Histology: The basis of histological classification of lung tumors is given by the classification of the WHO:

1. Epidermoid carcinoma including spindle cell carcinoma
2. Small cell carcinoma
   a. oat cell carcinoma
   b. intermediate cell type
   c. combined oat cell carcinoma
3. Adenocarcinoma
   a. acinar adenocarcinoma
   b. papillary adenocarcinoma
   c. bronchioloalveolar carcinoma
   d. solid carcinoma with mucus formation
4. Large cell carcinoma, variants:
   a. giant cell carcinoma
   b. clear cell carcinoma
5. Adenosquamous carcinoma
6. Carcinoid
7. Bronchial gland carcinoma
   a. adenoidcystic carcinoma
   b. mucoepidermoid carcinoma
   c. others
8. Others

From the clinical point of view it is important to distinguish between small cell anaplastic carcinoma and non-small cell carcinomas. Bronchioloalveolar carcinoma should be divided into diffuse and focal type. Histologic tumor heterogeneity causes difficulties for correct classification of large cell anaplastic carcinomas, which frequently show adenoid or epidermoid differentiation in a small portion of the tumor not present in biopsies performed prior to operation. In addition, major difficulties exist in attempts to separate primary lung tumors from metastases, especially in patients with a history of carcinomas of other organs and a long disease-free interval before the appearance of the carcinoma of the lung. Peripherally localized tumors do not necessarily have to be metastases; moreover, tumors infiltrating the bronchial mucosa may be of metastatic origin. The histomorphologic features of the different malignomas are described under the corresponding headings.

➤ *Descriptors:* Newly formed textures with metastasis potential:

- epithelial growth pattern
- mesenchymal growth pattern
- adenoid textures
- epidermoid textures
- solid textures
- endocrine textures
- sarcomatous textures
- lymphomatoid textures
- mucus production
- keratin production
- hormone production
- necrosis
- invasion of bronchial cartilage
- micrometastases (at margin of the tumor)
- frequent mitoses
- infrequent mitoses
- homogeneous nuclear and cellular size
- inhomogeneous nuclear and cellular size
- finely distributed nuclear chromatin
- prominent nucleoli
- oncogenes
- chromosome abnormalities
- micrometastases

■ *Special stains:* PAS, collagenous stains, Giemsa, immunohistochemistry for various markers including EMA, CEA, neuroendocrine markers, prostate-specific phosphatase, endogenous lectins, DNA analysis, syntatic structure analysis.

Hallmark of Diagnosis: See under corresponding headings.

Differential diagnosis: Metastatic tumor growth, severe dysplasia of epithelial cells.

Candidiasis

Definition: Infection of the lung with yeastlike fungi of the *Candida* genus.

Incidence/Epidemiology: The organisms live as part of the normal microflora of the mouth and oropharynx. *Candida* infections are worldwide and account for 50–70% of all opportunistic infections of the lung in immunocompromised patients such as those with leukemia, lymphoma, AIDS, solid malignancies, etc.

Etiology/Pathophysiology: Seven different species have been isolated and can be considered pathogenic: *C. albicans, C. tropicalis, C. parapsilosis, C. crusei, C. pseudotropicalis, C. guilliermondii,* and *C. stellatoidea.* Infections occur either superficially, involving the mucosal surface in preexistent bronchial alterations such as bronchiectasis, or as deep, disseminated forms after "barrier breaks" such as trauma, burns, surgical contamination, etc. Pulmonary involvement in these patients needs additional causative factors such as weakened immunodefence due to various reasons.

Clinical Presentation: The clinical symptoms are nonspecific and include fever, cough, chest pains, hemorrhage, etc. as seen in other opportunistic infections.

Prognosis: Usually defined by the underlying disease; however, infection with *candida* may force to discontinue therapeutic regimes necessary for the underlying disease.

Radiology: Chest radiographs usually show abnormalities which correlate with various pulmonary infections and are nonspecific.

Pathology:

Gross: Dependent upon the route of infection, circumscribed dense nodules with central hemorrhage and of grayish-yellowish color, either large and single or multiple, and of miliary manifestation can be recognized.

Histology: *Candida* infections usually cause a suppurative reaction of the lung parenchyma with predominantly neutrophilic granulocytes. Manifestations in preexisting infarcts are characterized by centrally localized organisms with necrotic lung tissue surrounded by neutrophilic granulocytes and an outer ring of hemorrhage. The fungi contain budding yeastlike organisms, pseudohyphae, and seldom true hyphae. The pseudohyphae present themselves as elongated cells with constrictions at the endpoints of attachment and are of ellipsoid configuration. In systemic candidiasis fungal thromboemboli in the smaller vessels are often detectable. The distinction between superficial and invasive candidiasis may be difficult and can be performed only on histological sections of lung parenchyma, requiring the demonstration of typical *candida* organisms in lung tissue with corresponding neutrophilic inflammatory reaction in addition to a clinical history of immunocompromise.

➤ *Descriptors:* Lung parenchyma with altered structure:
- necrosis and hemorrhage
- mixed inflammatory infiltrates
- fungus (*Candida*, hyphae);
- Lung parenchyma with preserved structure:
- intraalveolar fibrinoid material

■ *Special stains:* PAS, GMS, collagenous stains, immunofluorescence.

Hallmark of Diagnosis: Necrotizing pneumonia, demonstration of typical *candida* organisms, clinical history, chest radiographs.

Differential diagnosis: Other opportunistic infections, differentiation between superficial and invasive candidiasis.

Capillariasis

Definition: Infection of the lung with nematodes of the genus *Capillaria*.

Incidence/Epidemiology: Common parasite in dogs, cats, and foxes living in Europe, Asia, Australia, and North and South America. About 10 infected patients have been reported.

Etiology/Pathophysiology: The infective species are comprised of *C. philippinensis, C. hepatica*, and *C. aerophila*, which are not natural pathogens of man. The eggs become infective in warm soil and are ingested by animals. The larvae penetrate the intestinal wall and develop into adult worms in the lungs. Eggs are expectorated or swallowed and shed in the feces. The presence of an intermediate host is still unknown.

Clinical Presentation: The patients suffer from high fever, dyspnea, cough, and expectoration.

Prognosis: The natural course of infection is estimated to be 6–12 months. Mortality of infected patients is high and may reach 20% or even more.

Radiology: The chest radiographs usually display perihilar infiltrates and dense, miliary, reticular nodules.

Pathology:

Gross: The worms, measuring 2–6 mm, can be identified only with difficulty in the small bronchi and bronchioles or in the small intestines which show a thickened wall.

Histology: The worms measure about 20–30 μm in diameter. They contain embryonated, thin-shelled eggs in the center as well as small embryos without shell surrounded by a small muscular layer. The liver reacts mainly with granulomatous inflammation, whereas in the bronchioles a dense eosinophilic infiltrate can be observed destroying the bronchioles.

➤ *Descriptors:* Lung parenchyma with altered structure:
- parasites (worms, intrabronchiolar, degenerated)
- necrosis (bronchioles)
- eosinophils
- palisading histiocytes
- mononuclear inflammatory infiltrates

■ *Special stains:* PAS, collagenous stains, Movat stain.

Hallmark of Diagnosis: Necrotizing bronchiolitis, demonstration of the worms in the bronchioles and in the small intestines, or identification of the eggs in the stool, clinical history.

Differential diagnosis: Infection with other nematode species.

Caplan's Syndrome

Definition: Association of rheumatoid arthritis with coal pneumoconiosis and progression into massive fibrosis.

Incidence/Epidemiology: The increased prevalence of rheumatoid arthritis in men with coal pneumoconiosis and massive fibrosis was calculated to be 2.7% compared with 0.6% in men with simple pneumoconiosis. A similar increased prevalence was found for patients suffering from progressive systemic sclerosis and probably from systemic lupus erythematosus (SLE). The general prevalence of rheumatoid arthritis is in the same range in miners and nonminers.

Etiology/Pathophysiology: The massive fibrosis is assumed to be induced by rheumatoid factors which are triggered by inhalation of dust particles. Rheumatoid factors and labelled anti-IgM serum were identified in 80% of the rheumatic nodules but in only 18% in patients with massive fibrosis not showing vasculitis. Additional genetic or familial factors are suggested to play an important role in the etiology of the disease.

Clinical Presentation: Rheumatoid nodules in coal workers tend to develop suddenly and appear all over the lung, including peripheral lung zones. The patients suffer from increased shortness of breath, minor arthritic pains, dyspnea, cough. Progressive course of the disease is frequent.

Prognosis: Progression of respiratory failure is usually seen, leading to death after 5–10 years.

Radiology: Characteristic lesions show multiple, dense nodules 1–2 cm in diameter in the proximal and peripheral lung zones. Confluent nodules may be seen as well as interstitial fibrotic infiltrates.

Pathology:

Gross: Clear-cut nodules in the proximal and peripheral lung of black-yellowish color, in acute cases with central necrosis. They measure 5–15 mm in diameter and show a concentric arrangement of alternating black and yellowish rings.

Histology: Old nodules present massive, acellular, fibrotic masses in the center mixed with black dust particles which are not birefringent. The dark rings contain coal dust deposits, the yellowish rings fibrotic bundles with scattered mononuclear infiltrates. Active rheumatoid nodules contain central necrotic collagen surrounded by histiocytes, lymphocytes, plasma cells mixed with collagenous tissue, and multinucleated giant cells. Inflammatory mononuclear infiltrates in small arteries can often be detected near the active nodules.

➤ *Descriptors:* Lung parenchyma with altered structure:
- focal interstitial fibrosis (concentric)
- dust
- necrosis (central necrotic collagenous nodules)
- palisading histiocytes
- mixed inflammatory infiltrates
- multinucleated giant cells;
- Pulmonary vessels with preserved structure:
- mononuclear inflammatory infiltrates

■ *Special stains:* PAS, collagenous stains, Ziehl-Neelsen for excluding tuberculosis, immunohistochemistry (immunoglobulin deposits), endogenous lectins.

Hallmark of Diagnosis: Clinical history, chest radiographs, concentric arrangement of coal-silicotic nodules with alternating fibrotic "rings", rheumatoid nodules in active disease.

Differential diagnosis: Simple coal worker pneumoconiosis, severe damage of lung due to smoking, rheumatoid lung in heavy smokers.

Capsicum Lung

Definition: Lung damage associated with inhalation of capsicum pod dust.

Incidence/Epidemiology: Cases have been reported from Hungary and Eastern Europe. Paprika harvested during the damp season and stored in moldy rooms is polluted with various species of fungus, and the spores are released when the pods are split. The frequency of the disease has decreased remarkably after installation of ventilatory systems in the manufacturing plants.

Etiology/Pathophysiology: The disease is considered to be a chronic extrinsic allergic pneumonitis with still unidentified antigens.

Clinical Presentation: Usually subacute or chronic onset.

Prognosis: Usually good and without serious sequelae.

Radiology: Chest radiographs are normal or show diffuse, soft, interstitial infiltrates or fine granular densities.

Pathology:

Gross: The lungs are of normal color and consistency or may display small, firm, reddish-gray nodules.

Histology: The characteristic findings include nonnecrotizing epithelioid granulomas near the terminal bronchioles, desquamation, hypertrophy and hyperplasia of cells of the alveolar lining, marked eosinophilic inflammatory infiltrates, bronchiolitis obliterans and focal acute vasculitis. For details, see Allergic (Extrinsic) Alveolitis.

➤ *Descriptors:* Lung parenchyma with altered structure:
- noncaseous epithelioid granulomas
- eosinophils
- multinucleated giant cells
- intrabronchiolar fibrinoid material and histiocytes
- exulceration of bronchiolar mucosa;
- Lung parenchyma with preserved structure:
- macrophages
- desquamation, hypertrophy, hyperplasia and dysplasia of pneumocytes
- mononuclear inflammatory infiltrates
- intraalveolar serous fluid

■ *Special stains:* PAS, collagenous stains, Giemsa. For details, see Allergic (Extrinsic) Alveolitis.

Hallmark of Diagnosis: Clinical history, nonnecrotizing epithelioid granulomas, morphologic findings related to desquamative interstitial pneumonia, lymphoid interstitial pneumonia, bronchiolitis obliterans.

Differential diagnosis: Infectious and noninfectious granulomatous diseases such as sarcoidosis, fungal infections, or berylliosis. For details, see Allergic (Extrinsic) Alveolitis.

Carbamazepine

Definition: Alteration of the lung parenchyma associated with intake of carbamazepine (anticonvulsant), see Drug Toxicity.

Carborundum Pneumoconiosis

Definition: Disease of the lung caused by inhalation of silicon carbide particles.

Incidence/Epidemiology: Synthetic substance made by fusing high-grade sand, ground carbon, sodium chloride, and wood dust in an electric furnace. The substance is used for polishing and abrading various tools due to its hardness, which is similar to that of diamond. In a few cases, silicosis has been documented in carborundum workers.

Etiology/Pathophysiology: Animal experiments have given no indication of carborundum-induced pulmonary fibrosis. Carborundum itself is assumed to be inert to human lung tissue. The reported cases may have developed pneumoconiosis mainly due to exposure to silicon.

Clinical Presentation: Shortness of breath and cough may be present.

Prognosis: Usually good and without known sequelae.

Radiology: Chest radiographs have been reported to show bilateral reticulonodular densities and hilar masses.

Pathology:

Gross: Small, black to grayish nodules associated with proximal lung zones; fibrotic proximal lymph nodes may be present.

Histology: Dust-laden macrophages in the alveoli with peribronchiolar and perivascular distribution are characteristic. Birefringent particles and ferruginous bodies are visible. Fibrotic response of the lung parenchyma is mild.

➤ *Descriptors:* Lung parenchyma with preserved structure:
- dust (birefringent fibers, crystals)
- macrophages (dust-laden)
- ferruginous bodies

■ *Special stains:* Collagenous stains, Prussian blue, X-ray diffraction or related physical techniques for identification of carborundum.

Hallmark of Diagnosis: Clinical history, chest radiographs, dust-laden macrophages with birefringent particles, identification of the particles by physical techniques.

Differential diagnosis: Pneumoconiosis due to exposure to other dusts.

Carcinoid Tumor

Definition: Uncommon, low-grade, malignant tumor of neuroendocrine origin.

Incidence/Epidemiology: Carcinoids comprise 1% of all lung tumors and occur in both sexes with similar percentages at any age. The majority of patients are younger than patients with usual bronchial carcinoma. Association with risk factors such as smoking, asbestos, etc. is not known.

Etiology/Pathophysiology: Carcinoids are subclassified into the following types: tumorlets, peripheral carcinoids, central carcinoids, and atypical, highly malignant carcinoids. These tumors are histogenetically related to the so-called Kulchitsky's cell, which is of neuroendocrine origin and contains electron-dense granules, neuron-specific enolase with the subunits α, β, γ, chromogranins on the cellular surface (acidic proteins with glutamic acid), low and high weight neurofilaments (68, 160, 200 kD), synaptophysin (38-kD glycoprotein component of presynaptic vesicles), and various neuropeptides. These cells of the APUD (amine precursor uptake and decarboxylation) system have been identified in the submucosal glands of the major and smaller bronchi, and in the bronchioles. However, not all carcinoids express neuroendocrine markers to the same degree, and they grow in different patterns at the microscopic or submicroscopic level, indicating that they comprise a heterogeneous group of tumors.

Clinical Presentation: The clinical presentation depends upon the localization of the tumors. Central carcinoid tumors cause cough, hemoptysis and wheezing, usually with a history lasting for months or even years. Atelectasis or obstructive pneumonitis may be present. Peripheral carcinoids are usually silent, slowly growing tumors without characteristic symptoms.

Prognosis: Fair, about 80% of patients survive 5 years or longer. Local recurrence is frequently seen in patients with endobronchial resection of the tumors. Distant metastases occur only seldom.

Radiology: Normal chest radiographs may be obtained for central carcinoids if complications such as atelectasis or pneumonitis are absent. Endobronchial tumor masses may be detectable on chest tomograms. Peripherally localized carcinoids show dense, round nodules of various sizes.

Pathology:

Gross: Carcinoids are nonencapsulated, soft, yellowish-red tumors. A proximal carcinoid usually arises from one side of the bronchus and consists of a polypous oval tumor within the bronchial lumen with either an intact surface or one with circumscribed bleeding due to a previous biopsy. Most tumors measure 2–4 cm in diameter. Atypical carcinoids show multiple areas of hemorrhagic necrosis. Tumorlets measure 2–4 mm in diameter and are of a pale grayish color.

Histology: All carcinoids consist of small uniform cells with clear, slightly eosinophilic cytoplasm. The nuclei are of uniform size, show small unsuspicious nuclei or regularly distributed nuclear chromatin and are centrally placed within the cytoplasm. Variations in the staining intensity of the cytoplasm are seen. The typical growth patterns of carcinoids are adenoid structures with glandular appearance, solid nests or cords, trabeculae, or the so-called mosaic pattern which resembles solid nests separated by small fibrous stromal cords. Central carcinoids usually have a dense supply of small capillaries leading to bleeding during the performance of biopsies. Peripheral and atypical carcinoids are more variable in cellular size and arrangement and more often show mitotic figures. Spindle cells are more frequent, although the "endocrinoid" textures are still preserved. The cellular size is small compared with central carcinoids, and difficulty of differentiation from small cell anaplastic carcinomas may cause major problems. Tumorlets are small nests of round to ellipsoid cells which often lie within channels of fibrous tissue. Inflammatory tissue response is rare in all types of carcinoids. Central carcinoids have very rarely invaded the lung parenchyma at the time of diagnosis. Immunohistological features are positive staining to antibodies recognizing neuron-specific enolase (NSE), chromogranin A (Chrom A), synaptophysin (Sy38), bombesin, and serotonin. Carcinoembryonic antigen (CEA) is expressed in about 50% of the cases, and S-100 protein in about 30%.

➤ *Descriptors:* Newly formed structures with metastasis potential:
- epithelial growth pattern
- adenoid textures
- endocrine textures
- numerous capillaries
- hemorrhage
- homogeneous nuclear and cellular size
- small nuclei
- infrequent mitoses
- absent or weak inflammatory infiltrates

■ *Special stains:* PAS, silver stain, immunohistochemistry for NSE, Sy38, Chrom A, bombesin, DNA analysis.

Hallmark of Diagnosis: Characteristic adenoid and endocrine textures, cellular size and distribution of nuclear chromatin, macroscopic appearance, immunohistochemistry.

Differential diagnosis: Small cell anaplastic carcinoma, oncocytoma, adenocarcinoma, hyperplasia of Kulchitsky's cells, and minute pulmonary chemodectoma (for tumorlets).

Carcinoma of the Lung

Definition: Malignant lung tumor of epithelial origin.

Incidence/Epidemiology: Carcinomas of the lung comprise more than 90% of all lung tumors with an estimated incidence of 80–100/100 000 per year in men. the sex ratio (men:women) amounts to 8:1. Associated risk factors are smoking and various environmental elements such as exposition to asbestos, aluminum, cadmium, and radioactive particles.

Etiology/Pathophysiology: The majority of lung carcinomas arise from the proximal bronchi. Associated changes of bronchial mucosa include hyperplasia of goblet cells and basal cells and squamous cell metaplasia. Theories of histogenesis include multistep hits of bronchial mucosa leading to squamous cell metaplasia and various degrees of dysplasia, neuroendocrine origin of bronchial carcinoma (the majority if not all small cell anaplastic carcinomas and about 10% of non-small cell carcinomas), glandular cell origin, and alveolar lining cell origin (adenocarcinoma).

Clinical Presentation: The spectrum of clinical symptoms ranges from none to dyspnea, cough, loss of weight, and acute hemoptysis.

Prognosis: Usually poor. Patients with epidermoid carcinoma and adenocarcinoma have a better prognosis than those with large cell anaplastic carcinoma and small cell anaplastic carcinoma. Only 10–20% of patients survive 5 years or longer. (See also Cancer of the Lung).

Radiology: Centrally localized tumors are often unsuspicious, but peripherally localized tumors display circumscribed densities, often with characteristic peduncles.

Pathology:

Gross: Circumscribed grayish-white mass, often with central necrosis and hemorrhage. Diffuse, grayish infiltrations may suggest pneumonia.

Histology: The cell types are epidermoid carcinoma (40%), adenocarcinoma (25%), small cell anaplastic carcinoma (20%), large cell anaplastic carcinoma (10%), and mixed carcinoma, most frequently adenosquamous (5%). Small cell anaplastic carcinomas usually grow without inflammatory response of host tissue, whereas epidermoid carcinomas often show dense inflammatory infiltrates and evidence for enzymatic erosion of the bronchial cartilage. Diagnosis of large cell anaplastic carcinoma is performed after absolute exclusion of adenocarcinoma and of epidermoid carcinoma. Its frequency usually depends upon the amount of tissue available for histologic diagnosis. About 30% of adenocarcinomas involve extracellular mucus production.

➤ *Descriptors:* Newly formed textures with metastasis potential:
- epithelial growth pattern
- adenoid textures
- epidermoid textures
- solid textures
- endocrine textures
- mucus production
- keratin production
- hormone production
- necrosis
- invasion of bronchial cartilage
- micrometastases (at margin of the tumor)
- frequent mitoses
- infrequent mitoses
- homogeneous nuclear and cellular size
- inhomogeneous nuclear and cellular size
- finely distributed nuclear chromatin
- prominent nucleoli
- oncogenes
- growth factor receptors
- chromosome abnormalities
- micrometastases

■ *Special stains:* PAS, collagenous stains, immunohistochemistry for neuroendocrine markers, CEA, EMA, lymphocytic markers (small cell anaplastic carcinoma), DNA and syntactic structure analysis.

Hallmark of Diagnosis: Invasive, destructive growth of atypical cells with features of "epidermoid", "adenoid", "endocrine", or "not detectable" textures, clinical history.

Differential diagnosis: Cellular atypia, metastatic tumor growth, lymphoma.

Carcinosarcoma

Definition: Malignant tumor composed of both epithelial and mesenchymal tumor cells.

Incidence/Epidemiology: Rare tumor accounting for 0.3% of all pulmonary malignancies. More frequently seen in men than in women (5:1) and occurring in adult persons of any age. Associated risk factors are not exactly known but are assumed to be similar to those of the usual pulmonary carcinomas.

Etiology/Pathophysiology: Theories of the histogenetically different manifestations of tumorous growth include occurrence of two different tumors at the same time (carcinoma and sarcoma), manifestation of the "multipotentiality of the mother tissue", malignant transformation of hamartomas, and simultaneous expression of two extremes of cellular instability of tumor cells.

Clinical Presentation: Patients with carcinosarcoma present with the same symptoms as patients with ordinary malignant lung tumors.

Prognosis: Very poor, more than 90% of patients die within 2 years after diagnosis.

Radiology: The majority of the reported tumors, usually of large size (greater than 4 cm), were localized in the upper lobes.

Pathology:

Gross: Firm, grayish lesions with infiltrative growth into major bronchi, sometimes like intrabronchial polyps. Necrotic areas and hemorrhage are usually present.

Histology: Mixture of two different malignant components in different areas of the tumor. One area contains mainly epithelial cells, whereas the other contains mainly sarcomatous cells. Intermingling of the two portions is frequent and may resemble malignant epithelial growth with "atypical, predominant stromal reaction". The most common components are epidermoid differentiation of the epithelial part and fibrosarcomatous differentiation of the sarcomatous part. Other reported mesenchymal parts are chondrosarcoma or osteosarcoma. Necrotic areas are usually present as well as inflammatory infiltrates.

➤ *Descriptors:* Newly formed textures with metastasis potential:

- 1. epithelial tumor cells
- epithelial growth pattern
- epidermoid textures
- keratin production
- frequent mitoses
- inhomogeneous nuclear and cellular size
- adenoid textures
- mucus production
- moderate number of mitoses
- homogeneous nuclear and cellular size
- absent or weak inflammatory infiltrates
- necrosis
- 2. sarcomatous tumor cells
- mesenchymal growth pattern
- sarcomatous textures
- fragments of primitive bone
- fragments of primitive cartilage
- plump spindle cells
- moderate number of mitoses
- absent or weak inflammatory infiltrates
- necrosis and hemorrhage

■ *Special stains:* PAS, Giemsa, collagenous stains, immunohistochemistry for cytoskeleton, neuroendocrine markers, endogenous lectins.

Hallmark of Diagnosis: Two intermingling components of malignant epithelial and mesenchymal cells, usually epidermoid carcinoma and fibrosarcoma.

Differential diagnosis: Carcinoma with marked desmoplastic reaction, pulmonary blastoma, mixed malignant mesothelioma (in peripherally localized carcinosarcoma).

Carmustine

Definition: Alteration of the lung parenchyma associated with intake of carmustine, see Drug Toxicity.

Cartilage Atrophy

Definition: Degenerative disappearance of bronchial cartilage.

Incidence/Epidemiology: Rare disease seen in adult persons with emphysema and chronic airflow obstruction.

Etiology/Pathophysiology: The causes and observed associations of cartilage atrophy still remain unclear. The diminished amount of cartilage in patients with severe emphysema and chronic bronchitis reported by one author could not be confirmed by other authors, who found no relationship between the extent of cartilage atrophy and the Reid index.

Clinical Presentation: Symptoms of obstructive airway disease. Asthmoid collapsing segmental bronchus in severe cases.

Prognosis: Usually good. Sequelae are chronic inflammation and destruction of the associated peripheral lung parenchyma.

Radiology: No characteristic lesions except signs of emphysema and chronic obstructive bronchitis.

Pathology:

Gross: Floppy segmental or subsegmental bronchus with increased lumen and loss of characteristic circular segmentation of the bronchial mucosa.

Histology: Loss of cartilage with irregular boundaries and histiocytic cellular infiltrates in the submucosa.

➤ *Descriptors:* Bronchial mucosa with preserved structure:

- decreased size of cartilage
- erosion of cartilage
- mononuclear inflammatory infiltrates

■ *Special stains:* PAS, collagenous stains, Giemsa.

Hallmark of Diagnosis: Disappearance and fibrohistiocytic replacement of cartilage.

Differential diagnosis: Tracheobronchomalacia, Williams-Campbell syndrome.

Cat Lung Worm

Definition: Infection of cats with *Aelurostrongylus abstrusus.*

Incidence/Epidemiology: Infection of cats in Asia, Africa, and North and South America with the nematode species *A. abstrusus.* No human infections are known.

Etiology/Pathophysiology: The adult worm lives in the pulmonary arteries and terminal bronchioles. Infected eggs were passed with the sputum or feces. The life cycle of the nematodes includes snails and mice or birds as paratenic hosts. Infection with the lung worm results in severe hypertension with thickening of the muscular wall of the pulmonary arteries. The hypertrophy and hyperplasia are probably caused by toxic substances derived from the parasites.

Clinical Presentation: Severe hypertension with marked hypertrophy of the right heart.

Prognosis: The animals usually die from failure of the right heart.

Radiology: Enlargement of the main pulmonary arteries.

Pathology:

Gross: Multiple nodules several millimeters in diameter, of grayish-white color; thickening of the pulmonary artery walls.

Histology: Multiple granulomatous nodules containing eggs of various stages in the center, and histiocytes, lymphocytes, plasma cells, and multinucleated giant cells in the circumference. The media of the larger arteries are thickened and tortuous. The lumen of the vessels is narrowed by the hypertrophic and hyperplastic smooth muscle cells. The intima is usually unsuspicious.

➤ *Descriptors:* Lung parenchyma with altered structure:

- caseous epithelioid granulomas
- parasites (intragranulomatous, eggs)
- mononuclear inflammatory infiltrates
- multinucleated giant cells;
- Pulmonary vessels with altered structure:
- proliferating smooth muscle cells (medium-sized and larger arteries)
- stenosis (medium-sized pulmonary arteries)

■ *Special stains:* PAS, Giemsa, Movat, Prussian blue.

Hallmark of Diagnosis: Infectious necrotizing granulomas, identification of the worm, larvae, and eggs.

Differential diagnosis: Parasitic infections of other species.

Cement Disorders

Definition: Diseases of the lung associated with inhalation of cement particles.

Incidence/Epidemiology: Occasional development of circumscribed nodules observed on chest radiographs have been described in cement workers or in persons exposed to gypsum or limestone.

Etiology/Pathophysiology: The nonsiliceous dusts have little toxicity in man and other mammals. Gypsum, limestone, and cement do not induce pulmonary fibrosis in animal experiments and are mainly retained in the upper respiratory tract. Lung damage seen in the reported cases is probably caused by inhalation of additional amounts of quartz.

Clinical Presentation: Inhalation of high concentrations of cement may cause inflammation and swelling of the upper respiratory tract due to the hygroscopic cement particles. No specific symptoms of the lower respiratory tract are known.

Prognosis: Good and no sequelae are known.

Radiology: Dense peripheral nodules have been described in a few patients with additional exposure to quartz sand or dust.

Pathology:

Gross: No specific findings.

Histology: The findings are related to the quartz exposure and show small silicotic nodules with centrally whorled pattern of collagenous fibers surrounded by macrophages with ingested quartz particles. Inflammatory response is usually mild.

➤ *Descriptors:* Lung parenchyma with preserved structure:

- dust
- macrophages (dust-laden)
- absent inflammatory infiltrates

■ *Special stains:* PAS, collagenous stains, Prussian blue, X-ray diffraction techniques or related physical methods.

Hallmark of Diagnosis: Clinical history, dust and dust-laden macrophages, but no characteristic findings related to cement, limestone, or gypsum are known.

Differential diagnosis: Lung damage related to exposure to other agents, smoking.

Ceramic Fibers

Definition: Lung disease associated with inhalation of ceramic fibers.

Incidence/Epidemiology: Ceramic fibers consist of aluminum silicates, of which the principal ones are the kaolinite and montmorillonite (hydrated aluminum silicates). The fibers have a wide range of diameters, varying from 0.05–250 μm. They are used in materials requiring high thermal and chemical resistance, or in a broad variety of products such as toothpaste, vehicles for insecticides, cosmetics, pharmaceuticals, or as fillers in plastics, paints, and rubber. Lung damage ranging from simple radiologic findings to massive fibrosis have been reported in 5–10% of exposed workers.

Etiology/Pathophysiology: The hazard of man-made fibers including ceramic fibers depends strictly upon the diameter of the fibers due to the tendency of the fibers to be transported longitudinally with the air flow. The critical diameter of fibers which can reach the peripheral lung zones has been estimated to be 3.5 μm or less. The length of fibers penetrating the bronchioles or alveolar ducts can range up to 200 μm so long as their diameters measure less than 3.5 μm. The hazardous potential of the fibers depends upon the length, with special risk if long (> 8 μm) and thin (< 1.5 μm) ones are inhaled. Ceramic fibers are probably not as dangerous as fiberglass or asbestos fibers.

Clinical Presentation: Usually no or mild symptoms including cough, expectoration, shortness of breath.

Prognosis: Usually good; however, progressive massive fibrosis can occur. Patients have increased risk for lung cancer and probably for mesothelioma.

Radiology: Small peripherally located nodules or mild interstitial infiltrates. Signs of massive fibrosis in a few cases.

Pathology:

Gross: Thickened and fibrotic pleura, enlarged and fibrotic, dark hilar lymph nodes, several firm nodules of 4–6 mm in diameter and of grayish color, mostly occurring in the upper lung zones.

Histology: Fibrous "splitting" of the pleura with some scattered lymphocytes in the boundary, multiple dust-laden macrophages in the alveolar ducts and in the alveoli. Agglutination of kaolin surrounded by histiocytes, macrophages, lymphocytes, plasma cells, and multinucleated giant cells, and bundles of collagenous fibers. A fibrotic texture similar to silicotic nodules does not occur. The fibrosis is characterized by its diffuse pattern partly following the interalveolar septula.

➤ *Descriptors:* Lung parenchyma with altered structure:

- dust (kaolin, birefringent fibers, crystals))
- noncaseous epithelioid granulomas (ill-defined)
- mononuclear inflammatory infiltrates
- macrophages (dust-laden)
- multinucleated giant cells

- focal interstitial fibrosis (diffuse margins);
- Pleura with altered structure:
- acellular collagen (basket-weave)

■ *Special stains:* PAS, collagenous stains, Prussian blue, X-ray diffraction or similar physical techniques.

Hallmark of Diagnosis: Clinical history, identification of kaolin, noncaseous "diffuse-irregular" fibrosis.

Differential diagnosis: Pulmonary damage due to exposure to other agents, especially chalk, asbestos, fiberglass.

Cerium

Definition: Lung damage associated with exposure to cerium.

Incidence/Epidemiology: Element of the rare earth group used for polishing lenses and glassware, or as an additive for ceramics, tracer bullets, etc. No severe lung diseases related to exposure to cerium have been reported.

Etiology/Pathophysiology: Cerium belongs to the so-called inert metals. Animal experiments have failed to demonstrate major damage to the lung such as fibrosis.

Clinical Presentation: Associated symptoms are not known.

Prognosis: Good and no serious sequelae are known.

Radiology: A few cases with mild interstitial infiltrates have been reported.

Pathology:

Gross: No associated changes have been reported.

Histology: No specific reaction of the lung parenchyma has been reported.

➤ *Descriptors:* Lung parenchyma with preserved structure:

- dust (cerium)
- macrophages (dust-laden)
- absent inflammatory infiltrates

■ *Special stains:* PAS, collagenous stains, Prussian blue, X-ray diffraction or similar physical techniques.

Hallmark of Diagnosis: Clinical history, dust and dust-laden macrophages.

Differential diagnosis: Alterations of the lung parenchyma associated with other agents, smoking.

Cestodes

Definition: Infections of the lung with different genera of the subclass Cestodes, including sparganosis, cysticercosis, and echinococcosis.

Incidence/Epidemiology: The most important cestode infection in humans is caused by the *Echinococcus* worm which can be found worldwide, including Europe, North and South America, and Japan. *Taenia solium*, causing cysticercosis, is also distributed ubiquitously, whereas patients infected with a *Spirometra* species, causing sparganosis, have been most frequently reported from Malaysia, Taiwan, Paraguay, and North America.

Etiology/Pathophysiology: Sparganosis is acquired from snakes, frogs, fish, or copepods, cysticercosis most frequently by eating raw or undercooked pork, and echinococcosis from infected domestic dogs or cats. Subclassification and life cycles are discussed under the particular headings.

Clinical Presentation: Sparganosis is usually a disease of the subcutaneous fatty tissue, but three of four reported patients with pulmonary infections did not show subcutaneous nodules. Cysticercosis of the lung is usually an asymptomatic disease but may present with neurological symptoms, whereas infections with *Echinococcus* cause mechanically related symptoms due to large pulmonary cysts with pneumothorax, empyema, and recurring severe allergic reactions including anaphylactic shock.

Prognosis: Usually good; however, fatal cases have been reported which were associated with anaphylactic shock (echinococcosis), Jacksonian epilepsy, and meningitis (cysticercosis).

Radiology: Sparganosis may present with mediastinal masses with lateral shift of the heart; cysticercosis shows calcified nodules on chest X-radiographs, and echinococcosis usually produces larger cysts with sharply circumscribed orbs including smaller cysts within the larger sphere (*Echinococcus granulosus*) or multiple small dense foci of irregular shape in the peripheral lung zones or in the right lower lobe with attachment to the diaphragm and liver (*Echinococcus multilocularis*).

Pathology:

Gross: The parasite of sparganosis can be identified as a small, glistening, slowly moving, white, opaque worm between a few millimeters to some centimeters in length lying in an abscess or in a cyst. Cysticercosis usually leads to fibrotic or calcified nodules and scars of yellowish-white color without living parasites. *Echinococcus* cysts reach 20 cm in diameter and are surrounded by a 2–3 mm thick fibrotic layer. They contain a yellowish-white mucus, and are sometimes calcified.

Histology: Infections with sparganum cause the development of granulomatous reaction made up of neutrophilic granulocytes, lymphocytes, plasma cells, histiocytes, and absent or numerous eosinophilic granulocytes. The body of the worm consists of a tegument with microvilli, a double layer of smooth muscle cells, and tegumental cells. *Taenia solium* cysts are of milky-white color and up to 1 cm in diameter. The degenerated cysts are accompanied by a granulomatous reaction including histiocytes, lymphocytes, plasma cells, and numerous eosinophilic granulocytes. Residuals of cysts are fibrotic and calcified nodules. Hydatid cysts of *Echinococcus* show a surrounding layer of fibrotic tissue with some scattered lymphocytes and plasma cells. The scolices in the broad capsula have a double row of hooklets.

➤ *Descriptors:* Lung parenchyma with altered structure:
- parasites (thick tegument, two layers of smooth muscle cells, larval *Taenia solium*, cysticercosis) cysts (hydatid cysts, scolices and hooklets, intracystic, inner projections, *Echinococcus*)
- noncaseous epithelioid granulomas (*Spirometra*)
- mixed inflammatory infiltrates (*Spirometra*)
- focal interstitial fibrosis
- calcification

■ *Special stains:* PAS, collagenous stains, Movat, acid-fast stain, Giemsa.

Hallmark of Diagnosis: Clinical history, macroscopic appearance, infectious granulomas, intrapulmonary cysts, identification of parasites.

Differential diagnosis: Congenital cysts, fibrotic lesions of various causes, infections with other parasites.

Chagas Disease

Definition: Infectious disease with the protozoan *Trypanosoma cruzi* and less common with *T. rangeli*.

Incidence/Epidemiology: Human infection is common in all Central and South American countries, but rarely in the USA, Mexico, Aruba, or Trinidad. The parasites mostly infect poor people living in rural and suburban areas. About 10 million South Americans and several hundred thousand Central Americans are infected.

Etiology/Pathophysiology: The parasites circulating in the blood (trypomastigotes) invade many types of mammalian cells and live there, becoming amastigotes. Trypomastigotes are ingested by bloodsucking triatomid bugs (*Rhodnius prolixus*), and the parasites multiply in the alimentary tract of the bugs, which remain infected for life. After differentiation to metacyclic trypomastigotes, the latter are defecated onto the skin of mammals during blood sucking. Infection of mammals also occurs by ingestion of infected bugs, by contamination of mucous membranes, conjunctivae, and abraded skin. The mammalian reservoir includes marsupials, Edentata, bats, rodents, pigs, and primates. Pulmonary involvement is associated with (a) congenital infection of the lung parenchyma with amastigotes and (b) complications due to chagasic megaesophagus.

Clinical Presentation: Congenital infection causes meningoencephalitis, myocarditis, myositis, and pneumonitis with lethal outcome within the first few days of life. Usual infections cause myocarditis and encephalitis with the corresponding symptoms, including arrhythmias, hypotension, tachycardia, cardiomegaly, irritability, and drowsiness 15–25 days after contamination. Infection of the neuroglia of various organs causes massive dilatation most frequently seen in the esophagus and colon and less often in the bronchi, ureters, duodenum, and stomach. The consequences of megaesophagus are aspiration pneumonia, tuberculosis, pulmonary abscess, bronchiectasis, asthma, and pulmonary fibrosis.

Prognosis: Fatal outcome usually within 4 weeks is the general course of the disease. Pulmonary lesions are often a result of megaesophagus.

Radiology: Dilatation and loss of peristaltic movement of the esophagus, signs of pulmonary complications.

Pathology:

Gross: Enlarged and dilated heart with focal hemorrhagic and yellowish areas. The lungs show nodular grayish thickening besides possible pneumonic or necrotic areas due to aspiration.

Histology: The thickened interalveolar septula contain clusters of histiocytes and "foamy" cells with several ingested amastigotes. Scattered neutrophilic and eosinophilic granulocytes, acute edema, and endothelial swelling can be observed. In congenital infections, the amastigotes can be demonstrated in the Hofbauer cells and in the amniotic epithelial cells; in acute chagasic myocarditis, the parasites can be seen in the myofibers.

➤ *Descriptors:* Lung parenchyma with preserved structure:

- mononuclear inflammatory infiltrates (diffuse)
- macrophages (ingested amastigotes)
- histiocytes (ingested amastigotes)
- intraalveolar serous fluid
- mixed inflammatory infiltrates
- eosinophils (infrequent)

■ *Special stains:* Giemsa, reticulum stain, immunofluorescence.

Hallmark of Diagnosis: Clinical history, demonstration of amastigotes in histiocytes, myofibers, etc., or of trypomastigotes in the blood smear.

Differential diagnosis: Syphilis, hypothyroidism, primary cardiomyopathy, myocarditis of various causes.

Charcot-Leyden Crystals

Definition: Birefringent crystals related to degenerated eosinophils, see Asthma.

Cheese Washer's Lung

Definition: Allergic extrinsic alveolitis associated with inhalation of *Aspergillus clavatus.*

Incidence/Epidemiology: Rare disease seen in workers handling moldy cheese.

Etiology/Pathophysiology: Immune complex-mediated reaction of the lung parenchyma. For details, see Allergic (Extrinsic) Alveolitis.

Clinical Presentation: The disease may occur in the acute or chronic course.

Prognosis: Usually good and sequelae are rare.

Radiology: Usual signs of allergic extrinsic alveolitis, including mild diffuse alveolar infiltrates.

Pathology:

Gross: Findings of allergic extrinsic alveolitis including edema, consolidated lung tissue of grayish color.

Histology: Findings of allergic extrinsic alveolitis including interstitial mononuclear infiltrates, small nonnecrotizing granulomas, bronchiolitis obliterans.

➤ *Descriptors:* Lung parenchyma with altered structure:

- noncaseous epithelioid granulomas
- eosinophils
- multinucleated giant cells
- intrabronchiolar fibrinoid material and histiocytes
- ulceration of bronchiolar mucosa;
- Lung parenchyma with preserved structure:
- macrophages
- desquamation, hypertrophy, hyperplasia and dysplasia of pneumocytes
- mononuclear inflammatory infiltrates
- intraalveolar serous fluid

■ *Special stains:* PAS, collagenous stains, Giemsa, immunohistochemistry for immunoglobulins, endogenous lectins.

Hallmark of Diagnosis: Clinical history, noncaseating granulomatous interstitial pneumonia with additional pneumonitis (desquamation, hyperplasia, hypertrophy and dysplasia of the cells of the alveolar lining), bronchiolitis obliterans.

Differential diagnosis: Infectious granulomatous lung diseases, berylliosis, sarcoidosis.

Chemodectoma

Definition: Neoplasm of the intrapulmonary chemoreceptor organ (synonym paraganglioma).

Incidence/Epidemiology: Rare reports of neoplasms with microscopic appearance closely resembling paragangliomas, which are still controversial. So-called minute pulmonary chemodectoma are frequently multiple and occur in coincidence with other pulmonary abnormalities such as thromboembolism. These are often found incidentally in about 1:300 autopsies or surgical specimens.

Etiology/Pathophysiology: Chemoreceptor organs are reported to exist within the lung near the branching points of pulmonary arteries. The reported cases of large and so-called minute chemodectomas, however, have not shown neurosecretory granules and were ultrastructurally similar in appearance to meningiomas. Thus, the question arises whether they are actually variants of hemangiopericytomas. A few possibly true paragangliomas have been described as arising from pulmonary arteries or from small bronchioles.

Clinical Presentation: Minute chemodectomas do not cause clinically relevant symptoms, but large chemodectomas associated with pulmonary arteries yield cough and symptoms related to bronchial stenosis.

Prognosis: Usually good, local recurrence is rare, and distant metastases have not been reported.

Radiology: Minute chemodectomas are not visible on chest radiographs, but large chemodectomas show mediastinal nodules measuring 1–4 cm.

Pathology:

Gross: Minute chemodectomas measure 1–4 mm in diameter and are circumscribed, grayish-tan nodules. They are often located in the peripheral lung zones near the pleura or along the pulmonary septa. Large chemodectomas have a soft consistency and are yellowish.

Histology: The texture of both tumors is defined by nests of large tumor cells ("Zellballen") with abundant eosinophilic cytoplasm. Tumor growth seems to spread from the interalveolar septula into the alveoli with consequent occlusion of the airways in the tumor center and diffuse interstitial spread at the tumor boundaries. Necrotic areas and inflammatory response of host tissue are absent. The tumor cell nuclei contain finely dispersed chromatin located in spindle-shaped cells with indistinct cellular boundaries. The tumors contain numerous capillaries separating the tumor cells from the air spaces. Mitoses are rare.

➤ *Descriptors:* Newly formed textures without metastasis potential:
- epithelial growth pattern
- solid textures
- nests of tumor cells ("Zellballen")
- abundant cytoplasm (eosinophilic)
- spindle shaped tumor cells
- homogeneous nuclear and cellular size
- finely distributed nuclear chromatin
- absent or infrequent mitoses
- absent necrosis
- absent inflammatory infiltrates
- numerous capillaries

■ *Special stains:* PAS, collagenous stains, Giemsa, immunohistochemistry for vimentin, desmin, desmoplakin, cytokeratin, neurofilaments, neuroendocrine markers, endogenous lectins, DNA measurements, electron microscopy.

Hallmark of Diagnosis: For minute chemodectomas, size, characteristic cellular texture, "Zellballen"-grouping, features of nuclei and cytoplasm. For large chemodectomas, localization of origin, "Zellballen"-configuration, features of nuclei and cytoplasm, immunohistochemistry, electron microscopy.

Differential diagnosis: For minute chemodectomas, foci of bronchioloalveolar hyperplasia, tumorlet type of carcinoid tumors, hemangiopericytomas, metastatic paragangliomas. For large chemodectomas, metastatic paragangliomas, hemangiopericytomas, carcinoid tumors.

Chickenpox

Definition: Disease caused by primary infection with the herpes virus V-Z.

Incidence/Epidemiology: Pulmonary involvement is seen in less than 1% of primarily infected children, and in about 15% of primarily infected adults. Infection is more severe in immunocompromised patients.

Etiology/Pathophysiology: Infection with herpes virus V-Z usually occurs in the upper respiratory tract, inducing a primary viremia. A second viral replication takes place in the mononuclear phagocytic cells, leading to a second viremia with clinical symptoms. Humoral and cellular immunoresponse protect the patients against recurrence of varicella infection.

However, reactivation of latent viral inclusions in the nerve cells may lead to a painful vesicular rash in a dermatomal distribution (herpes zoster), observed more frequently in adults.

Clinical Presentation: After an incubation period of 14 days clinical symptoms of vesicular rash and mucosal vesicles appear. Pulmonary symptoms including cough, dyspnea, and hemoptysis arise 1–6 days after clinical onset of the disease. Varicella pneumonia may lead to secondary bacterial pneumonia and may heal without residual lesions or with numerous small calcified nodules, or it may develop into pulmonary fibrosis in some patients. Rare cases with sudden onset of pulmonary symptoms without preceding vesicular rash have been reported.

Prognosis: Usually good; sequelae are bacterial superinfection, chronic pneumonia and interstitial fibrosis.

Radiology: Chest radiographs are characterized by perihilar bilateral small nodules 5 mm in diameter, which may become confluent and may later calcify.

Pathology:

Gross: The lungs show multiple, small areas of necrosis and hemorrhage with denser clustering in the central zones. The trachea and larger bronchi may be red and have increased contents of mucus.

Histology: Small hemorrhagic and necrotic nodules are present near the small bronchi and bronchioles. The air spaces contain debris, fibrin, numerous neutrophilic granulocytes and in later stages lymphocytes, plasma cells, and macrophages. The interalveolar septa and cells of the alveolar lining are damaged and appear necrotic. Hyaline membranes are usually present as well as intranuclear inclusions in the alveolar lining cells which may show "ballooning", i.e., degenerative swelling with pale cytoplasm.

➤ *Descriptors:* Lung parenchyma with altered structure:
- necrosis and hemorrhage
- mixed inflammatory infiltrates
- multinucleated giant cells (inclusion bodies);
- Lung parenchyma with preserved structure:
- intraalveolar fibrinoid material
- hyaline membranes
- ballooning of pneumocytes

■ *Special stains:* PAS, Giemsa, Papanicolaou, immunofluorescence, electron microscopy.

Hallmark of Diagnosis: Clinical history, viral intranuclear inclusions, in Tzanck preparations (cytological analysis of basal cells in a dermal vesicle) multinucleated giant cells, virologic and microbiologic techniques.

Differential diagnosis: Infections with other viruses, especially herpes simplex virus.

Chlamydial Infections

Definition: Human pulmonary infection with the bacterium *Chlamydia psittaci* (psittacosis or ornithosis) or with *Chlamydia trachomatis* (infantile or adult pneumonia).

Incidence/Epidemiology: Endemic occurrences of psittacosis have been reported from Uster (Switzerland), and from the bayou region of the USA. *C. trachomatis* pneumonia develops in 10–20% of infected newborns with a favorable clinical course and in immunocompromised adults.

Etiology/Pathophysiology: Infection with *C. psittaci* occurs via the upper respiratory tract after contamination by a sick bird or carrier, usually a parrot, but also including other species. *C. trachomatis* is an infective agent of the genitourinary tract in adults. Intrapartum infection of babies is assumed to occur with a transmission rate of 50%. *Chlamydia* species are gram-negative bacteria with a different intracellular and extracellular appearance depending upon the presence of adenosine triphosphate and other metabolites in the environment. The metabolically inactive extracellular form develops into a metabolically active form after cellular ingestion. Intracellular multiplication of the active form produces multiple new organisms transducing into the inactive form prior to cell lysis.

Clinical Presentation: Incubation time with *C. psittaci* lasts approximately 7–14 days. Symptoms include headache, fever, cough. Besides the pulmonary manifestation, infections of the heart, liver, spleen, and the central nervous system have been reported. Infants infected with *C. trachomatis* usually present with mild symptoms of cough and tachypnea, similar to infected immunocompromised adults.

Prognosis: Usually good and without serious sequelae.

Radiology: Chest radiographs most often display unilateral, interstitial, patchy infiltrations within the lower lobes, a finding more dramatic than the clinical symptoms and findings.

Pathology:

Gross: Large, grayish-white areas most often located within the lower lobes.

Histology: The bronchioles and small bronchi contain dense inflammatory infiltrates made up of lymphocytes, plasma cells, and, less frequently neutrophilic granulocytes. The air spaces are filled with desquamated cells of the alveolar lining, macrophages, and edematous fluid. Hyaline membranes and diffuse alveolar damage can be observed only to a mild degree.

➤ *Descriptors:* Lung parenchyma with preserved structure:
- macrophages
- desquamation, hypertrophy, hyperplasia and dysplasia of pneumocytes
- intraalveolar serous fluid;
- Bronchial mucosa with preserved structure:
- mixed inflammatory infiltrates (dense)

■ *Special stains:* PAS, Giemsa, collagenous stains, immunofluorescence.

Hallmark of Diagnosis: Clinical history, serological examination, immunofluorescence, bronchiolitis with predominant mononuclear inflammatory infiltrates.

Differential diagnosis: Pulmonary infections with other organisms including *Mycoplasma, Rickettsia, Coxiella.*

Chlorambucil

Definition: Alteration of the lung parenchyma associated with intake of chlorambucil, see Drug Toxicity.

Chlordiazepoxide

Definition: Alteration of the lung parenchyma associated with intake of chlordiazepoxide, see Drug Toxicity.

Chlorine Gas

Definition: Lung damage associated with inhalation of chlorine gas.

Incidence/Epidemiology: Chlorine gas is used as a disinfectant and is usually conveyed in liquid form. It releases hydrochloric acid which acts as an oxidant. Accidental inhalations have been reported.

Etiology/Pathophysiology: Inhalation of toxic concentrations causes diffuse alveolar damage with acute pulmonary edema followed by hyaline membrane formation.

Clinical Presentation: Symptoms include cough, dyspnea, tachypnea, shortness of breath. Long-term damage of the lung probably does not occur.

Prognosis: Usually good; sequelae are rare but may present with chronic bronchitis, squamous metaplasia and dysplasia of the bronchial epithelial cells.

Radiology: Diffuse bilateral patchy densities of various degrees.

Pathology:

Gross: Edematous, swollen walls of the trachea and bronchi with an inflammatory red mucosa. Heavy, edematous lungs which may show areas of consolidation after several days.

Histology: Diffuse alveolar damage including intraalveolar edema, desquamation of cells of the alveolar lining, hyaline membranes, and neutrophilic granulocytes, later replaced by mononuclear infiltrates.

➤ *Descriptors:* Lung parenchyma with preserved structure:
- intraalveolar serous fluid
- hyaline membranes
- mixed inflammatory infiltrates;
- Bronchial mucosa with altered structure:
- squamous metaplasia and dysplasia
- mononuclear inflammatory infiltrates

■ *Special stains:* PAS, Giemsa, endogenous lectins.

Hallmark of Diagnosis: Clinical history, diffuse alveolar damage.

Differential diagnosis: Early onset of infectious pneumonia.

Chlorine Thiazole

Definition: Alteration of the lung parenchyma associated with intake of chlorine thiazole, see Drug Toxicity.

Chloromethylether

Definition: Patients exposed to chloromethylether have an increased risk of lung cancer, see Cancer of the Lung.

Chlorozotocin

Definition: Alteration of the lung parenchyma associated with intake of chlorozotocin, see Drug Toxicity.

Chlorphentermine

Definition: Alteration of the lung parenchyma associated with intake of chlorphentermine, see Drug Toxicity.

Chlorpromazine

Definition: Alteration of the lung parenchyma associated with intake of chlorpromazine, see Drug Toxicity.

Chlorpropamide

Definition: Alteration of the lung parenchyma associated with intake of chlorpropamide, see Drug Toxicity.

Chlorthalidone

Definition: Alteration of the lung parenchyma associated with intake of chlorthalidone, see Drug Toxicity.

Chondroblastoma

Definition: Benign tumor of cartilaginous origin of trachea or major bronchi.

Incidence/Epidemiology: Very rare tumor of the major airways.

Etiology/Pathophysiology: The detailed pathogenesis is unknown. It is suggested that the tumors have their origin from reticulohistiocytes or related cells or "as a reaction of normal cartilage cells to an altered local environment."

Prognosis: Usually good, but sequelae are related to the stenosis of the proximal airways.

Clinical Presentation: The symptoms are related to bronchial stenosis caused by the tumors.

Radiology: Chest radiographs may be unsuspicious. Tomograms usually show bronchial stenosis.

Pathology:

Gross: Firm, gray-yellowish tumors with partial occlusion of the bronchial lumen.

Histology: The characteristic cells (chondroblasts) are of spindle shape with oval to round nuclei. Nucleoli are usually present. These spindle cells grow in fiberlike textures and characteristically contain scattered giant cells and foci of calcification of individual cells. Mitoses are infrequent. Necroses and inflammatory infiltrations are usually lacking. The tumor cells have a broad connection to the original cartilage.

➤ *Descriptors:* Newly formed textures without metastasis potential:
- mesenchymal growth pattern
- chondromatous textures
- fibromatous textures
- chondroblasts (bronchial submucosa)
- spindle-shaped tumor cells (adjacent to original bronchus)
- prominent nucleoli
- absent or infrequent mitoses
- homogeneous nuclear and cellular size
- multinucleated giant cells
- calcification
- absent necrosis
- absent inflammatory infiltrates

■ *Special stains:* PAS, Giemsa, reticulin stain, DNA and syntactic structure analysis.

Hallmark of Diagnosis: Localization of the tumor, presence of chondroblasts with foci of calcified individual cells.

Differential diagnosis: Hamartoma, chondroma, chondrosarcoma, chondropathia osteoplastica, cartilaginous proliferation.

Chondroma

Definition: Benign tumor of the trachea and major bronchi arising from preexisting cartilage.

Incidence/Epidemiology: Very rare tumor occurring at any age. Manifestation of extraadrenal paraganglioma, gastric leiomyosarcoma, and pulmonary chondroma has been described in a young woman (Carney's triad).

Etiology/Pathophysiology: The tumors are assumed to develop from the perichondrium or preexisting cartilage and should not be confused with the much more common hamartomas.

Clinical Presentation: Symptoms are related to submucosal growth of the tumors within the trachea or proximal bronchi, causing stenosis of the proximal airways.

Prognosis: Good, as the slow increase in size usually takes years.

Radiology: Chest radiographs may be normal. Chest tomographs usually show the narrowing of the tracheal/bronchial lumen associated with a submucosal mass.

Pathology:

Gross: Firm, irregularly formed, white tumors with narrowing of the tracheal lumen and shiny surface. The tumors usually measure a few centimeters in diameter.

Histology: Proliferation of cartilaginous mature cells adjacent to the cartilage rings of the trachea/bronchus. Ossification and calcification may be present. Necrosis and inflammatory infiltrations as well as invasion with capillaries are lacking. Inclusion areas of mature fat cells or fibromatous cells cannot be observed. Mitoses are very rare or absent.

➤ *Descriptors:* Newly formed textures without metastasis potential:

- mesenchymal growth pattern
- chondromatous textures
- homogeneous nuclear and cellular size
- ossification (center)
- calcification (center)
- absent or infrequent mitoses
- absent necrosis
- absent inflammatory infiltrates

■ *Special stains:* PAS, Giemsa.

Hallmark of Diagnosis: Localization of the tumor, mature proliferation of cartilaginous cells with connection to the perichondrium of the cartilaginous rings.

Differential diagnosis: Chondroblastoma, hamartoma, cartilaginous proliferation, bronchopathia osteoplastica.

Chondromalacia

Definition: Degenerative disorder of bronchial/tracheal cartilage and that of other tissues with glycosaminoglycan content such as sclera, cornea, aorta, noncartilaginous ear parts (synonym relapsing polychondritis).

Incidence/Epidemiology: Rare disease affecting both sexes equally, most frequently in the 5th decade.

Etiology/Pathophysiology: The etiology of the disease is unknown. Immunologic studies have failed to demonstrate antibodies against cartilage. No congenital or familial disposition can be proven.

Clinical Presentation: The disease starts in the majority of cases with chondritis of the auricles and migratory arthritis (nonerosive, seronegative polyarthritis). Nasal chondritis, ocular inflammation, cochlear or vestibular complications, and tracheal or bronchial chondritis will follow. The disease is episodic, in periods lasting for 5–10 days, and slowly progressive. Pulmonary symptoms include stridor, asthmalike dyspnea, cough, and symptoms related to pulmonary complications such as pneumonia.

Prognosis: Fair, as slow progression lasting for decades is the usual course.

Radiology: Severe cases present with disappearance of tracheal air shadow and overinflation of the peripheral lung zones.

Pathology:

Gross: The trachea/bronchi/larynx are soft with diminished lumen due to dissolution of cartilage, which may be nearly complete.

Histology: The first morphological symptom is the loss of acid mucopolysaccharides in the cartilage followed by perichondrial inflammatory mononuclear infiltrates and loss of cartilaginous tissue beginning at the boundary. The border between the cartilage and the connective tissue becomes indistinct, and the width of the cartilage shrinks, leaving "ruins" of scattered islands of cartilaginous tissue. Dystrophic calcification or ossification are sometimes present.

➤ *Descriptors:* Bronchial mucosa with altered structure:

- decreased size of cartilage
- mononuclear inflammatory infiltrates
- erosion of cartilage
- fibrosis
- calcification (dystrophic)
- ossification (dystrophic)

■ *Special stains:* PAS, Giemsa, collagenous stains, immunohistochemistry for immunoglobulins and complement C3.

Hallmark of Diagnosis: Clinical history, loss of cartilage and replacement by connective tissue and chronic inflammatory infiltrates.

Differential diagnosis: Atrophy of cartilage, Williams-Campbell syndrome, tracheo/bronchomalacia, traumatic lesions.

Chondrosarcoma

Definition: Malignant tumor of the lung with chondromatous differentiation.

Incidence/Epidemiology: Rare malignancy occurring with equal frequency in males and females. No associated risk factors are known.

Etiology/Pathophysiology: The majority of these tumors arise in the peripheral lung zones; only a few cases have been related to tracheal/bronchial cartilage. Chondromatous differentiation may be found in a variety of other tumors such as epithelioid hemangioendothelioma of the lung.

Clinical Presentation: The tumors do not cause specific symptoms and may be detected accidentally due to their growth in the peripheral lung zones.

Prognosis: Poor, as more than 90% of patients die within the 1st year after diagnosis.

Radiology: Circumscribed peripheral nodules which may show calcification (ossification).

Pathology:

Gross: Firm, variegated, shiny, nodular, grayish-white tumors. Cysts, calcification, necrosis, and hemorrhage are usually present.

Histology: The tumors consist of large, oval cells with bizarre nuclei having one or more prominent nucleoli. The regular pattern of cartilage is lost. The nuclei and the tumor cells vary enormously in size and configuration. Immature ossification may be present. Necrotic areas and intratumorous hemorrhage can easily be demonstrated. Inflammatory infiltrations are inconspicuous. Mitotic figures are frequent.

➤ *Descriptors:* Newly formed textures with metastasis potential:

- mesenchymal growth pattern
- chondromatous textures
- sarcomatous textures
- large tumor cells (spindle-shaped)
- inhomogeneous nuclear and cellular size
- prominent nucleoli
- frequent mitoses
- necrosis and hemorrhage
- absent or weak inflammatory infiltrates
- micrometastases

■ *Special stains:* PAS, Giemsa, collagenous stains, DNA analysis, endogenous lectins, immunohistochemistry for Factor VIII or related endothelial markers.

Hallmark of Diagnosis: Clinical history (for excluding metastatic growth), sarcomatous tumor with cartilaginous differentiation.

Differential diagnosis: Metastatic chondrosarcoma, epithelioid hemangioendothelioma (formerly IVBAT, intravascular bronchioloalveolar tumor).

Choriocarcinoma

Definition: Metastases of choriocarcinoma into the lung may occasionally occur, see Metastases into the Lung.

Chromate

Definition: Patients with exposure to chromate have an increased risk of lung cancer, see Cancer of the Lung, Chromium Disorders.

Chromium Disorders

Definition: Lung disease associated with exposure to chromium (chromite).

Incidence/Epidemiology: Exposure to chromium (chromite) may occur in chromite mines (Russia, Turkey, South Africa), in manufacturing of dye, chrome pigment, or chromate sprays, or in metal polishing procedures. Associated risks include interstitial fibrosis and lung cancer, especially epidermoid carcinoma and undifferentiated carcinoma, with an estimated risk factor 30–50 times that of the population of nonsmokers.

Etiology/Pathophysiology: Exposure to bivalent chromium is assumed to be of special hazard, whereas exposure to trivalent chromium does not increase the risk of lung cancer. The etiology and pathophysiology of lung damage are not known.

Clinical Presentation: Contact with chromate causes sensitization of the skin and sometimes perforation of the nasal septum. Lung symptoms include cough, dyspnea, shortness of breath, and lung cancer-related alterations.

Prognosis: Fair, progressive respiratory failure and increased risk of lung cancer have been described.

Radiology: Diffuse interstitial densities indicate interstitial fibrosis which varies in its degree. Chromium-associated lung carcinomas are usually localized in the central lung zones.

Pathology:

Gross: Findings related to the degree of fibrosis ranging from inconspicuous lung parenchyma to honeycombing. Pleural plaques may be present.

Histology: Focal aggregations of extracellular birefringent black material surrounded by macrophages and histiocytes. The interstitial fibrosis is of the "diffuse" type and varies in degree. Squamous metaplasia of the bronchial epithelial cells with moderate to marked dysplasia indicate the carcinogenic potency, and lung carcinoma may be present.

➤ *Descriptors:* Lung parenchyma with altered structure:

- dust (birefringent crystals)
- macrophages (dust-laden)
- mononuclear inflammatory infiltrates
- diffuse interstitial fibrosis;
- Lung parenchyma with preserved structure:
- desquamation, hypertrophy, hyperplasia and dysplasia of pneumocytes;
- Bronchial mucosa with altered structure:
- squamous metaplasia and dysplasia (marked)

■ *Special stains:* PAS, collagenous stains, X-ray diffraction methods and related physical techniques, endogenous lectins.

Hallmark of Diagnosis: Clinical history, birefringent black extracellular deposits, interstitial fibrosis of various degrees, identification of chromium with physical techniques.

Differential diagnosis: Exposure to other metallic dusts, endogenous fibrosis, or tobacco-related lung cancer.

Chronic Airflow Obstruction

Definition: Lung damage associated with persistent abnormalities of expiratory flow.

Incidence/Epidemiology: The most important factor associated with obstructive air flow is tobacco smoke. Other factors are toxic gases (ammonia, sulfur dioxide, oxides of nitrogen), allergic agents including drugs (penicillamine), viral infections, metallic, carbonic, and silicotic dusts, and other environmental air pollutants. Related lung damage affects 10–25% of all adult persons and 5–10% of children.

Etiology/Pathophysiology: The flow of air or the amount of air exchange is determined by two factors: (a) the resistance of the system, and (b) the applied force. The expiratory airway resistance as measured by the forced expiratory volume in 1 s (FEV1) is 80–90% of that determined by the resistance of the proximal airways as predicted by the Weibel model. Obstructive damage of bronchioles and small bronchi will not contribute to the total resistance of airway flow to a considerable degree as long as it does not affect large areas of both lungs. Obstructive lesions of the small airways lead to mild chronic airflow obstruction with focal damage of the related alveoli. Consequences are mural inflammation, focal interstitial fibrosis, emphysematous changes, cor pulmonale. Obstruction of the larger bronchi leads to poststenotic bronchiectasis and emphysematous changes of larger portions of the lung including emphysematous cysts.

Clinical Presentation: Chronic airway obstruction includes a variety of different diseases such as nonspecific chronic bronchiolitis, rheumatoid bronchiolitis, bronchiolitis obliterans, chronic hypersecretive bronchitis, focal stenosis of proximal airways due to congenital disorders, chronic infectious diseases (tuberculosis), bronchial carcinoma, vascular abnormalities, parasitic infections. Related clinical symptoms and (emphysematous) changes of the lung parenchyma are described under their particular headings.

Prognosis: Slow progression of the disease is the common course.

Radiology: The characteristic changes are described under their particular headings.

Pathology:

Gross: The gross findings present enlarged peripheral lung zones (emphysema) with varying positional and structural distribution depending upon the degree and nature of the stenotic lesions and are described under their particular headings.

Histology: The degree of inflammatory infiltrates in the bronchioles is classified by the amount of mononuclear infiltrate in the bronchiolar wall, ranging from scattered lymphocytes/plasma cells to pseudofollicular arrangement, and by the degree of hypertrophic changes of the epithelial cells. Proximal stenotic lesions are best described by the percentage of the lumen with air passage and by the length of the lesion. Quantitative changes in the size of submucous glands seen on a histological cross-section are best computed by the Reid index, which is the ratio of the maximum thickness of a mucus gland internal to the cartilage divided by the bronchial wall thickness. The frequency distribution of the Reid index is unimodal with a broad peak (0.35–0.55) in nonbronchitic patients and a similar peak (0.5–65) in chronic bronchitic patients. A different approach measuring the volume fraction of submucosal glands or the absolute size of glands is superior to the Reid index, and the reported results correlate more strictly with the clinical situation.

➤ *Descriptors:* Bronchial mucosa with preserved structure:

- eosinophils
- mononuclear inflammatory infiltrates (bronchial and bronchiolar wall)
- hyperplasia of submucosal glands
- hyaline basal membrane
- increased number of goblet cells
- viscous mucus
- fungus (intrabronchial)
- parasites (intrabronchial);
- Bronchial mucosa with altered structure:
- squamous metaplasia and dysplasia
- noncaseous epithelioid granulomas (ill-defined);
- Lung parenchyma with altered structure:
- intrabronchiolar fibrinoid material and histiocytes
- ulceration of bronchiolar mucosa

■ *Special stains:* PAS, collagenous stains, Giemsa.

Hallmark of Diagnosis: Clinical history, lung function tests, quantitation of morphologic changes in the bronchioles or larger bronchi.

Differential diagnosis: According to the specific morphological alterations.

Churg-Strauss Syndrome

Definition: Chronic inflammatory disorder of the lung characterized by vasculitis, necrotizing granulomatous inflammation and eosinophilia, see Allergic Angiitis and Granulomatosis.

Chylothorax

Definition: Pleural effusion consisting of chylus.

Incidence/Epidemiology: Usually a rare disease. However, in thoracic hospitals it is not infrequently seen after extensive surgery of bronchial carcinoma with rupture of the ductus thoracicus, or in association with trauma. A frequent complication in lymphangioleiomyomatosis.

Etiology/Pathophysiology: Rupture of the thoracic duct causes penetration of chylus into the pleural cavity.

Clinical Presentation: Pleural effusion after surgical procedures, which may amount to several liters a day.

Prognosis: Usually good.

Radiology: Left- or right-sided pleural effusion with homogeneous shadowing of a complete lung.

Pathology:

Gross: Milky, grayish-white effusion.

Histology: Proteinous liquid with some scattered lymphocytes and plasma cells.

➤ *Descriptors:* Pleura with preserved structure:

- mononuclear inflammatory infiltrates
- proteinous pleural effusion

■ *Special stains:* Papanicolaou, PAS.

Hallmark of Diagnosis: Macroscopic appearance of effusion, clinical history.

Differential diagnosis: Due to underlying cause.

Clear Cell Carcinoma of the Lung

Definition: Malignant tumor of the lung, a subentity of large cell anaplastic carcinoma.
Incidence/Epidemiology: Clear cell carcinoma contributes less than 10% to all large cell carcinomas. It has the same association with carcinogenic risk factors as the other carcinomas of the lower respiratory tract.
Etiology/Pathophysiology: Tumor cells with "clear-cell" appearance are frequently seen in all types of non-small cell carcinoma of the lung. Clear cell carcinoma can be classified into undifferentiated adenocarcinoma or epidermoid carcinoma by electron microscopy, and thus presents a certain special cellular morphology among the more common lung carcinomas.
Clinical Presentation: The majority of clear cell carcinomas arise from the central lung zones and cause obstruction-related symptoms.
Prognosis: Similar to that of the common lung carcinomas.
Radiology: Centrally or peripherally localized dense masses with some necrotic features.
Pathology:
Gross: White or yellowish tumors measuring about 4 cm in maximum diameter with focal areas of necrosis.
Histology: The tumors consist of large, irregularly shaped tumor cells with abundant pale cytoplasm and small, round nuclei. Textural patterns are not visible. Mitotic figures are rare. The tumor cells tend to proliferate inside the air spaces with preserved interalveolar septula. Inflammatory response of the host tissue is not a predominant feature. Small foci of hemorrhage and necrosis are usually present. The tumors closely resemble metastatic hypernephroid carcinoma.

➤ *Descriptors:* Newly formed textures with metastasis potential:
- epithelial growth pattern
- solid textures
- large tumor cells (pale cytoplasm)
- small nuclei (round)
- homogeneous nuclear and cellular size
- finely distributed nuclear chromatin
- infrequent mitoses
- necrosis and hemorrhage
- absent or weak inflammatory infiltrates

■ *Special stains:* PAS, Giemsa, collagenous stains, immunohistochemistry for exclusion of hypernephroid carcinoma, DNA analysis, endogenous lectins.

Hallmark of Diagnosis: "Clear" large tumor cells, clinical history, thorough exclusion of metastatic hypernephroid carcinoma.
Differential diagnosis: Metastatic hypernephroid carcinoma, benign clear cell tumor of the lung (sugar tumor).

Coal Worker's Pneumoconiosis

Definition: Damage of the lung associated with inhalation of coal dust.
Incidence/Epidemiology: The prevalence was reported to range up to 10% in 1960 and decreased to 2% in 1983. The hazard for anthracite miners (14% with complicated diseases) is greater than that for bituminous miners (2.5%). In modern mines the risk for man working 35 years at a dust concentration of 4.3 mg/m^3 amounts to 3.4% for developing simple pneumoconiosis of radiologic category II. The prevalence depends, in addition, upon the individual coal-mine characteristics.
Etiology/Pathophysiology: The dust in coal mines is made up of a mixture of various substances such as lignite (brown coal), bituminous coal, and anthracite, and in addition, contains 2–8% quartz. The development of simple and complicated pneumoconiosis depends upon the balance between different components of stimuli and responses such as the composition of the dust, the inflammatory response, infectious factors, lipid involvement, and immunologic factors. Coal particles are ingested by macrophages which tend to agglutinate around the respiratory bronchioles, leaving inert deposits of coal particles. The deposits of dust particles are associated with emphysematous alterations of the respiratory bronchioles (proximal acinar emphysema). Induction of massive fibrosis in coal miners still remains unclear. Evidence exists that the amount of inhaled dust and a higher mineral content are directly associated with progressive radiologic changes in simple pneumoconiosis. However,

no association between the content of quartz particles and the degree of massive fibrosis has been established. Subclinical infection with tubercle bacilli in relation to the development of massive fibrosis is still discussed controversially. Coal-mine dust is less toxic to macrophages than silica. The defence system of the lung exposed to coal dust may thus be more effective for resistance to tubercular infection, and fibrotic lesions may develop by bacterially stimulated functional activity of the mononuclear phagocytic system. This concept has been confirmed in animal experiments but is questioned by various authors due to inconsistent epidemiologic findings. Immunologic analysis has shown increased serum levels of IgA and IgG in miners with massive fibrosis. Alterations of the T- and B-lymphocytic systems and of the histocompatibility antigens could not be observed. Increased risk of lung cancer in coal miners as well as a reduced length of survival could not be confirmed in epidemiologic studies. Still debated is the increased risk of stomach cancer in coal miners. Reported increased rates of lung cancer in gas and coke oven workers is believed to be related to exposure to polycyclic aromatic hydrocarbons.

Clinical Presentation: Clinical control of coal workers includes lung function tests measuring obstructive and restrictive changes in air flow, the physiologic dead space, etc., which are related to the amount of fibrosis and emphysematous changes in the lungs. Increase of breathlessness is not strictly related to the radiologic categories. Life expectancy is related to the amount of massive fibrosis and the magnitude of residual volume.

Prognosis: Usually good; however, slow progression of respiratory failure and sequelae (tuberculosis, rheumatoid involvement, and focal honeycombing) can occur.

Radiology: Dust lesions show up on chest radiographs as rounded (ranular) opacities superimposed with macular shadows. The ILO scheme differentiates between small nodules (p-nodules, less than 1.5 mm in diameter), intermediate nodules (q-nodules, measuring 1.5–3 mm in maximum diameter), and large nodules (r-nodules, measuring 3–10 mm in maximum diameter). The number of nodules is scaled with additional numbers ranging from 1 to 3. Large confluent masses with rare characteristics are divided into separate masses measuring 1–5 cm, confluent masses less than a whole upper lobe, and larger densities. Further abnormalities such as emphysema, tuberculous lesions, etc. are documented separately.

Pathology:

Gross: The alterations of lung parenchyma can be classified into simple and complicated pneumoconiosis. The same morphological changes are also seen in pneumoconiosis associated with exposure to graphite (graphite pneumoconiosis) and carbon (carbon pneumoconiosis). In simple pneumoconiosis, the lungs show multiple, small, deep black nodules (2–5 mm). In and around the nodules enlarged air spaces are seen, whereas the unaffected parts of the lungs are normal. The coal deposits are of firm consistency and palpable. In complicated pneumoconiosis, massive, hard, black lesions measuring several centimeters across are usually situated in the upper lobes, and some of them may show necrotic liquefaction. Reactive pleural fibrosis and adhesions are common. The hilar lymph nodes are enlarged and contain deposits of homogeneous black material. Emphysematous changes vary in degree and may even achieve honeycombing.

Histology: Four characteristic features of simple pneumoconiosis are found: (a) large deposits of black dust particles enclosing the respiratory bronchioles; (b) poor development of connective tissue and missing inflammatory response within and around these deposits; (c) emphysematous enlargement of the respiratory bronchioles that are surrounded by the deposits; (d) clear-cut boundaries of the lesions with adjacent unaltered lung parenchyma. Demonstration of birefringent crystals is usually not possible. The overall texture of the lung tissue is not altered except by focal proximal acinar emphysema. Dust-laden macrophages located within the alveoli are not a characteristic feature of coal worker's pneumoconiosis and are usually seen in heavy smokers. Complicated pneumoconiosis is characterized by large amounts of collagenous fibers intermingled with dust deposits. Focal colliquative necrotic areas are usually present. The emphysematous changes may result in complete alteration of the normal lung texture. The amount of inflammatory (mononuclear) infiltration is increased, but in general it is inconspicuous. The intrapulmonary lymph nodes are fibrotically altered by large amounts of dust deposits. The fibrotic changes affect the arteries and veins to the same degree as the involved smaller and larger bronchi and lead to complete occlusion of the lumens, partially caused by additional thrombotic lesions.

➤ *Descriptors:* Lung parenchyma with altered structure:
- dust
- macrophages (dust-laden)
- mononuclear inflammatory infiltrates (weak)
- necrosis (focal colliquative);
- Lung parenchyma with preserved structure:
- enlarged distant air spaces (adjacent)
- Bronchial mucosa with altered structure:
- fibrosis (bronchiolar and bronchial walls)
- dust (in lymphatic vessels)

■ *Special stains:* Collagenous stains, Prussian blue, X-ray diffraction techniques for identification of additional inhaled particles such as iron, calcium, etc.

Hallmark of Diagnosis: Macroscopic appearance of "black lung", clinical history, radiologic findings, deposits of black material ensheathing the respiratory bronchioles, proximal acinar emphysema, missing inflammatory infiltrations, irregular mixture of massive fibrosis with deposits of black material, colliquative necrosis.

Differential diagnosis: Silicopneumoconiosis, "heavy smoker's lung".

Cobalt Pneumoconiosis

Definition: Lung damage associated with exposure to cobalt.

Incidence/Epidemiology: Cobalt is used as a binder in the production of tungsten carbide and is usually involved in tungsten carbide pneumoconiosis. Cobalt concentrations above 500 $\mu g/m^3$ are considered to be related to the occurrence of fibrotic lung disease in tungsten carbide workers.

Etiology/Pathophysiology: It is assumed that cobalt interacts as a hapten with the lung tissue and consequently causes abnormalities of immunologic response related to the hypersensitivity reaction.

Clinical Presentation: Symptoms are related to obstructive airways disease and may resemble asthma. Progression to massive interstitial fibrosis has been reported.

Prognosis: Fair, but slow progressive respiratory failure is a common course.

Radiology: Diffuse small densities with additional signs of interstitial fibrosis of various degrees.

Pathology:

Gross: Heavy, firm lungs with small granular densities of grayish color.

Histology: The peripheral lung parenchyma contains noncaseating epithelioid granulomas with scattered multinucleated giant cells. Hyperplasia and cellular atypias of cells of the alveolar lining may be seen as well as squamous metaplasia of bronchial epithelial cells. The changes resemble hypersensitivity pneumonitis. Diffuse interstitial fibrosis with moderate amounts of inflammatory mononuclear infiltrates can be demonstrated in more advanced cases. Most particles cannot be identified by light microscopy due to their small size.

➤ *Descriptors:* Lung parenchyma with altered structure:
- noncaseous epithelioid granulomas
- multinucleated giant cells
- macrophages
- diffuse interstitial fibrosis;
- Lung parenchyma with preserved structure:
- desquamation, hypertrophy, hyperplasia and dysplasia of pneumocytes;
- Bronchial mucosa with altered structure:
- squamous metaplasia and dysplasia

■ *Special stains:* Collagenous stains, PAS, Prussian blue, X-ray diffraction techniques and related physical methods (mass spectrometry), endogenous lectins.

Hallmark of Diagnosis: Clinical history, morphological changes resembling allergic extrinsic alveolitis, identification of cobalt by physical techniques.

Differential diagnosis: Allergic extrinsic alveolitis, sarcoidosis, berylliosis, granulomatous infectious diseases.

Coccidioidomycosis

Definition: Infectious lung disease associated with the dimorphic saprophytic fungus *Coccidioides immitis*.

Incidence/Epidemiology: The fungus grows in dry warm soil and is endemic in the southwestern states of the USA, Mexico, Venezuela, Argentina, and Paraguay. Approximately 100 000 persons are infected each year in the USA, usually persons living in rural areas.

Etiology/Pathophysiology: The fungus replicates asexually in mammalian tissue by endosporulation in the form of spherules. The spherules measure 30–100 μm across and are surrounded by a 3 μm thick capsula. The spherules rupture, and the released endospores grow and repeat the cycle. Human infection is usually caused by inhalation of the organisms.

Clinical Presentation: The clinical course ranges from asymptomatic self-healing infection (60% of patients) with mild, nonspecific complaints to acute febrile pneumonia. The majority of patients recover after 6–8 weeks, but about 5% develop persistent pneumonia with fever, cough, chest pain, and hemoptysis. Extrapulmonary dissemination amounts to 1% of infected patients, especially in immunocompromised patients, blacks, Mexicans, Filipinos, American Indians, and pregnant women. Affected organs include the meninges, the liver, joints, bones, spleen, genitourinary tract.

Prognosis: Usually good; about 1 patient out of 1 000 newly infected cases has a fatal outcome.

Radiology: Chest radiographs show soft, patchy, or hazy infiltrates mimicking atypical pneumonia. Fibronodular lesions and multiple cavities are usually present in chronic persistent infections.

Pathology:

Gross: Noncaseating nodules measuring a few centimeters in diameter indicate chronic persistent infection. They are of soft consistency and grayish-brown. Primary pulmonary infections show dense, irregular, grayish-white areas of suppurative pneumonic infiltration.

Histology: In the acute stage one finds numerous spherules within inflammatory lung tissue mixed with neutrophilic and eosinophilic granulocytes, lymphocytes, plasma cells, and histiocytes. The fibrocaseous nodules of the persistent stage show central caseous necrosis and spherules at the boundary ensheathed with connective tissue, histiocytes, and focal multinucleated giant cells.

➤ *Descriptors:* Lung parenchyma with altered structure:

- caseous epithelioid granulomas
- fungus (intragranulomatous, numerous spherules)
- mixed inflammatory infiltrates
- eosinophils
- palisading histiocytes
- multinucleated giant cells
- focal interstitial fibrosis (at the margin)

■ *Special stains:* PAS, collagenous stains, Gomori's methenamine silver stains, immunofluorescence.

Hallmark of Diagnosis: Clinical history, skin and serologic tests, granulomatous inflammation with identification of *Coccidioides immites* spherules.

Differential diagnosis: Other granulomatous fungal infections such as histoplasmosis, cryptococcosis, blastomycosis.

Codeine

Definition: Alteration of the lung parenchyma associated with intake of codeine, see Drug Toxicity.

Coffee Worker's Lung

Definition: Lung damage associated with exposure to coffee bean dust.

Incidence/Epidemiology: Rare disease.

Etiology/Pathophysiology: Allergic extrinsic alveolitis with unknown antigen.

Clinical Presentation: Acute and chronic courses occur.

Prognosis: Usually good and without serious sequelae.

Radiology: Chest radiographs are normal or show diffuse, soft, interstitial infiltrates or fine granular densities.

Pathology:

Gross: The lungs are of normal color and consistency, or may display small, firm, reddish-gray nodules.

Histology: The characteristic findings include nonnecrotizing epithelioid granulomas near the terminal bronchioles, desquamation, hypertrophy and hyperplasia of cells of the alveolar lining, marked eosinophilic inflammatory infiltrates, bronchiolitis obliterans, and focal acute vasculitis. For details, see Allergic (Extrinsic) Alveolitis.

➤ *Descriptors:* Lung parenchyma with altered structure:

- noncaseous epithelioid granulomas
- eosinophils
- multinucleated giant cells
- intrabronchiolar fibrinoid material and histiocytes
- ulceration of bronchiolar mucosa;
- Lung parenchyma with preserved structure:
- macrophages
- desquamation, hypertrophy, hyperplasia and dysplasia of pneumocytes
- mononuclear inflammatory infiltrates
- intraalveolar serous fluid

■ *Special stains:* PAS, collagenous stains, Giemsa. For details, see Allergic (Extrinsic) Alveolitis.

Hallmark of Diagnosis: Clinical history, nonnecrotizing epithelioid granulomas, morphologic findings related to desquamative interstitial pneumonia, lymphoid interstitial pneumonia, bronchiolitis obliterans.

Differential diagnosis: Infectious and non-infectious granulomatous diseases such as sarcoidosis, fungal infections or berylliosis. For details, see Allergic (Extrinsic) Alveolitis.

Colchicine

Definition: Alteration of the lung parenchyma associated with intake of colchicine, see Drug Toxicity.

Community Acquired Pneumonias

Definition: Infectious lung diseases acquired outside the environment of hospitalization.

Incidence/Epidemiology: Not infrequently seen in persons with diminished defence mechanisms of the lung such as alcoholics, diabetics, persons with malnutrition or poor oral hygiene, aged persons, or persons with preexisting viral illnesses.

Etiology/Pathophysiology: The pneumonias usually include bacterial infections caused by *Pneumococcus pneumoniae, Klebsiella pneumoniae* (Friedländer pneumonia), *Legionella, Staphylococcus aureus, Streptococcus,* and *Hemophilus influenzae.* The infections progress through four stages: (a) congestive or edematous stage, (b) red hepatization stage, (c) gray hepatization stage, (d) resolution stage.

Clinical Presentation: Community acquired pneumonias usually have an acute onset with severe illness including high fever, malaise, dyspnea, headache, and chills. The mortality rate is high if the patient is not treated or inadequately so.

Prognosis: Fair, but it can be poor if sequelae develop such as adult respiratory distress syndrome (pneumococcal pneumonia), fibrosis (*Klebsiella* and *Legionella* pneumonia).

Radiology: Pneumonic infiltrations according to the extent and anatomy of the infection.

Pathology:

Gross: Depending upon the stage, heavy edematous and hyperemic lungs (stage 1), wet and firm lung areas red in color (stage 2), firm, consolidated, grayish areas (stage 3), and wet lungs of normal appearance with small grayish foci (stage 4).

Histology: Microscopically the four stages display (a) extensive intraalveolar edema with hemorrhage and invading neutrophilic granulocytes, (b) deposits of fibrin mixed with erythrocytes and scattered neutrophilic granulocytes in the air spaces, (c) massive numbers of neutrophilic granulocytes, plasma cells, lymphocytes and macrophages in the air spaces with cellular degeneration, (d) resolution of the exudate with decreasing number of granulocytes and restoration of the interalveolar septula. Pneumococcal pneumonia shows preservation of the lung texture during the acute phase with nearly obligatory bacteremia. *Klebsiella* pneumonias are usually characterized by increased numbers of macrophages during the acute stages with intracellular bacilli being demonstrable with methenamine silver stain. *Legionella* usually produces fibrinopurulent lung areas in which the bacilli can be demonstrated by the (nonspecific) Dieterle or Warthin-Starry procedure. *Staphylococcus* pneumonia may be accompanied by severe pleuritis and may manifest abscess formation. A special disease course associated with a chronic pneumonia syndrome called botryomycosis is accompanied by scarring, abscess formation, and histologically so-called sulfur granules (a mass of basophilic microorganisms embedded within hyaline material). Streptococcal bacteria are gram-positive and can be recognized in the infected lung zones by their typical arrangement into chains or pairs. *Hemophilus* pneumonia is destructive in nature and may lead to bronchiolitis obliterans. The bacilli are difficult to demonstrate on histological slides.

➤ *Descriptors:* Lung parenchyma with preserved structure:
- intraalveolar serous fluid
- hemorrhage
- bacteria
- neutrophils
- degeneration of pneumocytes
- mononuclear inflammatory infiltrates
- macrophages;
- Lung parenchyma with altered structure:
- necrosis and hemorrhage
- sulfur granules
- mixed inflammatory infiltrates

■ *Special stains:* PAS, Dieterle's, Warthin-Starry, Giemsa, collagenous stains, methenamine silver stain.

Hallmark of Diagnosis: Clinical history, serologic and bacteriologic findings, inflammatory exudate of various degrees and stages.

Differential diagnosis: Infectious lung diseases with other agents and various underlying causes.

Conchoidal Bodies

Definition: Irregular, partly laminated calcopherites (Schaumann bodies) which occur in multinucleated giant cells, see Sarcoidosis, Tuberculosis, Berylliosis.

Congenital Abnormalities

Definition: Morphologic alterations of the lower respiratory tract occurring during the developmental period.

Incidence/Epidemiology: Minor alterations are quite frequent, whereas severe malformations are usually rare events. Detailed information is given under the particular headings.

Etiology/Pathophysiology: The developmental period of the lung starts in the 4th week of gestation when the right and left mainstem bronchi form the basis of the later lungs. The pseudoglandular period forming evenly distributed primitive conducting airways lasts from the 6th to the 16th week. Acinar differentiation of the lung parenchyma with development of primitive bronchioles and alveolar ducts is estimated to develop in the interval 17–28 weeks followed by the saccular period during 28–34 weeks with the development of small saccules and invasion of capillaries into the interstitium. The alveolar period occurs during the interval 28–36 weeks and into the childhood. The following malformations of the lower respiratory tract have been reported:

Trachea: Agenesis, stenosis, malacia, megaly, fistulas (to the esophagus, which are often associated with malformations of other organs: VATER, VACTER, VACTERL (vertebral, anal, cardiac, tracheo-esophageal, renal, limb)).

Bronchus: Abnormalities of origin or location (tracheal bronchus, additive bronchus, bridging bronchus, bronchogenic cysts); abnormal size or component (atresia, stenosis, malacia, ectasis); abnormal connection (fistula).

Lung parenchyma: Ectopic lung, agenesis, hypoplasia (scimitar syndrome), sequestration, infantile lobar emphysema, polyalveolar lobe, congenital pulmonary lymphangiectasis, congenital cystic adenomatoid malformation.

Diaphragm: Agenesis, accessory diaphragm, hernia.

Clinical Presentation: The malformations of the lower respiratory tract are often associated with malformations of other organs, especially the heart, the kidneys, and nervous system. For details, see under the particular headings.

Prognosis: Depends upon the malformation, see under the particular headings.

Radiology: See under the particular headings.

Pathology:

Gross: Depends upon the malformation, see under the particular headings.

Histology: The microscopic findings are usually superimposed by morphologic changes due to chronic infections. For details, see under the particular headings.

➤ *Descriptors:* Lung parenchyma with preserved structure:
- no morphological abnormalities
- desquamation, hypertrophy, hyperplasia and dysplasia of pneumocytes
- mixed inflammatory infiltrates;
- Lung parenchyma with altered structure:

- cysts
- mixed inflammatory infiltrates;
- Bronchial mucosa with preserved structure:
- viscous mucus
- increased number of goblet cells
- mixed inflammatory infiltrates
- increased number of smooth muscle cells;
- Bronchial mucosa with altered structure:
- squamous metaplasia and dysplasia
- mixed inflammatory infiltrates;
- Pulmonary vessels with preserved structure:
- stenosis
- intimal fibrosis
- thrombosis
- ectatic lumen;
- Pulmonary vessels with altered structure:
- proliferating smooth muscle cells
- mononuclear inflammatory infiltrates

■ *Special stains:* Usually PAS, collagenous stains, Giemsa. For details, see under the particular headings.

Hallmark of Diagnosis: Usually gross findings, clinical history. For details, see under the particular headings.

Differential diagnosis: Congenital infections, hamartomas. For details, see under the particular headings.

Coniosporosis

Definition: Allergic extrinsic alveolitis associated with *Coniosporidium*, see Maple Bark Stripper's Disease.

Contraceptives

Definition: Alteration of the lung parenchyma associated with intake of contraceptives, see Drug Toxicity.

Contrast Media

Definition: Alteration of the lung parenchyma associated with exposure to contrast media, see Drug Toxicity.

Copper

Definition: Patients with exposure to copper have an increased risk of lung cancer, see Cancer of the Lung.

Coptic Lung

Definition: Alterations of the lung parenchyma seen in persons who perform cloth wrapping of mummies.

Incidence/Epidemiology: Rare disease.

Etiology/Pathophysiology: Allergic extrinsic alveolitis with unknown antigen.

Clinical Presentation: Acute and chronic courses occur.

Prognosis: Usually good and without serious sequelae.

Radiology: Chest radiographs are normal or show diffuse, soft, interstitial infiltrates or fine granular densities.

Pathology:

Gross: The lungs are of normal color and consistency, or may display small, firm, reddish-gray nodules.

Histology: The characteristic findings include nonnecrotizing epithelioid granulomas near the terminal bronchioles, desquamation, hypertrophy and hyperplasia of cells of the alveolar lining, marked eosinophilic inflammatory infiltrates, bronchiolitis obliterans and focal acute vasculitis. For details, see Allergic (Extrinsic) Alveolitis.

➤ *Descriptors:* Lung parenchyma with altered structure:

- noncaseous epithelioid granulomas
- eosinophils
- multinucleated giant cells
- intrabronchiolar fibrinoid material and histiocytes
- ulceration of bronchiolar mucosa;
- Lung parenchyma with preserved structure:
- macrophages
- desquamation, hypertrophy, hyperplasia and dysplasia of pneumocytes
- mononuclear inflammatory infiltrates
- intraalveolar serous fluid

■ *Special stains:* PAS, collagenous stains, Giemsa. For details, see Allergic (Extrinsic) Alveolitis.

Hallmark of Diagnosis: Clinical history, non-necrotizing epithelioid granulomas, morphologic findings related to desquamative interstitial pneumonia, lymphoid interstitial pneumonia, bronchiolitis obliterans.
Differential diagnosis: Infectious and noninfectious granulomatous diseases such as sarcoidosis, fungal infections, or berylliosis. For details, see Allergic (Extrinsic) Alveolitis.

Cor Pulmonale

Definition: Hypertrophy of the right ventricle resulting from diseases which affect the function and/or structure of the lung (increasing the intrapulmonary vascular resistance), see Hypertension Pulmonary, Asbestos-Associated Diseases, Chronic Airflow Obstruction, Paracoccidiomycosis, Schistosomiasis.

Corpora Amylacea

Definition: Intraalveolar, PAS-positive, laminated, spherical and ellipsoidal bodies (protein condensates, birefringent, Maltese cross), see Desquamative Interstitial Pneumonia, Pneumonia.

Coxsackievirus

Definition: Infection of the lung with coxsackievirus, see Viral Infection.

Creola Bodies

Definition: Clusters of columnar cells in the sputum, see Asthma.

Crocidolite Fibers

Definition: Asbestos-related mineral fibers, see Asbestos-Associated Diseases.

Crohn's Disease

Definition: Alterations of the lung parenchyma associated with Crohn's disease.

Incidence/Epidemiology: Patients suffering from Crohn's disease over a long period of time present in about 50% of cases with restrictive and diffusion abnormalities in lung function tests.
Etiology/Pathophysiology: The etiology of Crohn's disease is still unknown, although disturbances of the immune system are probably involved. The disease is characterized by granulomas of the epithelioid cell type in the intestines resembling sarcoidosis. Lung involvement may be present if Crohn's disease develops into a generalized disorder.
Clinical Presentation: Patients with Crohn's disease frequently show additional rheumatoid lesions such as erythema nodosum or rheumatoid arthritis. Pulmonary involvement is usually detected by lung function tests which evoke restrictive and diffusive abnormalities with and without radiologic evidence. Symptoms include cough, dyspnea, and expectoration.
Prognosis: Fair, but slow progression of respiratory failure is the common course.
Radiology: Chest radiographs may be normal but can also show mediastinal or hilar lymph nodes, multiple, usually subpleural, spotty shadows, or interstitial infiltrates.
Pathology:
Gross: The lungs are of firm consistency and show multiple, grayish-white spots or fibrous areas.
Histology: Lung tissue abnormalities are characterized by (a) granulomatous interstitial lymphocyte infiltrates; (b) acute alveolitis with dysplasia of pneumocytes; (c) moderate interstitial fibrosis. Additional findings include angiitis, intraalveolar exudation of fibrinoid material, deposits of IgA, and expression of HLA-DR receptors in pneumocytes. Necrosis, cytoplasmic inclusions, cholesterol clefts, and calcified bodies have not been reported.

➤ *Descriptors:* Lung parenchyma with altered structure:

- lymphoid granulomas
- desquamation, hypertrophy, hyperplasia and dysplasia of pneumocytes
- focal interstitial fibrosis
- mononuclear inflammatory infiltrates;
- Pulmonary vessels with preserved structure:
- mononuclear inflammatory infiltrates;
- Lung parenchyma with preserved structure:
- intraalveolar fibrinoid material

- *Special stains:* PAS, collagenous stains, methenamine silver stain, immunohistochemistry for immunoglobulins, endogenous lectins.

  Hallmark of Diagnosis: Clinical history, lymphocytic granulomatous interstitial infiltrates, acute alveolitis, interstitial fibrosis of mixed, usually mild, degree.

  Differential diagnosis: Sarcoidosis, infectious granulomatous diseases, allergic extrinsic alveolitis.

Cromoglycate

Definition: Alteration of the lung parenchyma associated with intake of cromoglycate, see Drug Toxicity.

Cromolyn

Definition: Alteration of the lung parenchyma associated with intake of cromolyn, see Drug Toxicity.

Cryoglobulinemia

Definition: Alteration of lung associated with mixed essential cryoglobulinemia.

Incidence/Epidemiology: Essential mixed cryoglobulinemia is a rare disease exhibiting purpura, arthralgias, weakness, serum cryoglobulins, and rheumatoid factor activity. Pulmonary involvement has been reported in 20–30% of patients.

Etiology/Pathophysiology: The disease is characterized by an abnormal globulin (cryoglobulin) which causes increased blood viscosity below normal body temperature leading to disturbances of microcirculation in the capillaries.

Clinical Presentation: Pulmonary symptoms include cough, dyspnea, asthmoid complaints, pleurisy, and hemoptysis.

Prognosis: Pulmonary involvement may show a slow progression but has no influence on the outcome of the disease.

Radiology: Chest radiographs may be normal or show signs of mild interstitial fibrosis.

Pathology:

Gross: No data are known.

Histology: No data are known. Histological changes are probably similar to those seen in usual interstitial pneumonia (UIP). Patients with UIP often have an increase in circulating cryoglobulins.

➤ *Descriptors:* Lung parenchyma with preserved structure:
  - mononuclear inflammatory infiltrates
  - intraalveolar serous fluid;
  - Pulmonary vessels with preserved structure:
  - microthrombosis (capillaries)

- *Special stains:* PAS, collagenous stain, immunohistochemistry for immunoglobulins, endogenous lectins.

  Hallmark of Diagnosis: Clinical history, identification of serum cryoglobulins.

  Differential diagnosis: Usual interstitial pneumonia, secondary cryoglobulinemia, collagenous diseases.

Cryptococcus

Definition: Infection of the lung with *Cryptococcus neoformans* (synonyms: torulosis, European blastomycosis).

Incidence/Epidemiology: Worldwide distributed mycosis with exogenous source of fungal growth in soil or bricks contaminated with pigeon droppings. Pulmonary infection is rare.

Etiology/Pathophysiology: A remarkable percentage of patients (40–80%) have diminished immunodefence mechanisms, either as defects of cellular immunity or as severe underlying diseases. After pulmonary entry of the fungus, hematogenous spread may occur, most frequently affecting the cerebromeninges.

Clinical Presentation: The clinical spectrum ranges from transient asymptomatic infection of the tracheobronchial tree via a self-limiting or progressive course to chronic cryptococcosis with circumscribed pulmonary nodules. The clinical onset is usually subacute to chronic. Besides the meninges, dissemination occurs into the skin, bones, joints, kidneys, prostate, liver, and spleen. The symptoms include cough, low grade fever, chest pain, malaise, loss of weight.

Prognosis: Cryptococcosis is usually a self-limited disease with self-healing or formation of pulmonary nodules (cryptococcoma).

Chronic invasive cryptococcosis can be fatal, usually with cerebromeningeal infection.

Radiology: Chest radiographs demonstrate a broad spectrum of signs, including alveolar or interstitial infiltrates, segmental or lobar consolidation, hilar adenopathy, pleural effusions, or circumscribed nodules which may show calcification.

Pathology:
Gross: Heavy fluid lungs with areas of grayish consolidation or circumscribed, firm, yellowish-white nodules with central necrosis and hemorrhage.

Histology: The cryptococcosis organisms grow either intraalveolarly or interstitially. They proliferate in yeastlike cells or in small round cells having a mucinous capsula. Interstitial inflammation and multiple giant cells containing the organisms are usually present. Clusters of fungi may show central caseous necrosis surrounded by epithelioid cells, lymphocytes, plasma cells, and multinucleated giant cells, thus forming a caseous epithelioid granuloma. Central calcification seldom occurs and only in older lesions. *Cryptococcus* organisms are difficult to see on HE sections.

➤ *Descriptors:* Lung parenchyma with altered structure:
- caseous epithelioid granulomas
- fungus (intragranulomatous capsule-defined yeast)
- palisading histiocytes
- multinucleated giant cells (capsule defined yeast)
- necrosis
- mixed inflammatory infiltrates
- eosinophils
- focal interstitial fibrosis (at the margin)

■ *Special stains:* PAS, Mayer's mucicarmine stain, GMS stain, methenamine silver stain, collagenous stains, immunofluorescence.

Hallmark of Diagnosis: Clinical history, identification of the organisms in mucicarmine stain, latex agglutination test for capsular polysaccharide antigen in serum, immunofluorescence, microbiology culture.

Differential diagnosis: Other fungal infections, especially histoplasmosis, paracoccidioidomycosis, *Pneumocystis carinii.*

Cryptosporidiosis

Definition: Infection of the lung with the protozoan parasite *Cryptosporidium.*

Incidence/Epidemiology: Infection of the intestines is frequent in patients with AIDS. Infection of the lung has been reported in a few immunocompromised children. It has also been demonstrated in healthy people.

Etiology/Pathophysiology: The infectious organisms have their reservoir in birds, calves, pigs, and rodents. Infection is probably acquired by eating raw or poorly cooked meat. The oocysts of the parasites are passed with the feces.

Clinical Presentation: Chronic, profuse, watery diarrhea is usually present. Pulmonary symptoms such as cough and dyspnea develop after the gastrointestinal manifestation.

Prognosis: Pulmonary infection in immunocompromised children is usually fatal.

Radiology: Chest radiographs are normal or show multiple, diffuse densities.

Pathology:
Gross: The lungs are heavy and wet, and show multiple, grayish-white densities with firm consistency.

Histology: The infective organisms are small and measure 4–5 μm in diameter. They are highly refractile. Ingested tachyzoites may be seen in interstitial and intraalveolar histiocytes and foamy macrophages. Areas of hemorrhage and necrosis may be present.

➤ *Descriptors:* Lung parenchyma with altered structure:
- infectious organisms (oocysts, *Cryptosporidium*)
- macrophages (foamy, ingested tachyzoites)
- necrosis and hemorrhage

■ *Special stains:* PAS, Movat, collagenous stain, immunofluorescence.

Hallmark of Diagnosis: Clinical history, identification of the protozoa, necrotizing pneumonia, foamy macrophages.

Differential diagnosis: Infections with other protozoa, bacterial and viral infections.

Cryptostromosis

Definition: Allergic extrinsic alveolitis associated with *Cryptostroma corticale*, see Maple Bark Stripper's Lung.

Crystalline Bodies

Definition: Lucent birefringent calcium oxalate crystals seen in multinucleated giant cells, see Sarcoidosis, Berylliosis.

Curschmann's Spirals

Definition: Dense mucus plugs of the sputum, see Asthma.

Cyclophosphamide

Definition: Alteration of the lung parenchyma associated with intake of cyclophosphamide, see Drug Toxicity.

Cylindroma

Definition: Carcinoma of the lung with a specific histomorphological appearance, see Adenoid Cystic Carcinoma.

Cyst

Definition: Encapsulated or pseudoencapsulated, structureless formation of the lung parenchyma filled with air, mucus, or mucoid substances.

Incidence/Epidemiology: Frequent observation related to various underlying diseases. These include (a) congenital cysts such as bronchogenic cyst, congenital cystic adenomatoid malformation (type l), lymphangioleiomyomatosis, intralobar sequestration, and (b) acquired cysts such as parasitic (*Echinococcus* (hydatid, paragonimiasis), emphysema, postinfarction, postinfection, and postneoplastic (teratoma). Other classifications of lung cysts are based upon the macroscopic appearance or the localization.

Etiology/Pathophysiology: Congenital cysts do not necessarily have to be genetic in nature. They may have developed as a result of intrauterine infection or local disturbance of growth of the lung parenchyma. Other theories include agenesis of bronchiolar ducts, malformation of lymph spaces, and stenosis of airways. Acquired cysts may be caused by local alteration of interstitial lung tissue and differences in tensional forces leading to the development of cysts. Infections destroy lung parenchyma, which cannot be entirely reconstituted.

Clinical Presentation: Cysts can be asymptomatic or can cause severe clinical problems such as dyspnea, bacterial and fungal infections, or hemorrhage.

Prognosis: According to the underlying disease, slow increase in size can be seen in most of the cases.

Radiology: Cysts present different images on chest X-radiographs depending upon localization and degree of filling. Peripheral lung cysts in older patients are usually transparent due to their emphysematous origin, and postinfectious cysts have a marked circumference of fibrous tissue or are filled with dense material (fungus).

Pathology:

Gross: Cysts are either large empty air spaces or homogeneous, mucinous (firm) areas surrounded by white tissue. Fungal cysts are of crumbly consistency, grayish-yellow, and measure a few centimeters in diameter. Parasitic cysts are usually large and can measure up to 20 cm in diameter. They are filled with greenish, viscous mucus and have a thin or fibrous outer layer. Postinfarction cysts contain a broad, dark red-brown wall. Postneoplastic cysts are often filled with serous transparent mucus and have a fibrous wall varying greatly in thickness.

Histology: Emphysematous cysts are empty air spaces without detectable structure. The surrounding lung tissue may be normal or focally fibrotic. Postinfectious cysts have thick fibrous layers around their circumference, often with palisading histiocytes and multinucleated giant cells. Parasitic cysts may be of similar appearance or still possess the parasitic membrane with protoscolices. Postinfarction cysts are made up of a central colliquative necrosis and dense layers of hemosiderin-laden macrophages in the circumference. Postneoplastic cysts have a thick wall consisting of acellular collagenous fibers with scattered lymphocytes and plasma cells. Other areas contain dense clusters of foamy macrophages, often with ingested hemosiderin.

➤ *Descriptors:* Lung parenchyma with altered structure:
- cysts (air, serous fluid, exudate, debris, fungus, parasites, hemorrhage)
- focal interstitial fibrosis (fibrous layer)

■ *Special stains:* PAS, collagenous stains, methenamine silver stain, immunohistochemistry for residual tumor cells, endogenous lectins.

Hallmark of Diagnosis: Macroscopic appearance, clinical history, empty air space, compartments of the cystic wall.

Differential diagnosis: Due to the underlying disease.

Cystadenoma

Definition: Benign epithelial neoplasm of the lung, see Adenoma.

Cystic Adenomatoid Malformation

Definition: Congenital cystic lesion of the lung characterized by the presence of abnormal bronchiolar structures of hamartous character, see Adenomatoid Cystic Malformation of the Lung.

Cysticercosis

Definition: Infectious disease caused by the larval stage of the tapeworm *Taenia solium.*

Incidence/Epidemiology: The parasite has a worldwide distribution and can infect humans who eat raw or inadequately cooked pork. People living in poor areas or those with poor personal hygiene experience a higher risk.

Etiology/Pathophysiology: Man is the only definite host of this tapeworm which lives in the intestines. Gravid proglottids are passed with the stool. Excreted eggs contaminate the soil and are eaten by pigs which are the intermediate host. The eggs release oncospheres in the pig's intestines, which enter into the blood stream and invade the muscles, where they become encysted. The cysticerci are eaten by man and develop to the adult tapeworm in the intestines. Serious infection of various organs including the lung occur when the intermediate cysticerci infect man.

Clinical Presentation: Intestinal tapeworm usually causes no symptoms. Cysticerci may enter into the brain, eyes, skin, or lung, causing meningitis, hydrocephalus, loss of vision, and cough. Symptoms of pulmonary infection are absent or mild.

Prognosis: Usually good; however, cerebromeningeal infection can be fatal.

Radiology: Chest X-radiographs may present calcified nodules.

Pathology:

Gross: The cysticerci measure 1 cm in diameter and are of milky-white color. The worm measures several centimeters in length and about 1 cm in diameter. Necrotic calcified nodules in lung tissue correspond to dead cysticerci.

Histology: The cysticerci have four suckers with several birefringent hooklets. The cystic wall measures 100–200 μm in thickness. The tegumentum is thin and covered with microvilli. An inflammatory tissue response is usually not present. Dead cysticerci cause a granulomatous reaction with histiocytes and multinucleated giant cells and may later calcify.

➤ *Descriptors:* Lung parenchyma with altered structure:
- parasites (absent inflammation in viable parasites)
- cysts (thin tegument covered with microvilli)
- noncaseous epithelioid granulomas
- parasites (intragranulomatous, degenerated)
- multinucleated giant cells
- mononuclear inflammatory infiltrates
- focal interstitial fibrosis (at the margin)
- calcification

■ *Special stains:* PAS, Movat.

Hallmark of Diagnosis: Clinical history, identification of cysticerci and of the tapeworm.

Differential diagnosis: Other parasitic infections.

Cystic Fibrosis

Definition: Alteration of the lung parenchyma associated with cystic fibrosis (mucoviscidosis).

Incidence/Epidemiology: Cystic fibrosis is an autosomal recessive disorder of eccrine mucus production. It is the most frequently observed congenital disorder within the Caucasian race. Changes in the conducting airways occur in patients older than 6 months.

Etiology/Pathophysiology: The abnormal composition of the mucus affects its viscosity and results in sluggish material blocking the glandular ducts and the subsequent mucus passages. Bronchiectasis, seen in practically all affected children after 1 year of age, combined with recurrent infection of the airways is the result.

Clinical Presentation: Patients suffer from asthmoid bronchitis, atelectasis with recurrent pneumonias, dyspnea, and cyanosis and usually die due to respiratory insufficiency.

Prognosis: Usually poor, most of the patients die during adolescence. The clinical situation may change with progress in genetic engineering.

Radiology: Chest X-radiographs show severe bronchiectases and mucus-filled bronchi, atelectases, pneumonic areas.

Pathology:

Gross: Dilated large and smaller bronchi filled with sluggish, greenish mucus. The bronchial walls are thickened. The peripheral lung tissue displays areas of dense consistency filled with mucus plugs. Additional pneumonic changes are usually present.

Histology: The larger and smaller bronchi and the bronchioles are dilated and filled with homogeneous mucus. The walls are edematous, and enlarged and contain mononuclear inflammatory infiltrates. Mucus plugs spread focally into the alveolar ducts and alveoli which are the origin of subsequent bacterial infection. Interstitial fibrosis and granulomatous reaction of the lung parenchyma are not a sign of cystic fibrosis.

➤ *Descriptors:* Bronchial mucosa with preserved structure:
- ectatic lumen
- viscous mucus
- mononuclear inflammatory infiltrates;
- Bronchial mucosa with altered structure:
- fibrosis (peribronchial);
- Lung parenchyma with preserved structure:
- viscous mucus
- mononuclear inflammatory infiltrates

■ *Special stains:* PAS, methenamine silver stain.

Hallmark of Diagnosis: Clinical history, bronchiectasis with viscous mucus plugs, spread of mucoid impactions into the peripheral lung tissue.

Differential diagnosis: Bronchiectasis and mucoid impactions due to other underlying diseases.

Cystine Storage Disease

Definition: Alteration of the lung parenchyma associated with cystine storage disease (Lignac-Fanconi disease).

Incidence/Epidemiology: Very rare disease of simple recessive inheritance. Two forms of the disease appear: (a) the early onset or infantile nephropathic form and (b) late onset or adolescent nephropathic form.

Etiology/Pathophysiology: The enzymatic storage disease causes increased storage of cystine in the reticuloendothelial cells due to a disorder of protein anabolism. The principally affected organs are the spleen, the bones, kidneys, lymph nodes, and liver. However, other organs may also be affected, including the lung.

Clinical Presentation: Patients suffer from kidney disorders (ranging from simple proteinuria to renal failure), dwarfism, retinopathia pigmentosa, and headache. Lung function tests may show decreased diffusion values. Symptoms include shortness of breath, tachypnea, dyspnea.

Prognosis: Outcome of patients is not defined by pulmonary involvement.

Radiology: Chest X-radiographs are normal or show diffuse interstitial infiltrates of mild degree.

Pathology:

Gross: Normal lung tissue with some mild interstitial fibrosis.

Histology: Birefringent cystine crystals may be detected within reticuloendothelial cells of small vessels (endothelial cells). Severe mononuclear or granulocytic inflammatory infiltrates are usually not present.

➤ *Descriptors:* Lung parenchyma with preserved structure:
- hyaline material (birefringent crystals, in histiocytes and endothelial cells of small vessels)
- mononuclear inflammatory infiltrates (weak)

■ *Special stains:* Kossa stain with prior alcohol fixation of the lung parenchyma.

Hallmark of Diagnosis: Clinical history, identification of cystine crystals in reticuloendothelial cells.

Differential diagnosis: Von Gierke's disease, foreign body deposits, other storage diseases.

Cytomegalovirus

Definition: Infection of the lung parenchyma with cytomegalovirus.

Incidence/Epidemiology: Congenital infections with cytomegalovirus (CMV) are estimated to occur in 1% of infants and about 1% of congenitally infected infants present with CMV pneumonia. Antibodies against CMV are detectable in 40–70% of the west European population. Infection occurs transplacentally and in adult persons by aerosol droplets, blood transfusion, organ transplantation, or contact with semen, cervical secretions, or milk. A special risk attends immunocompromised patients, especially those with AIDS.

Etiology/Pathophysiology: The virus replicates in the nuclei of infected cells, presenting with characteristic herpesvirus nucleocapsids. CMV infects the cells of the alveolar lining and cells of the reticuloendothelium. The virus itself is of low virulence, and infected cells are usually recognized by the cellular immunodefence system and destroyed by lysis. The severity of infections is highly dependent upon the status of the cellular immune system.

Clinical Presentation: The infection period lasts for 14 days, after which patients present with symptoms of pneumonia including nonproductive cough, fever, tachypnea, dyspnea, hypoxemia. Immunocompromised patients have a high fatality risk and are in danger of superinfections with bacteria or protozoa.

Prognosis: Usually good in immunocompetent patients; however, infection of immunocompromised patients is often fatal.

Radiology: CMV pneumonia usually starts with bilateral peripheral diffuse shadows in the lower lobes with central propagation.

Pathology:

Gross: The fluid-laden lungs are red to grayish and present diffuse changes in consistency and color from the peripheral to the central zones.

Histology: The air spaces contain fibrin, debris, macrophages, and mononuclear inflammatory cells. The interalveolar septulae are edematous, and widened and show scattered inflammatory cells made up of lymphocytes and plasma cells. Cells of the alveolar lining are hyperplastic and contain large, isolated cells with characteristic virus inclusion bodies. Intracytoplasmic inclusion bodies are also present. Rarely, macrophages containing two or three nuclei with corresponding inclusion bodies can be observed.

➤ *Descriptors:* Lung parenchyma with preserved structure:
- intraalveolar fibrinoid material
- mononuclear inflammatory infiltrates
- macrophages
- desquamation, hypertrophy, hyperplasia and dysplasia of pneumocytes
- inclusion bodies (intracytoplasmic, in large isolated pneumocytes);
- Bronchial mucosa with preserved structure:
- mononuclear inflammatory cells (bronchi, bronchioles)
- desquamation, hypertrophy, hyperplasia and dysplasia of epithelial cells

■ *Special stains:* PAS, Feulgen, collagenous stains, DNA hybridization (in situ hybridization), immunofluorescence.

Hallmark of Diagnosis: Intranuclear and intracytoplasmic inclusion bodies, identification of the virus by DNA hybridization, immunofluorescence, isolation of the virus from the urine or sputum, clinical history.

Differential diagnosis: Pneumonia stemming from other viruses, especially herpes simplex, adenovirus, or measles.

Cytosine arabinoside

Definition: Alteration of the lung parenchyma associated with intake of cytosine arabinoside, see Drug Toxicity.

Dantrolen –
Extrauterine Transition Disorders

Dantrolen

Definition: Alteration of the lung parenchyma associated with intake of dantrolen, see Drug Toxicity.

Dengue Hemorrhagic Fever

Definition: Alteration of the lung parenchyma seen in patients infected with dengue virus (type 1, 2, 3, 4).

Incidence/Epidemiology: The disease is endemic in Southeast Asia, especially Cambodia, Singapore, India, Thailand, Malaysia, and the Philippines. Children and persons living in a poor social environment are frequently infected as well as tourists with a nonadapted immune system.

Etiology/Pathophysiology: At least 4 (possibly 6) different types of dengue and chikungunya virus have been identified. Man is infected by mosquito bites (*Anopheles aegypti*). The mosquito breeds in urban water containers. Epidemic outbreaks are usually seen during or at the end of the rainy season. Man-mosquito-man transmission is the common cause of urban epidemics.

Clinical Presentation: The patients (usually children) present with symptoms of a common cold including fever, cough, pharyngitis, headache, nausea, and vomiting. After 3–4 days abrupt deterioration with high fever, weakness, hypotension, and tachycardia occurs. Macular or maculopapular rash is seen in about 50% of the cases and is usually followed by recovery. Patients with a fatal outcome develop coma, hematemesis, cyanosis, dyspnea, and convulsions.

Prognosis: Fair, as fatal cases are seen in about 10–30% of the patients. Death occurs usually on the 4th or 5th day of the disease.

Radiology: Chest radiographs are normal or show diffuse interstitial densities.

Pathology:

Gross: The lungs are heavy, wet and present with large areas of hemorrhage.

Histology: The distant air spaces are filled with extravasated erythrocytes and show focal areas of necrosis. The interalveolar septula contain numerous mononuclear inflammatory infiltrates. Intraalveolar fibrinoid material may be present.

➤ *Descriptors:* Lung parenchyma with preserved structure:
- intraalveolar fibrinoid material
- mononuclear inflammatory infiltrates;
- Lung parenchyma with altered structure:
- necrosis and hemorrhage

■ *Special stains:* PAS, collagenous stains, immunofluorescence.

Hallmark of Diagnosis: Clinical history, hemorrhage, usual interstitial pneumonia, identification of the virus.

Differential diagnosis: Pneumonia due to other infectious organisms, pulmonary edema, diffuse alveolar damage.

Dermatomyositis

Definition: Alteration of the lung parenchyma associated with dermatomyositis.

Incidence/Epidemiology: The frequency of patients having primary changes of the lung parenchyma in association with dermatomyositis amounts to 5–10% of patients suffering from polymyositis/dermatomyositis.

Etiology/Pathophysiology: Pulmonary involvement of collagenosis is most frequently due to complications of the disease such as aspiration and consecutive pneumonias. Primary changes affect the interstitial tissue with chronic interstitial inflammatory infiltrates. The etiology of the disease is still unknown.

Clinical Presentation: Usually slow progress with restrictive lung functions, dyspnea, almost never pleural effusions.

Prognosis: Usually slow, seldom rapid progression of respiratory failure. About 50% of patients die of respiratory failure within 10 years, 15% of patients develop lung cancer.

Radiology: Diffuse interstitial infiltrates without pleural thickening or pleural effusions.

Pathology:

Gross: Normal findings or (seldom) diffuse fibrotic changes with mild increase of consistency.

Histology: Nonspecific inflammatory interstitial infiltrates comprising lymphocytes, plasma cells, and rarely polymorphonuclear cells. Interstitial fibrosis is infrequent and mild. Obliterative bronchiolitis may occur.

➤ *Descriptors:* Lung parenchyma with preserved structure:
- mononuclear inflammatory infiltrates;
- Lung parenchyma with altered structure:
- intrabronchiolar fibrinoid material and histiocytes
- ulceration of bronchiolar mucosa
- diffuse interstitial fibrosis

■ *Special stains:* Collagenous stains, endogenous lectins, immunohistochemistry for HLA-DR, immunoglobulins.

Hallmark of Diagnosis: Clinical history, careful exclusion of changes associated with complications of dermatomyositis (aspiration).

Differential diagnosis: Usual interstitial pneumonia, changes of the lung parenchyma due to aspiration, pulmonary involvement of other collagenous diseases.

Desquamative Interstitial Pneumonia (DIP)

Definition: Chronic pneumonitis with hyperplasia of type II alveolar lining cells.

Incidence/Epidemiology: Rare disease occurring in adults and children but the majority of patients are over 40 years old. Special risk factors are not known.

Etiology/Pathophysiology: The relation of the disease to cryptogenic collagen vascular disease is still under discussion. There is a close relation to the usual interstitial pneumonia. Etiology and pathogenesis are not known. Similar histomorphologic changes occur in obstructed lung areas.

Clinical Presentation: The symptoms are nonspecific and usually consist of dry cough, insidious onset of dyspnea, and progressive shortness of breath with exertion. Pulmonary function tests show abnormal gas exchange with decreased diffusion capacity. Serological findings include the demonstration of nuclear-specific antibodies, rheumatoid factors, cryoglobulins, elevated erythrocyte sedimentation rate (all findings in about 10–20% of patients).

Prognosis: Median survival of patients with DIP has been calculated to be 10–14 years. Slow progression of respiratory failure causes death in 20–30% of patients.

Radiology: Chest radiographs show bilateral reticular or noduloreticular infiltrates which are denser at the bases of the lungs. Advanced stages show honeycombing.

Pathology:

Gross: Early stages of the disease are associated with normal macroscopic findings. Late stages show various areas of honeycombing, with polycystic and scarred areas separated from each other by nearly normal lung portions.

Histology: The characteristic finding of DIP is the uniform distribution of macrophages filling the distant air spaces. The majority of macrophages have a slightly pigmented cytoplasm, and some of them contain small amounts of iron or PAS-positive deposits. The cells of the alveolar lining are nearly uniformly hyperplastic and may also exhibit mild dysplasia. The interstitial tissue contains a small to moderate number of mononuclear cells consisting of lymphocytes and plasma cells. Hyaline membranes or exudation of fibrin are not a feature of DIP. Laminated conchoidal bodies (blue bodies) can be seen within the macrophages.

➤ *Descriptors:* Lung parenchyma with preserved structure:
- macrophages
- multinucleated giant cells
- desquamation, hypertrophy, hyperplasia and dysplasia of pneumocytes
- mononuclear inflammatory cells

■ *Special stains:* PAS, Prussian blue, collagenous stains, immunohistochemistry for immunoglobulins, endogenous lectins.

Hallmark of Diagnosis: Hyperplasia of cells of the alveolar lining, type II, filling of alveoli with macrophages, blue bodies, mononuclear interstitial infiltrate, clinical history.

Differential diagnosis: Obstructive pneumonitis, usual interstitial pneumonia, giant cell interstitial pneumonia, bronchioloalveolar carcinoma, eosinophilic granuloma, pneumoconiosis due to hard metals, talc, silica, aluminum, or asbestos.

Dextran

Definition: Alteration of the lung parenchyma associated with intake of dextran, see Drug Toxicity.

Diabetic Xanthogranuloma

Definition: Xantholomatous storage of lipids in the lung associated with diabetes mellitus.
Incidence/Epidemiology: Some 6% of diabetic patients show these alterations compared with 2% of nondiabetic patients.
Etiology/Pathophysiology: Disturbance of sugar pathways leads to increased deposits of lipoid substances, especially in macrophages.
Clinical Presentation: No characteristic symptoms regarding the lung are described.
Prognosis: Not associated with pulmonary involvement.
Radiology: No specific findings.
Pathology:
Gross: No specific findings.
Histology: Perivascular agglutinations of foamy macrophages arranged into pseudonodular structures. Hyalinosis of the media of small arteries.

➤ *Descriptors:* Lung parenchyma with preserved structure:
- macrophages (perivascular agglutinations, foamy);
- Pulmonary vessels with altered structure:
- hyaline material (arteries)
- lipoid material
- stenosis

■ *Special stains:* PAS, collagenous stains, Prussian blue.

Hallmark of Diagnosis: Cluster of foamy macrophages, hyalinosis of arterial walls, clinical history.
Differential diagnosis: Lipid storage diseases, nonspecific (obstructive) alterations of the lung parenchyma.

Dialysis

Definition: Alteration of the lung parenchyma associated with dialysis.
Incidence/Epidemiology: Involvement of the lung is seen in 50–80% of dialysis patients.
Etiology/Pathophysiology: Chronic renal failure causes disturbances in calcium/phosphate metabolism leading to deposits of calcium crystals.
Clinical Presentation: Lung function tests remain normal for a long period of time. Specific symptoms are not present.
Prognosis: Not associated with pulmonary involvement.
Radiology: Diffuse granular infiltrations of various degree may be present; however, normal lung chest radiographs are the usual findings.
Pathology:
Gross: Focal areas of dry, firm changes within the lung tissue, sometimes accompanied by grittiness.
Histology: Diffuse deposits of calcium crystals in severe cases without major inflammatory response of host tissue. Mild interstitial fibrosis may be present.

➤ *Descriptors:* Lung parenchyma with preserved structure:
- calcium deposits (intraalveolar)
- absent inflammatory infiltrates

■ *Special stains:* PAS, Kossa stain, immunohistochemistry for immunoglobulins, endogenous lectins, X-ray diffraction or similar physical techniques.

Hallmark of Diagnosis: Clinical history, deposits of calcium crystals.
Differential diagnosis: Dystrophic calcification, pulmonary ossification.

Diaphragm, Accessory

Definition: Congenital malformation with aberrant muscular tissue in the diaphragm.
Incidence/Epidemiology: Rare disease, usually seen in children, and incidentally in adults.
Etiology/Pathophysiology: The malformation is considered to be a result of incomplete descent of the septum transversum which divides a hemithorax into upper and lower compartments.
Clinical Presentation: Patients may be asymptomatic or may show respiratory distress. The malformation is always unilateral and is right-sided in about 90% of patients.
Prognosis: Usually good and without serious sequelae.
Radiology: Posterolateral and lateral chest radiographs show an abnormal position of the right diaphragm.
Pathology:
Gross: Aberrant flat muscular tissue in the right diaphragm.

Histology: Normal striated muscular fibers with connective tissue.

➤ *Descriptors:* Lung parenchyma with preserved structure:

- no morphological abnormalities;
- Diaphragm with preserved structure:
- no morphological abnormalities

■ *Special stains:* None.

Hallmark of Diagnosis: Macroscopic findings, chest radiographs.

Differential diagnosis: Diaphragmatic hernia.

Diaphragm, Agenesis

Definition: Congenital malformation with complete absence of one compartment of the diaphragm.

Incidence/Epidemiology: Rare disease usually seen in newborn children.

Etiology/Pathophysiology: Malformation of the septum transversum. An autosomal recessive disorder is discussed in the literature.

Clinical Presentation: Agenesis of the diaphragm usually occurs on the left side and causes severe respiratory problems. Hypoplasia of the lung is a common associated malformation.

Prognosis: Death related to cardiopulmonary problems occurs frequently.

Radiology: Chest radiographs show intrathoracic abdominal contents and herniation.

Pathology:

Gross: Absence of the left diaphragm and consequent herniation of intraabdominal contents into the thorax.

Histology: None.

➤ *Descriptors:* Lung parenchyma with preserved structure:

- no morphological abnormalities

■ *Special stains:* None.

Hallmark of Diagnosis: Macroscopic findings, chest radiographs.

Differential diagnosis: Diaphragmatic hernia.

Diaphragmatic Eventration

Definition: Congenital immobile diaphragm.

Incidence/Epidemiology: Rare disease, more frequently seen in men.

Etiology/Pathophysiology: Aplasia of the striated muscles of the diaphragm causes immobility.

Clinical Presentation: Usually unilateral malformation seen on the right side of the thorax. Symptoms are mild to absent and may include an increased number of infections of the lower respiratory tract.

Prognosis: Usually good; however, sequelae related to recurrent pulmonary infections are frequent.

Radiology: Posterolateral or lateral chest radiographs show an abnormal position of the right diaphragm.

Pathology:

Gross: The diaphragm is usually fibrotic and white-yellowish. Muscular tissue is absent or rare.

Histology: Absent or only scattered skeletal muscle cells and an increased number of collagenous fibers.

➤ *Descriptors:* Diaphragm with altered structure:

- absent or decreased number of striated muscle cells
- fibrosis

■ *Special stains:* None.

Hallmark of Diagnosis: Chest radiographs, absent or nearly absent striated muscle fibers.

Differential diagnosis: Diaphragmatic hernia.

Diaphragmatic Hernia

Definition: Congenital abnormality with defect of the diaphragm.

Incidence/Epidemiology: One of the most frequent abnormalities of the lung and the thorax. The estimated frequency ranges from 1/2 000 to 1/5 000 births.

Etiology/Pathophysiology: The malformation occurs during the 9th week of gestation when the posterolateral pleuroperitoneal folds are closing. As a result, abdominal contents penetrate into the thoracic cavity and cause pulmonary hypoplasia. Several additional abnormalities are associated with diaphragmatic herniation such as trisomy 18, 21; meningomyelocele, fetal alcohol syndrome, pulmonary hypoplasia, extralobar sequestration, congenital cystic adenomatoid malformation, tracheoesophageal fistula; cardiovascular involvement (tetralogy of Fallot, atrial and ventral defects, coarctation of the aorta, stenosis of the pulmonary arteries); gastrointestinal involvement (pyloric stenosis, stomach duplication, malrotation of the bowel, omphalocele, imperforate anus); genitourinary involvement (hydronephrosis, multicystic kidneys, duplication of ureters).

Clinical Presentation: Left-sided herniation is more frequent than right-sided. The abdominal contents found in the thoracic cavity may include the liver, intestines, or spleen, depending upon the side of herniation. Pulmonary symptoms are usually severe and include respiratory distress or recurrent respiratory infections. Diaphragmatic hernia may be mimicked by Chilaiditi's syndrome (interposition of the colon between the liver and diaphragm).

Prognosis: About 10–20% of children die due to the severe respiratory distress within the first hours after birth.

Radiology: Various abdominal contents in the thoracic cavity.

Pathology:

Gross: Fragments of the affected diaphragm surround the defect.

Histology: Normal appearance of skeletal muscle fibers.

➤ *Descriptors:* Lung parenchyma with preserved structure:

- no morphological abnormalities

■ *Special stains:* None.

Hallmark of Diagnosis: Clinical history, macroscopic findings, normal appearance of striated muscle fibers.

Differential diagnosis: Agenesis of the diaphragm, diaphragmatic eventration.

Diazepam

Definition: Alteration of the lung parenchyma associated with intake of diazepam, see Drug Toxicity.

Diethylcarbamazine

Definition: Alteration of the lung parenchyma associated with intake of diethylcarbamazine, see Drug Toxicity.

Diffuse Alveolar Damage

Definition: Clinical syndrome that results from damage to the alveolar capillary membranes and subsequent (severe) respiratory failure, see Adult Respiratory Distress Syndrome.

Digitalis

Definition: Alteration of the lung parenchyma associated with intake of digitalis, see Drug Toxicity.

Diphenylhydantoin

Definition: Alteration of the lung parenchyma associated with intake of diphenylhydantoin, see Drug Toxicity.

Dirofilariasis

Definition: Infection of the lung with the dog heartworm *Dirofilaria immitis*.

Incidence/Epidemiology: The parasite lives in the southern and temperate areas of America and infects both dogs and humans. Increasing frequency of infected humans has been reported within the past few years. Men aged 40–60 years are at highest risk. Ownership of dogs has no special influence on infection.

Etiology/Pathophysiology: The adult worms live in the hearts of infected mammals (dog, wolf, coyote, fox, bear, seal, otter, muskrat, beaver, domestic cat) and release microfilariae into the peripheral blood, where they are ingested by blood-sucking mosquitos (*Aedes* genus). Within the mosquito the larvae molt twice and become infectious larvae which migrate through the subcutaneous fatty tissue when retransmitted to humans or other mammals. After molting they enter the blood stream and stay in the heart. In humans the parasites die in the right heart and are swept into the system of pulmonary arteries provoking thrombosis and granulomatous inflammation in the peripheral lung parenchyma.

Clinical Presentation: The majority of infected patients have no symptoms. Others present with cough, hemoptysis, chest pain, fever, chills, and malaise. Eosinophilia is rare.

Prognosis: Usually good and without sequelae.

Radiology: Chest radiographs usually show peripheral circumscribed "coin lesions".

Pathology:
Gross: Circumscribed grayish-white necrotic areas 1–3 cm in diameter, usually in the subpleural lung parenchyma.

Histology: The coagulative necrotic lung parenchyma contains intact or degenerative immature parasites measuring 100–350 μm in diameter. The multilayered cuticle measuring 25 μm in diameter surrounds the cuticular ridge, intestines, and focal muscle cells. The dead parasites are embedded in granulomatous inflammatory tissue consisting of lymphocytes, plasma cells, histiocytes, and multinucleated giant cells, resembling tuberculosis.

➤ *Descriptors:* Lung parenchyma with altered structure:
- caseous epithelioid granulomas
- parasites (ghost outlines, immature, in pulmonary vessels)
- mononuclear inflammatory infiltrates
- multinucleated giant cells
- necrosis
- focal interstitial fibrosis (perigranulomatous)
- calcification

■ *Special stains:* PAS, Movat, methenamine silver stain, collagenous stain.

Hallmark of Diagnosis: Clinical history, identification of parasites within coagulative necrotic areas surrounded by epithelioid granulomatous tissue resulting from an inflammatory reaction. Serologic tests are not diagnostic.

Differential diagnosis: Tuberculosis, granulomatous fungal infection, Wegener's disease, lung infarction.

Disodium Chromoglycate

Definition: Alteration of the lung parenchyma associated with intake of disodium chromoglycate, see Drug Toxicity.

L-Dopa

Definition: Alteration of the lung parenchyma associated with intake of L-dopa, see Drug Toxicity.

Down's Syndrome

Definition: Alterations of the lung parenchyma associated with Down's syndrome.

Incidence/Epidemiology: About 5–15% of patients with Down's syndrome show pulmonary abnormalities, especially pulmonary hypoplasia and diaphragmatic hernia.

Etiology/Pathophysiology: The etiology of the observed associations is still unknown.

Clinical Presentation: Patients usually present with severe respiratory distress syndrome.

Prognosis: Poor; if infants survive the first hours after birth recurrent infections may cause severe clinical problems.

Radiology: Chest radiographs show a shift of the mediastinum and/or invagination of abdominal contents into the thoracic cavity.

Pathology:
Gross: Absent or hypoplasia of the lung parenchyma and/or central defect of the diaphragm.

Histology: Pulmonary hypoplasia in Down's syndrome is associated with a reduced number of alveoli per alveolar duct. Diaphragmatic hernia shows normal striated muscle fibers around the defect.

➤ *Descriptors:* Lung parenchyma with altered structure:
- reduced number of distant air spaces
- decreased size of distant air spaces;
- Bronchial mucosa with preserved structure:
- reduced number of bronchial generations

■ *Special stains:* PAS, collagenous stains, chromosomal analysis, morphometric analysis of the lung parenchyma.

Hallmark of Diagnosis: Clinical history, identification of chromosomal abnormality, macroscopic findings, identification of skeleton muscle fibers (diaphragmatic hernia).

Differential diagnosis: Agenesis of the diaphragm, eventration of the diaphragm.

Drowning

Definition: Filling of the lungs with fresh or sea water.

Incidence/Epidemiology: More frequently observed during warm periods of the year.

Etiology/Pathophysiology: Cells of the alveolar lining act as semipermeable membranes. Fresh water drowning causes movement of fluid into the interstitial lung parenchyma due to the lower osmotic pressure of the fluid. Sea water acts in the reversed direction and causes movement of interstitial fluid into the air spaces.

Clinical Presentation: Near drowning in fresh water is usually complicated by late onset of pulmonary edema-"secondary drowning".

Prognosis: Depends upon the severity of the injury. Patients with "secondary drowning" can suddenly die several hours after the first event.

Radiology: Diffuse pulmonary infiltrates on chest films.

Pathology:

Gross: Edematous lungs.

Histology: Interstitial or intraalveolar edema with high protein concentrations. Polymorphonuclear leukocytes are increased in number in "near drowning patients" and may cause signs of an adult respiratory distress syndrome.

➤ *Descriptors:* Lung parenchyma with preserved structure:

- intraalveolar serous fluid
- interstitial edema
- neutrophils

■ *Special stains:* PAS, collagenous stains.

Hallmark of Diagnosis: Clinical history, pulmonary edema (interstitial edema in fresh water drowning, and intraalveolar edema in sea water drowning).

Differential diagnosis: Acute pulmonary edema, adult respiratory distress syndrome, drug toxicity.

Drug Abuse

Definition: Alteration of the lung parenchyma associated with intravenous application of drugs.

Incidence/Epidemiology: Intravenous drug abuse is a common behavior of drug dependent persons. The incidence of drug-dependent persons is steadily increasing and can be estimated to be 0.1% of young adults.

Etiology/Pathophysiology: Intravenous drug application frequently causes right-sided infectious endocarditis. The infectious emboli are sluiced out into the peripheral lung parenchyma and may cause severe pneumonia (*Staphylococcus* pneumonia). Drugs containing starch, lactose, talc, or insoluble fibers cause emboli in the pulmonary vasculature, which induce a granulomatous inflammatory reaction of the lung parenchyma around small arteries or capillaries.

Clinical Presentation: The symptoms range from mild decrease in lung function test to severe bacterial pneumonia.

Prognosis: Depends upon the severity of the pulmonary infection. Drug emboli can induce slow progressive respiratory failure.

Radiology: The findings of chest radiographs reflect the underlying disease. Granulomatous reactions due to foreign body emboli measure 0.1–1 cm in diameter and are thus visible on chest radiographs.

Pathology:

Gross: Multiple, small, firm, grayish-white nodules (foreign body granulomas) or necrotic, brown-red areas of the lung parenchyma (bacterial pneumonic abscess).

Histology: Septic emboli cause destruction of capillary walls which are predominantly infiltrated with neutrophilic granuloctyes and less frequently with lymphocytes and plasma cells. Foreign body emboli cause extended inflammatory reaction of the lung parenchyma with multinucleated giant cells, histiocytes, lymphocytes, and plasma cells. Talc and fiber deposits can be recognized by their birefringent appearance and are usually intermingled with collagenous fibers.

➤ *Descriptors:* Lung parenchyma with altered structure:

- necrosis (focal, perivascular)
- mixed inflammatory infiltrates
- emboli (foreign body, birefringent crystals, intracapillary)
- multinucleated giant cells (foreign body)

■ *Special stains:* PAS, collagenous stains, polarized light.

Hallmark of Diagnosis: Clinical history, infectious arteritis, foreign body granulomas.

Differential diagnosis: Infectious emboli from other causes, noncaseating granulomatous diseases such as sarcoidosis, talcosis, berylliosis, allergic extrinsic alveolitis.

Drug Toxicity

Definition: Alteration of the lung parenchyma associated with intake of drugs.

Incidence/Epidemiology: Alteration of the lung parenchyma associated with drug regimes is not a rare event. Patients suffering from intrapulmonary metastases and being treated with cytostatic multidrug regimes show changes in lung tissue in 30–60% of cases. The intake of the following drugs is reported to be associated with lung parenchyma alterations:

- acetoaminophen, α-adrenergic nasal sprays, althesin, aminorex, aminosalicylic acid, amiodarone, amitriptyline, ampicillin, antacids, antibiotics, anticoagulants, antitetanus serum, acetylsalicylic acid, azathioprine;
- baygon, BCG therapy, BCNU (carmustine), beclomethasone, bleomycin, bromocarbamide, busulfan,
- calcium salts, carbamazepine, carmustine, chlorambucil, chlordiazepoxide, chlorine thiazole, chloromethyl ether, chlorophentermine, chlorozotocin, chlorphentermine, chlorpromazine, chlorpropamide, chlorthalidone, codeine, colchicine, contraceptives, contrast media, cromoglycate, cromolyn, cyclophosphamide, cytosine arabinoside,
- dantrolene, dextran, diazepam, diethylcarbamazine, digitalis, diphenylhydantoin, disodium chromoglycate, L-dopa,
- epinephrine, estrogens, ethosuximide, ethylchlorvynol, ethylenglycol, ethyl ether,
- fluorescein, fluphenazine, formalin,
- gold, griseofulvin, guanoxan,
- haloperidol, halothane, heroin/morphine, hexamethonim, hydralazine, hydrochlorothiazide, hypaque,
- ibuprofen, imipramine, indomethacin, intravenous (illegal) drugs, iodine, iodinized oils (lipiodol), isoguanazepam, isoniazid, isoproteronol, isoquinzepam,
- levodopa, librium, lidocain, lipiodol, lymphangiographic dyes,
- mecamylamine, mefenamic acid, meglumine diatrizoate, melphalan, mephenesin, mephenytoin, 6-mercaptopurine, metaraminol, methacholine, methadone, methotrexate, methyl-dopa, methylphenidate, methylthiouracil, methysergide, mineral oil, mitomycin, monocrotaline,
- naloxone, narcotics, neocarcinostatin, neostigmine, niridazole, nitrofurantoin, nitrogen dioxide, nitrogen mustard,
- oral contraceptives, oxygen, oxyphenisatin, oxyprenolol, ozone,
- pancreatin, paraaminosalicylic acid, paraquat, penicillamine, penicillin, pentazocine, pentolinium, phenylbutazone, phosgene, phosphorus, pindolol, piperazine, pituary snuff, practolol, primidone, procainamide, procarbazine, propanolol, propoxur, propoxyphene, propylthiouracil, prostaglandin F3a, pyrrolizidine alkaloids,
- quinicrine talc, quinidine,
- reserpine,
- salicylates, salicylazosulfapyridine, saline (hypertonic), samustine, serrapeptase, sodium diatrizoate, streptomycin, succinylcholine, sulfachrysceidine, sulfadimethoxine, sulfanilamide, sulfasalazine, sulfonamides,
- tacainide, talc, tartrazine, tetracyclin, thiozides, tolazamide, tolbutamide, tranylcypromine, trimethadione, triphenamines, trypsin, tween,
- vinblastine, visciodol, vitamin D.

Etiology/Pathophysiology: The mechanisms of drug-induced lung diseases can be classified into three different types:

(a) Oxidant lung injury or direct toxicity, which is a dose-dependent injury with cumulative effect and possibly irreversible changes.

(b) Allergic (hypersensitivity) reaction, which is usually of acute onset after an induction period.

(c) Individual susceptibility, which is of acute onset without induction period due to idiopathic conditions.

The related morphological tissue alterations consist of:

allergic extrinsic alveolitis, alveolar proteinosis, angiitis, bronchiolitis obliterans, desquamative interstitial pneumonitis, diffuse alveolar damage, eosinophilic pneumonia, edema, fibrosis, foreign body granulomas, hemorrhage, lipoid pneumonia, lymphoid interstitial pneumonia, metastatic calcification, microgranulomatosis, parenchymal necrosis, pleuritis, pulmonary hypertension, usual interstitial pneumonia.

Clinical Presentation: Diffuse alveolar damage is the most common drug reacton of the lung and yields symptoms like cough, dyspnea, malaise, or respiratory distress. Similar symptoms are seen in idiosyncratic drug reaction and in hypersensitivity pneumonitis. Frequently, changes of lung parenchyma are only mild, and no corresponding clinical symptoms exist.

Prognosis: Usually good; however, progressive respiratory failure can occur.

Radiology: Diffuse interstitial infiltrates and mild fibrosis are the most common findings, but in many cases chest radiographs are normal.

Pathology:

Gross: The lungs may be macroscopically normal or altered due to the specific individual reaction, showing edema, fibrosis, and areas of consolidation.

Histology: In early stages the microscopic findings show focal alterations of the lung parenchyma made up of one or several of the following changes: intraalveolar edema, interstitial edema, desquamative intraalveolar macrophages, dysplasia of alveolar lining cells, interstitial lymphocytic infiltrates, intraalveolar macrophages, lymphocytes, fibrin exudate combined with interstitial mononuclear infiltrates, eosinophilic granulocytes, noncaseating granulomas, dense foamy macrophages in the air spaces, colliquation necrosis, focal fibrosis, and honeycombing in the late stages. The macrophages and cells of the alveolar lining have altered sugar receptors.

➤ *Descriptors:* Lung parenchyma with preserved structure:

- intraalveolar serous fluid
- interstitial edema
- macrophages
- desquamation, hypertrophy, hyperplasia and dysplasia of pneumocytes
- multinucleated giant cells
- mononuclear inflammatory infiltrates (interstitial, intravascular, arterial walls)
- hyaline membranes
- eosinophils;
- Lung parenchyma with altered structure:
- noncaseous epithelioid granulomas
- necrosis (colliquation)
- focal interstitial fibrosis
- enlarged distant air spaces

■ *Special stains:* PAS, collagenous stains, Prussian blue, immunohistochemistry for immunoglobulins, HLA-DR receptor, endogenous lectins.

Hallmark of Diagnosis: Clinical history, diffuse alveolar damage, granulomatous lung tissue reaction, interstitial pneumonia (desquamative interstitial pneumonia, lymphoid interstitial pneumonia, usual interstitial pneumonia), dysplasia of alveolar lining cells, hemorrhage, eosinophilic granulocytic infiltrates.

Differential diagnosis: Corresponding (idiopathic) lung diseases not associated with drug intake.

Dust, Organic

Definition: Alteration of the lung parenchyma associated with exposure to organic dust. The lesion is also known as allergic extrinsic alveolitis.

Incidence/Epidemiology: Organic dust causes extrinsic allergic reactions of the lung parenchyma in 2–6% of exposed persons, especially among farmers or persons working with agricultural products or activities including cheese production, pigeons, chicken breeding, grain mills, tobacco, tea and coffee plants, hay harvesting. The following agents are related to allergic extrinsic alveolitis:

Bacteria: *Micropolyspora faeni, Thermoactinomyces candidus, sacchari*, and *vulgaris*.

Fungi: *Aspergillus clavatus, clavus*, and *fumigatus, Cryptostroma corticale, Alternaria, Graphium, Penicillum casei, Mucor stolinifer, Trichosporum cutaneum.*

Animal proteins from birds, bovines, swine, fish, bats, fur.

Insect proteins from mites, fleas, ants, bugs.

The agents leading to allergic extrinsic alveolitis in grain workers, coffee workers, tea workers, or tobacco growers are not known.

Etiology/Pathophysiology: Reaction of the lung parenchyma due to exposure to organic dust is related to a combination of type III and type IV immune complex mechanisms. Precipitating antibodies against the causative agent can

be demonstrated 4–6 h after exposure. Cell-mediated immunoresponse is probably involved in view of the formation of granulomas.
Clinical Presentation: Two courses may occur, (a) an acute or subacute course with fever, malaise, dyspnea, etc., and (b) a chronic course with inconspicuous onset and prolonged duration or progress into respiratory failure. For details, see Allergic (Extrinsic) Alveolitis.

Prognosis: Usually good; however, slow progressive respiratory failure can occur.

Radiology: Chest radiographs may be normal or show diffuse interstitial bilateral infiltrates.

Pathology:
Gross: Normal lung tissue or consolidated, firm, and rubbery lung parenchyma. For details, see Allergic (Extrinsic) Alveolitis.

Histology: Diffuse interstitial noncaseating epithelioid granulomas combined with reactive hyperplasia of cells of the alveolar lining. For details, see Allergic (Extrinsic) Alveolitis.

➤ *Descriptors:* Lung parenchyma with altered structure:
- noncaseous epithelioid granulomas
- eosinophils
- multinucleated giant cells
- intrabronchiolar fibrinoid material and histiocytes
- ulceration of bronchiolar mucosa;
- Lung parenchyma with preserved structure:
- macrophages
- desquamation, hypertrophy, hyperplasia and dysplasia of pneumocytes
- mononuclear inflammatory infiltrates
- intraalveolar serous fluid

■ *Special stains:* PAS, collagenous stains, silver stain, immunohistochemistry for OKT8 and OKT4, endogenous lectins.

Hallmark of Diagnosis: Noncaseating granulomas combined with alveolitis (hyperplasia and dysplasia of cells of the alveolar lining), clinical history.

Differential diagnosis: Sarcoidosis, granulomatous infections, berylliosis, drug reaction, usual interstitial pneumonia, desquamative interstitial pneumonia, lymphocytic interstitial pneumonia.

Dysplasia, Bronchopulmonary

Definition: Disease of the newborn during the "transition period" which results in bronchiolar epithelial dysplasia, necrotizing bronchiolitis, and peribronchiolar edema, see Bronchopulmonary Dysplasia.

Echinococcosis

Definition: Infection of the lung with the cestodes *Echinococcus granulosus, multilocularis*, and *vogeli* (oligarthrus).
Incidence/Epidemiology: *E. granulosis* has a worldwide distribution; about 100 infections per year are reported from various European countries. *E. multilocularis* lives in North America, Alaska, Europe as far south as Switzerland, and Siberia. *E. vogeli* has been reported from Columbia, Ecuador, Venezuela, Panama, and Costa Rica.
Etiology/Pathophysiology: Dogs, sheep, wolves, and moose are the definite hosts of *E. granulosis* (cystic hydatid disease), foxes are the definite hosts of *E. multilocularis*, and dogs and paca are the definite host of *E. vogeli*. Humans become infected upon ingesting the live soil-borne eggs of the parasites, which hatch into invasive onchospheres in the intestines. The onchospheres enter the venous blood stream and lodge in organs and subsequently capillary systems, especially in the liver, spleen, and lung. *E. granulosis* develops into a spherical cyst measuring 1–20 cm in diameter after 5–10 months, containing a thin, living, inner membrane with broad capsules of infectious protoscolices. The alveolar hydatid cyst of *E. multilocularis* is sterile, whereas the polycystic hydatid cyst of *E. vogeli* is infectious.
Clinical Presentation: Pulmonary *Echinococcus* cysts usually do not produce clinical symptoms and may remain undetected for several years. Ruptured cysts, however, may cause severe anaphylactic shock. The sputum contains protoscoleces, hooklets, or compartments of the cystic wall. Cysts of *E. vogeli* grow faster than cysts of *E. granularis* or *E. multilocularis*.
Prognosis: Slow asymptomatic growth of the hydatid cysts is the common course; however, rupture can induce severe anaphylactic shock with fatal outcome.

Radiology: *E. granulosis* cysts have the appearance of sharply circumscribed balls with smaller inclusion cysts within the large orbit. *E. multilocularis* infection results in multiple small dense masses of irregular shape and peripheral localization, or in dense masses in the lower right lobe with connection to the diaphragm and liver (penetration of the parasites through the diaphragm).

Pathology:

Gross: Cysts of *E. granulosus* and *E.vogeli* are embedded in a 2–4 mm thick fibrous layer of the host tissue, whereas cysts of *E. multilocularis* are embedded in necrotic debris or cavities. *E. granulosis* cysts are filled with transparent fluid, but *E. multilocularis* cysts have a rather solid consistency.

Histology: The walls of *E. granulosis* cysts have a laminated membrane 1 mm in thickness without nuclei. It is covered by a germinal layer with embedded nuclei, which is 10–25 μm broad. Attached to the germinal layer multiple invaginated scolices about 100 μm in maximum diameter can be detected, containing a sucker, a double crown of hooklets, and calcareous bodies. *E. multilocularis* cysts do not contain scolices and consist of a laminated membrane without nuclei. The multiple locules are usually embedded in broad fibrous tissue or in necrotic areas consisting of debris, neutrophilic and eosinophilic granulocytes, lymphocytes, and plasma cells. The microscopic appearance of *E. vogeli* cysts resembles that of *E. granulosis* cysts.

➤ *Descriptors:* Lung parenchyma with altered structure:
- parasites (*Echinococcus*, invaginated scolices)
- cysts (fibrous, attached germinal layer)
- necrosis
- mixed inflammatory infiltrates
- eosinophils

■ *Special stains:* PAS, Ziehl-Neelsen, collagenous stains.

Hallmark of Diagnosis: Clinical history, macroscopic appearance, identification of cystic walls and scolices.

Differential diagnosis: Noninfectious cysts, infections with other cestodes (cysticercosis).

Echo Virus

Definition: Infection of the human lung with Echo virus.

Incidence/Epidemiology: Characteristic summer-autumn peaks in incidence of infections, usually in children. Ubiquitous in the moderate zones.

Etiology/Pathophysiology: Enteric cytopathogenic human orphan virus (RNA virus) is transmitted by smears, droplets, or direct contact and causes acute infections of the upper and lower respiratory tract (types E 6,8,11,20,28).

Clinical Presentation: Acute febrile onset of the disease with symptoms of bronchopneumonia.

Prognosis: Usually good and without sequelae.

Radiology: Chest radiographs can be normal or may show diffuse pneumonic infiltrates.

Pathology:

Gross: Inflammation of the larger bronchi, signs of pneumonic infiltrations of various degrees.

Histology: Hyperplasia and dysplasia of cells of the alveolar lining, mononuclear inflammatory infiltrate, but virus inclusion bodies are usually not striking.

➤ *Descriptors:* Lung parenchyma with preserved structure:
- mononuclear inflammatory infiltrates
- desquamation, hypertrophy, hyperplasia and dysplasia of pneumocytes

■ *Special stains:* PAS, Giemsa, collagenous stains, electron microscopy.

Hallmark of Diagnosis: Clinical history, characterization of the virus with tissue cultures, electron microscopy.

Differential diagnosis: Bronchopneumonia caused by other organisms.

Ectopic Lung

Definition: Herniation of the lung outside the thoracic cavity.

Incidence/Epidemiology: Rare diesease seen in adults with emphysema, asthma, or chronic bronchitis. Unusual disease in newborns occurring in cri du chat syndrome (autosomal chromosome aberration, deletion of chromosome B5 with microencephalus, epicanthus, etc.) and in the Klippel-Feil syndrome (familial hereditary disturbance of development with short neck, spina bifida, arthropathia neurotropica).

Etiology/Pathophysiology: Herniation may occur through the diaphragm, intercostal spaces, and into the neck (newborn period).

Clinical Presentation: Symptoms range from mild dyspnea to severe respiratory distress syndrome.

Prognosis: Usually good if infants survive the newborn period.

Radiology: Chest radiographic findings depend upon the localization and the degree of herniation.

Pathology:

Gross: Atelectatic lung tissue outside the pleural cavity.

Histology: Atelectatic lung parenchyma with normal textures. Chronic inflammatory infiltrates may be present in older lesions.

➤ *Descriptors:* Lung parenchyma with preserved structure:

- atelectatic distant air spaces
- macrophages
- mononuclear inflammatory infiltrates

■ *Special stains:* None.

Hallmark of Diagnosis: Clinical history, macroscopic findings.

Differential diagnosis: Due to underlying disease, extralobar sequestration.

Ectopic Tissue in the Lung

Definition: Occurrence of normal tissue in the lung deriving from organs located outside the lung.

Incidence/Epidemiology: Rare abnormality seen in infants with multiple malformations, in adults after traumatic lesions, or in postpartum women.

Etiology/Pathophysiology: Ectopic tissue in the lung can derive from embryologic remnants, from traumatic implantation or from embolic fragments of other organs.

Clinical Presentation: Clinical symptoms depend upon the amount and source of ectopic tissue in the lung. Repeated chest pain and recurrent pneumothoraces are reported to be symptoms of endometriosis in lung.

Prognosis: Usually good and without sequelae.

Radiology: Chest radiographs are usually normal.

Pathology:

Gross: Congenital ectopic tissue in the lung may be of macroscopically detectable size, but the majority of cases show an unsuspicious macroscopic appearance.

Histology: There have been reported intrapulmonary ectopias of the endometrium, striated muscle fibers, adrenals, liver, exocrine and endocrine pancreatic tissue of normal appearance.

➤ *Descriptors:* Lung parenchyma with altered structures:

- ectopic tissue (endometrium, exocrine and endocrine pancreatic tissue, striated muscle cells, adrenals and liver)

■ *Special stains:* PAS, collagenous stains.

Hallmark of Diagnosis: Normal parenchyma of nonrespiratory organs within the lung tissue.

Differential diagnosis: Intrapulmonary teratoma.

Edema

Definition: Pulmonary disease caused by movement of fluid from the cardiovascular space into the interstitium and alveoli.

Incidence/Epidemiology: Frequent disease seen in aged patients, in children with abnormalities of the cardiovascular system or with oxygen dependency, in persons exposed to toxins or drugs, and in patients suffering from various diseases such as cancer, silicosis, lung transplant, etc.

Etiology/Pathophysiology: The lung is called edematous when its amount of extravascular water exceeds 4–5 ml/g of dry tissue. The extravasation of fluid into the interstitium and into the air spaces is controlled by the 4 Starling forces (intravascular and extravascular hydrostatic pressure, intravascular and extravascular colloidal osmotic pressure). These forces are also influenced by the permeability of the capillary endothelial cells, by properties of the alveolar epithelial cells (permeability to small and larger proteins), and by lymphatic drainage. Arterioles and venules less than 100 μm in external diameter lack smooth muscle fibers and consist of a single elastic lamina with lined epithelial cells. The pulmonary capillaries are located at the meeting points of three alveolar walls and over the length of the interalveolar septula and comprise approximately 80 capillaries per 100 μm of interalveolar septula. If the pressure inside the air spaces exceeds the pulmonary artery pressure, the capillaries over the length of the alveolar walls opposite those located in the corners collapse. Between neighboring endothelial cells tight junctions exist, making possible the exchange of fluids and solutions. The capillaries within the interalveolar septula show a thick and a thin side adjacent to the air spaces. The interstitial space is defined to be the space between the basement lamina of the epithelial cells and the capillary endothelial cells on the thick side. This space between the epithelial cells and the endothelial cells is 1 μm in width, is normally filled with fluid, elastin, collagen fibrils, proteoglycans, fibroblasts, and macrophages, and does not usually contain lymphocytes. The interstitial space communicates continuously with the interstitial spaces of the corner capillaries and merges with the connective tissue that surrounds the pulmonary lobules, arteries, and veins. The following pathophysiologic mechanisms are of clinical importance:

(a) Increased intravascular hydrostatic pressure: left-heart failure (myocardial infarction), mitral stenosis, hypertensive left-heart cardiomyopathy, obliteration of pulmonary veins, increased intracapillary flow by overtransfusion;

(b) Decreased interstitial hydrostatic pressure: acute atelectasis, rapid reexpansion of pneumothorax (hydrothorax);

(c) Increased permeability of microvascular membrane:

a. infectious agents: bacterial toxins, malaria, mycoplasma, virus;
b. inhaled substances: nitrogen dioxide, oxygen, smoke, sulfur dioxide;
c. aspiration: fresh and salt water drowning, gastric contents;
d. drug reaction: amphotericin B, azathioprine, BCNU, bleomycin, busulfan, chlorambucil, colchicine, cytosine arabinoside, cytoxan, ethylchlorvynol, gold, heroin, hexamethonium, hydrochlorothiazide, kerosone, melphalan, methotrexate, mitomycin, nitrofurantoin, paraquat, penicillamine, phenylbutazone, practolol, salicylate;
e. radiation;
f. acute disturbance: shock, trauma;
g. side reaction in diseases: acute pancreatitis, pregnancy, sepsis, systemic lupus erythematosus, uremia;
h. decreased lymphatic drainage: lung transplant, pneumoconioses with scarring, tumors;
i. other: high altitude, neurogenic.

Clinical Presentation: The clinical signs and symptoms depend upon the degree and the timely development of the edema which is usually subclassified into an acute and a chronic stage. Mild symptoms are dyspnea on exertion, dry cough, paroxysmal nocturnal dyspnea. In severe stages frothy, blood tinged cough and respiratory distress appear. Chronic pulmonary edema is usually caused by cardiac insufficiency and may result in progressive dyspnea. The special signs and symptoms are discussed under Adult Respiratory Distress Syndrome.

Prognosis: Depends upon the cause and severity of the disease. Acute edema can be fatal, especially if induced by toxic agents, acute cardiac failure, shock, or trauma. Chronic edema can proceed to progressive interstitial fibrosis and progressive respiratory failure.

Radiology: The characteristic findings on chest radiographs are short subpleural linear septal markings, called Kerley B lines. Prominent pulmonary vessels and patchy alveolar densities with a "butterfly or bat-wing" distribution indicate more severe stages.

Pathology:

Gross: Heavy lungs with large amounts of tan to blood-tinged fluid exuding from the cut surface. Chronic edematous lungs are orange-brown with randomly distributed grayish-white spots ("leopard spots").

Histology: Widened interstitial septula with preserved lung texture and scattered granulocytic and mononuclear intraalveolar and interstitial infiltrates. Within the air spaces homogeneous fluids of "light appearance" are found. Chronic pulmonary edema is usually combined with hypertensive changes in the arterial walls such as thickening of the fibrointimal and medial layer. A fine interstitial fibrosis is a common finding.

➤ *Descriptors:* Lung parenchyma with preserved structure:

- intraalveolar serous fluid
- mononuclear inflammatory infiltrates;
- Lung parenchyma with altered structure:

- diffuse interstitial fibrosis;
- Pulmonary vessels with altered structure:
- fibrosis (arteries)
- increased number of smooth muscle cells
- stenosis
- thrombosis

■ *Special stains:* PAS, collagenous stains, Grocott's (for exclusion of *Pneumocystis carinii*), Prussian blue (chronic congestion).

Hallmark of Diagnosis: Clinical history, macroscopic findings, preserved lung texture with interstitial and intraalveolar "protein-light" fluids, mild inflammation.

Differential diagnosis: Alveolar proteinosis, *Pneumocystis carinii* infection, drowning, classification of the edema due to the underlying cause.

Effusion, Pleural

Definition: Serous or sanguinous fluid in the pleural cavity exceeding 20 ml.

Incidence/Epidemiology: Common disease, especially in the elderly. The diagnostic frequency depends upon the nature of the underlying disease and the specialty of the physician.

Etiology/Pathophysiology: The pleural cavity contains about 20 ml of transudative fluid in healthy persons which has a high turnover of transudation and reabsorption. Disturbance of the balance may cause pleural effusions. Common causes are:

(a) Decreased reabsorption (cardiac failure, renal failure, nephrotic syndrome, cirrhosis, superior vena cava syndrome, Meigs' syndrome);

(b) Increased (exudative) production: infections, collagen vascular diseases, neoplasms, endometriosis;

(c) Eosinophilic effusions: drug sensitivity, idiopathic, pneumothorax, pulmonary infarction, pneumonia;

(d) Hemorrhagic effusions: trauma, neoplasms, tuberculosis, infarction, pneumothorax.

Clinical Presentation: Symptoms include fever, chest pain, dyspnea, respiratory distress.

Prognosis: Depends upon the underlying disease, infections, parapneumonic and parainfarctious effusions carry a good prognosis, whereas those induced by endometriosis are usually recurrent, and those induced by neoplasms, cardiac or renal failure, and liver cirrhosis are difficult to cure.

Radiology: Chest radiographs present homogeneous densities of one complete lung.

Pathology:

Gross: Yellowish to bloody fluid.

Histology: Pleural effusions contain few lymphocytes and plasma cells and a few to a moderate number of mesothelial cells. Metastatic cancer cells are absent if the cancerous growth is predominantly in the lymphatic and venous vessels of the pleura. Mitotic figures in mesothelial cells are not necessarily characteristic of a malignant growth.

➤ *Descriptors:* Pleura with preserved structure:
- mononuclear inflammatory infiltrates
- mixed inflammatory infiltrates
- fibrinoid material (pleural surface)
- hypertrophy and hyperplasia of mesothelial cells;
- Pleura with altered structure:
- caseous epithelioid granulomas
- noncaseous epithelioid granulomas
- multinucleated giant cells
- eosinophils
- fibrosis
- Newly formed textures with metastasis potential:
- epithelial growth pattern
- mesenchymal growth pattern
- adenoid textures
- solid textures
- infrequent mitoses
- vascular and pleural invasion

■ *Special stains:* PAS, Papanicolaou.

Hallmark of Diagnosis: Clinical history, macroscopic findings, cellular pattern of the effusion.

Differential diagnosis: Depends on the underlying disease.

Ehlers-Danlos Syndrome

Definition: Alteration of the lung parenchyma seen in patients with Ehlers-Danlos syndrome.

Incidence/Epidemiology: Ehlers-Danlos syndrome is an autosomal dominant (type I–III) or recessive (type IV–VII) nonhereditary disease with disturbance of synthesis and network of collagenous fibers. The disease rarely affects the lungs.

Etiology/Pathophysiology: Abnormalities of the collagenous network cause cystic spaces within the interstitium and abnormalities within the walls of arteries, leading to circumscribed stenoses.

Clinical Presentation: Usually no pulmonary symptoms.

Prognosis: The prognosis is not associated with pulmonary involvement.

Radiology: Chest radiographs may be normal. Angiographies may show stenotic lesions in the peripheral pulmonary arteries.

Pathology:

Gross: Usually no abnormal findings.

Histology: Stenotic lesions in the peripheral pulmonary arteries with abnormal texture of the collagenous network within the intimal and medial layer.

➤ *Descriptors:* Pulmonary vessels with altered structure:

- fragmentation of elastic fibers
- stenosis
- hyaline material

■ *Special stains:* Collagenous stains, methenamine silver stain.

Hallmark of Diagnosis: Clinical history, peripheral stenotic lesions of the pulmonary arteries.

Differential diagnosis: Stenotic lesions of the pulmonary arteries due to other causes such as Down's syndrome, cutis laxa, von Recklinghausen's disease.

Elastic Tissue Encrustation with Iron

Definition: Deposits of iron in the elastic tissue of the lung.

Incidence/Epidemiology: Frequently seen in children with congestive heart failure or in adults with chronic or persistent hemorrhages such as primary pulmonary hemosiderosis or venoocclusive disease.

Etiology/Pathophysiology: Disintegration of erythrocytes leads to iron deposits within macrophages or multinucleated giant cells, and in the extracellular spaces near small venules and arteries.

Clinical Presentation: Symptoms due to the underlying disease (chronic hemorrhage).

Prognosis: Usually slow progressive respiratory failure.

Radiology: Signs due to the underlying disease.

Pathology:

Gross: Thickened and brittle, grayish-yellow connective tissue.

Histology: Accumulation of iron in the elastic tissues around small veins and arteries. Iron crystals ingested by macrophages and multinucleated giant cells in the peribronchial alveoli.

➤ *Descriptors:* Lung parenchyma with preserved structure:

- dust (iron)
- macrophages (iron crystals)
- multinucleated giant cells (iron crystals)

■ *Special stains:* Prussian blue, collagenous stains.

Hallmark of Diagnosis: Iron deposits in elastic periarterial and perivenous tissue and in macrophages and multinucleated giant cells.

Differential diagnosis: Asbestos bodies, encrustation with other agents (calcium, organic and mineral dust).

Embolism, Pulmonary

Definition: Acute occlusion of a pulmonary artery with an embolus.

Incidence/Epidemiology: Pulmonary embolism is a frequent event and includes thrombotic and nonthrombotic emboli. Thrombotic emboli seen in older immobile patients may arise in 20–40% of patients. Increased thromboembolic risk exists in patients under estrogen treatment (birth control, prostatic carcinoma) or those with hereditary abnormalities of the blood clotting mechanism (protein C, protein S, etc.). Emboli from extravascular sources are usually rare and include air emboli, infectious emboli, tissue emboli, amniotic fluid emboli, foreign body emboli, and emboli in drug abusers.

Etiology/Pathophysiology: Peripheral veins of the body such as those of the legs (deep venous thrombosis) may form thromboses adjacent to the intima in the periphery of the vessel and growing towards the center. This part of the thrombosis may tear off, and the embolus is then carried into the pulmonary artery system via the right heart. Immobilized patients with low venous return (fractures of the femoral and pelvic bones, surgery, heart infarction, etc.) are particularly at risk of forming thromboses. Emboli from the extravascular system are associated with a variety of special conditions such as head and neck surgery, trauma of the great veins, inadequate intravenous infusions, etc. that may lead to air embolism; delivery that may lead to amniotic fluid embolism; trauma, fractures, and malignancies that may lead to tissue emboli, including bone marrow emboli; infectious endocarditis, parasites, and infectious dermatitis that may lead to infectious emboli; and invasive iatrogenic procedures or intravenous drug abuse that may lead to foreign body emboli. Intrapulmonary emboli are usually small and lodge in arteries of corresponding size. They cause acute death if the cardiac output from the right heart is decreased by 75% or more. Thromboemboli become organized after 4–6 weeks. Small emboli are removed from the lobar arteries within four weeks. The lung parenchyma distal to the occluded artery undergoes temporary (by hemorrhage) or permanent (by infarction) ischemia, if the collateral circulation from the bronchial arteries or pulmonary arteries is insufficient.

Clinical Presentation: Patients with pulmonary emboli seldom present with symptoms such as brief chest pain or shortness of breath. Sudden massive thromboembolism, however, is fatal in the majority of cases due to right heart failure.

Prognosis: Massive thrombosis is usually fatal, while smaller emboli usually heal without serious sequelae.

Radiology: Chest radiographs may be normal or show peripheral wedge-shaped infiltrations.

Pathology:

Gross: The premortem emboli have a rubbery surface, are firm and blunt-ended, and may be infolded. Fresh emboli are pale-red, while older emboli are hardened and may be calcified. Postmortem emboli are soft in consistency, have a smooth glittery surface, and are dark red.

Histology: Fresh premortem emboli have a certain circular regularity in structure with layers of fibrin strands between degenerated red cells. Organized emboli display multiple channels of recanalization with channel walls composed of fibroelastic tissue. The walls are continuously attached to the intima of the artery which shows a fibroelastic reaction. The structure of postmortem clots is related to one layer of the artery caused by sedimentation of red cells separated by a layer consisting of leucocytes and fibrin. Nonthrombotic emboli are recognized by their tissue within the pulmonary arteries, which may undergo degeneration and histiocytic inflammatory reaction of the arterial wall. Air embolism causes pulmonary edema and pleural effusion.

➤ *Descriptors:* Lung parenchyma with preserved structure:
- intraalveolar serous fluid;
- Pulmonary vessels with preserved structure:
- emboli (small and large arteries, fresh, organized)
- mononuclear inflammatory infiltrates;
- Pleura with preserved structure:
- pleural effusion

■ *Special stains:* PAS, Collagenous stains.

Hallmark of Diagnosis: Clinical history, macroscopic findings, identification of the embolic structures or tissue.

Differential diagnosis: Postmortem clots, veno-occlusive disease.

Emphysema

Definition: Permanent enlargement of distal air spaces (with destruction of their walls).

Incidence/Epidemiology: Emphysematous changes of lung parenchyma are closely related to the age of the patients, with an increase in frequency of about 60% from the 3rd to the 7th decade of life. The degree is related to smoking and air pollution. Its prevalence has been calculated to be 60% in men and 15% in women. Centrilobular emphysema is the most common type, followed by the panacinar form. Hereditary forms of emphysema have been reported to occur in α_1-antitrypsin deficiency (familial emphysema).

Etiology/Pathophysiology: In the adult, 4 types of emphysema can be distinguished morphologically: (a) Centrilobular emphysema involves the respiratory bronchioles and the proximal part of the acinus. It is a gradually progressive disease seen in smokers or those with simple coal pneumoconiosis and associated with chronic airflow obstruction. (b) Panacinar emphysema involves the air spaces from the center to the periphery of an acinus in a nearly uniform distribution. It is associated with α_1-antitrypsin deficiency (familial emphy-

sema) and the corresponding exhibition of co-dominant alleles for proteinase inhibitors (Pi) such as PiZ, PiMZ, PiS. It is also associated with atresia of the bronchioles especially in the Swyer-James or MacLeod syndrome (unilateral pulmonary emphysema). (c) Localized (distal acinar) emphysema involves the peripheral part of the acinus. It is usually localized in the lung periphery, may cause pneumothorax (mantel emphysema) and is frequently seen in young adults. (d) Perifocal (irregular) emphysema is always associated with scars such as postinfectious or pneumoconiotic lung parenchyma alterations. Congenital lobar overinflation (infantile lobar emphysema) and interstitial emphysema involving the interstitial and subpleural connective tissue describe emphysematous changes in lung parenchyma without significant destruction of air spaces.
Smoking produces inflammation in lung parenchyma, for example respiratory bronchiolitis, which may activate the proteolytic activity of macrophages and decrease the activity of α_1-antitrypsin. Other proteolytic enzymes such as leukocyte-derived elastase also participate in disturbance of the proteolysis-antiproteolysis balance, which is assumed to be of major importance for emphysematous destruction of lung parenchyma. Disturbance of the homogeneity of tensional forces associated with scars produces reactive inflammation leading to similar disturbances of the proteolytic balance.

Clinical Presentation: Clinically, emphysematous changes of lung parenchyma are closely related to chronic airflow obstruction. Patients with emphysema have cor pulmonale more frequently than patients without emphysematous changes. Syndromes associated with severe emphysematous lung parenchyma alterations are "blue bloaters" (patients with severe hypoxemia, frequently hypercarbia, polycythemia, and right ventricular failure), and the "pink buffers" (thin patients with increased forced vital capacity). Lung function tests are important for diagnosis of emphysema, for example, increased total lung capacity, increase in functional residual lung capacity, and decreased expiratory flow rate, or carbon monoxide diffusion capacity. Clinical history reveals any association with cigarette smoking and chronic bronchitis.

Prognosis: Usually slow progressive respiratory failure.

Radiology: Radiologic signs of severe emphysema are diaphragmatic flattening, deficiency of peripheral arteries, and increased translucence.

Pathology:

Gross: (a) In centrilobular emphysema, the connective tissue of the lobular septa is usually well demarcated. Close to the center of the lobules, empty air spaces measuring several millimeters to 1 cm in diameter are present. The distribution of the emphysematous changes is nearly uniform. (b) In panacinar emphysema, enlargement of the acini arises in a uniformly distributed manner measuring a few millimeters in diameter. The lower zones of the lung are more frequently affected. (c) Localized emphysema is usually limited to the posterior and anterior parts of the upper lung zones. The size of the emphysematous cysts may reach several centimeters. (d) In perifocal emphysema there are widespread scars in the lung with adjacent larger empty air spaces. The scars are usually dark brown-black and contain dust deposits or may show calcified areas.

Histology: (a) In centrilobular emphysema one sees destruction of the terminal bronchioles with preserved terminal air spaces in the acinar periphery, at least in some areas (criteria for distinguishing centrilobular emphysema from panacinar emphysema). The degree of emphysematous changes varies very considerably within one lobule. (b) In panacinar emphysema, enlarged and flattened alveoli appear in the early stages. Progressive emphysematous changes affect all distant air spaces to a nearly homogeneous degree within the same lobule. (c) In localized emphysema, there are large empty air spaces below and adjacent to the pleura. The pleura itself is focally fibrotic and may be atrophic in other portions. (d) In perifocal emphysema, central scars are surrounded by empty enlarged air spaces involving the acini and bronchioles. The scars may consist of granulomatous tissue, calcified parenchyma, or deposits of dust intermingled with collagenous fibers.

➤ *Descriptors:* Lung parenchyma with altered structure:

- enlarged distant air spaces
- focal interstitial fibrosis

- macrophages
- mononuclear inflammatory infiltrates

■ *Special stains:* Collagenous stains, barium sulfate impregnation of the specimen (for demonstration of panacinar emphysema).

Hallmark of Diagnosis: Macroscopic findings, distribution of emphysematous changes.

Differential diagnosis: Cysts and pseudocysts of various origins.

Emphysema, Interstitial

Definition: Presence of air within the interstitial connective tissue of the lung.

Incidence/Epidemiology: Frequently seen in premature infants with artificial ventilation for respiratory distress syndrome (in about 20% of cases) and having a high negative correlation with body weight at birth. In 75% of these infants, interstitial emphysema develops within the 1st day of life.

Etiology/Pathophysiology: Ventilation of the lung causes ruptures of the alveolar walls near their bases with direct connection to the interstitial tissue surrounding the blood vessels. Positive pressure of ventilation forces the air into the interstitium and directs it along the connective tissue of the vessels to the mediastinum, pericardium, and pleura with subsequent pneumomediastinum, pneumopericardium or pneumothorax. Rapid reabsorption of the air may follow, as well as long-lasting persistence, eliciting a fibroblastic inflammatory reaction, including foreign-body giant cells.

Clinical Presentation: The infants show progressive respiratory distress the more they receive enforced artificial ventilation.

Prognosis: Mortality of infants is closely associated with birth weights, and about 50% of patients with a birth weight less than 1 500 g die. More than 50% of survivors develop bronchopulmonary dysplasia.

Radiology: Chest radiographs show lucent linear streaks, interstitial markings, cystic spaces with a tendency to hilar radiation. Mediastinal shift, depression of the diaphragm, and atelectasis of noninvolved lobes may occur.

Pathology:
Two different stages have to be distinguished: (a) acute diffuse stage and (b) persistent localized or diffuse stage.

Gross: (a) In the acute stage, round to oval air-filled (empty) spaces 0.2–0.4 mm in diameter, present around the bronchovascular structures and beneath the interlobar septa. Atelectatic compression of the peripheral lung tissue. (b) In the chronic stage, large cysts 0.2–2 cm in size arise along the interlobar septula having a thin fibrous wall 0.1–0.2 mm thick. The adjacent lung parenchyma is usually atelectatic.

Histology: (a) In the acute stage, the bronchi and arteries are surrounded by clear empty spaces which are also present along the interlobular septa. The adjacent lung parenchyma is characterized by atelectatic alveoli with mild inflammatory mononuclear infiltrates. (b) The persistent stage shows large, irregular, air-filled (empty) spaces limited to the interlobular septa. These air spaces are surrounded by a thin layer of fibroblasts and densely packed, multinucleated, foreign-body giant cells. The adjacent lung parenchyma shows mild to moderate interstitial inflammatory infiltrations and a moderate hyperplasia of cells of the alveolar lining.

➤ *Descriptors:* Lung parenchyma with preserved structure:

- enlarged distant air spaces (clear, empty, around the bronchi and vessels)
- atelectatic distant air spaces
- mononuclear inflammatory infiltrates
- multinucleated giant cells
- macrophages
- desquamation, hypertrophy, hyperplasia and dysplasia of pneumocytes;
- Lung parenchyma with altered structure:
- proliferating fibroblasts

■ *Special stains:* PAS, collagenous stains, Giemsa.

Hallmark of Diagnosis: Empty air spaces around the broncho-vascular structures and along the interlobular septa (multinucleated giant cells in the persistent stage).

Differential diagnosis: Bronchopulmonary dysplasia, congenital lymphangiectasis.

Emphysema, Lobar Infantile

Definition: Overinflation of lung parenchyma associated with congenital malformation of the lung.

Incidence/Epidemiology: More frequently seen in boys than in girls (8:1), and most frequently occurring before 6 months of age. Usually associated with cardiovascular abnormalities such as Fallot's tetralogy, ventricular septal defect, and patent ductus arteriosus.

Etiology/Pathophysiology: Overinflation occurs secondary to bronchial obstruction caused by stenosis, atresia of a bronchus or the trachea, external compression due to anomalous vessels, rotation of a lobe, bronchogenic cysts in the mediastinum, or scars secondary to infection, trauma, or aspiration of meconium.

Clinical Presentation: The children present with mild respiratory distress, progressive dyspnea, vomiting, cyanosis, feeding difficulties, or respiratory infections.

Prognosis: Usually good and related to the associated congenital abnormalities.

Radiology: Chest radiographs reveal a hyperlucent lobe with mediastinal shift, herniation of the lung across the mediastinum, compression of uninvolved lobes.

Pathology:

Gross: Enormous enlarged lobe with smooth surface and tan color. In about 80% of cases the upper lobes are involved.

Histology: Enormous widened alveolar ducts and alveoli with preserved structures. The interalveolar septula may be focally disrupted. Necrosis, alveolar fibrosis, or marked interstitial inflammation are not features of infantile lobar emphysema.

➤ *Descriptors:* Lung parenchyma with preserved structure:

- enlarged distant air ways

■ *Special stains:* PAS, collagenous stains.

Hallmark of Diagnosis: Clinical history, macroscopic findings, enlarged terminal airways with preserved structures.

Differential diagnosis: Polyalveolar lobe, congenital pulmonary lymphangiectasis, adenomatoid cystic (congenital) malformation, pulmonary sequestration.

Empyema

Definition: Pus in the pleural cavity.

Incidence/Epidemiology: Relatively uncommon disease with declining frequency. Spontaneously infectious empyemas are secondary to iatrogenic and traumatic empyema.

Etiology/Pathophysiology: Bacteria causing spontaneous empyemas include *Pneumococcus, Staphylococcus, Streptococcus* and any of those organisms causing abscess formation in pneumonia. Tuberculous empyema is rare but not really uncommon in immunocompromised patients.

Clinical Presentation: Severe disease with high fever, chills, and a high mortality (25%).

Prognosis: High mortality, especially in immunocompromised patients (up to 50%).

Radiology: Chest radiographs display extensive densities in one lung.

Pathology:

Gross: Pus. Shaggy exudate on the pleural surface.

Histology: Cellular debris, fibrin; the biopsies exhibit dense granulocytic inflammatory infiltrates and layers of fibrin. Severe atypias of mesothelial cells may mimic mesothelioma.

➤ *Descriptors:* Pleura with altered structure:

- fibrinoid material
- mixed inflammatory infiltrates
- necrosis
- hyperplasia and hypertrophy of the mesothelial cells

■ *Special stains:* PAS, collagenous stains, Ziehl-Neelsen.

Hallmark of Diagnosis: Macroscopy, exclusion of malignancy.

Differential diagnosis: Due to underlying cause.

Endometriosis

Definition: Ectopic tissue of endometrium in the lung parenchyma and pleura.

Incidence/Epidemiology: Rare disease seen in postpartum women.

Etiology/Pathophysiology: Fragments of endometrial tissue are transported into the lung after gaining access to the venous system.

Clinical Presentation: Most patients suffer from bloody pleural effusions or pneumothorax. Periodical hemoptysis associated with menstruation has been reported.

Prognosis: Usually good and without sequelae.

Radiology: Most patients present with signs of pleural effusions.

Pathology:
Gross: Bloody pleural effusions with focally thickened pleura or occasionally circumscribed, tan-grayish nodules within the lung tissue.
Histology: Benign columnar cells which may show a decidual reaction.

➤ *Descriptors:* Pleura with altered structure:
- decidual reaction in the pleura
- benign columnar cells
- hemorrhage

■ *Special stains:* PAS, Prussian blue, collagenous stains, Giemsa.

Hallmark of Diagnosis: Clinical history, identification of endometrial cells.

Differential diagnosis: Obstructive lung disease (clusters of macrophages or reactive mesothelial cells), pleural effusions due to other causes.

Enterobiasis

Definition: Infection of the lung with the nematode *Enterobius vermicularis*.

Incidence/Epidemiology: A parasite with worldwide distribution, especially in temperate or cold regions. Well adapted to man and usually causes infections of the colon and rectum; only three cases with parasites detected in the lung have been described.

Etiology/Pathophysiology: The male and female parasites live in the colon of man, where the male dies shortly after copulation. The female worm moves to the anus, and the embryonated infectious eggs are deposited into the perianal and perineal skin. No intermediate host is required for the infectious eggs which are transmitted to new hosts through fingernails, clothing, etc.

Clinical Presentation: Besides some asymptomatic patients, most frequently intense, nocturnal anal pruritus caused by the migrating female worm has been reported. Other symptoms are nasal pruritus (retrograde migration of worms), rectal colic, convulsions, anorexia.

Prognosis: Usually good and without serious sequelae.

Radiology: The pulmonary lesions are peripherally located, circumscribed, centrally necrotic nodules.

Pathology:
Gross: The white worms measure 8–13 × 0.3–0.5 mm (female) and 2–5 × 0.1–0.2 mm (male). In the lungs, the worms produce necrotic grayish-red nodules measuring several centimeters in diameter.
Histology: The cuticle of the worms surrounds a small noncontinuous layer of smooth muscle cells. Two opposing alae are attached to the cuticle. Invasion of the lung causes a severe granulomatous inflammatory reaction with central necrosis and numerous eosinophilic granulocytes.

➤ *Descriptors:* Lung parenchyma with altered structure:
- caseous epithelioid granulomas
- parasites (intragranulomatous)
- eosinophils (numerous)

■ *Special stains:* PAS, Movat.

Hallmark of Diagnosis: Clinical history, caseous epithelioid granulomas, identification of the parasites.

Differential diagnosis: Infections with other parasites.

Enterovirus Infection

Definition: Infection of the lung with enterovirus.

Incidence/Epidemiology: Usually infection of the intestines and the upper respiratory tract, seldom of the lung.

Etiology/Pathophysiology: The virus can multiply in various tissues and may produce a systemic infection including pneumonia, myocarditis, and meningitis.

Clinical Presentation: Symptoms of pneumonia or viremia.

Prognosis: Usually good; however, cardiac infection and bacterial superinfection may cause severe clinical problems.

Radiology: Chest X-radiographs correspond to pneumonic infection and may show diffuse densities.

Pathology:
Gross: Nonspecific pneumonic findings including heavy, wet, red-grayish lungs.
Histology: Nonspecific pulmonary damage with hyperplasia and dysplasia of cells of the alveolar lining, fibrinoid exudation, mononuclear interstitial infiltrates.

➤ *Descriptors:* Lung parenchyma with preserved structure:
- desquamation, hypertrophy, hyperplasia and dysplasia of pneumocytes
- mononuclear inflammatory infiltrates
- intraalveolar fibrinoid material

■ *Special stains:* PAS, Giemsa, collagenous stains, immunofluorescence.

Hallmark of Diagnosis: Immunologic or serologic identification of the virus.

Differential diagnosis: All kinds of pneumonitis, including other viruses, usual interstitial pneumonia, desquamative interstitial pneumonia, collagenous disorders, etc.

Eosinophilia, Tropical Pulmonary

Definition: Infection of the lung with *Wuchereria bancrofti* or *Brugia malayi*.

Incidence/Epidemiology: So-called elephantiasis caused by *W. bancrofti* is distributed in several countries south of 40° N latitude and can be found in West and East Africa, India, China, Japan, Taiwan, the Philippines, the East Indies, and northern Australia. The parasites are transmitted by various species of mosquitoes including *Culex*, *Anopheles*, and *Aedes*. Eosinophilia and microfilaremia occur during the acute stage of human infection.

Etiology/Pathophysiology: The adult worm lives in the lymph nodes for many years. The female discharges microfilariae into the peripheral blood that are ingested by a mosquito. The microfilariae metamorphose into third stage larvae within the mosquitos and are retransmitted to man during a mosquito bite. Tropical eosinophilia (Weingarten's syndrome) can occur in occult or cryptic filariasis or in filarial hypereosinophilia (circulating antibodies against filaria without demonstrable parasites).

Clinical Presentation: Patients present with cough, wheezing, dyspnea, and chest pain, usually at night.

Prognosis: Good and usually without sequelae; recurrence – even after years – may occur.

Radiology: Chest X-radiographs show diffuse interstitial infiltrates with variable intensity or multiple, small, circumscribed nodules.

Pathology:

Gross: Wet grayish-yellowish lungs or multiple, small, circumscribed, necrotic nodules measuring several millimeters in maximum diameter.

Histology: Identification of the parasites surrounded by dense infiltrates of eosinophilic granulocytes. At a later stage dead parasites can be found embedded in granulomatous tissue with palisading histiocytes, macrophages, and multinucleated giant cells. Other areas of the lung may contain dense interstitial eosinophilic granulocytes and scattered mononuclear infiltrates.

➤ *Descriptors:* Lung parenchyma with preserved structure:
- eosinophils (numerous);
- Lung parenchyma with altered structure:
- parasites (surrounded by numerous eosinophils)
- caseous epithelioid granulomas
- parasites (intragranulomatous, degenerated)
- multinucleated giant cells

■ *Special stains:* PAS, Movat, collagenous stains, Giemsa.

Hallmark of Diagnosis: Clinical history, eosinophilic pulmonary infiltrates (occasionally with parasites and necrotic nodules), high serum titers of filarial antibodies.

Differential diagnosis: Pulmonary infections with other parasites, eosinophilic pneumonia, histiocytosis X.

Eosinophilic Granuloma

Definition: Alteration of the lung parenchyma of unknown origin, caused by infiltration of histiocytes resembling Langerhans cells, see Histiocytosis X.

Eosinophilic Pneumonia

Definition: Alteration of the lung parenchyma defined by dense, intrapulmonary, eosinophilic granulocytes associated with various diseases.

Incidence/Epidemiology: Eosinophilic pneumonia is associated with the following clinical entities: (a) Löffler's syndrome or simple pulmonary eosinophilia, (b) chronic eosinophilic pneumonia, (c) Churg-Strauss syndrome, (d) tropical eosinophilia, (e) hypereosinophilic syndrome, (f) periartheritis nodosa and polyarthritis. Löffler's syndrome is often associated with infection caused by *Ascaris lumbricoides* or by other parasites or with drug intake (sulfonamides), fungal infections, metallic dusts, or pollen allergens. Löffler's syndrome or acute eosinophilic pneumonia is not a rare disease, but the chronic form is relatively less common.

Etiology/Pathophysiology: Eosinophilic pulmonary infiltrates in acute and chronic eosinophilic pneumonia are probably caused by release of the mast-cell-derived eosinophilic chemotactic factor of anaphylaxis (ECF-A), which is a component of the slow reacting substance of anaphylaxis (SRS-A). The eosinophils contain an alkaline "major basic protein" which is suggested to be involved in killing parasites. Other enzymes contained in eosinophils are thought to modulate mast cell enzymes such as histamine, chemotactic factors, heparin, and chymotrypsin.

Clinical Presentation: Acute eosinophilic pneumonia is usually associated with blood eosinophilia. The symptoms are mild, and a spontaneous cure after 2–3 weeks is normal. Chronic eosinophilic pneumonia is a severer disease and may appear with and without asthma. Patients present with dyspnea, cough with mucoid sputum, and severe loss of weight. Mild hemoptysis and night sweats may occur. The duration of the disorder is correlated with the intensity of the symptoms and may last for several months.

Prognosis: Usually good and without severe sequelae.

Radiology: Chest radiographs reflect diffuse pulmonary infiltrates with changing localization within a few days. Peripheral, nonsegmental, ground-glass like opacifications are characteristic in chronic eosinophilic pneumonia.

Pathology:

Gross: Heavy, wet lungs; intrapulmonary parasites may be recognized.

Histology: Dense, diffuse eosinophilic granulocytes within the alveoli and in the interstitial spaces, usually accompanied by macrophages and scattered multinucleated giant cells. Small foci of necroses are usually present, surrounded by palisading histiocytes. The overall structure of the lung parenchyma is usually intact. The microscopic appearance of acute and chronic eosinophilic pneumonia is identical, and the division into the two stages has to be performed by use of clinical data.

➤ *Descriptors:* Lung parenchyma with preserved structure:
- eosinophils (numerous)
- multinucleated giant cells;
- Lung parenchyma with altered structure:
- necrosis
- palisading histiocytes
- eosinophils

■ *Special stains:* PAS, Giemsa, Movat, collagenous stains, immunohistochemistry for S-100 protein, OKT6, endogenous lectins.

Hallmark of Diagnosis: Clinical history, chest radiographs, dense eosinophilic intraalveolar and interstitial infiltrates.

Differential diagnosis: Desquamative interstitial pneumonia, usual interstitial pneumonia, eosinophilic granuloma, sarcoidosis, infectious and noninfectious granulomas.

Epidermoid Carcinoma

Definition: Malignant epithelial tumor of the lung with "epidermoid" features, (synonym squamous cell carcinoma).

Incidence/Epidemiology: Most frequent malignant tumor of the lower respiratory tract in Europe; in the USA, second most frequent one after adenocarcinoma. The incidence of the tumor is associated with certain risk factors such as smoking and chronic inflammatory lung tissue alterations leading to squamous metaplasia. It occurs more frequently in men and amounts to about 45% of all malignant lung tumors in men and about 25% of all malignant lung tumors in women.

Etiology/Pathophysiology: Epidermoid carcinomas arise in 75% of cases from the main, segmental, or subsegmental bronchi, and in 25% from the peripheral lung tissue commonly related to chronic inflammatory changes such as scars or honeycombing. Precursors of epidermoid carcinoma are well documented and include squamous cell metaplasia with various degrees of metaplasia and carcinoma in situ.

Clinical Presentation: The growth of epidermoid carcinoma can be divided into a preclinical stage and a clinical stage with manifest symptoms. Tumors of the preclinical stage can be detected by sputum cytology. They may already have grown, however, to massive invasive carcinomas or still be at the stage of carcinoma in situ. The symptoms commonly include cough, expectoration, signs of obstructive pneumonia, hemoptysis, malaise, fever, and loss of weight. Peripherally located tumors may be detected accidentally by chest radiographs.

Prognosis: About 20–30% of patients are still alive after 5 years. Prognosis depends upon lymph node invasion (N stage), size and localization of the tumor (T stage), inflammatory response of host tissue, invasion of bronchial cartilage.

Radiology: Chest radiographs usually show centrally localized tumor masses with consequent obstructive pneumonia.

Pathology:

Gross: Epidermoid carcinomas are firm tumor masses with irregular shape and grayish-white. The tumors tend to spread along the bronchi and often create polypoid masses in the bronchial lumen. Multiple separated tumor "implantations" within the bronchial mucosa may be present.

Histology: The microscopic requirements of the WHO for epidermoid carcinoma contain at least one of the three features: (a) formation of intracellular keratin, (b) formation of keratin pearls, (c) intercellular bridges. Epidermoid carcinoma can be graded as well differentiated, moderately differentiated, poorly differentiated, and anaplastic carcinoma. Poorly differentiated or anaplastic carcinoma seldom shows one of the above-mentioned features and can be recognized only by the "flattened" cells growing in textures resembling squamoid growth, i.e., long stretched tumor bundles with tumor cells oriented in a "basal membrane" and nonisotropic growth pattern. Epidermoid carcinomas commonly have a high mitotic rate and are accompanied by dense inflammatory infiltrates of lymphocytes and plasma cells. About 50% of these tumors erode the bronchial cartilage, a stage considered to be an indicator of poor prognosis. PAS stain is useful for distinguishing these tumors from small cell anaplastic carcinomas which are usually PAS-negative. About 10% of epidermoid carcinomas express antigens against neuroendocrine markers (bombesin, synaptophysin, chromogranin A, NSE).

➤ *Descriptors:* Newly formed textures with metastasis potential:

- epithelial growth pattern
- epidermoid textures
- keratin production
- intercellular bridges
- frequent mitoses
- prominent nucleoli
- inhomogeneous cellular and nuclear size
- dense inflammatory infiltrates

■ *Special stains:* PAS, Giemsa, immunohistochemistry for cytokeratins, neuroendocrine markers, CEA, endogenous lectins, DNA analysis.

Hallmark of Diagnosis: Formation of keratin, intercellular bridges, "epidermoid growth textures".

Differential diagnosis: Small cell anaplastic carcinoma, adenocarcinoma, large cell anaplastic carcinoma, squamous metaplasia with severe dysplasia.

Epinephrine

Definition: Alteration of the lung parenchyma associated with intake of epinephrine, see Drug Toxicity.

Epithelioid Hemangioendothelioma

Definition: Peculiar tumor of the lung with various degrees of malignancy, see Hemangioendothelioma, Epithelioid.

Epstein-Barr Virus

Definition: Infection of the lung with the Epstein-Barr virus, see Viral Infection.

Erionite Fibers

Definition: Alteration of the lung parenchyma associated with inhalation of erionite fibers, see Nonasbestos Mineral Fibers, Zeolite (Asbestos Fibers).

Escherichia coli

Definition: Infection of the lung with *Escherichia coli.*
Incidence/Epidemiology: Not uncommon in hospitalized patients with reduced immunity.
Etiology/Pathophysiology: Infection of the lung usually follows infection of other organs, especially pyelonephritis, or gastrointestinal surgery.
Clinical Presentation: Most frequently severe infection of the lung with bronchopneumonic symptoms, bacteremia, and high mortality.
Radiology: Chest X-radiographs show findings of severe necrotizing pneumonia with dense, usually diffuse infiltrations.
Prognosis: High mortality (20–40%) in immunocompromised patients; good prognosis in young children (about 70% of infections heal without sequelae if treated with antibiotics).
Pathology:
Gross: Heavy, red-grayish lungs. Necrotic areas (abscess) are relatively uncommon.
Histology: Dense granulocytic infiltrates in the peripheral lung and in the walls of the small and large bronchi.
➤ *Descriptors:* Lung parenchyma with preserved structure:
- intraalveolar fibrinoid material
- neutrophils (intraalveolar, numerous)

■ *Special stains:* PAS, collagenous stains, Giemsa.
Hallmark of Diagnosis: Clinical history, bacterial pneumonia, identification of *E. coli* in cultures.
Differential diagnosis: Infectious pneumonias with other organisms, abscess, neonatal disorders.

Esophageal Atresia

Definition: Occlusion (blind end) of the proximal or distal part of the esophagus, see Fistula, Tracheoesophageal, Chagas Disease.

Estrogens

Definition: Alteration of the lung parenchyma associated with intake of estrogens, see Drug Toxicity.

Ethosuximide

Definition: Alteration of the lung parenchyma associated with intake of ethosuximide, see Drug Toxicity.

Ethylchlorvynol

Definition: Alteration of the lung parenchyma associated with intake of ethylchlorvynol, see Drug Toxicity.

Ethyleneglycol

Definition: Alteration of the lung parenchyma associated with intake of ethyleneglycol, see Drug Toxicity.

Ethyl Ether

Definition: Alteration of the lung parenchyma associated with intake of ethyl ether, see Drug Toxicity.

Extrauterine Transition Disorders

Definition: Abnormal alterations of the lung parenchyma associated with transition from intrauterine life to the air-breathing state.
Incidence/Epidemiology: Inflation of the lung with air and adequate lung stability is closely related to the maturation of cells of the alveolar lining and thus associated with gestational age. Complications associated with functional immaturity of the lung include (a) Hyaline membrane disease (HMD), (b) bronchopulmonary dysplasia (BPD), (c) interstitial emphysema (IE), (d) pulmonary hemorrhage, (e) meconium aspiration, and (f) perinatal pneumonia. Bronchopulmonary dysplasia is the most frequent extrauterine transition disorder followed by hyaline membrane disease (HMD) and interstitial emphysema (IE). Interstitial hemorrhage is freqently seen in infants with HMD, BPD, or IE. Perinatal pneumonia is often associated with ascending infections of the amniotic fluid, contaminated from a vaginal source.

Etiology/Pathophysiology: Adequate extension and stability of the lung depends upon the presence of a surfactant released from mature alveolar type II cells. Disorders during the perinatal period may develop either due to insufficient expansion of the airways and subsequent iatrogenic interaction (HMD, BPD, IE) or due to aspiration or ascendant infection during delivery (meconium aspiration, perinatal pneumonia). Delayed clearance of fetal lung fluid may cause transient tachypnea or more severe symptoms.

Clinical Presentation: Details are discussed under the particular headings.

Prognosis: Usually poor, severe sequelae may develop if the patients survive.

Radiology: Details are discussed under the particular headings.

Pathology:

Gross: Usually firm atelectatic lungs. For details see under particular headings.

Histology: The findings include hyaline membranes, interstitial emphysema, severe inflammatory infiltrates or hypertrophy and hyperplasia of cells of the alveolar lining. For details see under particular headings.

➤ *Descriptors:* Lung parenchyma with preserved structure:

- hyaline membranes
- enlarged distant air spaces
- hemorrhage
- intraalveolar fibrinoid material
- mixed inflammatory infiltrates
- desquamation, hypertrophy, hyperplasia and dysplasia of pneumocytes;
- Lung parenchyma with altered structure:
- necrosis
- focal interstitial fibrosis
- proliferating smooth muscle cells
- meconium
- caseous epithelioid granulomas
- intraalveolar amniotic fluid

■ *Special stains:* PAS, Giemsa, collagenous stains, endogenous lectins, immunohistochemistry for surfactant.

Hallmark of Diagnosis: Clinical history, microscopic findings as discussed under the particular headings.

Differential diagnosis: Congenital disorders, see under particular headings.

Fabry's Disease – Gypsum

Fabry's Disease

Definition: Alteration of the lung parenchyma associated with angiokeratoma corporis diffusum universale.

Incidence/Epidemiology: Hereditary X-linked recessive disorder of glycolipid metabolism. The existence of pulmonary involvement still remains unclear.

Etiology/Pathophysiology: Disturbance of glycolipid metabolism may include cells lining the alveoli and endothelial cells of pulmonary vessels as well as smooth muscle fibers.

Clinical Presentation: Obstructive disorders have been reported in some patients with Fabry's disease. Other patients have shown only minimal or no symptoms.

Prognosis: Death of patients is usually related to cardiac, renal, or cerebrovascular failure; involvement of the lung is of minor influence.

Radiology: No specific findings have been reported.

Pathology:
Gross: No specific findings have been reported.

Histology: The deficiency of α-galactosidase leads to deposits of crystalline glycosphingolipid, which is birefringent (Maltese cross type). The crystals can be seen in endothelial cells, smooth muscle cells, histiocytes, and perithelial cells.

No detailed histomorphologic findings in the lung parenchyma have been published.

➤ *Descriptors:* Lung parenchyma with preserved structure:
- hyaline material (birefringent crystals, endothelial cells, histiocytes, smooth muscle cells);
- Bronchial mucosa with preserved structure:
- mononuclear inflammatory infiltrates

■ *Special stains:* PAS, Giemsa, collagenous stains, endogenous lectins.

Hallmark of Diagnosis: Clinical history, identification of the enzyme deficiency, Maltese cross crystals in histiocytes, smooth muscle cells, and endothelial cells.

Differential diagnosis: Alterations of the lung parenchyma associated with environmental habits such as smoking.

Farber's Disease

Definition: Alteration of the lung parenchyma associated with disseminated lipogranulomatosis.

Incidence/Epidemiology: Rare storage disease associated with lipomatoid granulomas in the reticular tissue.

Etiology/Pathophysiology: Hereditary disease with abnormal storage of fatty acids.

Clinical Presentation: A patient with severe respiratory distress and lethal outcome at the age of 21 months has been reported.

Prognosis: Pulmonary involvement is associated with poor prognosis.

Radiology: Chest radiographs showed diffuse interstitial infiltrates.

Pathology:
Gross: The lungs showed multiple, dense, grayish-yellowish granulomas.

Histology: Noncaseating granulomas consisting of histiocytes and foamy macrophages surrounded by lymphocytes and plasma cells.

➤ *Descriptors:* Lung parenchyma with altered structure:
- noncaseous epithelioid granulomas
- macrophages (foamy)
- mononuclear inflammatory infiltrates

■ *Special stains:* PAS, collagenous stains, endogenous lectins, immunohistochemistry for various fatty acids.

Hallmark of Diagnosis: Clinical history, lipoid granulomas.

Differential diagnosis: Other lipid storage diseases, noncaseating granulomatous diseases including sarcoidosis or berylliosis, infectious granulomatous diseases.

Farmer's Lung Disease

Definition: Alteration of the lung parenchyma (allergic extrinsic alveolitis) associated with inhalation of *Micropolyspora faeni*.

Incidence/Epidemiology: Rare disease seen in persons exposed to moldy hay.

Etiology/Pathophysiology: Hypersensitivity reaction in a combination of type III (immune complex) and type IV (cell-mediated immunologic reaction) immune response. For details, see Allergic (Extrinsic) Alveolitis.

Clinical Presentation: The hypersensitivity reaction can be acute or chronic.

Prognosis: Usually good; however, slow progressive respiratory failure can occur.

Radiology: Chest radiographs are normal or show diffuse, soft, interstitial infiltrates or fine granular densities.

Pathology:

Gross: The lungs are of normal color and consistency, or may display small, firm, reddish-gray nodules.

Histology: The characteristic findings include non-necrotizing epithelioid granulomas near the terminal bronchioles, desquamation, hypertrophy and hyperplasia of cells of the alveolar lining, marked eosinophilic inflammatory infiltrates, bronchiolitis obliterans and focal acute vasculitis. For details, see Allergic (Extrinsic) Alveolitis.

➤*Descriptors:* Lung parenchyma with altered structure:

- noncaseous epithelioid granulomas
- eosinophils
- multinucleated giant cells
- intrabronchiolar fibrinoid material and histiocytes
- ulceration of bronchiolar mucosa;
- Lung parenchyma with preserved structure:
- macrophages
- desquamation, hypertrophy, hyperplasia and dysplasia of pneumocytes
- mononuclear inflammatory infiltrates
- intraalveolar serous fluid

■ *Special stains:* PAS, collagenous stains, Giemsa. For details, see Allergic (Extrinsic) Alveolitis.

Hallmark of Diagnosis: Clinical history, nonnecrotizing epithelioid granulomas, morphologic findings related to desquamative interstitial pneumonia, lymphoid interstitial pneumonia, bronchiolitis obliterans.

Differential diagnosis: Infectious and noninfectious granulomatous diseases such as sarcoidosis, fungal infections or berylliosis. For details, see Allergic (Extrinsic) Alveolitis.

Fasciitis, Eosinophilic

Definition: Alteration of the lung parenchyma associated with eosiniphilic fasciitis.

Incidence/Epidemiology: Patients suffering from scleroderma may develop eosinophilic fasciitis which is a syndrome with eosinophilic infiltrates in various fasciae. The incidence of pulmonary parenchyma changes is not clear.

Etiology/Pathophysiology: The causes of the scleroderma and eosinophilic fasciitis are not clear. The involvement of the immune system and disturbance of collagen metabolism are under discussion.

Clinical Presentation: A patient suffering from eosinophilic fasciitis with pulmonary involvement has been described. The clinical symptoms included cough, malaise, and dyspnea.

Prognosis: Involvement of the lung is of minor influence to the prognosis.

Radiology: Chest X-radiographs show diffuse, microgranular, interstitial infiltrates.

Pathology:

Gross: Heavy wet lungs with multiple, small granulomas.

Histology: Diffuse interstitial mononuclear infiltrates and bronchiolitis obliterans.

➤*Descriptors:* Lung parenchyma with altered structure:

- intrabronchiolar fibrinoid material and histiocytes
- ulceration of bronchiolar mucosa;
- Lung parenchyma with preserved structure:
- mononuclear inflammatory infiltrates

■ *Special stains:* PAS, collagenous stains, immunohistochemistry for immunoglobulins, endogenous lectins.

Hallmark of Diagnosis: Clinical history, bronchiolitis obliterans.

Differential diagnosis: Bronchiolitis obliterans associated with other diseases.

Fat Emboli

Definition: Emboli of fatty tissue in the small arteries and capillaries, usually associated with (severe) trauma, see Embolism, Pulmonary.

Feldspar Fibers

Definition: Alteration of the lung parenchyma associated with inhalation of Feldspar fibers, see Nonasbestos Mineral Fibers.

Ferruginous Bodies

Definition: Deposition of fibers coated with iron-protein mucopolysaccharide substances in the lung.

Incidence/Epidemiology: Most frequently seen in persons with exposure to asbestos. Counting of ferruginous bodies can be used to define the degree of dust exposure. Fibers of various origins can become coated such as talc, fiberglass, ceramic fibers, silicon carbide, diatomaceous earth, sheet silicates, iron oxide, chromium, rutile, zeolite (sometimes called pseudoferruginous bodies).

Etiology/Pathophysiology: The inhaled fibers become phagocytized by macrophages and are transported into the phagolysozyme system, where they become coated. Coated fibers are not oncogenic or fibrogenic. The reasons that fibers become coated in some exposed persons while others do not have coated fibers are not known.

Clinical Presentation: No specific symptoms, only histomorphological features.

Prognosis: Ferruginous bodies are usually associated with exposure to asbestos. Patients have a high risk of development of asbestos-associated diseases (diffuse interstitial fibrosis, fibrosis of the pleura, mesothelioma, and lung cancer).

Radiology: No specific findings.

Pathology:

Gross: No specific findings.

Histology: The average length of coated fibers is estimated to 30–50 μm. They present a distinct microscopic appearance with pearl-like configuration of proteins along the fiber and dumbbell-like thickening at the ends of the fiber. Ferruginous bodies are usually located within the alveoli or may be identified within fibrotic interstitial tissue.

➤ *Descriptors:* Lung parenchyma with preserved structure:
- asbestos bodies (birefringent fibers)
- macrophages (birefringent fibers, asbestos bodies)

■ *Special stains:* Prussian blue.

Hallmark of Diagnosis: Iron-protein-coated mineral fibers.

Differential diagnosis: Pseudoferruginous bodies, noncoated deposits of dust particles.

Fiberglass Workers

Definition: Alteration of the lung parenchyma in persons exposed to fiberglass.

Incidence/Epidemiology: Borosilicate and alkaline silicate glasses mixed with various amounts of silica, lime, aluminum, or titanium are used for manufacturing fiberglass. Persons working in the application of fiberglass have a higher risk of inhalation than persons working in the production of fiberglass as they are unaware of the hazard.

Etiology/Pathophysiology: The clearance of inhaled fibers in the lung depends mainly upon the physical properties of the fibers, i.e., their size and their geometry. Glassfibers have a high resistance to heat, cold, and chemicals and cannot be dissolved in the macrophagocytic system of man. Their surface acts as a stimulant for fibrotic activity similar to asbestos fibers.

Clinical Presentation: Usually no or mild symptoms such as cough and progressive dyspnea.

Prognosis: Usually good; however, slow progressive respiratory failure may occur. Increased risk for diffuse interstitial fibrosis, fibrosis of the pleura, mesothelioma, and lung cancer is still being discussed controversially, and is less than that of asbestos fibers.

Radiology: Chest radiographs are normal or may show mild diffuse interstitial fibrosis.

Pathology:

Gross: Usually normal appearance or mild fibrosis.

Histology: Usually noncoated fibers are seen which may be broken into smaller units, and which are located within the terminal airways. Diffuse interstitial fibrosis can be seen depending upon the amount of inhaled fibers.

➤ *Descriptors:* Lung parenchyma with preserved structure:
- dust (birefringent fibers, crystals)
- macrophages
- mononuclear inflammatory infiltrates;
- Lung parenchyma with altered structure:
- diffuse interstitial fibrosis

■ *Special stains:* Prussian blue, collagenous stains, X-ray diffraction or related physical techniques, endogenous lectins.

Hallmark of Diagnosis: Clinical history, identification of glass fibers.

Differential diagnosis: Exposure of the lung to other dust particles.

Fibrobullous Disease

Definition: Circumscribed subpleural emphysematous changes, usually of the upper lobes (apex), associated with rheumatoid diseases.

Incidence/Epidemiology: Large emphysematous cysts with perifocal fibrosis are seen in 2–20% of patients suffering from ankylosing spondylitis, in 2–5% of patients with rheumatoid diseases, in patients with Marfan's syndrome, and in coal pneumoconiosis. Most of the patients are adult men.

Etiology/Pathophysiology: In ankylosing spondylitis the chest wall restriction leads to chronic hypoventilation and chronic interstitial infiltrates in the upper lobes. Pleural thickening and fibrosis causes emphysematous changes, usually in the apex, followed by honeycombing which may spread to the middle and lower parts of the lung. A similar mechanism is discussed in other diseases associated with fibrobullous changes of the lung.

Clinical Presentation: Patients are usually asymptomatic or may show shortness of breath or complications such as pneumothorax, fever, cough, or hemoptysis.

Prognosis: Slow progression of the disease is the course most frequently seen.

Radiology: Chest radiographs show a bilateral increase in interstitial marking, pleural thickening of the upper lobes, and cysts or cavities, sometimes filled with fungus balls.

Pathology:

Gross: Thickened pleura and subpleural bullae with fibrotic chains or honeycombing are the gross findings.

Histology: Fibrosis of the pleura with scattered mononuclear infiltrates and large subpleural air spaces surrounded by irregularly arranged fibrous tissue. Squamous metaplasia of bronchial epithelial cells, bronchiectasis, and interstitial smooth muscle fibers may be present as well as secondary bacterial or fungal infection.

➤ *Descriptors:* Lung parenchyma with altered structure:

- enlarged distant air spaces
- focal interstitial fibrosis (at the boundary)
- proliferating fibroblasts
- proliferating smooth muscle cells
- squamous metaplasia and dysplasia of the pneumocytes;
- Bronchial mucosa with altered structure:
- ectatic lumen
- squamous metaplasia and dysplasia

■ *Special stains:* Collagenous stains.

Hallmark of Diagnosis: Macroscopic findings, emphysematous changes of the upper lobes, clinical history of associated diseases such as ankylosing spondylitis, rheumatoid diseases, Marfan's syndrome, or coal pneumoconiosis, focal interstitial fibrosis, proliferating fibroblasts, and smooth muscle cells.

Differential diagnosis: Honeycombing of the lung associated with other diseases, chronic obstructive airways disease.

Fibroma

Definition: Benign tumors of the lung of specific fibromatous cell type.

Incidence/Epidemiology: Rare intrapulmonary tumor of the lung most frequently associated with a major bronchus. It usually occurs in adult men (sex ratio 2:1), and may suffer a myxomatoid change (fibromyxoma).

Etiology/Pathophysiology: These tumors arise from fibromatous tissue and have to be distinguished from hamartomas (chondrofibrolipomas) which are more frequent.

Clinical Presentation: Fibromas may arise in connection with the pleura, a major bronchus, or within the peripheral lung parenchyma. The symptoms are associated with the localization of the tumors and may include recurring obstruction.

Prognosis: Usually good and without known sequelae.

Radiology: Chest radiographs show either a circumscribed peripheral nodule, a nodule connected to the pleura, or an obstruction of a bronchial lumen.

Pathology:

Gross: Solid, white-grayish, firm tumors measuring 1–3 cm in diameter.

Histology: The tumors are characterized by dense hyalinized tissue with some scattered mononuclear infiltrates and some spindle cells mostly located at the periphery of the tumor.

Entrapped air spaces can usually be detected near the boundary of the tumor. Necrotic areas and mitotic figures are not present. The center of the tumor is acellular and hyalinized.

➤ *Descriptors:* Newly formed textures without metastasis potential:

- mesenchymal growth pattern
- fibromatous textures
- plump spindle cells
- homogeneous nuclear and cellular size
- finely distributed nuclear chromatin
- absent or infrequent mitoses
- absent necrosis
- absent inflammatory infiltrates

■ *Special stains:* PAS, collagenous stains, immunohistochemistry for vimentin, desmin, desmoplakin, lysozyme, endogenous lectins, DNA analysis, texture analysis.

Hallmark of Diagnosis: Circumscribed tumor consisting of collagenous matrix with scattered spindle cells resembling fibroblasts. Missing are mitotic figures, necroses and inflammatory infiltrates.

Differential diagnosis: Fibrous histiocytoma, hamartoma, sclerosing hemangioma, fibrous scar.

Fibromatosis of the Lung

Definition: Alteration of the lung parenchyma associated with congenital generalized fibromatosis.

Incidence/Epidemiology: Rare disease in young children. About 20 cases with pulmonary involvement have been reported.

Etiology/Pathophysiology: The disease is considered to be a congenital generalized tumorous disorder of low malignancy.

Clinical Presentation: Pulmonary involvement is associated with a poor prognosis in children. They present with dyspnea, cyanosis, and recurring bronchopneumonia.

Prognosis: Usually poor, with progressive respiratory failure.

Radiology: Usually diffuse increase of markings in both lungs.

Pathology:

Gross: Small fibrous nodules in both lungs and firm fibrous lung parenchyma.

Histology: Multiple nodules of spindle cells usually bound to small bronchi and bronchioles or small artery walls. In addition diffuse, interstitial, cellular fibrosis.

➤ *Descriptors:* Newly formed textures without metastasis potential:

- mesenchymal growth pattern
- fibromatous textures
- plump spindle cells (multiple small foci around central bronchi, bronchioles, or small vessels)
- mononuclear inflammatory infiltrates (scattered)
- Lung parenchyma with altered structure:
- diffuse interstitial fibrosis
- squamous metaplasia and dysplasia of the pneumocytes

■ *Special stains:* Collagenous stains, immunohistochemistry for vimentin, desmin, desmoplakin, lysozyme, endogenous lectins, DNA analysis, texture analysis.

Hallmark of Diagnosis: Clinical history, multiple nodules of proliferating spindle cells bound to bronchioles, small bronchi, and small artery walls.

Differential diagnosis: Inflammatory pseudotumor, histiocytosis X, neurofibroma.

Fibromyxoma

Definition: Benign mesenchymal tumor of the lung, see Fibroma.

Fibrosarcoma

Definition: Malignant mesenchymal tumor of the lung composed of spindle cells resembling fibroblasts.

Incidence/Epidemiology: Uncommon tumor of the lung. It has been reported in both sexes. Endobronchial fibrosarcomas occur more frequently in young adults whereas fibrosarcomas of the peripheral lung tissue occur more often in middle-aged to elderly persons.

Etiology/Pathophysiology: These tumors may have their origin in fibroblasts present in the walls of the bronchi, arteries, veins, and bronchioles. No precancerous lesions related to pulmonary sarcomas are known. Smoking is not related to the occurrence of sarcomas.

Clinical Presentation: Symptoms are dependent on the location of the tumor. About 30%

arise from proximal bronchi with symptoms and a radiological appearance similar to proximally located bronchial carcinomas. Peripheral lesions are usually detected accidentally.

Prognosis: Poor prognosis, death occurs usually within 2 years after clinical manifestation.

Radiology: Chest radiographs reflect either dense proximal lesions, usually with signs of obstruction, or circumscribed solid peripheral masses.

Pathology:

Gross: Polypoid yellowish lesions with ulceration and hemorrhage or necrotic areas measuring 10–40 mm in maximum diameter. Peripherally located tumors may range up to 20 cm in diameter. Very large peripheral lung tumors are always suspected to be sarcomatous lesions.

Histology: Dense clusters of proliferating atypical tumorous spindle cells with numerous mitotic figures, rather large necrotic areas. Palisading may be present. The interstitial lung parenchyma is completely destroyed and an inflammatory response of the host tissue is rare. Fibromatous tumors measuring 3 cm or more in maximum diameter are always suspected to be malignancies.

➤ *Descriptors:* Newly formed textures with metastasis potential:
- mesenchymal growth pattern
- sarcomatous textures
- plump spindle cells
- frequent mitoses
- necrosis
- inhomogeneous nuclear and cellular size

■ *Special stains:* Collagenous stains, Congo, Giemsa, immunohistochemistry for vimentin, lysozyme, desmin, and desmoplakin, endogenous lectins, DNA analysis.

Hallmark of Diagnosis: Size of the tumors, composition of the tumors with spindle cells, necrosis, numerous mitoses.

Differential diagnosis: Malignant fibrous histiocytoma, leiomyosarcoma, spindle cell amelanotic melanoma, metastatic tumor into the lung, fibroma, benign fibrous histiocytoma.

Fibrosis

Definition: Circumscribed or diffuse increase of collagenous fibers in lung parenchyma.

Incidence/Epidemiology: Common finding in lung parenchyma associated with various risk factors or disorders. Focal fibrosis may occur in relation to preceding inflammation, infarction, or metastatic lesions altered by cytostatic regimes. Diffuse interstitial fibrosis may occur in connection with exposure to asbestos, beryllium, coal or silica, in allergic extrinsic alveolitis, fuller's earth lung, hematite miner's lung, histiocytosis X, bronchopulmonary dysplasia, emphysematous changes of the lung, or in association with familial susceptibility, drug intake, or as so-called idiopathic fibrosis.

Etiology/Pathophysiology: Chronic inflammatory lesions are related to increase of histiocytes and fibroblasts and subsequent deposits of collagen. In addition to the above associated disorders, smoking, virus infection, oxygen toxicity, and a genetic disposition are mentioned as potential causes. Fibrin extravasation may not resolve and can thus be organized into inert collagen fibers (type I).

Clinical Presentation: Focal fibrosis usually does not produce clinically relevant symptoms, whereas diffuse interstitial fibrosis usually causes progressive pulmonary dysfunction with shortness of breath, dyspnea, and finally severe restriction of oxygen exchange.

Prognosis: Diffuse fibrosis is usually slowly progressive and causes fatal respiratory failure after several years. Focal fibrosis is usually a self-healing disorder without any major clinical importance.

Radiology: Focal fibrosis may calcify and be the basis of circumscribed densities, whereas diffuse fibrosis is related to interstitial bilateral infiltrates that are usually more prominent at the basal parts of the lungs.

Pathology:

Gross: Either circumscribed, white-grayish densities measuring 8–30 mm in diameter or diffuse fibrotic bundles several millimeters in diameter with corresponding enlargement of the terminal air spaces. The pleural surface is characterized by a granular "cirrhotic" pattern.

Histology: Dense collagen fibers either in foci of various sizes or in a diffuse pattern with complete destruction of the normal lung texture. The amount of enclosed inflammatory infiltrates is associated with the progression of the fibrotic alteration of the lung parenchyma.

➤ *Descriptors:* Lung parenchyma with altered structure:
- diffuse interstitial fibrosis
- proliferating smooth muscle cells
- mononuclear inflammatory infiltrates
- focal interstitial fibrosis
- calcification
- ossification
- squamous metaplasia and dysplasia of the pneumocytes

■ *Special stains:* Collagenous stains, Prussian blue, endogenous lectins, immunohistochemistry for immunoglobulins, HLA-DR.

Hallmark of Diagnosis: Increase of collagen in the lung parenchyma with subsequent destruction of normal lung textures.

Differential diagnosis: Fibroma, fibrosarcoma, lymphangioleiomyomatosis.

Fibrous Xanthoma

Definition: Benign mesenchymal tumor of the lung, see Histiocytoma.

Filariasis

Definition: Infection of the lung with filarial nematodes.

Incidence/Epidemiology: Three species of filarial nematodes have been reported to invade human lungs: *Wuchereria bancrofti, Brugia malayi,* and *Onchocerca volvulus*. The species are found between 40° N latitude and 20° S latitude in Asian and African countries and in coastal parts of Central and South America. Persons living in poor suburbs or in rural areas of these regions are at special risk.

Etiology/Pathophysiology: The parasites have a length of 50–200 mm and are between 150–450 μm thick. The life cycle of Bancroftian and Malayan filariae are identical, and man is the only known definite host. The adult worms invade the lymphatic vessels (lymph nodes of the testis, epididymis) and may live there for years. The female worms, which have two uteri in the midbody, discharge microfilariae into the peripheral blood. Mosquitoes (*Culex, Aedes, Anopheles*) ingest the microfilariae which metamorphose into infective filariform larvae (third stage larvae). These larvae are retransmitted to man when the mosquitoes bite. *Onchocerca volvulus* is transmitted from person to person by black flies of the genus *Simulium*. Both infective larvae and adult filariae have been found in human lungs.

Clinical Presentation: Clinical symptoms usually develop months or years after infection and include fever, lymphadenitis, orchitis, epididymitis, funiculitis, headache, changes in the skin, and if infected by *O. volvulus*, blindness. Infection of the lung by adult worms causes pulmonary infarctions; infection of the lung with infectious third stage larvae causes tropical pulmonary eosinophilia. Symptoms may include hemoptysis, chest pain, cough, wheezing, or peripheral eosinophilia.

Prognosis: Usually good; sequelae are scars in the peripheral lung parenchyma.

Radiology: Chest X-radiographs show diffuse, patchy, pulmonary infiltrates or circumscribed pulmonary masses.

Pathology:

Gross: The parasites can be seen in the larger pulmonary arteries embedded in granulomatous necrotic lesions. Peripheral hemorrhagic infarctions may be present.

Histology: The degenerating parasites are surrounded by polymorphonuclear leukocytes and histiocytes and are usually embedded in a caseation necrosis. Infectious larvae are accompanied by eosinophilic granulocytes and can be seen in capillaries. Multinucleated giant cells and palisading epithelioid cells mark the central necrotic lesions.

➤ *Descriptors:* Lung parenchyma with altered structure:
- caseous epithelioid granulomas
- parasites (intragranulomatous, degenerated, nematodes)
- mixed inflammatory infiltrates
- eosinophils (pericapillary)
- multinucleated giant cells;
- Pulmonary vessels with preserved structure:
- parasites (intracapillary, larvae)

■ *Special stains:* Giemsa, Movat, collagenous stains.

Hallmark of Diagnosis: Clinical history, identification of adult worms or infectious larvae, caseous necrosis with palisading epithelioid histiocytes, infarction, and thrombosis of the pulmonary arteries.

Differential diagnosis: Infection with other species of nematodes, infective and noninfective granulomatous lung diseases, pulmonary infarction.

Fish Meal Worker's Lung

Definition: Alterations of the lung parenchyma associated with exposure to fish meal dust.

Incidence/Epidemiology: Rare disease seen in persons working in fish meal manufacture.

Etiology/Pathophysiology: Hypersensitivity reaction of the lung due to exposure to fish proteins inhaled during preparation of crushed fish meat.

Clinical Presentation: The inhalation of fish protein may cause an acute or chronic clinical form as described under Allergic (Extrinsic) Alveolitis.

Prognosis: Usually good; however, slow progressive respiratory failure may occur.

Radiology: Chest radiographs show soft, diffuse, interstitial infiltrates or fine granulomatous pattern. For details, see Allergic (Extrinsic) Alveolitis.

Pathology:

Gross: Normal appearance of the lung or edematous changes. Seldom seen are severe chronic changes such as interstitial fibrosis.

Histology: Usually diffuse edema with some interstitial eosinophilic infiltrates. Noncaseating epithelioid granulomas, bronchiolitis obliterans, and hyperplasia of cells of the alveolar lining may be present. Honeycombing of the lung may be observed in the end stage of the disease. For details, see under the heading Allergic (Extrinsic) Alveolitis.

➤ *Descriptors:* Lung parenchyma with altered structure:

- noncaseous epithelioid granulomas
- eosinophils
- multinucleated giant cells
- intrabronchiolar fibrinoid material and histiocytes
- ulceration of bronchiolar mucosa;
- Lung parenchyma with preserved structure:
- macrophages
- desquamation, hypertrophy, hyperplasia and dysplasia of pneumocytes
- mononuclear inflammatory infiltrates
- intraalveolar serous fluid

■ *Special stains:* PAS, collagenous stains, immunohistochemistry for immunoglobulins, endogenous lectins.

Hallmark of Diagnosis: Clinical history, noncaseating epithelioid granulomas associated with interstitial pneumonitis and hyperplasia of cells of the alveolar lining , bronchiolitis obliterans, diffuse interstitial fibrosis with honeycombing.

Differential diagnosis: Infectious and non-infectious granulomatous diseases, allergic extrinsic alveolitis due to other agents.

Fistula

Definition: Abnormal connection of a bronchus or the trachea with adjacent structures such as the esophagus, pleura, or stomach.

Incidence/Epidemiology: Fistulae are either congenital disorders or acquired anomalies due to chronic inflammatory processes or malignancies. Congenital fistulae are rare, with an incidence of approximately 1/1 000 births and include bronchobiliary fistula and bronchoesophageal fistula in connection with tracheal agenesis. Acquired bronchoesophageal or tracheoesophageal fistulae are a common finding in proximally localized advanced bronchial carcinomas or esophageal carcinomas. Bronchopleural fistulae may be seen in cavernous tuberculosis.

Etiology/Pathophysiology: Congenital fistulae are usually associated with maldevelopment of the forward gut. Chronic inflammation or malignant growth destroy the surrounding connective tissue of the bronchus or trachea.

Clinical Presentation: In addition to symptoms caused by the underlying disease patients suffer from frequent substance aspirations (bronchoesophageal fistula) or collapsing lung (bronchopleural fistula).

Prognosis: Depends upon the underlying disease, chronic fistulae are usually fatal due to recurrent pulmonary infections if surgical treatment is not successful.

Radiology: Chest X-radiographs usually display indirectly related symptoms such as collapsing lung, necrotizing pneumonia, etc.

Pathology:

Gross: Congenital fistulae are usually associated with additional malformations and may be difficult to detect. Acquired fistulae are often of large size. Hemorrhage and abscess are frequently present.

Histology: The histomorphological image is characterized by severe chronic inflammation and/or tumor cells.

➤ *Descriptors:* Bronchial mucosa with altered structure:
- ulceration
- mixed inflammatory infiltrates
- squamous metaplasia and dysplasia

■ *Special stains:* PAS, collagenous stains.

Hallmark of Diagnosis: Clinical history, macroscopic findings.

Differential diagnosis: Due to the underlying disease.

Flatworm

Definition: Infection of the lung with flatworms, see Trematodes.

Flax Worker's Disease

Definition: Alteration of the lung parenchyma associated with inhalation of flax dust (byssinosis), see Byssinosis.

Fluorescein

Definition: Alteration of the lung parenchyma associated with intake of fluorescein, see Drug Toxicity.

Fluphenazine

Definition: Alteration of the lung parenchyma associated with intake of fluphenazine, see Drug Toxicity.

Formalin

Definition: Alteration of the lung parenchyma associated with exposure to formalin, see Drug Toxicity.

Friedländer's Pneumonia

Definition: Infection of the lung with the bacteria *Klebsiella pneumoniae.*

Incidence/Epidemiology: About 1% of all bacterial pneumonias are caused by infection with *Klebsiella pneumoniae.* The infection, with a high mortality (about 50%), is frequently seen in young children, in the elderly, or in persons with decreased immunodefences such as diabetics, alcoholics, chronic pulmonary disease, or malignant tumors.

Etiology/Pathophysiology: The gram-negative bacillus is commonly found in the oral cavity and on the surface of the tonsils. Reduced immunity or aspiration gives the organisms access to the lung, where they multiply rapidly.

Clinical Presentation: The clinical picture is characterized by a sudden onset of the disease with high fever, chills, tachypnea, cyanosis, cough, and gelatinous bloody sputum. Leukopenia is a common finding.

Prognosis: Acute *Klebsiella* pneumonia is seldom fatal but may proceed to the chronic form which usually induces severe fibrosis with progressive respiratory failure.

Radiology: Chest radiographs show necrotizing densities usually in the upper and lower lobes of the right lung. Abscess formation is common. Late stages may show encapsulated cavities or fibrosis associated with bronchiectasis.

Pathology:

Gross: The infected lobe presents a firm, consolidated parenchyma with a purulent exudate on the pleura. The cut surface exudes a bloody, gelatinous, slimy, pink-yellowish fluid.

Histology: In early stages the air spaces are filled with neutrophilic and eosinophilic granulocytes and less commonly with lymphocytes and plasma cells. The fibrin deposits are usually scarce compared with the dense inflammatory infiltrates. Very soon the granulocytes are replaced by macrophages which usually predominate. The bacteria can usually be demonstrated within the macrophages by Dieterle's silver stain. The interalveolar walls are destroyed. Consolidation and granulomatous organization of the necrotic areas usually start at the boundary of the lesion after 4–6 days, leading to encapsulation and cavitation. Metastatic abscess formation in the close neighborhood of the infected areas is common, i.e., several lesions in various stages of organization can be observed. Final stages include scarring, bronchiectasis, focal fibrosis, and honeycombing.

➤ *Descriptors:* Lung parenchyma with altered structure:
- necrosis and hemorrhage (massive)
- macrophages
- mixed inflammatory infiltrates
- focal interstitial fibrosis

■ *Special stains:* PAS, Dieterle's, Warthin-Starry stain, collagenous stain.

Hallmark of Diagnosis: Clinical history, abscess formation with gram-negative bacteria, predominant macrophages with ingested bacteria, rare deposits of fibrin.

Differential diagnosis: Infection of the lung caused by other organisms.

Fuller's Earth Lung

Definition: Alteration of the lung parenchyma associated with inhalation of the calcium derivative of montmorillonite.

Incidence/Epidemiology: Fuller's earth, a clay mineral with adsorbent properties has been used as a base for cosmetic and pharmaceutical powders, as a mud in oil wheel drilling, and as a stabilizer of emulsion paints. The greatest number of patients suffering from disorders of the lung have been reported from Surrey, UK where the clay is mined. The risk of exposure has only been reported for persons working in mining and bagging the clay, and not for those working in application of the clay.

Etiology/Pathophysiology: Inhalation of the dust leads to deposits of the mineral fibers within or close to the respiratory bronchioles. The fibers cause a granulomatous reaction of the lung parenchyma. They are considered to be a nonfibrogenic agent or at most a mild one.

Clinical Presentation: The clinical picture is unsuspicious or includes mild symptoms such as shortness of breath during exercise or mild chest pain.

Prognosis: Good and without serious sequelae.

Radiology: Chest radiographs are normal or may show a mild diffuse granular infiltrate and pleural thickening.

Pathology:
Gross: Normal appearance of the lung or slight increase of consistency with diffuse, black, granular infiltrates a few millimeters in diameter.
Histology: The small granulomas with black deposits of birefringent dust particles near the terminal bronchioles consist of dust-laden macrophages and diffuse embedded reticulin fibers. The surrounding lung parenchyma is unsuspicious. Massive fibrosis or superinfected tuberculosis is not a sign of fuller's earth lung.

➤ *Descriptors:* Lung parenchyma with preserved structure:
- macrophages (dust-laden)
- focal interstitial fibrosis (peribronchiolar)
- dust (birefringent fibers, crystals)

■ *Special stains:* PAS, collagenous stains, endogenous lectins, identification of the clay with X-ray diffraction or similar physical techniques.

Hallmark of Diagnosis: Clinical history, dust-laden macrophages with birefringent fibers agglutinated to small granulomas near the terminal bronchioles.

Differential diagnosis: Exposure to other silicates such as shale, bentonite, nepheline, volcanic ash, micas, talc; heavy smoking.

Fumes, Metal

Definition: Alteration of the lung parenchyma associated with inhalation of metal fumes.

Incidence/Epidemiology: Metal fumes usually include those of cadmium, vanadium, osmium, mercury, manganese, and arsenic. However, only exposure to cadmium fumes is of some clinical importance. Only a few cases exposed to the other fumes have been reported.

Etiology/Pathophysiology: Both dust and fumes consist of the same particles, but they are of different size. Fume particles, being smaller than dust particles, tend to deposit in the terminal airways, are usually of submicroscopic size, and tend to aggregate within the alveoli. Inhalation of dense fumes causes acute intoxication with disturbance of the fluid-air barrier and acute edema. Restitutio ad integrum usually follows if the patient survives the acute poisoning. Chronic exposure may lead to chronic bronchitis with bronchiectasis, to emphysema, or very infrequently to honeycombing.

Clinical Presentation: The clinical symptoms include recurrent fever (Monday fever) and shortness of breath, or acute dyspnea, cyanosis, and tachypnea in severe poisoning. Chronic exposure is characterized by chronic dry cough and progressive decrease in restrictive lung function tests accompanied by obstructive dysfunction.

Prognosis: Usually good even in regularly recurrent events; sequelae are interstitial fibrosis, chronic bronchitis, and bronchiectases.

Radiology: Chest radiographs show diffuse edematous infiltrates, subpleural emphysematous changes, or bronchiectasis.

Pathology:

Gross: Edematous lungs in acute poisoning. Enlargement of the smaller bronchi and subpleural focal emphysema.

Histology: No specific findings have been reported. Acute poisoning is associated with intraalveolar transudate, fibrin exudation, and possible bacterial superinfection. In chronic stages one sees chronic bronchitis with bronchiectasis, subpleural emphysema, and small foci of scarring. The metal particles are not visible by light microscopy.

➤ *Descriptors:* Lung parenchyma with preserved structure:

- intraalveolar serous fluid
- intraalveolar fibrinoid material
- mononuclear inflammatory infiltrates;
- Bronchial mucosa with preserved structure:
- mononuclear inflammatory infiltrates
- ectatic lumen
- atrophy

■ *Special stains:* PAS, collagenous stains, electron microscopy, X-ray diffraction method and related physical techniques.

Hallmark of Diagnosis: Clinical history, identification of the metal particles by physical techniques.

Differential diagnosis: Acute respiratory distress syndrome, alterations of the lung parenchyma due to other agents.

Fungus

Definition: Infection of the lung with fungal organisms.

Incidence/Epidemiology: Fungal infections can occur in healthy, immunologically intact persons and in immunocompromised persons (opportunistic infections). Opportunistic fungal infections are of greater clinical importance than primary fungal infections.

Etiology/Pathophysiology: Fungal infections can be classified into three clinical categories: (a) cutaneous, (b) subcutaneous, and (c) systemic infections. In the lower respiratory tract invasive and noninvasive mycotic infections have to be distinguished. Noninvasive fungal infections occur in damaged airways such as bronchiectasis, obstructive airway disease, and preformed cavities. They may develop into invasive fungal infections if the immunity decreases. The following fungal organisms are of importance in the human lower respiratory tract: *Aspergillus, Blastomyces, Candida albicans, Coccidioidomyces, Cryptococcus, Emmonsia, Fusarium, Geotrichum candidum, Histoplasma, Mucor, Paracoccidioides, Penicillus marnefei, Pseudallescheria, Rhinosporidium, Sporotrichum, Torulopsis, Trichosporon.*

Clinical Presentation: The clinical manifestation of fungal infections varies considerably. They may be detected accidentally, may cause chronic cough with expectoration, or may develop into a life-threatening disease with fungosemia and sepsis.

Prognosis: Pulmonary fungal infections are noninvasive or encapsulated disorders in the majority of patients; however, they are often fatal in immunocompromised patients.

Radiology: The characteristic findings on chest radiographs are medium-sized cavities with intracavitary masses separated from the boundaries by crescents of air. Other findings include solid circumscribed calcified nodules, bulky mediastinal lymphadenopathy with diffuse peripheral infiltrates, granulomatous miliary densities, patchy bilateral infiltrates, or dense areas of consolidation.

Pathology:

Gross: The gross findings include circumscribed, calcified nodules, yellowish necrotic abscesses, cavities filled with grayish-yellowish, firm masses, multiple, small, firm, miliary nodules, heavy lungs with consolidating areas, ectatic bronchi with mucoid impactions, and solitary, caseous nodules mimicking tuberculosis.

Histology: The characteristic histomorphological findings include central caseating epithelioid granulomas with multinucleated giant cells, calcified nodules surrounded by collagen fibers, mononuclear interstitial inflammation, mixtures of multinucleated giant cells and neutrophilic granulocytes in the distant air spaces, suppurative alveolar exudate with increased number of eosinophilic granulocytes, infarct-like necrotic areas. The histomorphological findings are characteristic of the specific infective fungi and are described under the corresponding headings.

➤ *Descriptors:* Lung parenchyma with altered structure:
- caseous epithelioid granulomas
- fungus (intragranulomatous, yeast, spores)
- multinucleated giant cells
- eosinophils
- mixed inflammatory infiltrates
- necrosis (infarctlike);
- Lung parenchyma with preserved structure:
- intraalveolar fibrinoid material
- eosinophils
- fungus

■ *Special stains:* PAS, Gomori's methenamine silver stain (GMS), Gridley's fungus stain, Mayer's mucicarmine stain, direct immunofluorescence. For screening purposes, PAS and GMS stain are widely used. GMS stain can be counterstained with HE for demonstration of host tissue response.

Hallmark of Diagnosis: Demonstration and identification of fungus (spores and yeast).

Differential diagnosis: Infectious granulomas of other organisms, especially tuberculosis, noninfectious granulomas.

Furrier's Lung

Definition: Alteration of the lung parenchyma associated with inhalation of dust of animal pelts.

Incidence/Epidemiology: Rare disease seen in persons working with animal pelts.

Etiology/Pathophysiology: Allergic extrinsic alveolitis due to exposure to animal proteins. For details, see Allergic (Extrinsic) Alveolitis.

Clinical Presentation: Acute, subacute or chronic hypersensitivity reaction may occur.

Prognosis: Usually good and without serious sequelae.

Radiology: Chest radiographs may be normal or may exhibit mild, diffuse, patchy infiltrates.

Pathology:

Gross: The lungs may show mild edema or mild increase in consistency.

Histology: No specific changes have been reported except those as described under the heading Allergic (Extrinsic) Alveolitis.

➤ *Descriptors:* Lung parenchyma with altered structure:
- noncaseous epithelioid granulomas
- eosinophils
- multinucleated giant cells
- intrabronchiolar fibrinoid material and histiocytes
- ulceration of bronchiolar mucosa;
- Lung parenchyma with preserved structure:
- macrophages
- desquamation, hypertrophy, hyperplasia and dysplasia of pneumocytes
- mononuclear inflammatory infiltrates
- intraalveolar serous fluid

■ *Special stains:* PAS, collagenous stains, immunohistochemistry for immunoglobulins, HLA-DR, endogenous lectins.

Hallmark of Diagnosis: Clinical history, noncaseating epithelioid granulomas with additional hyperplasia of cells of the alveolar lining, diffuse interstitial inflammatory infiltrates, increased number of eosinophilic granulocytes.

Differential diagnosis: Infectious and noninfectious granulomas such as tuberculosis, sarcoidosis, or berylliosis. For details, see Allergic (Extrinsic) Alveolitis.

Fusariosis

Definition: Infection of the lung with the fungus *Fusarium* spp.

Incidence/Epidemiology: *Fusarium* species are widely distributed and live in soil or on plants. They cause severe human infections in the skin of burned patients or act as opportunistic organisms in immunocompromised patients suffering from lymphoma or acute leukemia or renal transplant recipients.

Etiology/Pathophysiology: Infection of the lower respiratory tract is usually an invasive infectious disorder and occurs as a secondary infection with preceding necrotic skin lesions or ulcers of the skin. Coexisting pulmonary infections with *Candida*, herpes simplex, or bacteria have been reported.

Clinical Presentation: Patients are usually in poor condition. The fungal pulmonary infection provokes the symptoms of necrotizing pneumonia.

Prognosis: Infection with *Fusarium* spp is often fatal.

Radiology: Chest radiographs show either circumscribed, necrotizing densities or diffuse patchy and usually progressive infiltrates.

Pathology:

Gross: The lungs contain several centrally necrotized, brownish-grayish nodules mimicking older infarctions.

Histology: The fungus can be seen in the air spaces and also in the small pulmonary arteries. It consists of branched septated hyphae measuring 3–7 μm in diameter.The branches often arise perpendicular to the parent hyphae and may be difficult to distinguish from *Aspergillus*. Granulomatous reaction of the host tissue with surrounding fibrosis can be seen in older lesions.

➤ *Descriptors:* Lung parenchyma with altered structure:
- necrosis and hemorrhage (massive)
- mixed inflammatory infiltrates
- eosinophils
- caseous epithelioid granulomas
- fungus (intragranulomatous, septated hyphae)

■ *Special stains:* PAS, GMS, collagenous stains.

Hallmark of Diagnosis: Clinical history, especially skin lesions, identification of the fungus, necrotizing epithelioid granulomas with multinucleated giant cells.

Differential diagnosis: Infections by other fungal species, especially *Aspergillus* and *Trichosporon*.

Gastric Acid Aspiration

Definition: Alteration of the lung parenchyma associated with aspiration of gastric acid, see Acid Gastric Aspiration.

Gaucher's Disease

Definition: Alteration of the lung parenchyma associated with Gaucher's disease (sphingolipodosis).

Incidence/Epidemiology: Rare autosomal recessive disorder with abnormal storage of cerebrosides. Three different clinical courses can be distinguished: (a) a chronic course without neurological symptoms in adults, (b) a subacute course with neurological symptoms in juvenile patients, (c) a massive acute course with neurological symptoms in infants. Abnormal storage of glucocerebrosides has been described, mainly in the juvenile and adult diseases.

Etiology/Pathophysiology: Deficiency or lack of glucocerebrosidase causes abnormal storage of glucocerebrosides in macrophages and histiocytes of the lung. Accumulation of macrophages causes interstitial fibrosis and chronic pneumonitis.

Clinical Presentation: Clinical symptoms include enlargement of the spleen, liver, and lymph nodes, osteoporosis, hypochromic anemia, and hypercalcemia. Patients may suffer from dyspnea, recurrent infectious pneumonia, shortness of breath and tachypnea.

Prognosis: Poor, as patients with pulmonary involvement usually die during early childhood (4–10 years old).

Radiology: Chest radiographs are normal or may show patchy or miliary interstitial infiltrations.

Pathology:

Gross: The lungs may show increased consistency with small grayish areas of consolidation.

Histology: The distant air spaces are filled with agglutinations of foamy macrophages measuring 20–100 μm in diameter. The foamy cytoplasm is of pink color in HE stains. Some of the macrophages have a shrunken shape which has been named "wrinkled tissue paper", "crumpled silk" and "striated small rod-like". The cells of alveolar lining are unsuspicious. The alveolar walls may be thickened and show slight fibrosis.

➤ *Descriptors:* Lung parenchyma with preserved structure:
- macrophages (foamy, "wrinkled tissue paper");
- Lung parenchyma with altered structure:
- diffuse interstitial fibrosis (mild)

- *Special stains:* PAS, Giemsa, Prussian blue, Sudan black, collagenous stains, endogenous lectins.

Hallmark of Diagnosis: Clinical history, foamy macrophages in the distant airways with "shrunken shape", monocytic interstitial infiltrates.

Differential diagnosis: Other storage disorders such as Fabry's or Niemann-Pick disease; desquamative interstitial pneumonia, aggressive autoimmune disorders.

Genetic Systemic Disorders

Definition: Alteration of lung parenchyma associated with systemic genetic disorders.

Incidence/Epidemiology: The lung is frequently involved in systemic genetic disorders. The lung damage may be directly due to inborn errors in cells of the lung parenchyma, such as enzymatic deficiency in the cells of the reticulohistiocytic system, or secondary to infections caused by alterations of the air conducting system, or both. Pulmonary involvement may reach 100% in various systemic genetic disorders.

Etiology/Pathophysiology: Systemic genetic disorders usually affect the immune system, reticulohistiocytic cells, or cells of the exocrine-endocrine glands. The defence mechanisms of the lung are based upon all three categories of cells and are very vulnerable to their disturbance. Besides alterations characteristic of the underlying disease, additional bacterial and viral pulmonary infections are common.

The following genetic disorders usually affect the lung: cystic fibrosis, α_1-antitrypsin deficiency, autoimmune disorders, congenital storage diseases, metabolic disorders.

Clinical Presentation: The symptoms are usually related to recurrent severe infections.

Prognosis: Usually poor, with serious sequelae inducing honeycombing.

Radiology: The chest radiographs usually show increased interstitial markings after cure of the acute infection.

Pathology:

Gross: Increased consistency and usually completely destroyed lung with honeycombing.

Histology: Complete alteration of the lung texture with secondary interstitial fibrosis. The characteristic findings (for example, foamy macrophages in the distant airways, angiitis, etc.) are usually present in lung areas that have preserved their texture, i.e., it is necessary to analyze the "unsuspicious" areas of the lung parenchyma.

➤ *Descriptors:* Lung parenchyma with altered structure:
- mononuclear inflammatory infiltrates
- macrophages
- focal interstitial fibrosis
- enlarged distant air spaces;
- Bronchial mucosa with altered structure:
- viscous mucus
- ectatic lumen
- mixed inflammatory infiltrates
- squamous metaplasia and dysplasia

- *Special stains:* PAS, Prussian blue, collagenous stains, Giemsa, endogenous lectins, immunohistochemistry for immunoglobulins.

Hallmark of Diagnosis: Clinical history, characteristic findings as described under the specific headings.

Differential diagnosis: Chronic idiopathic pulmonary infections.

Geotrichosis

Definition: Infection of lung with *Geotrichum candidum.*

Incidence/Epidemiology: Rare infection of the lung with an opportunistic fungus which is not as aggressive as *Candida albicans*. The organism is a ubiquitous saprophyte living in soil, contaminated food, and decomposing organic substances. Only infections in patients with strongly decreased immunodefence mechanisms have been reported.

Etiology/Pathophysiology: The organisms can enter the body through the oropharynx and may proliferate in the distant airways, bronchi, or gastrointestinal tract. Cutaneous infections with consequent transient fungemia and invasive pulmonary infections are rare. The organisms tend to stay in preformed cavities such as bronchiectases, necrotic bronchial carcinomas, necrotic infarctions, pulmonary cysts, etc.

Clinical Presentation: Patients present with persistent cough, expectoration of grayish, purulent, or blood-tinged mucus, mild fever.

Prognosis: Usually good and without serious sequelae.

Radiology: Chest radiographs are either normal or show pre-existing cavities with dense material, rarely patchy interstitial infiltrates.

Pathology:

Gross: Grayish, gelatinous mucus in bronchiectases or pulmonary cavities.

Histology: The fungus consists of short hyphae with some branching intermingled with dissociated, rectangular or oval arthroconidiae (spores). The hyphae measure 3–6 μm and vary widely in diameter. The organisms stain only weakly with HE; they can be best demonstrated with GMS or PAS stain. The inflammatory response of the host tissue either consists of neutrophilic and eosinophilic granulocytes, lymphocytes, and central necrosis or takes the form of a granulomatous epithelioid reaction with multinucleated giant cells. Invasive intrapulmonary geotrichosis is extremely rare.

➤ *Descriptors:* Bronchial mucosa with preserved structure:

- ectatic lumen
- mixed inflammatory infiltrates
- fungus (intrabronchial, hyphae and spores);
- Bronchial mucosa with altered structure:
- caseous epithelioid granulomas
- fungus (intragranulomatous, spores)
- eosinophils
- multinucleated giant cells

■ *Special stains:* PAS, GMS, immunofluorescence.

Hallmark of Diagnosis: Necrotizing granulomatous bronchitis, identification of the fungus, agar colonization of the fungus.

Differential diagnosis: Other fungal infections, especially those with *Candida albicans* or *Aspergillus*.

Germ Cell Tumor

Definition: Metastasis of a germ cell tumor into the lung.

Incidence/Epidemiology: Metastasis of germ cell tumors into the lung is a common finding in advanced tumors of the testes and may even occur years after potentially curative surgery of the primary tumor.

Etiology/Pathophysiology: The spread of tumor cells into the lung may occur via the lymphatic system or the veins. Liver metastases do not usually exist.

Clinical Presentation: Patients may be asymptomatic or may present with shortness of breath, chest pain, or chronic cough.

Prognosis: Usually poor, most patients die within 2 years after clinical evidence of pulmonary metastases.

Radiology: Chest radiographs show multiple, usually small (a few millimeters in diameter), circumscribed, peripheral densities intermingled with some larger nodules. Necrosis and cystic appearance may be seen, especially after cytostatic therapy.

Pathology:

Gross: The gross appearance varies from solid, firm, grayish nodules to central necrotic masses with hemorrhage. Cysts filled with mucoid fluid may also be seen.

Histology: The histomorphological appearance depends upon the response to preceding cytostatic therapy and may present the following images:

(a) Central hyaline masses with surrounding pale tumor cells of abundant cytoplasm and small dense nuclei mimicking macrophages.

(b) Solid tumor masses of various histological cell types surrounded by dense collagen fibers.

(c) Tubular and papillary tumor textures with "blastomatous" epithelial tumor cells and central necrosis and hemorrhage.

(d) Cysts with epithelial cells of "normal appearance" filled with serous fluid and surrounded by dense collagen fibers.

Inflammatory response of host tissue is usually absent. Multiple metastases – if present – may vary considerably in their morphology.

➤ *Descriptors:* Newly formed textures with metastasis potential:

- epithelial growth pattern
- adenoid textures
- large tumor cells
- prominent nucleoli
- acellular hyaline areas (large)
- necrosis and hemorrhage
- cysts (serous fluid)
- absent or weak inflammatory infiltrates

- *Special stains:* PAS, collagenous stains, Giemsa, immunohistochemistry for various tumor markers, endogenous lectins, DNA analysis.

  Hallmark of Diagnosis: Clinical history (including details of cytostatic therapy), identification of viable tumor cells.

  Differential diagnosis: Healed infectious lesions, primary lung carcinomas such as adenocarcinoma.

Ghon Focus

Definition: Circumscribed primary manifestation of tuberculous infection in the middle part of the lungs, subpleural, see Tuberculosis.

Giant Cell Interstitial Pneumonia

Definition: Specific chronic interstitial pneumonitis with characteristic tissue reaction (multinucleated giant cells in the distant air spaces).

Incidence/Epidemiology: Unusual disease seen in some persons exposed to cobalt and other hard metals, especially tungsten carbide. It may be seen in young children with aggressive autoimmune disorders (autoimmune hepatitis).

Etiology/Pathophysiology: The characteristic tissue reaction has been provoked experimentally with cobalt. It has been suggested that the multinucleated giant cells are composed of type II pneumocytes and macrophages.

Clinical Presentation: The symptoms include nonproductive cough, restrictive lung function in relevant tests, dyspnea, and tachypnea.

Prognosis: Fair and comparable to that of desquamative interstitial pneumonia, i.e., respiratory failure occurs after several years.

Radiology: Chest radiographs show diffuse, usually bilateral interstitial infiltrates running from the pulmonary hila down to the peripheral diaphragm.

Pathology:

Gross: The lungs are of slightly grayish color and have a denser consistency. Circumscribed nodules are absent.

Histology: The characteristic findings are those of desquamative interstitial pneumonitis with numerous or predominant multinucleated giant cells in the distant airways. The giant cells measure 30–60 µm in diameter. The cytoplasm may contain asteroid bodies but no viral inclusion bodies. The cells of the alveolar lining surrounding the multinucleated giant cells are unsuspicious and not hyperplastic. Some interstitial monocytic infiltrates and a weak fibrosis are present. Fibrin deposits and hyaline membranes are absent.

➤ *Descriptors:* Lung parenchyma with preserved structure:
  - multinucleated giant cells
  - macrophages
  - mononuclear inflammatory infiltrates (scattered)
  - unsuspicious pneumocytes
  - absent hyaline membranes

- *Special stains:* PAS, collagenous stains, immunohistochemistry for immunoglobulins, endogenous lectins.

  Hallmark of Diagnosis: Identification of characteristic giant cells, histomorphology of desquamative interstitial pneumonia, exposure to cobalt or hard metal fumes.

  Differential diagnosis: Measles pneumonia.

Glanders

Definition: Infection of the lung with *Malleomyces mallei*.

Incidence/Epidemiology: Rare disease in humans working with horses or mules or with their carcasses.

Etiology/Pathophysiology: The gram-negative bacteria are highly infective in horses, mules, asses, or cats. Human infection may occur as a localized or generalized disease process.

Clinical Presentation: The localized form appears as a chronic ulcerative lesion with suppurative exudation and involvement of the regional lymph nodes. Bacteremia may follow and may cause a severe, fatal, necrotizing pneumonia with foul suppurative expectoration, high fever, and chest pain.

Prognosis: Infection of the lung is often fatal.

Radiology: Chest radiographs show circumscribed necrotic areas which may consolidate.

Pathology:

Gross: Multiple, hemorrhagic-necrotic, yellowish-pink nodules of various sizes with surrounding rings of consolidation.

Histology: The nodules are made up of large necrotic masses intermingled with neutrophilic granulocytes, lymphocytes, and relatively many macrophages. The areas of consolidation are of inflammatory cellular appearance and indicate only a weak fibrous tissue reaction.

➤ *Descriptors:* Lung parenchyma with altered structure:

- necrosis
- mixed inflammatory infiltrates

■ *Special stains:* PAS, collagenous stains, silver methenamine stain.

Hallmark of Diagnosis: Clinical history, lung abscess.

Differential diagnosis: Infection of the lung by other organisms, aspiration pneumonia.

Glass Fibers

Definition: Alteration of the lung parenchyma associated with inhaled glass fibers.

Incidence/Epidemiology: Glass fibers may be inhaled by persons working in the production or use of rock wool or fiberglass wool used for insulation of buildings, to reinforce plastics, in chemical filters, or in rubber and paper manufacture. Epidemiologic studies have not been able to confirm an increased risk of obstructive lung disease in exposed workers; however, evidence exists for an increased risk of mesothelioma.

Etiology/Pathophysiology: The glass fibers have a broad range of size and can be inhaled and deposited in the distant airways. Long fibers are suggested to be more fibrinogenic than short fibers. In animal experiments glass fibers have been proven to initiate mesothelioma and interstitial fibrosis.

Clinical Presentation: No specific symptoms have been reported.

Prognosis: Fair, but slow progression into respiratory failure can occur. Patients have an increased risk of mesothelioma and lung cancer.

Radiology: Chest radiographs are usually normal or may show mild interstitial fibrosis or indicate mesothelioma.

Pathology:

Gross: No specific findings exist.

Histology: Long glass fibers may break into smaller ones, and can be detected by birefringent techniques. Coating may be present. Interstitial fibrosis related to glass fibers is of diffuse nature and usually mild. Macrophages may ingest glass fibers. Agglutination of glass fibers is commonly seen in or close to the respiratory bronchioles.

➤ *Descriptors:* Lung parenchyma with preserved structure:

- dust (birefringent fibers, crystals)
- ferruginous bodies
- macrophages (ingested glass fibers);
- Lung parenchyma with altered structure:
- diffuse interstitial fibrosis (mild)

■ *Special stains:* Collagenous stains, X-ray diffraction techniques or related physical techniques, Prussian blue, polarization.

Hallmark of Diagnosis: Clinical history, identification of glass fibers by physical techniques.

Differential diagnosis: Asbestos fibers, silica.

Glial Tissue

Definition: Heterotopic glial tissue in the lung parenchyma.

Incidence/Epidemiology: Glial tissue may be found in the lung parenchyma of anencephalic infants.

Etiology/Pathophysiology: Malformation of the central nervous system provokes the development of islands of nervous tissue in the lung.

Clinical Presentation: No specific symptoms.

Prognosis: Intrapulmonary glial tissue has no prognostic influence.

Radiology: No specific symptoms.

Pathology:

Gross: No specific findings.

Histology: Small areas of glia surrounded by unsuspicious lung parenchyma.

➤ *Descriptors:* Lung parenchyma with altered structure:

- glial tissue (small foci)
- absent inflammatory infiltrates

■ *Special stains:* None.

Hallmark of Diagnosis: Glial tissue in the lung, usually in anencephalic infants.

Differential diagnosis: Emboli of nervous tissue in the pulmonary arteries due to trauma.

Glomus Tumor

Definition: Low-grade tumor of the lung derived from the cells of the Sucquet-Hoyer canal.
Incidence/Epidemiology: About ten cases of tumors arising in the trachea or lung have been reported. They may occur at any age or in either sex but most frequently in young adults. Some of the reported cases were benign, whereas others showed metastases shortly after resection.
Etiology/Pathophysiology: The tumors are thought to derive from a special cell of the arteriovenous shunt, the Sucquet-Hoyer canal. The glomus apparatus which is responsible for control of blood flow is located in this area; however, it is not well-defined in the lung. Outside the lung glomus tumors are usually benign lesions and are frequently seen in the extremities (around the fingernails) or in the gastrointestinal tract.
Clinical Presentation: Symptoms are related to the location of the tumors and may mimic asthmoid bronchitis or may be detected incidentally.
Prognosis: No features of the glomus tumors are known to predict the prognosis which can be fatal in 30–50% of patients.
Radiology: Solid, noncalcifying mass in the peripheral lung or findings related to tracheal stenosis.
Pathology:
Gross: The tumors are well-circumscribed masses grayish-tan to red-brown in color and of soft consistency. They may show multiple proliferative centers. Necrosis, a capsula, or hemorrhage are not signs of glomus tumors.
Histology: The tumors are composed of nests of small- to medium-sized cells with uniform, small nuclei and pale, relatively abundant cytoplasm. The tumor nests have small venioles in their center. Molding, severe inflammatory response of host tissue and numerous mitoses are absent. The tumors resemble hemangiopericytomas. Immunohistochemistry for various neuroendocrine markers (NSE, bombesin, synaptophysin, chromogranin) is negative. They stain positively with vimentin.

➤ *Descriptors:* Newly formed textures with metastasis potential:
- mesenchymal growth pattern
- solid textures (small central venioles)
- small tumor cells
- abundant cytoplasm (pale)
- homogeneous nuclear and cellular size
- finely distributed nuclear chromatin
- infrequent mitoses

■ *Special stains:* PAS, collagenous stains, immunohistochemistry for neuroendocrine markers, cytokeratin, vimentin, desmin, desmoplakin, endogenous lectins, DNA analysis.

Hallmark of Diagnosis: Highly vascularized tumor without necrosis and hemorrhage consisting of small tumor cells with homogeneous nuclei and pale cytoplasm. Negative staining with neuroendocrine markers, positive with vimentin, low DNA index.
Differential diagnosis: Small cell carcinoma of the lung, carcinoid, hemangiopericytoma, leiomyoblastoma, epithelioid leiomyosarcoma, benign clear cell tumor of the lung, chemodectoma.

Gnathostomiasis

Definition: Infection of the lung with the nematode *Gnathostoma spinigerum.*
Incidence/Epidemiology: Gnathostomiasis is endemic in southeast Asia including India, Thailand, Japan, the Philippines, and China. The nematode is a form of "larva migrans", and a definite host location is the stomach wall of tigers, leopards, and domestic cats and dogs.
Etiology/Pathophysiology: The parasite requires passage through two aquatic hosts before it reaches the land host. The first host is the minute cyclops which is eaten by the second host, fresh water fish. Infection of man is caused by eating raw, marinated, or poorly cooked fresh water fish. The parasite cannot mature in man and migrates through various tissues causing a variety of symptoms of larva migrans. The immature parasites can survive in man for a period of 12 years. Infection of man can also occur by eating raw flesh of infected animals such as chicken or pork. The regular sequence of migration is through the stomach wall into the peritoneal cavity, followed by transmigration through the liver and finally into the skeletal muscle and connective tissue. In the final stage the larva reenters the proximal part of the stomach and embeds its cephalic end into the mucosa.

Clinical Presentation: The symptoms start with nausea, vomiting, salivation, pruritus, and urticaria within 2–4 days after eating infected fish or meat. The movement of the parasite may provoke brief sharp pains. Blood-tinged sputum or acute cough and chest pain indicate pulmonary infection. Pneumothorax may occur if the larva penetrates through the pleura.

Prognosis: Usually good, although infection of the central nervous system or massive pulmonary infection may cause severe clinical problems.

Radiology: Chest radiographs may be normal or may display irregularly shaped, diffuse densities.

Pathology:

Gross: The immature parasites measure less than 1 cm in length and 2–4 mm in diameter. Their wake may be seen as small disrupted areas filled with blood.

Histology: The cephalus of the parasite is covered with multiple small spikes measuring about 30 μm in length and 10 μm in diameter. The parasites are usually embedded in normal tissue which shows only a weak inflammatory reaction of edema, eosinophilic granulocytes, lymphocytes, and plasma cells.

➤ *Descriptors:* Lung parenchyma with altered structure:
- parasites (living)
- mononuclear inflammatory infiltrates (weak)
- eosinophils;
- Pleura with altered structure:
- parasites (living)
- mononuclear inflammatory infiltrates (weak)
- eosinophils

■ *Special stains:* PAS, Movat, connective tissue stains.

Hallmark of Diagnosis: Clinical history, viable parasites in the pleura, identification of the parasites.

Differential diagnosis: Infection with other nematodes.

Gold

Definiton: Alteration of the lung parenchyma associated with gold therapy (gold salts).

Incidence/Epidemiology: Toxic effects of gold salts on the lung parenchyma have been described in a limited number of patients.

Etiology/Pathophysiology: Gold may provoke a hypersensitivity reaction of the lung or may induce diffuse alveolar damage that may progress to the usual interstitial pneumonia. It has also been proven to induce a systemic lupus erythematosus (SLE)-like syndrome with involvement of the lung and pleura.

Clinical Presentation: Patients suffer from shortness of breath, dyspnea, chest pain, pleural or pericardial effusions, and cough.

Prognosis: Usually good and without serious sequelae.

Radiology: Chest radiographs reflect diffuse interstitial infiltrates suggesting pulmonary edema, interstitial pneumonia, or consolidated areas of atelectasis.

Pathology:

Gross: Edematous lungs. Chronic exposure may provoke honeycombing.

Histology: Findings indicate diffuse alveolar damage, usual interstitial pneumonia, hypersensitivity reaction of the lung, or (SLE)-like findings with lymphoid aggregates around the bronchioles and pulmonary arteries. Fibrinoid necrosis of the bronchial walls may be present.

➤ *Descriptors:* Lung parenchyma with altered structure:
- noncaseous epithelioid granulomas
- eosinophils
- multinucleated giant cells
- intrabronchiolar fibrinoid material and histiocytes
- ulceration of bronchiolar mucosa;
- Lung parenchyma with preserved structure:
- macrophages
- desquamation, hypertrophy, hyperplasia and dysplasia of pneumocytes
- mononuclear inflammatory infiltrates
- (peribronchiolar)
- intraalveolar serous fluid

■ *Special stains:* PAS, collagenous stains, Giemsa, immunohistochemistry for immunoglobulins, endogenous lectins.

Hallmark of Diagnosis: Clinical history, radiologic findings, histomorphology of usual interstitial pneumonia, diffuse alveolar damage, allergic extrinsic pneumonitis, (SLE)-like syndrome.

Differential diagnosis: Corresponding lung findings associated with other agents.

Goodpasture's Syndrome

Definition: Disease with diffuse pulmonary hemorrhage caused by glomerular basement membrane-specific antibody with or without additional nephropathy, see Antiglomerular Basement Membrane Disease.

Granular Cell Tumor of the Lung

Definition: Benign tumor of the lung with specific histomorphologic appearance (synonym granular cell myoblastoma).
Incidence/Epidemiology: Rare tumor of the lower trachea and bronchi with about 60 reported cases. It occurs most frequently in young adults and rarely during childhood.
Etiology/Pathophysiology: The tumors are believed to originate from Schwann cells.
Prognosis: Usually good and without recurrence or sequelae.
Clinical Presentation: The patients suffer from airway obstruction or irritation and present with cough, dyspnea, and hemoptysis.
Radiology: Chest radiographs show a solitary mass in the trachea or in the proximal bronchi. Rarely, the tumors arise in the peripheral lung parenchyma.
Pathology:
Gross: The tumors are soft to rubbery in consistency and yellow-tan to grayish. They measure about 2 cm in diameter.
Histology: The tumors grow without any detectable microscopic texture and are composed of large tumor cells with relatively small nuclei of homogeneous nuclear chromatin. The tumor cells and their nuclei vary little in their size and present a uniform picture. Necrotic areas, mitotic figures, and inflammatory response of the host tissue are unsuspicious. The cytoplasm contains small eosinophilic granules. The tumor cells stain positively with S-100 protein.

➤ *Descriptors:* Newly formed textures without metastasis potential:

- mesenchymal growth pattern
- solid textures
- lymphomatoid textures
- abundant cytoplasm (small granules)
- small nuclei (condensed)
- homogeneous nuclear and cellular size
- absent or infrequent mitoses
- absent necrosis
- absent inflammatory infiltrates

■ *Special stains:* PAS, Giemsa, immunohistochemistry for neurosecretory markers, S-100 protein, DNA analysis.

Hallmark of Diagnosis: Large uniform tumor cells with granular cytoplasm, small uniform nuclei; absence of necrotic areas and specific growth textures.
Differential diagnosis: Carcinoid, oncocytoma, malacoplakia, Whipple's disease, infection with *Mycobacterium avium intracellulare.*

Granuloma

Definition: Focal chronic inflammation of the lung parenchyma with peculiar (granulomatous) texture, see Granulomatosis, Granulomatous Disease in Childhood Chronic, Sarcoidosis, Tuberculosis, Berylliosis, Fungus, Parasites.

Granulomatosis

Definition: Specific (granulomatous) alteration of the lung parenchyma associated with different intrapulmonary structures.
Incidence/Epidemiology: The lesions include pulmonary angiitides and granulomatoses, i.e., Wegener's granulomatosis, allergic angiitis and granulomatosis, necrotizing sarcoid granulomatosis, lymphomatoid granulomatosis, and bronchocentric granulomatosis. In addition, a genetic X-linked chromosomal disorder produces a chronic granulomatous disease of childhood. Each disease is a distinct clinicopathological entity and is described under the specific headings. All pulmonary angiitides and granulomatoses occur less frequently than other granulomatous diseases (infectious or noninfectious such as sarcoidosis). Most of the patients suffering from pulmonary angiitis and granulomatosis are young to middle-aged adults.
Etiology/Pathophysiology: True angiitis can be seen in Wegener's granulomatosis, allergic angiitis and granulomatosis, and possibly in

necrotizing sarcoid granulomatosis. It is probably a secondary phenomenon in lymphomatoid granulomatosis and in bronchocentric granulomatosis. The etiology of the diseases is still unknown, although bronchocentric granulomatosis is frequently associated with allergic bronchopulmonary aspergillosis.

Clinical Presentation: Patients can be grouped clinically into asthmatic and nonasthmatic cases. Asthma and eosinophilia are frequently seen in patients with Wegener's granulomatosis, allergic angiitis and granulomatosis, and bronchocentric granulomatosis. Patients with necrotizing sarcoid granulomatosis or lymphomatoid granulomatosis often show chest pain, cough, dyspnea, and occasionally hemoptysis. Patients with Wegener's granulomatosis or allergic angiitis and granulomatosis may commonly or occasionally develop glomerulonephritis, whereas patients with necrotizing sarcoid granulomatosis or with bronchocentric granulomatosis do not show extrapulmonary involvement. The prognosis of patients with lymphomatoid granulomatosis is poor compared with that of patients with other granulomatous diseases.

Prognosis: Most of the patients die within 10 years after clinical diagnosis.

Radiology: Chest radiographs usually show multiple, circumscribed nodules in patients with Wegener's granulomatosis, necrotizing sarcoid granulomatosis, and lymphomatoid granulomatosis. Those of patients with bronchocentric granulomatosis show areas of consolidation, and those of patients with allergic angiitis and granulomatosis show transient diffuse densities which may change their location within a few days.

Pathology:

Gross: The lungs usually contain firm, hemorrhagic to yellowish, irregular formed masses which may reach several centimeters in diameter.

Histology: Histomorphological details are described under the specific headings. The general findings are necrotic infarctlike areas with surrounding histiocytes, lymphocytes, plasma cells, and multinucleated giant cells.The granulomas are bronchocentric in patients with bronchocentric granulomatosis and angiocentric in the other disorders. Palisading histiocytes are a characteristic feature of Wegener's granulomatosis, allergic angiitis and granulomatosis, and bronchocentric granulomatosis. Dense infiltrates of eosinophilic granulocytes are a characteristic feature of bronchocentric granulomatosis and of allergic angiitis and granulomatosis. Atypical lymphoreticular cells are usually seen in lymphomatoid granulomatosis.

➤ *Descriptors:* Lung parenchyma with altered structure:
- necrosis and hemorrhage (infarctlike, angiocentric and bronchocentric)
- palisading histiocytes
- mononuclear inflammatory infiltrates
- multinucleated giant cells
- eosinophils (numerous)
- atypical lymphoid cells

■ *Special stains:* PAS, collagenous stains, immunohistochemistry for immunoglobulins, endogenous lectins, DNA analysis (lymphomatoid granulomatosis).

Hallmark of Diagnosis: Clinical history, central necrotized granulomatous lesions with either angiocentric or bronchocentric appearance, exclusion of infectious disorders or lymphoma.

Differential diagnosis: Infectious disorders such as tuberculosis, fungus, parasites, lymphoma, sarcoidosis.

Granulomatous Disease in Childhood, Chronic

Definition: Inherited disorder in which macrophages cannot phagocytize.

Incidence/Epidemiology: Rare X-linked chromosomal disorder.

Etiology/Pathophysiology: Inability to phagocytize results in an inability to kill microorganisms and consequently to chronic infection with specific histomorphologic appearance.

Clinical Presentation: Children suffer from recurrent pulmonary infections with cough, fever, malaise, and expectoration.

Prognosis: Fair, common sequelae are chronic pulmonary infections with final honeycombing.

Radiology: Chest radiographs present multiple ill-defined densities.

Pathology:

Gross: The lungs contain multiple hemorrhagic yellowish necrotic nodules which may reach several centimeters in diameter.

Histology: Large areas of massive necrosis surrounded by pigmented histiocytes, lymphocytes, plasma cells, and multinucleated giant cells. The necrotic infection usually starts close to terminal bronchioles or small pulmonary arteries.

➤ *Descriptors:* Lung parenchyma with altered structure:
- necrosis (large areas)
- mononuclear inflammatory infiltrates
- multinucleated giant cells
- macrophages (pigmented)
- reduced number of granulocytes

■ *Special stains:* PAS, collagenous stains, GMS.

Hallmark of Diagnosis: Clinical history, chromosome analysis, histiocytic granulomas with central infarctlike necrosis.

Differential diagnosis: Infectious and noninfectious granulomas (tuberculosis, fungus, necrotizing sarcoidlike granulomatosis).

Graphite Pneumoconiosis

Definition: Alteration of the lung parenchyma associated with inhalation of graphite dust.

Incidence/Epidemiology: Graphite is a mineral mined as lumps or flakes in Korea, Austria, USSR, China, and Mexico. Graphite contains small amounts of free silica which are removed by solution in hydrofluoric acid. The risk to miners is related to the percentage of quartz in the air: If the percentage of quartz ranges within 5–10% no prediction of progressive pneumoconiosis arising can be made. If, however, the percentage of quartz exceeds 20% in respirable airborne dust, silicotic features of pneumoconiosis will develop.

Etiology/Pathophysiology: After exposure to graphite or carbon either simple or complicated pneumoconiosis may develop. The inhaled dust will be deposited near the respiratory bronchioles and will be removed by macrophages only to a small degree. Some 2.5–45 g of dust can be stored in the lung in the case of simple pneumoconiosis. Complicated pneumoconiosis or massive progressive fibrosis occurs in persons with a greater amount of dust deposit and higher mineral content. Additional factors have been seen in infective conditions (tuberculosis) and in elevation of IgA and IgG levels. Graphite pneumoconiosis can be associated with increased risk of influenza virus infection due to suppression of interferon induction and a consequent higher risk of bacterial infection. The risk of tuberculosis and the lung cancer seems not to be increased in graphite workers. The development of cor pulmonale is associated with both simple and complicated pneumoconiosis.

Clinical Presentation: The symptoms include shortness of breath, progressive dyspnea, and chronic cough.

Prognosis: Fair; patients have an increased risk for viral and bacterial infections; slow or rapid progressive respiratory failure can occur.

Radiology: Chest radiographs may show either well-defined nodules or diffuse granular infiltrates. The lesions are classified and graded according to the ILO classification.

Pathology:

Gross: Circumscribed black nodules in simple pneumoconiosis or honeycombing with firm black nodules in complicated pneumoconiosis.

Histology: The lesions may be similar to coal worker's pneumoconiosis with dense deposits of black amorphous material in the terminal bronchioles mixed with histiocytes and macrophages. The presence of giant cells in the distant airways of graphite worker's lung has been described as characteristic. Massive fibrosis with dissolution of the original lung texture intermingled with nodules of dust deposits are the alterations of the lung tissue in complicated pneumoconiosis.

➤ *Descriptors:* Lung parenchyma with preserved structure:
- dust (coal)
- macrophages (coal-laden)
- multinucleated giant cells;
- Lung parenchyma with altered structure:
- focal interstitial fibrosis (massive, coal)
- mononuclear inflammatory infiltrates
- enlarged distant air spaces

■ *Special stains:* PAS, Prussian blue, collagenous stains.

Hallmark of Diagnosis: Clinical history, deposits of black dust with admixed macrophages, and interstitial fibrosis of various degrees.

Differential diagnosis: Alterations of the lung parenchyma due to smoking or other inhaled substances.

Griseofulvin

Definition: Alteration of the lung parenchyma associated with intake of griseofulvin, see Drug Toxicity.

Guanoxan

Definition: Alteration of the lung parenchyma associated with intake of guanoxan, see Drug Toxicity.

Gypsum

Definition: Alteration of the lung tissue associated with exposure to gypsum.

Incidence/Epidemiology: Gypsum is an important component of cement and is used worldwide. Chemically it consists of hydrated calcium sulfate and is mined in the USA, Europe, and Russia.

Etiology/Pathophysiology: Gypsum is an inert substance and induces no fibrosis or malignancies.

Clinical Presentation: Patients are usually asymptomatic or may present with mild chronic cough and shortness of breath.

Prognosis: Good and no serious sequelae are known.

Radiology: Chest radiographs are usually normal or may show mild interstitial markings.

Pathology:

Gross: No specific findings have been reported.

Histology: Small silicotic lesions may be seen near the terminal bronchioles.

➤ *Descriptors:* Lung parenchyma with preserved structure:

- dust (deposits of gypsum)
- macrophages
- mononuclear inflammatory infiltrates

■ *Special stains:* PAS, Prussian blue, collagenous stains.

Hallmark of Diagnosis: Clinical history, small deposits of silica.

Differential diagnosis: Silicotic lesions of other origin.

Haemophilus Influenzae – Juvenile Cirrhosis

Haemophilus Influenzae

Definition: Infection of the lung with *Haemophilus influenzae.*

Incidence/Epidemiology: Common community-acquired pathogen of the lower respiratory tract, usually in combination with anaerobic bacteria. It is capable of necrosis and with some regularity is found in bronchiectasis or secondary to measles infection.

Etiology/Pathophysiology: It is considered to be a saprophyte which becomes infective after damage to the lung parenchyma or bronchial mucosa by viral infection or preexisting damage such as bronchiectasis, cavitation, tumor necrosis. It causes extensive destruction of the bronchial mucosa and may be associated with bronchiolitis obliterans.

Clinical Presentation: Patients suffer from high fever, dyspnea, malaise, large quantities of sputum, i.e., symptoms of the more common bacterial pneumonias.

Prognosis: Usually good; however, progressive damage of bronchi and lung parenchyma can occur.

Radiology: Chest radiographs show diffuse, dense infiltrates in both lungs.

Pathology:

Gross: The lung may display areas of consolidation, necrosis, and enlarged bronchi filled with yellowish mucus.

Histology: Extensive destruction of the larger and smaller bronchi with surrounding necrotic lung parenchyma containing neutrophilic and eosinophilic granulocytes, lymphocytes, and plasma cells. Bronchiolitis obliterans may be present as well as bronchiectasis and ulceration of the bronchial mucosa.

➤ *Descriptors:* Lung parenchyma with altered structure:
- necrosis and hemorrhage
- mixed inflammatory infiltrates
- intrabronchiolar fibrinoid material and histiocytes
- ulceration of bronchiolar mucosa
- macrophages;
- Bronchial mucosa with altered structure:
- necrosis (bronchioles and smaller bronchi)
- ulceration

■ *Special stains:* PAS, Gram (*Haemophilus* stains positively), collagenous stains, GMS.

Hallmark of Diagnosis: Bacterial pneumonia, identification of the organisms.

Differential diagnosis: Bacterial pneumonia due to other organisms.

Haloperidol

Definition: Alteration of the lung parenchyma associated with intake of haloperidol, see Drug Toxicity.

Halothane

Definition: Alteration of the lung parenchyma associated with inhalation of halothane, see Drug Toxicity.

Halzoun

Definition: Clinical symptoms characterized by discomfort in the throat, cough, sneezing, and occasionally dysphagia, and vomiting, see Leeches, Pentastomiasis, Trematodes.

Hamartoma

Definition: Tumorlike malformation in the lung.

Incidence/Epidemiology: Hamartomas are the most common benign tumor of the lung, and are observed in 1/400 autopsies. Peripheral lesions are more common in women (sex ratio 1:3, men:women), but central lesions have an equal sex ratio. It occurs at any age (except in babies and children below 9 years old), and is seen in children sometimes associated with extraadrenal paragangliomas and gastric leiomyosarcomas (Carney's triad). Central hamartomas account for 10–15% of all hamartomas.

Etiology/Pathophysiology: The lesions have been considered to be mesenchymal neoplasms with extraordinarily slow growth. Other authors consider the lesions to be hamartomatous malformations which reach their detectable size after some decades of growth. Malignant transformation is unusually rare.

Clinical Presentation: Most lesions are asymptomatic and are detected incidentally. Centrally localized hamartomas can constrict the central airways and cause obstructive symptoms.

Prognosis: Good and no serious sequelae are known.

Radiology: Chest radiographs show peripheral, sharply defined nodules 3 cm in diameter or less often with lobulated borders, sometimes with a "popcorn" type of calcification. Centrally localized hamartomas show air-displacing masses within the air shadows of the bronchi.

Pathology:

Gross: Circumscribed, firm, grayish masses, often with a loose connection to the surrounding lung tissue. They measure from a few millimeters to several centimeters in maximum diameter. Calcification and ossification may occur. Endobronchial hamartomas are usually of polypoid shape with chondroid appearance.

Histology: Hamartomas consist of a mixture of various mature mesenchymal components such as cartilage, fat, fibrous tissue, and myxomatoid tissue. The proportions of the components vary considerably. The mesenchymal components are surrounded by an epithelial layer consisting of ciliated cells resembling bronchial epithelium. Inflammatory infiltrates are usually scarce. However, agglutinations of mononuclear cells may be seen. Mitotic figures and necroses are absent. The lesions completely destroy the basic lung parenchyma and have an indistinct boundary with the surrounding lung tissue, which may be altered by interstitial fibrosis.

➤ *Descriptors:* Newly formed structures without metastasis potential:

- myxomatoid textures
- fibromatous textures
- fragments of cartilage (mature)
- fatty tissue
- absent or infrequent mitoses
- absent necrosis
- absent inflammatory infiltrates

■ *Special stains:* PAS, collagenous stains.

Hallmark of Diagnosis: Mixture of various mature mesenchymal tissue components, lack of necrosis and (usually) mitoses.

Differential diagnosis: Metastases of teratomas into the lung, especially after cytostatic therapy, so-called benign metastasizing leiomyoma, bronchial chondroma, adenomatoid cystic malformation of the lung.

Hamazaki-Wesenberg Bodies

Definition: Intracytoplasmic inclusion bodies seen in macrophages and multinucleated giant cells, see Sarcoidosis.

Hamman-Rich Syndrome

Definition: Progressive idiopathic interstitial fibrosis, see usual interstitial pneumonia.

Hand-Schüller-Christian Disease

Definition: Alteration of the lung parenchyma caused by infiltration of histiocytes resembling Langerhans' cells, see Histiocytosis X.

Hard Metal Lung

Definition: Alteration of the lung tissue associated with inhalation of metal fumes.

Incidence/Epidemiology: Employees working in the machine-tool industry or technicians in dental laboratories may be exposed to dusts of various rare or inert metals such as hafnium, niobium, titanium, tungsten with carbon, cobalt, or nickel. A few persons have developed progressive interstitial fibrosis with fatal outcome.

Etiology/Pathophysiology: Metallic fumes can be divided into those irritative to the lung parenchyma and inert ones. Irritative are nickel, chromium, and cobalt. Inert are titanium, iron, zirconium, hafnium, niobium, tin, antimony, and barium. Irritative fumes are fibrogenic mainly by virtue of macrophage involvement and an impaired defence mechanism against infective organisms.

Clinical Presentation: Patients suffer from shortness of breath, progressive dyspnea, and chronic cough or may present with only mild radiologic changes.

Prognosis: Usually good; however, slow progressive interstitial fibrosis may occur after inhalation of irritative fumes.

Radiology: Chest radiographs may show diffuse interstitial markings or signs of honeycombing in severe cases.

Pathology:
Gross: No specific findings have been reported in patients with mild symptoms. The lungs may be grayish to black with small nodules situated subpleurally or larger cysts with bundles of fibrous tissue (honeycomb lung).

Histology: The common finding in severe cases is diffuse interstitial fibrosis around the small bronchi, bronchioles, and small arteries. Epithelial hyperplasia and dysplasia of the terminal airways may be combined with marked desquamative interstitial pneumonia. Dust-laden macrophages can be detected. The inhaled particles measure 1–2 μm in length.

➤ *Descriptors:* Lung parenchyma with preserved structure:
- macrophages (dust-laden)
- dust (birefringent fibers)
- mononuclear inflammatory infiltrates (mild);
- Lung parenchyma with altered structure:
- diffuse interstitial fibrosis (mild)

■ *Special stains:* PAS, Prussian blue, collagenous stains, immunohistochemistry for immunoglobulins, endogenous lectins, X-ray diffraction or related physical techniques.

Hallmark of Diagnosis: Clinical history, histomorphologic findings of desquamative interstitial pneumonia, peribronchial, peribronchiolar, and perivascular fibrosis, honeycomb lung, identification of dust particles.

Differential diagnosis: Idiopathic desquamative interstitial pneumonia, alterations of the lung tissue due to exposure to other agents.

Heerfordt's Syndrome

Definition: Clinical triad of facial nerve palsy, parotid enlargement, anterior uveitis, see Sarcoidosis.

Hemangioendothelioma, Epithelioid

Definition: Peculiar tumor of the lung with various degrees of malignancy.

Incidence/Epidemiology: Unusual tumor of the lung (a series of 20 cases and several single cases have been described). It occurs more frequently in women (sex ratio 1:4, men:women) at any age (4–93 years). It is probably not associated with external risk factors.

Etiology/Pathophysiology: The tumor is believed to arise from endothelial cells. Similar tumors have been reported in the liver, skin (Kimura's disease, i.e., histiocytoid hemangioma of the skin), heart, bones, and pleura. Involvement of the tumor in multiple organs has been documented in a few cases.

Clinical Presentation: The tumors are localized in the peripheral lung tissue and may cause chronic cough, shortness of breath, fever, malaise.

Prognosis: Usually good and without known sequelae.

Radiology: Chest radiographs record diffuse peripheral, sometimes bilateral nodules of various sizes with a predominance in the lower lobes.

Pathology:
Gross: Multiple, peripherally localized lesions of firm consistency measuring 1–2 cm in diameter and grayish-white and translucent.

Histology: The tumor has a specific growth texture which is characterized by polypoid tumor cell nodules in the alveoli, connected through the pores of Kohn. The medium-sized tumor cells predominantly contain a pale, densely hyalinized or fine granular cytoplasm and round nuclei with unsuspicious nucleoli. Central necrosis is commonly present, but a marked inflammatory reaction of the host tissue is usually missing. The original texture of the lung tissue is preserved. The tumor spreads into the lymphatic and venous vessels. Low-grade tumors have clearly detectable growth textures and few mitotic figures; high-grade tumors have more frequent mitoses, larger areas of necrosis, and a higher variability of nuclear features.

➤ *Descriptors:* Newly formed textures without metastasis potential:
- mesenchymal growth pattern
- vascular textures
- nests of tumor cells (connected with the pores of Kohn)
- granular cytoplasm
- small nuclei
- homogeneous nuclear and cellular size
- absent or infrequent mitoses
- necrosis
- absent inflammatory infiltrates

■ *Special stains:* PAS, Giemsa, collagenous stains, immunohistochemistry for Factor VIII, Ulex Europaeus I (UEA) lectin (α-L-fucose binding specificity), endogenous lectins.

Hallmark of Diagnosis: Clinical history, chest radiographs, microscopic tumor growth texture, positive staining to Factor VIII, electron microscopy.

Differential diagnosis: Metastatic sarcoma, (leiomyosarcoma, chondrosarcoma, osteosarcoma), sclerosing hemangioma.

Hemangioma, Cavernous

Definition: Vascular malformation (abnormally large vessels) within the lung.

Incidence/Epidemiology: Unusual disorder of early childhood either related to hereditary hemorrhagic telangiectasis (Osler-Weber-Rendu disease) or occurring as a sporadic disease.

Etiology/Pathophysiology: The lesions are abnormal arteriovenous fistulae of congenital origin.

Clinical Presentation: Depending upon the nature of the arteriovenous shunt, severe clinical symptoms may be present including cyanosis, dyspnea, polycythemia, hemoptysis, clubbing of the fingers.

Prognosis: Depends upon the shunt volume, usually good or fair.

Radiology: Chest radiographs may show circumscribed mass lesions which can be multiple.

Pathology:

Gross: Ectatic, irregularly arranged blood vessels with thin walls, usually associated with larger bronchi.

Histology: Ectatic venous vessels with unusual outer shape of the vessel and thin wall which may vary in thickness within its circumference. Nearby, similarly enlarged vessels.

➤ *Descriptors:* Newly formed textures without metastasis potential:

- mesenchymal growth pattern
- vascular textures
- clusters of venous vessels (ectatic)
- mononuclear inflammatory infiltrates (focal)
- macrophages (hemosiderin-laden)

■ *Special stains:* Collagenous stains.

Hallmark of Diagnosis: Clinical history, macroscopic findings, dilated vessels with abnormal shape and thin walls.

Differential diagnosis: Lymphangioleiomyomatosis, lymphangiectasis.

Hemangioma, Sclerosing

Definition: Benign neoplasm of the lung with a variable but characteristic histology.

Incidence/Epidemiology: Rare neoplasm most frequently seen in women (sex ratio 1:5, men:women) of any age after early childhood. External risk factors are not known.

Etiology/Pathophysiology: The nature of the lesion is not known. Most of the investigators believe that the tumors are of endothelial origin. However, others have found cells of epithelial origin (similar to type II pneumocytes), whereas still others have concluded, based on electron microscopic findings, that the tumors are of mesothelial origin.

Clinical Presentation: The most common symptom is hemoptysis. Some patients may complain of fever, anorexia, and chest pain, but the majority are without symptoms (50–70%).

Prognosis: Usually good and without known sequelae.

Radiology: Chest radiographs show sharply demarcated peripheral lesions with no or very slow growth.

Pathology:

Gross: The tumors measure from a few millimeters to a few centimeters in maximum diameter (mean 2.8 cm). They are hemorrhagic to yellowish in color, of firm consistency, and often surrounded by a fibrous capsula. They are usually subpleural and may bulge into the pleural cavity.

Histology: The tumors consist of a marked focal proliferation of small blood vessels, large blood lakes, broad areas of large mononuclear cells with pale or eosinophilic cytoplasm, and a predominant fibroepithelial papillary proliferation resembling bronchiolo-alveolar carcinoma. The small vessels have densely fibrotic walls with obliterated lumen. Calcification may occur as well as focally mature fat. Mitoses and necrotic areas are absent.

➤ *Descriptors:* Newly formed textures without metastasis potential:

- mesenchymal growth pattern
- fibromatous textures

- clusters of venous vessels (small, obliterated lumen)
- hemorrhage
- large tumor cells
- abundant cytoplasm (pale to eosinophilic)
- small nuclei
- homogeneous nuclear and cellular size
- epithelial growth pattern
- adenoid textures (papillary)
- homogeneous nuclear and cellular size
- absent or infrequent mitoses
- calcification (focal)
- absent necrosis
- absent inflammatory infiltrates

■ *Special stains:* PAS, collagenous stains, Giemsa, hyaluronic acid with digestion, immunohistochemistry for Factor VIII (negative), ulex (negative), low molecular weight cytokeratin (negative), vimentin (positive), actin (negative), EMA (positive), endogenous lectins.

Hallmark of Diagnosis: Focal areas with small hyalinized vessels, fibroepithelial papillary projections, blood lakes, solid areas with mononuclear cells.

Differential diagnosis: Inflammatory pseudotumor, adenocarcinoma, pulmonary blastoma, epithelioid hemangioendothelioma, benign sugar tumor of the lung, histiocytoma, metastatic tumors such as paraganglioma, carcinoid tumor, thyroid and renal adenocarcinoma.

Hemangiopericytoma

Definition: Low-grade (benign) or high-grade (malignant) pulmonary neoplasms arising from pericytes that lie around the smaller vessels.

Incidence/Epidemiology: Unusual tumor arising with equal frequency in both sexes with somewhat earlier onset in men (40 years) than in women (50 years). No external risk factors are known.

Etiology/Pathophysiology: The tumors derive from the pericytes that are localized around the smaller vessels.

Clinical Presentation: About half of the patients are asymptomatic. The remainder complain of hemoptysis, chest pain, dyspnea, and cough.

Prognosis: Good and without known sequelae for patients with low-grade tumors; poor for patients with high grade tumors.

Radiology: Chest radiographs show circumscribed dense masses which may occur either in peripheral lung tissue or in central regions. Calcification does not occur.

Pathology:

Gross: The tumors measure a few centimeters in diameter and are yellow-tan to gray-white. They possess characteristic vascular spaces and may be encapsulated.

Histology: The texture is characterized by "antlerlike" (empty) vascular spaces with narrow and elongated caliber. The sinusoidal spaces are surrounded by uniform spindle cells with round nuclei. Mitotic figures are rare. Round, medium-sized cells with eosinophilic cytoplasm may be intermingled. Reticulin stain may show characteristic circles of small reticulin fibers arranged around small vessels. Necrotic areas and numerous mitotic figures as well as being over 5 cm in size are features of high-grade (malignant) tumors. Inflammatory response of host tissue is usually scarce and infrequent.

➤ *Descriptors:* Newly formed textures without metastasis potential:

- mesenchymal growth pattern
- vascular texture (antlerlike spaces)
- plump spindle cells (surrounding)
- small nuclei (round)
- homogeneous nuclear and cellular size
- absent or infrequent mitoses
- weak or absent inflammatory infiltrates;
- Newly formed textures with metastasis potential:
- mesenchymal growth pattern
- vascular texture (antlerlike spaces)
- plump spindle cells (surrounding)
- inhomogeneous nuclear and cellular size
- frequent mitoses
- necrosis
- moderate or dense inflammatory infiltrates

■ *Special stains:* PAS, collagenous stains, reticulin stain, immunohistochemistry for keratin, vimentin, lysozyme, actin, desmin, desmoplakin, endogenous lectins, DNA analysis.

Hallmark of Diagnosis: Sinusoidal spaces with surrounding uniform spindle cells, texture of reticulin fibers.

Differential diagnosis: Fibroma, peripheral carcinoid, metastastic sarcoma.

Hematite Miner's Lung

Definition: Alteration of the lung tissue associated with inhalation of hematite.

Incidence/Epidemiology: Hematite or iron sesquioxide (Fe_2O_3) is mined in Belgium, Sweden, UK, and the USA. Alterations of the lung tissue (siderosilicosis) have been reported in several studies.

Etiology/Pathophysiology: Iron oxide is inert in the human lung, and large numbers of the particles can accumulate in the interstitial lung parenchyma. The additional presence of crystalline silica may result in various degrees of fibrosis, i.e., a mild diffuse, nodular, or massive fibrosis may develop. Complications are increased risk for tuberculosis, cor pulmonale, and (in West Cumberland where additionally radon gas exposure is present) lung cancer.

Clinical Presentation: Exposed persons may complain of shortness of breath on exercise, dyspnea, and chronic cough. Slow progression may occur.

Prognosis: Usually fair; however, slow progressive respiratory failure may occur. Patients with hematite exposure have increased risk of tuberculosis, chronic pulmonary infections, and lung cancer.

Radiology: Chest radiographs show mild, diffuse, interstitial markings, dense circumscribed nodules, or massive fibrosis with emphysematous changes (honeycomb lung).

Pathology:

Gross: The lungs may show a mild form of diffuse fibrosis with focal subpleural emphysema, or firm nodules of black to brick-red color measuring 5–20 mm in maximum diameter. Central necrosis may occur. Massive fibrosis is most severe in the upper lobes which are of red-brown color and show large cystic alterations (cavitation) with fibrotic nodules and strings.

Histology: The interstitial lung tissue has a large number of black dust particles which are also present in macrophages and in distant airways. Birefringent particles correspond to silicotic crystals. Whorled interstitial fibrosis can be seen in relation to the agglutinations of dust particles. Necrotic areas may be present or may indicate additional tuberculosis. Hematite does not stain with Prussian blue.

➤ *Descriptors:* Lung parenchyma with altered structure:
- dust (hematite, birefringent fibers, crystals)
- macrophages (dust-laden)
- focal interstitial fibrosis ("whorled")
- necrosis (focal)

■ *Special stains:* PAS, collagenous stains, Prussian blue (for hemosiderin deposits), polarization, X-ray diffraction methods or related physical techniques.

Hallmark of Diagnosis: Clinical history, pneumoconiosis with iron deposits and a few birefringent crystals.

Differential diagnosis: Other forms of pneumoconiosis, additional infection with tubercle bacteria.

Hemorrhage

Definition: Intrapulmonary hemorrhage due to various agents.

Incidence/Epidemiology: Common pathologic findings in autopsies and surgical specimens due to various agents such as intraoperative manipulations, trauma, collagen vascular diseases, fungal infections (*Aspergillus*, candidiasis), Goodpasture's syndrome, *Pseudomonas* pneumonia, thrombosis of the pulmonary arteries, parasites (strongyloidiasis), granulomatous diseases (Wegener's granulomatosis). In infants it is seen most frequently in idiopathic pulmonary hemosiderosis and in bronchopulmonary dysplasia.

Etiology/Pathophysiology: Disturbance of the blood/air barrier may be associated with infections, collagenous diseases, increase or decrease in blood pressure, inflammation, and destruction of the vascular walls.

Clinical Presentation: Patients may be asymptomatic or present with "bleeding" from the bronchial tree.

Prognosis: Usually fair but depends upon the underlying disease and upon the volume of affected lung parenchyma. Sequelae are bacterial superinfection and scarring.

Radiology: Chest radiographs of massive pulmonary hemorrhage show large fluffy densities usually predominant on one side. Focal pulmonary hemorrhage produces chest radiographs with circumscribed, ill-defined, peripheral densities.

Pathology:
Gross: The lungs exhibit confluent areas filled with blood. Their size may vary, and single or multiple lesions may be present.
Histology: The terminal air spaces are filled with fresh blood. The interalveolar septula are preserved. A mild inflammatory response can be seen. Older lesions contain agglutinations of hemosiderin-laden macrophages.

➤ *Descriptors:* Lung parenchyma with preserved structure:
- hemorrhage (massive)
- mononuclear inflammatory infiltrates
- macrophages (hemosiderin-laden)

■ *Special stains:* Prussian blue, collagenous stains, PAS (to exclude fungal infection), immunohistochemistry for immunoglobulins (collagenous disorders).

Hallmark of Diagnosis: Intraalveolar and partly interstitial agglutinations of blood with preserved architecture of the lung.
Differential diagnosis: Pulmonary infarction, classification of the disease due to the underlying disorder.

Hemorrhagic Fever

Definition: Alteration of the lung parenchyma seen in arbovirus and arenovirus infections presenting with hemorrhagic manifestations.
Incidence/Epidemiology: The disease is endemic in southeast Asia, especially the Philippines, Thailand, Vietnam, Cambodia, Malaysia and India (dengue hemorrhagic fever, virus types 1, 2, 3, 4), and in Argentina and Bolivia (Junin virus, Machupo virus, zoonotic hemorrhagic fever). Young children, unadapted foreigners, and persons under poor social conditions have a high risk of infection. Epidemics usually occur during or at the end of the rainy season.
Etiology/Pathophysiology: The virus is transmitted by mosquitoes (*Aedes aegypti*, Dengue fever), the vector and the reservoir of arenoviral infection are unknown.
Clinical Presentation: The symptoms are similar to those of a common cold in the beginning: fever, cough, pharyngitis, headache, anorexia, vomiting. After 3–5 days petechiae (forehead, distal extremities, dengue fever) or bleeding from the gums, hematemesis, melena (Bolivian fever), hypotension, tachycardia, and coma occur.
Prognosis: Fair. About 10–20% of patients die, usually during day 4–8.
Radiology: Chest radiographs are normal or show diffuse interstitial densities.
Pathology:
Gross: The lungs are heavy and wet and present with large areas of hemorrhage or massive edema.
Histology: The distant air spaces are filled with extravasated erythrocytes and show focal areas of necrosis. A massive pulmonary edema is usually present.

➤ *Descriptors:* Lung parenchyma with preserved structure:
- intraalveolar serous fluid
- intraalveolar fibrinoid material
- mononuclear inflammatory infiltrates
- hemorrhage;
- Lung parenchyma with altered structure:
- necrosis

■ *Special stains:* PAS, collagenous stains, immunofluorescence.

Hallmark of Diagnosis: Clinical history, hemorrhage, massive pulmonary edema, usual interstitial pneumonitis, identification of the virus.
Differential diagnosis: Pneumonia due to other infectious organisms, pulmonary edema, diffuse alveolar damage.

Hemosiderosis

Definition: Alterations of the lung parenchyma associated with increased intrapulmonary deposits of hemosiderin.
Incidence/Epidemiology: Idiopathic hemosiderosis (IPH) is a rare disease seen in young children or with a mild course in young adults (age 20 years, or sometimes age 40–60 years). The incidence in children is estimated to be 1/50 000 000 children per year; about 100 cases in adults have been documented. The sex ratio is 1:1 in children and 1:3 (men:women) in adults.
Etiology/Pathophysiology: The etiology is still unclear. Some associations with gluten-sensitive enteropathy or cow's milk hypersensitivity (Heiner's syndrome) have been reported. Goodpasture's syndrome is related to IPH but

exhibits antibodies to alveolar basement membranes, which are absent in IPH. Immunologic alterations in patients with IPH have not been identified.

Clinical Presentation: The symptoms are nonspecific and include cough, lethargy, dyspnea, and sometimes hemoptysis. Eosinophilia can be demonstrated in 10–20% of patients, elevated serum IgA in 50%. Hypochromic microcytic anemia is usually present.

Prognosis: Usually poor as most of the children die within 2–5 years after clinical diagnosis. Adults have a more favorable diagnosis with silent periods lasting for 20 years between two attacks of the disease.

Radiology: Chest radiographs are nonspecific and may show multiple diffuse densities in both lungs which may resolve after several weeks.

Pathology:

Gross: The lungs are firm in consistency and red-brown.

Histology: The distant air spaces contain blood, free hemosiderin, and agglutinations of hemosiderin-laden macrophages. The interalveolar septula are slightly thickened. The cells of the alveolar lining are hyperplastic in some areas but often unsuspicious. Diffuse fibrosis indicates a long course and the late stage of disease. Fibrin deposits, hyaline membranes, necrosis, interstitial or intraalveolar edema and dense granulocytic infiltrates are not signs of IPH.

➤ *Descriptors:* Lung parenchyma with preserved structure:

- macrophages (hemosiderin-laden)
- hyaline material (thickened interalveolar septula)
- desquamation, hypertrophy, hyperplasia and dysplasia of pneumocytes;
- Lung parenchyma with altered structure:
- diffuse interstitial fibrosis (mild)

■ *Special stains:* PAS, Prussian blue, collagenous stains, immunohistochemistry for IgA, endogenous lectins.

Hallmark of Diagnosis: Clinical history, laboratory findings, agglutinations of hemosiderin-laden macrophages within the distant air spaces with mild interstitial inflammatory infiltrates.

Differential diagnosis: Goodpasture's syndrome, Legionnaires' disease, uremic lung bleeding, lupus erythematosus, acute lupus pneumonitis, immune complex-associated "systemic vasculitis", traumatic lung lesions, mitral stenosis, aspiration of blood, side effects of drugs (anticoagulant use, etc).

Herbicides

Definition: Alteration of the lung parenchyma associated with inhalation of herbicides.

Incidence/Epidemiology: Most such accidents have been reported in persons using paraquat (spot weed and grass killer). Small amounts of inhaled aqueous solutions or of sprays may cause severe symptoms.

Etiology/Pathophysiology: The substance is assumed to mediate the formation of free (oxygenic) radicals in the lung, which are thought to be responsible for the formation of diffuse alveolar damage.

Clinical Presentation: The initial symptoms include burning in the upper respiratory tract followed by nausea, vomiting, dyspnea, and chest pain, which may develop several days later. Progression into honeycomb lung is frequent.

Prognosis: Usually poor with progression into respiratory failure after a few years.

Radiology: Chest radiographs show diffuse densities in both lungs, which may organize into small nodules and areas with increased transparency.

Pathology:

Gross: The lungs are heavy and exhibit usually greater consistency and mild interstitial fibrosis even in early stages.

Histology: The alveoli are filled with fibrin deposits, macrophages, mononuclear infiltrates, and in lesser amount, with neutrophilic and eosinophilic granulocytes. Hyaline membranes are present as well as interstitial mononuclear infiltrates, hypertrophy, hyperplasia of the cells of the alveolar lining. Marked interstitial fibrosis indicates the late stage of intoxication.

➤ *Descriptors:* Lung parenchyma with preserved structure:

- intraalveolar fibrinoid material
- hyaline membranes
- macrophages
- mononuclear inflammatory infiltrates
- desquamation, hypertrophy, hyperplasia and dysplasia of pneumocytes;

- Lung parenchyma with altered structure:
- diffuse interstitial fibrosis

■ *Special stains:* PAS, collagenous stains, immunohistochemistry for HLA-DR, endogenous lectins.

Hallmark of Diagnosis: Clinical history, diffuse alveolar damage and diffuse interstitial fibrosis in various degrees.

Differential diagnosis: Diffuse alveolar damage due to other agents, desquamative interstitial pneumonia, usual interstitial pneumonia, adenocarcinoma.

Hermansky-Pudlak Syndrome

Definition: Alteration of the lung parenchyma in the oculocutaneous albinism syndrome, see Albinism Oculocutaneus.

Herniation of the Lung

Definition: Displacement of the lung outside the thoracic cavity.

Incidence/Epidemiology: Rare disease seen in adults with severe emphysema or asthma or in infants with anencephalus (Klippel-Feil syndrome, cri du chat syndrome).

Etiology/Pathophysiology: Increased intrathoracic pressure associated with atrophic surrounding connective tissue results in displacement of the lung parenchyma into the neck, through the diaphragm, or into the intercostal spaces.

Clinical Presentation: The patient may be asymptomatic or may present with chest pain, shortness of breath, recurrent infections.

Prognosis: Usually good; sequelae are recurrent infection and chronic damage of the herniated lung parenchyma.

Radiology: Chest radiographs are usually normal.

Pathology:

Gross: Atelectatic compression of herniated lung parenchyma.

Histology: The lung parenchyma is altered by recurrent infections and atelectatic compression. Long-lasting herniation may result in fibrosis.

➤ *Descriptors:* Lung parenchyma with preserved structure:

- atelectatic distant air spaces
- macrophages
- mononuclear inflammatory infiltrates;
- Lung parenchyma with altered structure:
- enlarged distant air spaces
- focal interstitial fibrosis;
- Bronchial mucosa with altered structure:
- ectatic lumen
- ulceration
- squamous metaplasia and dysplasia

■ *Special stains:* None.

Hallmark of Diagnosis: Macroscopic findings, reports of thoracic surgery.

Differential diagnosis: Extralobular sequestration in infants, recurrent infections due to other agents.

Heroin/Morphine

Definition: Alteration of the lung parenchyma associated with intake of heroin/morphine, see Drug Toxicity.

Herpes Simplex Infection

Definition: Infection of the lung with herpex simplex virus.

Incidence/Epidemiology: The infection occurs in neonates with an approximate frequency of 3–40/100 000 births, especially among the lower socioeconomic classes. In adults herpes simplex infections are associated with immunosuppressive disorders or treatments. Both types are spread by contaminated secretions.

Etiology/Pathophysiology: HSV is only infective in man. The virus can be transmitted even by asymptomatic persons from either the oral cavity or the genital tract. It may grow in various tissues such as epithelial cells, nervous tissue, and endothelial cells. Pulmonary infection occurs most frequently by aspiration of oral secretions.

Clinical Presentation: Cutaneous vesicles or perioral ulcerations are usually the first sign followed by cough, chest pain, high fever, dyspnea, and sometimes by multisystem failure.

Prognosis: Usually good; serious sequelae are rare and include necrotic pneumonia with bacterial superinfection and chronic necrotizing bronchitis. Poor in newborns who have a mortality 40–70% if the lung is involved.

Radiology: Chest radiographs display patchy diffuse densities, areas of necrotizing pneumonia, or signs of tracheobronchitis.

Pathology:

Gross: The lungs are heavy and consolidated. Small focal areas of necrosis may be present or miliary grayish-white nodules.

Histology: Herpetic inclusion bodies are present in pneumocytes and intraalveolar macrophages. Multinucleated giant cells also contain inclusion bodies with a sharply delineated acidophilic structure surrounded by a halo. Focal necrosis, ulceration of bronchial mucosa, fibrinopurulent exudate, and formation of pseudomembranes can usually be demonstrated. Neutrophils are the predominant inflammatory cell population.

➤ *Descriptors:* Lung parenchyma with preserved structure:
- macrophages (viral inclusion bodies)
- desquamation, hypertrophy, hyperplasia and dysplasia of pneumocytes
- inclusion bodies (viral)
- multinucleated giant cells
- neutrophils (dense)
- intraalveolar fibrinoid material;
- Lung parenchyma with altered structure:
- necrosis;
- Bronchial mucosa with altered structure:
- ulceration
- necrosis (bronchial and bronchiolar walls)
- neutrophils (dense)

■ *Special stains:* PAS, Giemsa, collagenous stain, immunohistochemistry for HSV, DNA probe for HSV.

Hallmark of Diagnosis: Clinical history, necrotizing pneumonia, macrophages and multinucleated giant cells with inclusion bodies, identification of the virus.

Differential diagnosis: Other viral infections such as cytomegalovirus, varicella zoster, rubella, respiratory syncytial virus, measles virus.

Heterotopia

Definition: Ectopic tissue resembling other organs within the lung.

Incidence/Epidemiology: Rare disorder, most frequently seen in infants with additional severe malformations such as anencephaly.

Etiology/Pathophysiology: Congenital disorder thought to be related to "leftovers" of corresponding tissue in the lung during maturation and separation of organs.

Clinical Presentation: Usually no specific symptoms.

Prognosis: Good.

Radiology: Chest radiographs are usually normal.

Pathology:

Gross: Small, circumscribed, firm, grayish nodules in normal lung parenchyma, accidental findings.

Histology: Islands of striated muscle fibers (rhabdomyomatous dysplasia), tissue of the adrenal cortex or of glia within normal lung parenchyma.

➤ *Descriptors:* Lung parenchyma with altered structure:
- ectopic tissue (striated muscle cells, cells of the adrenal cortex, central nervous system)

■ *Special stains:* PAS, collagenous stains, silver methenamine.

Hallmark of Diagnosis: Identification of heterotopic tissue within the lung.

Differential diagnosis: Traumatic embolism of extrapulmonary tissue into the lung.

Hexamethonium

Definition: Alteration of the lung parenchyma associated with intake of hexamethonium, see Drug Toxicity.

Hirudiniasis

Definition: Infection of the pharynx/trachea with leeches.

Incidence/Epidemiology: Rare disorder caused by *Limnati nilotica*. The organism lives in fresh water throughout the world.

Etiology/Pathophysiology: Infection of man occurs by drinking fresh water which contains the organisms.

Clinical Presentation: The symptoms are related to infection of the air-conducting system and include cough, hemoptysis, loss of speech, and chest pain. Sometimes halzoun may exist (pain, dyspnea, headache, facial edema, hemoptysis, and vomiting).

Prognosis: Usually good with natural expectoration of the leeches.

Radiology: Chest radiographs are normal or may show peribronchiolar infiltrates.

Pathology:

Gross: Ulceration and necrosis of the trachea and the major bronchi, which are red.

Histology: Acute ulceration of the epithelial cells and fibrinopurulent exudate comprising neutrophilic and eosinophilic granulocytes, lymphocytes, plasma cells, fibrin, and debris are the common findings. The leeches are usually expectorated.

➤*Descriptors:* Bronchial mucosa with altered structure:

- leeches
- fibrinoid material
- ulceration
- mixed inflammatory infiltrates (dense)

■ *Special stains:* None.

Hallmark of Diagnosis: Clinical history, acute tracheitis and bronchitis.

Differential diagnosis: Acute tracheitis, pharyngitis, or bronchitis due to other agents.

Histiocytoma

Definition: Benign tumor of histiocytoid appearance (synonyms inflammatory pseudotumor, plasma cell granuloma, fibroxanthoma, mast cell granuloma).

Incidence/Epidemiology: Unusual tumor in young or very old adults (60% of patients were under 40 years, and a second peak is described in the elderly, 70 years old) and in children (1 year or older). About 400 cases have been described. Although no association with smoking could be demonstrated, a high percentage of patients (50%) had a history of pulmonary infections.

Etiology/Pathophysiology: The etiology of the lesion is still unclear. Most investigators consider the tumors to be reactive postinflammatory lesions. A true neoplasm or altered immune response of host tissue cannot be excluded. Similar lesions have been described in the trachea, heart, liver, pancreas, stomach, spleen, kidneys, soft tissue, and orbit.

Clinical Presentation: The majority of patients are asymptomatic. Others may suffer from chest pain, cough, or dyspnea.

Prognosis: Usually good and without serious sequelae.

Radiology: Chest radiographs usually show circumscribed, well-defined peripheral nodules, sometimes with calcification or cavitation. Pleural effusions are rare.

Pathology:

Gross: The majority of tumors measure 1–5 cm in maximum diameter and have well defined margins without true fibrous capsula. Depending upon the predominant cell type they are of firm, rubbery or soft consistency and grayish, tan, or yellow-orange. Hemorrhage, calcification, and cavitation may be seen infrequently.

Histology: The original lung texture is completely destroyed by different cell populations, and only entrapped bronchi or bronchioles may be identified. The predominant cell population are usually plump spindle cells intermingled with plasma cells. The spindle cells form cellular bundles like those usually seen in fibrous soft-tissue tumors. Russell's bodies can be identified within the plasma cells. At the tumor boundary lymphocytic cells are more frequent as well as eosinophilic and neutrophilic granulocytes. Necrotic areas are, if existent, small and usually hemorrhagic. The walls of small arteries and veins are fibrotic and occluded by the reactive proliferation of intima cells and organized thrombosis. Mitotic figures may be present but are usually rare. Within the spindle cells and the mononuclear infiltrates, cellular atypias of mild degree or scattered multinucleated giant cells may be identified.

➤*Descriptors:* Newly formed textures without metastasis potential:

- mesenchymal growth pattern
- lymphomatoid textures
- plump spindle cells
- homogeneous nuclear and cellular size
- absent or infrequent mitoses
- plasma cells (intermingled)
- multinucleated giant cells
- absent necrosis
- fibrosis (arterial and venous walls)
- mixed inflammatory infiltrates

■ *Special stains:* PAS, Giemsa, collagenous stains, immunohistochemistry for subtypes of lymphocytes, lysozyme, vimentin, desmin, desmoplakin, keratin, DNA analysis.

Hallmark of Diagnosis: Circumscribed tumor with bundles of plump spindle cells intermingled with plasma cells, lymphocytes, scattered granulocytes, a few giant cells.

Differential diagnosis: Hodgkin's disease, sclerosing hemangioma, lymphoma, fibrous histiocytoma.

Histiocytosis X

Definition: Alteration of the lung tissue caused by infiltration of histiocytes resembling Langerhans' cells. Patients with lesions entirely confined to the lung have been reported (synonym eosinophilic granuloma).

Incidence/Epidemiology: Four forms of histiocytosis X occur: (a) localized disorder in the bone; (b) disseminated chronic histiocytosis X (Hand-Schüler-Christian); (c) disseminated acute/subacute histiocytosis X (Letterer-Siwe); (d) sole involvement of the lung. Pulmonary involvement in histiocytosis X is assumed to occur in 2–5% of patients presenting with chest radiographs showing miliary nodules. Patients are usually children or young to middle-aged adults (10–40 years old) with approximately equal sex distribution. The majority of adult patients are heavy cigarette smokers.

Etiology/Pathophysiology: The etiology of histiocytosis X is unknown. Associated risk factors are cigarette smoking, exposure to external fumes (cement, lime kilns, horse serum, sawdust, bird droppings), i.e., the disease may be interpreted to represent a form of hypersensitivity pneumonitis. Elevated serum immune complexes (IgG and C3) have also been demonstrated along the interalveolar walls. In addition, C-virus like particles have been identified within the Langerhans' precursor cells (interdigitating reticulum cells of the lymph nodes). These findings suggest a close relation of histiocytosis X to mycosis fungoides and Sezary syndrome. A decreased number of histamine receptors in the the T lymphocytes suggest a suppressor T-cell deficiency. In premature infants those below 1 year of age vaccination of the mother during pregnancy or congenital rubella infection have been noted (viral etiology?). The evolution of the disease starts with a cellular phase predominantly including histiocytosis X cells and eosinophilic granulocytes followed by an aproliferative phase with fibrosis and a reduced number of histiocytosis X cells and eosinophilic granulocytes. The end stage is defined by scarring, honeycombing, or bronchiolitis obliterans with organizing pneumonia.

Clinical Presentation: The common symptoms are chronic cough, dyspnea, chest pain, fever, hemoptysis, loss of weight, or flulike illness. About 25% of patients are asymptomatic. Lung function tests show restrictive and obstructive disorders.

Prognosis: Fair, about 50% of patients remain stable or heal with minimal scarring. Others may show slow progressive respiratory failure or rapid progression with honeycombing.

Radiology: Chest radiographs vary considerably and show nodular, reticulonodular, interstitial, and cystic densities or may reflect bilateral symmetric infiltrates with circumscribed nodules measuring up to 15 mm in diameter. The majority of nodules measure less than 5 mm and present a typical stellate configuration. The lesions can be localized in the center or in the peripheral lung parenchyma. Cysts and honeycombing may occur in old lesions.

Pathology:

Gross: Depending upon the stage of the disease the macroscopic findings indicate well-circumscribed, irregularly shaped nodules of grayish-white color measuring 1–2 cm in maximum diameter, honeycombing or soft yellowish nodules measuring a few millimeters in maximum diameter. Pleural scarring and focal fibrosis may occur.

Histology: Morphologically, pulmonary histiocytosis X is a progressive disorder with corresponding changes in histologic appearance. The following stages can be distinguished: (a) cellular stage (eosinophilic granulocytes, lymphocytes, plasma cells, histiocytosis X cells, neutrophilic granulocytes); (b) proliferative stage (dense intraalveolar macrophages around the nodules, interstitial fibrosis with chronic interstitial inflammation, alveolitis with hypertrophy, hyperplasia and atypia of cells of the alveolar lining, decreasing number of histiocytosis X cells); (c) fibrotic phase (scarring, bronchiolitis obliterans, organizing pneumonitis, interstitial fibrosis with honeycombing). The lesions are usually not all of the same age, and the stages may overlap. The characteristic histiocytosis X cells are spindle shaped and have highly convoluted nuclei and poorly defined cytoplasmic borders. These medium-sized to large cells are usually accompanied by various inflammatory cells, especially eosinophilic granulocytes but also (in older lesions) predominantly lymphocytes and plasma cells. A characteristic feature of the granulomatous lesions is the "diffuse arrangement" of the boundaries with several small pedicules. This feature allows a histological diagnosis at low microscopic magnification. Older "healed" lesions show only fibrosis with corresponding honeycombing. The histiocytosis X cells contain S-100 protein antibodies and stain positively with OKT6.

➤*Descriptors:* Lung parenchyma with altered structure:

- atypical cells (spindle-shaped, histiocytosis X)
- lymphocytic granulomas
- eosinophils
- mixed inflammatory infiltrates
- macrophages
- focal interstitial fibrosis (irregularly)
- proliferating fibroblasts
- honeycombing

■ *Special stains:* PAS, Giemsa, collagenous stains, Prussian blue, immunohistochemistry for S-100 protein, OKT6, endogenous lectins, electron microscopy.

Hallmark of Diagnosis: Clinical history, identification of histiocytosis X cells, eosinophilic granulomatous infiltrates, and indistinct boundaries of the granulomatous lesions.

Differential diagnosis: Usual interstitial pneumonia, allergic extrinsic alveolitis, granulomatous infectious lesions, desquamative interstitial pneumonia, virus pneumonia, sarcoidosis, Hodgkin's disease, Wegener's granulomatosis, pulmonary hemosiderosis, pulmonary alveolar proteinosis.

Histoplasmoma

Definition: Circumscribed fungal infection of the lung, see Histoplasmosis.

Histoplasmosis

Definition: Infection of the lung with *Histoplasma capsulatum.*

Incidence/Epidemiology: The organisms live in soil and are distributed worldwide. The highest incidence of human infections has been reported from the eastern and central states of the USA. Infections occur both in immunocompetent and immunocompromised persons.

Etiology/Pathophysiology: Infection usually occurs by inhalation of the organisms, which multiply in cells of the reticuloendothelial system. They grow abundantly in macrophages and other phagocytic cells in immunocompromised patients and form epithelioid granulomas in resistant persons. Fungemia may be present and may result in metastases into the liver, kidneys, spleen, and other organs.

Clinical Presentation: A large number of infections are self-limiting disorders which may be recognized by peripheral calcified nodules. Only 5–15% of patients present with clinical symptoms such as (a) acute pulmonary infection with fever, cough, malaise, chest pain, (b) a disseminated disorder with hematogenous dissemination into various organs, occurring most frequently in immunocompromised patients (fever, chest pain, hemoptysis, headache, drowsiness, diarrhea, all of which often mimic progressive lymphoma), (c) a chronic pulmonary infection clinically indistinguishable from other chronic progressive pulmonary infections (cough, low grade fever, progressive dyspnea).

Prognosis: Usually good; however, immunocompromised patients have a high risk of fungemia.

Radiology: Old lesions show circumscribed peripheral nodules that are usually calcified. Chest radiographs of younger lesions show dense patchy infiltrations, circumscribed nodules with cavitation, fibrosis with associated emphysema, or "coin" lesions resembling carcinoma. Enlargement and calcification of the mediastinum or calcified miliary nodules may occur.

Pathology:

Gross: Circumscribed, firm or calcified, grayish-yellowish nodules measuring 0.5–3 cm in maximum diameter.

Histology: The organisms cause caseating or noncaseating epithelioid granulomas with multinucleated giant cells in immunocompetent patients and large areas of necrosis with consolidation in immunocompromised patients. The organisms are uniform yeastlike cells measuring 2–4 μm in diameter, identifiable in macrophages, giant cells, and terminal air spaces. The nuclei and a clear halo can be seen in the organisms under high magnification.

➤ *Descriptors:* Bronchial mucosa with altered structure:

- fungus (uniform yeastlike cells)
- squamous metaplasia and dysplasia
- caseous epithelioid granulomas
- eosinophils
- mononuclear inflammatory infiltrates
- multinucleated giant cells;
- Lung parenchyma with altered structure:
- caseous epithelioid granulomas
- fungus (intragranulomatous, yeastlike cells)
- eosinophils
- mononuclear inflammatory infiltrates
- multinucleated giant cells
- necrosis
- focal interstitial fibrosis
- calcification

■ *Special stains:* PAS, GMS, Grocott.

Hallmark of Diagnosis: Clinical history, granulomatous epithelioid lesions or necrotic areas with consolidation, identification of the organisms in macrophages or in necrotic areas.

Differential diagnosis: Leishmaniasis, *Histoplasma capsulatum* var. *duboisii*, toxoplasmosis, *Pneumocystis carinii*, *Cryptococcus neoformans*, *Blastomyces*.

Histoplasmosis, African

Definition: Infection of the lung with *Histoplasma capsulatum* var. *duboisii*.

Incidence/Epidemiology: African histoplasmosis is endemic in African countries between Rhodesia and the Sahara. The organisms live in the soil. As opposed to infections with *Histoplasma capsulatum*, primary pulmonary lesions are rare. The organisms manifest in the bones and skin in the majority of the reported cases.

Etiology/Pathophysiology: Infected patients may present two different clinical courses: (a) a localized infection with lymphadenopathy, ulceration of the skin, and osteolytic lesions (cranium, ribs, sternum, vertebrae, long bones); (b) a disseminated form involving the lungs, liver, spleen, and intestines.

Clinical Presentation: The symptoms of the localized form include multiple skin ulcers with subcutaneous abscess, formation of fistulae, and regional osteitis. Patients suffering from the disseminated form are fatally ill and present with high fever, cough, chest pain, and hemoptysis if the lungs are involved.

Prognosis: Poor, and involvement of the lung is usually associated with systemic infections.

Radiology: Chest radiographs show patchy infiltrates with cavitation, fibrosis and rarely calcification.

Pathology:

Gross: Usually multiple hemorrhagic-necrotic nodules with cavitation, and surrounding fibrosis.

Histology: The organisms can be demonstrated in huge multinucleated giant cells which measure 10–15 μm in diameter. They cause caseous granulomas with surrounding fibrosis. Calcification is rare. The fungus often forms characteristic attached parent-daughter cells with a larger "hour-glass" cell and a smaller "dark" daughter cell. They can be demonstrated less often in macrophages than in cases of *Histoplasma capsulatum*.

➤ *Descriptors:* Lung parenchyma with altered structure:

- caseous epithelioid granulomas
- fungus (uniform, double-cell formation)
- eosinophils
- mononuclear inflammatory infiltrates
- multinucleated giant cells
- focal interstitial fibrosis
- calcification

■ *Special stains:* PAS, GMS, Grocott's.

Hallmark of Diagnosis: Clinical history, caseous granulomas, multinucleated giant cells containing the organisms, "double-cell" formation of the organisms.

Differential diagnosis: *Histoplasma capsulatum*, leishmaniasis, toxoplasmosis, *Pneumocystis carinii*, *Cryptococcus neoformans*, *Blastomyces*.

Hodgkin's Disease

Definition: Involvement of the lung in cases of Hodgkin's disease.

Incidence/Epidemiology: Primary pulmonary Hodgkin's disease is extremely rare. However, cases of disseminated or mediastinal Hodgkin's disease not infrequently elicit pulmonary involvement. Primary Hodgkin's disease of the lung is seen more frequently in older women (40–60 years; sex ratio 1:2, men:women), than in men (25–45 years). Patients suffering from secondary pulmonary involvement of Hodgkin's disease usually have had the disease for several years.

Etiology/Pathophysiology: Hodgkin's disease is a malignant tumor developing from undifferentiated cells of the reticuloendothelial system which may occur in any organ, especially lymph nodes. Primary Hodgkin's disease of the lung is considered to develop from cells of the bronchially associated lymphatic tissue (BALT). Secondary pulmonary involvement may develop in widely disseminated cases or by extension from hilar or mediastinal lymph nodes.

Clinical Presentation: Patients with primary Hodgkin's disease present with cough, fever, loss of weight, dyspnea, chest pain, or may be asymptomatic. Patients with secondary pulmonary involvement are usually asymptomatic or may present with mild dyspnea, chest pain, or cough. Secondary pulmonary involvement usually can not be distinguished from alterations of the lung parenchyma due to previous cytostatic therapy and radiation.

Prognosis: Fair; patients with pulmonary Hodgkin's disease still have a median survival of 2–5 years.

Radiology: Chest radiographs usually show solid, circumscribed, single or multiple nodules (primary Hodgkin's disease) or diffuse reticular or reticulonodular infiltrates (secondary Hodgkin's disease).

Pathology:

Gross: The lungs reveal single or multiple firm nodules with indistinct boundaries of grayish-white color or diffuse grayish-white infiltrates of increased consistency.

Histology: Hodgkin's and Reed-Sternberg cells are usually easy to identify in pulmonary involvement of Hodgkin's disease, as are atypical histiocytes. The texture of the basic lung parenchyma is completely destroyed, and eosinophilic granulocytes are often present. About half of the cases can be classified as a nodular sclerosing type, and the remainder as mixed cellular type. In our experience, the lymphocytic type is less frequent. Involvement of hilar lymph nodes is present in the majority of cases of secondary pulmonary involvement, but not in all.

➤ *Descriptors:* Newly formed textures with metastasis potential:

- mesenchymal growth pattern
- lymphomatoid textures
- Hodgkin's cells
- multinucleated giant cells (Reed-Sternberg cells)
- histiocytes (atypical)
- eosinophils
- mononuclear inflammatory infiltrates
- infrequent mitoses
- absent necrosis
- fibrosis

■ *Special stains:* PAS, collagenous stains, Giemsa, immunohistochemistry for identification of Reed-Sternberg and Hodgkin's cells (Ki1).

Hallmark of Diagnosis: Clinical history, malignant histiocytic lymphoma with Hodgkin's and Reed-Sternberg cells.

Differential diagnosis: Lymphomatoid granulomatosis of the lung, alteration of the lung parenchyma due to previous cytostatic therapy/radiation.

Honeycombing of the Lung

Definition: Complete destruction of the lung by fibrosis and emphysematous alterations.

Incidence/Epidemiology: Honeycombing of the lung is an end stage of multiple disorders affecting the lung, including infectious diseases, inhaled agents such as asbestos, idiopathic fibrosis, sarcoidosis, drug reactions, congenital disorders such as cystic fibrosis, etc. It may affect one or several lobes in one or both lungs. It occurs more frequent in men than women and is usually seen in aged patients.

Etiology/Pathophysiology: The lung is exposed to various agents and infective organisms during human life. It is also a complicated organ with permeable texture allowing gas exchange between two different liquid systems and a gas phase. Steady movement increases the risk of local disturbance of normal textures. Focal areas of abnormal function caused by various agents may result in focal fibrosis and alteration of the lung texture, with increased volume of airways and obliterated capillaries. Additional damage increases volume and number of such areas, leading to functionally dead parts which may grow in size by additional damage such as infections or infarctions. Independent of the primary damage the end stage of the lung parenchyma alteration results in complete loss of function and of healthy, normal texture that is, so-called honeycombing.

Clinical Presentation: Symptoms include dyspnea, chest pain, recurrent infections, loss of gas exchange.

Prognosis: Fair or poor, depending upon the volume of destroyed lung parenchyma. Progression is usually caused by recurrent bacterial infections which spread into healthy parts of the lung.

Radiology: Chest radiographs show abnormal densities close to areas with increased transparency, enlarged hilar lymph nodes, diffuse interstitial infiltrates, and enlarged terminal air spaces.

Pathology:

Gross: Large emphysematous cysts are clustered with firm, fibrotic nodules or strings, enlarged bronchi usually filled with purulent or viscous mucus.

Histology: Normal distant air spaces are rare and are replaced by enlarged cystic emphysematous bubbles surrounded by fibrotic nodules or strings. The connective tissue may contain mononuclear infiltrates indicating an active disorder. The cells of the alveolar lining are replaced by ciliated bronchial epithelial cells or metaplastic squamous epithelial cells. The lumina of smaller blood vessels are occluded by old thrombotic lesions, and the walls may be thickened and hyalinized. Bronchiectasis and mucus plaques are usually present.

➤ *Descriptors:* Lung parenchyma with altered structure:

- enlarged distant air spaces (cystic)
- focal interstitial fibrosis
- diffuse interstitial fibrosis
- mononuclear inflammatory infiltrates
- desquamation, hypertrophy, hyperplasia and dysplasia of pneumocytes;
- Pulmonary vessels with altered structure:
- hyaline material
- increased number of smooth muscle cells
- thrombosis (organized, occlusive);
- Bronchial mucosa with altered structure:
- ectatic lumen (cystic)
- squamous metaplasia and dysplasia
- mononuclear inflammatory infiltrates

■ *Special stains:* PAS, collagenous stains, Giemsa.

Hallmark of Diagnosis: Complete disturbance of the lung texture with increased fibrous tissue and enlarged terminal air spaces.

Differential diagnosis: Due to underlying cause of the disorder.

Horseshoe Lung

Definition: Congenital abnormality of both lungs with fusion of the right and left lungs behind the heart.

Incidence/Epidemiology: Rare congenital disease observed with equal frequency in boys and girls.

Etiology/Pathophysiology: The maldevelopment of the lungs is usually associated with additional abnormalities of arterial supply and venous drainage of the lungs, suggesting an early onset during development of the lung parenchyma (6–12 weeks of gestation).

Clinical Presentation: Patients may be asymptomatic or may show increased rates of recurrent infections.

Prognosis: Usually good; however, recurrent infection may spread to noninvolved healthy parts of the lung.

Radiology: The chest radiographs may be normal or may reflect anomalous arterial or venous supply, sometimes suggesting a scimitar syndrome.

Pathology:

Gross: Fusion of the right and left lungs behind the heart.

Histology: No specific findings have been reported.

➤ *Descriptors:* Lung parenchyma with preserved structure:

- no morphological abnormalities

■ *Special stains:* None.

Hallmark of Diagnosis: Macroscopic findings, sometimes associated with abnormalities in arterial supply or venous drainage.

Differential diagnosis: Intralobular sequestration, scimitar syndrome.

Hughes-Stovin Syndrome

Definition: Symptom complex comprised of aneurysms of the pulmonary arteries, recurrent thrombophlebitis, increased intracranial pressure.

Incidence/Epidemiology: Rare disease occurring in younger adults (20–40 years old).

Etiology/Pathophysiology: The etiology is not known. The clinical and histopathological findings are similar to those seen in patients suffering from Behçet's disease (oral aphthous ulcers, genital ulcerations, relapsing iritis, thrombophlebitis migrans, arthritis, erythema nodosum).

Clinical Presentation: Patients suffer from recurrent pulmonary infarctions, hemoptysis, dyspnea, and chest pain.

Prognosis: Chronic progression of the pulmonary involvement is the natural course.

Radiology: Chest radiographs show diffuse interstitial densities with peripherally circumscribed nodules.

Pathology:

Gross: The lungs exhibit several smaller hemorrhagic lesions of various ages.

Histology: The walls of the small arteries and veins are infiltrated by lymphocytes and plasma cells, leading to complete destruction of the arterial and venous walls (necrotizing angiitis). Fresh and partly organized hemorrhagic infarctions are associated with the angiitic lesions as well as perivascular fibrosis. The larger arteries and veins evolve aneurysms covered by thrombotic adhesions.

➤ *Descriptors:* Lung parenchyma with altered structure:

- necrosis and hemorrhage
- focal interstitial fibrosis (perivascular);
- Pulmonary vessels with altered structure:
- mononuclear inflammatory infiltrates (vascular walls)
- thrombosis (small arteries and veins)
- ectatic lumen
- necrosis

■ *Special stains:* Collagenous stains, Giemsa, endogenous lectins.

Hallmark of Diagnosis: Clinical history, necrotizing angiitis, pulmonary infarctions, arterial and venous aneurysms.

Differential diagnosis: Behçet's disease, periarteritis nodosa, hypersensitivity vasculitis, angiocentric large cell lymphoma, benign lymphocytic angiitis and granulomatosis, Wegener's granulomatosis, Churg-Strauss syndrome.

Hyaline Membrane Disease

Definition: Specific morphologic findings in premature infants with idiopathic respiratory distress syndrome.

Incidence/Epidemiology: Infrequent disease seen in stillborn or premature infants dying as early as 3–4 h after birth. Infants surviving for more than 2–4 days will usually develop the morphological changes classified as bronchopulmonary dysplasia.

Etiology/Pathophysiology: Hyaline membranes are a mixture of degenerating cells, fibrin and serum protein deposits covering the surface of the distant airways. Immaturity (deficiency of pulmonary surfactant) or damage of the cells of the alveolar lining causes disturbance of the blood/air barrier and exudation of fibrin and serum proteins associated with cellular death.

Clinical Presentation: The infants present with tachypnea, hypoxemia, and intercostal retractions.

Prognosis: Fair; infants with "uncomplicated hyaline membrane disease" (not requiring high oxygen tension) usually survive without serious sequelae. Those with "complicated hyaline membrane disease" develop bronchopulmonary dysplasia if they survive for more than 3–4 days.

Radiology: Chest radiographs show the ground-glass appearance of the lungs associated with diffusely scattered reticulogranular densities.

Pathology:

Gross: Heavy, atelectatic lungs of firm consistency resembling liver more than lung parenchyma.

Histology: The distant airways are atelectatic, containing some ectatic and dilated bronchioles and smaller bronchi. The surface of the alveoli is covered by a pink hyaline membrane which undergoes resorption and organization by macrophages, histiocytes, and regenerating cells of the alveolar lining after a couple of days. The hyaline membranes may be infected by bacteria such as streptococci, *Escherichia coli*, pneumococci.

➤ *Descriptors:* Lung parenchyma with preserved structure:
- hyaline membranes
- macrophages
- mononuclear inflammatory infiltrates
- atelectatic distant air spaces;
- Bronchial mucosa with preserved structure:
- ectatic lumen (bronchioles and small bronchi)

■ *Special stains:* PAS, Gram's stain, GMS.

Hallmark of Diagnosis: Clinical history, presence of hyaline membranes covering the alveolar surface.

Differential diagnosis: Bronchopulmonary dysplasia, bacterial infection.

Hyalinosis Cutis et Mucosae

Definition: Congenital (recessive) storage disease with abnormal storage of lipoproteins (PAS-positive) in the cutis and mucosa, see Urbach-Wiethe Syndrome, Alveolar Proteinosis.

Hydatid Disease

Definition: Infection of the lung with hydatid parasites (*Echinococcus*), see Echinococcosis.

Hydralazine

Definition: Alteration of the lung parenchyma associated with intake of hydralazine, see Drug Toxicity.

Hydrochlorothiazide

Definition: Alteration of the lung parenchyma associated with intake of hydrochlorothiazide, see Drug Toxicity.

Hypaque

Definition: Alteration of the lung parenchyma associated with intake of hypaque, see Drug Toxicity.

Hyperlucent Lung

Definition: Increased transparency of the lung parenchyma on chest X-radiographs, see Adenovirus Infection, Respiratory Syncytial Virus Infection.

Hypernephroma, Metastatic

Definition: Metastasis of hypernephroid carcinoma into the lung.
Incidence/Epidemiology: Hypernephroid carcinomas frequently metastasize into the lung. About 20–40% of cases develop metastatic lesions in the lung prior to detection of the kidney tumor. Metastasis into the lung may occur several years after curative resection of the kidney tumor (5–25 years). Men and women are equally involved.
Etiology/Pathophysiology: Metastasis of renal tumors into the lung parenchyma may occur via the lymphatic or the venous vessels without passing through the liver. Growth conditions of kidney tumors in the lung parenchyma are equivalent to those in renal tissue, allowing a slow but continuous development of hypernephroid carcinomas.
Clinical Presentation: The majority of patients present with hilar masses, chronic cough, and dyspnea. The symptoms may be confused with signs of sarcoidosis.
Prognosis: Poor, as most of the patients die within 2 years after clinical manifestation of metastases.
Radiology: Chest radiographs show hilar or bihilar masses suggesting sarcoidosis in the majority of patients. Other findings include pe-

ripherally circumscribed densities, subpleural nodules, or multiple reticular lesions.

Pathology:

Gross: The metastases are grayish-yellow and usually seen in the hilar lymph nodes with invasion of the adjacent bronchi, simulating primary bronchial carcinoma. Focal areas of hemorrhagic necrosis are present.

Histology: The tumors are composed of large "clear" cells with abundant cytoplasm and small nuclei located at the cellular periphery. Mitoses are rare, and an adenoid growth pattern can be recognized in some areas, usually at the tumor boundary. The tumors usually grow without destruction of the interalveolar septula and show – if at all – only a weak inflammatory response of the host tissue. Necrotic areas are small; however, they can be recognized by the naked eye. The PAS stain is negative or only weakly positive.

➤ *Descriptors:* Newly formed textures with metastasis potential:
- epithelial growth pattern
- adenoid textures
- solid textures
- large tumor cells ("clear")
- homogeneous nuclear and cellular size
- small nuclei (round)
- infrequent mitoses
- micrometastases
- necrosis
- absent or weak inflammatory infiltrates

■ *Special stains:* PAS, Giemsa, immunohistochemistry for renal-specific antibodies, DNA analysis.

Hallmark of Diagnosis: Clinical history, "clear cell" carcinoma with adenoid growth pattern.

Differential diagnosis: Clear-cell carcinoma of the lung, large cell anaplastic carcinoma, benign sugar tumor.

Hypersensitivity Pneumonitis

Definition: Alteration of the lung parenchyma associated with extrinsic antigens, see Allergic (Extrinsic) Alveolitis.

Hypertension, Pulmonary

Definition: Increase of systolic arterial intrapulmonary pressure to 30 mm Hg or more.

Incidence/Epidemiology: Pulmonary hypertension is not infrequently seen in patients suffering from a variety of diseases such as pretricuspid shunts, posttricuspid shunts, mitral (rheumatic) stenosis, chronic hypoxemia (caused by chronic bronchitis, emphysema, kyphoscoliosis, pickwickian syndrome), pulmonary fibrosis, recurrent pulmonary embolisms, liver cirrhosis, congenital malformations, parasites (*Schistosoma*), idiopathic pulmonary hypertension.

Etiology/Pathophysiology: Increased intravascular pressure, it is believed, stimulates the growth of smooth muscle fibers, leading to medial hypertrophy. The size and the number of smooth muscle cells in the media is increased. These changes are followed by changes of the intima, usually cellular (smooth muscle cell) proliferation. These changes induce a deposition of collagen and elastic fibers (intima fibrosis) with consecutive narrowing of the lumen of the vessels. However, other vessels may become dilated with veinlike branches and large variation in the thickness of the walls (angiomatoid lesions). The most advanced stage is the hyalinization of smooth muscle fibers (fibrinoid necrosis), which may be associated with organized recanalized thromboemboli. Increased pulmonary pressure usually leads to atherosclerotic lesions in the larger arteries. Pulmonary hypertension can be induced by pyrrolizidine alkaloids in animal experiments. The development of morphological changes in the pulmonary vessels only takes a few weeks.

Clinical Presentation: Symptoms include chest pain, hypoxemia, shortness of breath on exercise.

Prognosis: Depending upon the cause, patients with idiopathic pulmonary hypertension usually present with progression leading to death within 2 years. Patients with mechanically induced pulmonary hypertension present with a prolonged clinical course which may become stable, whereas drug abusers usually show slow progressive respiratory failure.

Radiology: Chest radiographs reveal increased size of the right heart and diffuse interstitial densities or reticulonodular patterns.

Pathology:

Gross: The large pulmonary arteries may be ectatic and may show intima plaques, increased size of walls, and thrombotic adhesions. The peripheral lung parenchyma has increased consistency and reticular-fibrotic areas.

Histology: The earliest changes of the walls of small arteries can be detected by morphometric measurement of the thickness of the media and intima by the formula $m = (m_1+m_2)/2d_1$ and $i = (i_1+i_2)/2d_2$, where m_1, m_2 are the thickness of the media on both sides of a transverse section of the vessel, and i_1, i_2 are the corresponding thickness of the intima, and d_1, d_2 are the inner and outer diameters of the vessel. Medial hyperplasia is present if m or i exceeds 7% of the corresponding diameter. The histomorphologic changes can be classified and graded as follows:

(a) increase of smooth muscle cells in the media (width > 7%);

(b) increase of width of the intima with cellular proliferation;

(c) concentric laminar proliferation of smooth muscle cells and obliteration of the lumen;

(d) formation of plexiform lesions with dilatation and focal thickening of the arterial walls (occluded small vessels associated with ectatic small vessels);

(e) focal rupture of ectatic small vessels associated with hemorrhage and hemosiderin-laden macrophages, perifocal fibrosis;

(f) fibrinoid necrosis, either with invasion of neutrophilic granulocytes, lymphocytes, and plasma cells or with hyalinized areas containing fragments of the elastic laminas.

➤ *Descriptors:* Lung parenchyma with altered structure:
- focal interstitial fibrosis (perivascular)
- necrosis and hemorrhage
- macrophages (hemosiderin-laden);
- Pulmonary vessels with altered structure:
- fibrosis (intimal, patchy eccentric, arteries)
- proliferating smooth muscle cells (small arteries)
- stenosis (small and medium-sized arteries)
- thrombosis
- fibrinoid material
- necrosis
- mixed inflammatory infiltrates
- ectatic lumen (large pulmonary arteries)

■ *Special stains:* Collagenous stains, Prussian blue, morphometry.

Hallmark of Diagnosis: Thickening of the arterial walls, vascular thrombosis, clinical history.

Differential diagnosis: Angiitis, atherosclerosis, thrombosis, pulmonary hemosiderosis, pulmonary hypertension due to the underlying disorder.

Hypervitaminosis D

Definition: Alteration of the lung parenchyma associated with hypervitaminosis D.

Incidence/Epidemiology: Unusual disease reported to occur after intake of dietary vitamin D (calciferol).

Etiology/Pathophysiology: Excessive intake of vitamin D causes an increase of serum calcium and phosphorus associated with resorption by osteoclasts. Calcium phosphate will deposit in areas of alkaline pH.

Clinical Presentation: The symptoms include shortness of breath, chest pain, and disorders of the kidneys.

Prognosis: Usually good and without progression.

Radiology: Chest radiographs show diffuse granular "stony" infiltrates.

Pathology:

Gross: The lungs are heavy and firm in consistency and feel gritty when cut.

Histology: The calcium salts form a thin layer along the basement membrane of the alveoli and bronchioles. Small clusters of salt deposits may be seen within the distant air spaces in advanced cases.

➤ *Descriptors:* Lung parenchyma with preserved structure:
- calcium deposits (salts)
- mononuclear inflammatory infiltrates (weak)

■ *Special stains:* Collagenous stains, Kossa's stain, Prussian blue, polarization, morphometry, X-ray diffraction or related physical techniques.

Hallmark of Diagnosis: Clinical history, identification of calcium salt deposits.

Differential diagnosis: Pulmonary ossification, deposits of other crystals, diffuse alveolar calcification due to other disorders.

Hypoplasia, Pulmonary

Definition: Incomplete or defective development of the lung with a reduced number of terminal air spaces.

Incidence/Epidemiology: Pulmonary hypoplasia has been reported to occur in 5–10% of autopsied stillborn or infants. It is frequently associated with additional lesions such as diaphragmatic hernia, renal agenesis, diaphragmatic hypoplasia, chromosomal abnormalities (trisomy 13, 18, 21), anencephaly, scimitar syndrome, and cardiovascular, gastrointestinal, or neuromuscular malformations.

Etiology/Pathophysiology: Several factors may induce pulmonary hypoplasia including abnormal extrapulmonary pressure prohibiting normal growth and expansion of the lung parenchyma, malnutrition due to decreased blood flow into the lung, diminished stimuli for lung parenchyma growth (abnormal fetal breathing movements), abnormalities in the proliferating mesodermal cells.

Prognosis: Usually poor, depending upon the volume of involved lung parenchyma and associated malformations.

Clinical Presentation: The infants develop a respiratory distress syndrome minutes after delivery. Artificial ventilation due to progressive hypoxemia may induce interstitial emphysema or pneumothorax.

Radiology: Chest radiographs may show additional dense masses in the hemithorax, shift of the mediastinum, diffuse densities.

Pathology:

Gross: One or both lungs are diminished in size and weight. Normal lung weight to body weight ratio is 0.022 ± 0.002.

Histology: The number of alveoli per square unit (centimeter) is diminished as well as the number of intersections of subpleural interalveolar septula. Alterations in the number of the branches of the conducting airways may occur as well as a reduction in the length of the branches. The normal architecture is preserved. An accurate technique for estimation of the hypoplasia is the measurement of the total DNA content of the lung (normal lung measures more than 100 mg/kg of body weight).

➤ *Descriptors:* Lung parenchyma with preserved structure:
- reduced number of distant air spaces;
- Bronchial mucosa with preserved structure:
- reduced number of bronchial generations
- decreased length of bronchi

■ *Special stains:* Collagenous stains, latex injection for airway branching count, DNA measurement, morphometry, measurement of size and weight of the total lung.

Hallmark of Diagnosis: Diminished size, weight, number of alveoli, number of airway branches, DNA content of the lung.

Differential diagnosis: Atelectasis, ectopic lung.

Hypothyroidism

Definition: Alterations of the lung parenchyma associated with hypothyroidism.

Incidence/Epidemiology: Unusual disorder of the lung parenchyma seen in only 10–20% of untreated patients with hypothyroidism.

Etiology/Pathophysiology: Hypothyroidism may induce the deposition of mucoproteins attached to basement membranes (myxedema).

Clinical Presentation: Patients may present with chronic cough, shortness of breath and dyspnea, indicating pulmonary manifestation of the myxedema.

Prognosis: Usually good and without serious sequelae.

Radiology: Chest radiographs may show diffuse patchy densities in both lungs.

Pathology:

Gross: The lungs are heavy with an increased consistency.

Histology: Deposits of pale hyaline layers along the basement membranes of the small vessels and the alveolar septula can be seen. Inflammatory infiltrates, hypertrophy, hyperplasia of cells of the alveolar lining, alteration of the lung texture, and interstitial fibrosis are missing or rare.

➤ *Descriptors:* Lung parenchyma with preserved structure:
- hyaline material (along the basement membranes)
- hyaline membranes

- *Special stains:* PAS, Congo, collagenous stains, GMS, endogenous lectins.

Hallmark of Diagnosis: Clinical history, hyaline deposits in the interalveolar septula and around the smaller vessels.

Differential diagnosis: Amyloidosis, interstitial fibrosis, hyaline necrosis in pulmonary hypertension.

Hypoxemic Pulmonary Hypertension

Definition: Alteration of the lung parenchyma associated with chronic hypoxemia.

Incidence/Epidemiology: The morphological changes in the walls of the pulmonary vessels of patients with chronic hypoxemia occur frequently independently of the underlying disorder. The causes of chronic hypoxemia include congenital disorders and enlarged tonsils in children and chronic obstructive diseases, interstitial fibrosis, high altitudes, pickwickian syndrome, kyphoscoliosis, and muscular disorders (atrophy of the thoracic muscles) in adults.

Etiology/Pathophysiology: Alveolar hypoxemia induces vasoconstriction and consequent increased intraarterial pressure with hypertrophy of the right heart.

Clinical Presentation: Patients may be asymptomatic or present with chest pain, shortness of breath on exercise, or dyspnea in severe cases.

Prognosis: Usually good; however, slow progression of the disease can occur.

Radiology: Chest radiographs show an enlarged right heart and occasionally diffuse patchy densities.

Pathology:

Gross: The large pulmonary vessels are usually normal. Slight interstitial fibrosis (perivascular) may be seen.

Histology: The small arteries (below 100 μm in diameter) show thickened media with hyperplasia of the smooth muscle cells and muscularization of small (usually nonmuscularized) branches. The intima is usually normal or only mildly altered. Mild perivascular fibrosis is a common finding. Inflammatory infiltrates and severe vascular changes are not a feature of chronic hypoxemia.

➤ *Descriptors:* Lung parenchyma with altered structure:
  - focal interstitial fibrosis (mild, perivascular);
  - Pulmonary vessels with altered structure:
  - fibrosis (intimal, small arteries)
  - proliferating smooth muscle cells (small arteries)

- *Special stains:* Collagenous stains, reticulin stain.

Hallmark of Diagnosis: Clinical history, mild hypertrophic changes of small arteries and muscularization of the media of small arterial branches, normal appearance of larger arteries.

Differential diagnosis: Pulmonary hypertension due to other agents, normal lung.

Ibuprofen

Definition: Alteration of the lung parenchyma associated with intake of ibuprofen, see Drug Toxicity.

Idiopathic Interstitial Fibrosis

Definition: Nonspecific reaction of lung tissue with a predominantly inflammatory process due to unknown cause (synonyms idiopathic fibrosing alveolitis, usual interstitial pneumonia, diffuse interstitial pulmonary fibrosis, Hamman-Rich syndrome, cryptogenic fibrosing alveolitis).

Incidence/Epidemiology: The prevalence of idiopathic interstitial fibrosis has been estimated to be 5–10/100 000 in Western countries. It is most frequently seen in middle-aged men and women. Cigarette smoking is suggested to be an important risk factor. Other patients suffer from collagen vascular diseases such as Sjögren's syndrome, scleroderma, mixed connective tissue disease, systemic lupus erythematosus (SLE), rheumatoid arthritis, polymyositis-dermatomyositis.

Etiology/Pathophysiology: The etiology of the disease is not known. Several factors have been associated such as cigarette smoking, hepatitis B, liver cirrhosis, genetic disorders (high risk in certain families), virus infection (Epstein-Barr virus antigens), drugs (bleomycin). The pathogenesis includes a chronic form following acute onset caused by shock, oxygen toxicity, radiation, infection (acute respiratory distress syndrome) and a chronic onset without recognizable cause. Immunopathogenesis is characterized by increased infiltrations of inflammatory cells (neutrophils, lymphocytes, macrophages) and their interaction. Pulmonary macrophages originating in the bone marrow release a chemotactic factor responsible for migration of neutrophils into the lung, a second factor that stimulates the production of granulocytes and monocytes in the bone marrow, a third factor, fibronectin, that attracts fibroblasts and stimulates their invasion into the collagenous matrix, and a fourth factor that stimulates the growth of fetal fibroblasts in tissue cultures (alveolar macrophage growth factor). The alveolar macrophage growth factor is not produced by macrophages in healthy persons. Its release is associated with the presence of activated T lymphocytes; however, the ratio of helper/suppressor cells in fibrotic lungs is normal. In addition, the release of lymphokines has been suggested to be responsible for the proliferation of fibroblasts, inducing the deposits of collagen fibers.

Clinical Presentation: Symptoms include progressive dyspnea, clubbing of the digits, fatigue, loss of weight and arthralgias. Pulmonary function tests indicate decrease of total lung volume, diffusion capacity, forced vital capacity, and residual volume.

Prognosis: Poor with progressive repiratory failure; the median survival time is approximately 4–5 years. Only 20% of patients show response to therapy.

Radiology: Chest radiographs usually show bilateral diffuse densities with increased involvement in the lower lobes and sparing of the apices. Diffuse alveolar infiltrates, patchy densities mimicking atelectasis, or reticulonodular patterns are also observed.

Pathology:

Gross: The pleural surface is of granular appearance and dull finish, the weight of the lungs is increased, and the size of the terminal airways is enlarged and grayish-white fibrotic tissue is intermingled.

Histology: The histologic findings depend upon the degree of the disease. Early lesions show acute, diffuse alveolar damage with desquamated pneumocytes, fibrin exudates, lymphocytes and plasma cells in the interalveolar septula, hypertrophy, hyperplasia and dysplasia of the cells of the alveolar lining. More advanced stages show disorganization of the lung architecture and fibrotic and widened interalveolar septula, sometimes containing smooth muscle cells. Fibrin deposits contain fibroblasts and histiocytes. The walls of small arteries and veins are thickened and show some degree of muscular hypertrophy and intimal fibrosis.

➤ *Descriptors:* Lung parenchyma with preserved structure:
- degeneration of pneumocytes
- desquamation, hypertrophy, hyperplasia and dysplasia of pneumocytes
- intraalveolar fibrinoid material
- mononuclear inflammatory infiltrates;
- Lung parenchyma with altered structure:
- enlarged distant air spaces
- proliferating fibroblasts
- diffuse interstitial fibrosis;
- Pulmonary vessels with altered structure:
- fibrosis (intimal, small arteries)
- proliferating smooth muscle cells (small arteries)

■ *Special stains:* PAS, collagenous stains, immunohistochemistry for immunoglobulins, HLA-DR, desmin, vimentin, desmoplakin, lymphocytic subpopulations, endogenous lectins.

Hallmark of Diagnosis: Clinical history, distortion of normal lung texture, fibrin deposits, interstitial mononuclear infiltrates, hypertrophy, hyperplasia and dysplasia of pneumocytes, fibrosis.

Differential diagnosis: Allergic extrinsic alveolitis, histiocytosis X, postobstructive pneumonitis, organizing pneumonia, AIDS, sarcoidosis.

Illite Fibers

Definition: Alteration of the lung parenchyma associated with inhalation of illite fibers.

Incidence/Epidemiology: Illite fibers are a component of wollastonite which is a fire-resistant nonasbestos insulating mineral mined in Austria, Finland, Mexico and USA. The quartz content range is 2–5%.

Etiology/Pathophysiology: Animal experiments have proven that illite fibers can induce pleural mesothelioma in rats. However, in man exact data about the pathogenicity are not available. The amount of quartz in the mineral may be of importance.

Clinical Presentation: Exposed people exhibit an increased prevalence of chronic bronchitis.

Prognosis: Usually good; however, exact data about increased risk of interstitial fibrosis, mesothelioma, and lung cancer are not known.

Radiology: Chest radiographs show increased interstitial markings, pleural thickening, and calcification.

Pathology:

Gross: No spe(ific findings are known.

Histology: The inhaled fibers measure 0.2–0.3 μm in length and can only just be detected by light microscopy. Details on microscopic findings have not been reported.

➤ *Descriptors:* Lung parenchyma with preserved structure:

- dust (fibers)
- macrophages (dust-laden);
- Lung parenchyma with altered structure:
- diffuse interstitial fibrosis (mild)

■ *Special stains:* Electron microscopy, scanning electron microscopy, X-ray diffraction or related physical techniques.

Hallmark of Diagnosis: Clinical history, findings of chest radiographs, identification of illite fibers.

Differential diagnosis: Alterations of the lung parenchyma due to other inhaled agents, especially other nonasbestos fibers.

Imipramine

Definition: Alteration of the lung parenchyma associated with intake of imipramine (tricyclic antidepressant), see Drug Toxicity.

Immotile Cilia Syndrome

Definition: Hereditary abnormalities of the ciliated epithelial cells of the bronchial mucosa. Subclassification of the disease is possible according to the defects of the dynein arms (electron microscopy).

Incidence/Epidemiology: Rare disease occurring in equal proportions in men and women.

Etiology/Pathophysiology: A variety of abnormalities in the axonemes of the ciliated cells are known. The absence of both dynein arms is most common, followed by the absence of the inner or outer arms or by supernumerary microtubules. The patients may present, in addition, with an incomplete situs inversus, dextrocardia, bronchiectasis (Kartagener's triad); men are usually sterile. The absence of abnormal movements of the cilia of the bronchial mucosa induces recurrent sinobronchial infections and bronchopneumonias.

Clinical Presentation: The patients present with recurrent bronchopulmonary infections, otitis media, and nasal polyps starting in early childhood. About 50% have situs inversus or dextrocardia. Bronchiectases develop in later life.

Prognosis: Fair; recurrent infections induce chronic bronchitis and bronchiectasis after 10–30 years.

Radiology: Chest radiographs show diffuse interstitial infiltrates, peribronchiolar densities, and saccular or cylindrical bronchiectases.

Pathology:

Gross: No specific findings have been reported except for postinfectious lung parenchyma alterations such as scarring or saccular and cylindrical bronchiectases.

Histology: The usual tissue processing yields no specific findings. However, wet mounts of live bronchial mucosa cells maintained at 37° C display no or uncoordinated beats of the cilia. Electron microscopy is necessary to examine the microtubules in the ciliated cells.

➤ *Descriptors:* Bronchial mucosa with preserved structure:

- mononuclear inflammatory cells
- noncoordinated beats of cilia

■ *Special stains:* Wet mounts at 37° C, electron microscopy.

Hallmark of Diagnosis: Clinical history, chronic bronchitis, bronchiectasis, demonstration of abnormalities (dyskinesia) of ciliated bronchial epithelial cells.

Differential diagnosis: Chronic bacterial infections of the lower respiratory tract due to other causes.

Immunodeficiency

Definition: Alteration of the lung parenchyma associated with immunodeficiency (acquired immunodeficiency syndrome), see Acquired Immunodeficiency Syndrome (AIDS).

Impaction, Mucoid

Definition: Bronchiectasis and impaction of the major (second to fourth order) bronchi with viscous mucus.

Incidence/Epidemiology: Not infrequently seen in older persons who may suffer from asthmoid bronchitis, allergic bronchopulmonary aspergillosis, or chronic bronchitis. The majority of cases have been reported from UK and the USA.

Etiology/Pathophysiology: The etiology of the disease is not known. The mucous impactions induce bronchiectasis. The mucus may be infected by *Aspergillus* or retention of small amounts of mucus may cause allergic bronchopulmonary aspergillosis with consequent bronchiectasis and retention of mucus.

Clinical Presentation: Patients present with chronic cough and dyspnea and expectorate plugs of viscous mucus.

Prognosis: Usually good, or related to the underlying disease.

Radiology: Chest radiographs show bronchiectases and usually poststenotic atelectases.

Pathology:

Gross: The major bronchi are dilated and filled with ropey, putty-like, yellowish-brown mucus. The peripheral lung parenchyma is atelectatic or fibrotic.

Histology: The ectatic bronchi have a thin fibrotic wall with a diminished number of bronchial glands and atrophic epithelial cells. Squamous metaplasia is usually present. The lumen of the ectatic bronchi is filled with PAS-positive, whorled mucus containing degenerative eosinophils, lymphocytes, plasma cells. Fragments of fungus (*Aspergillus*) may be present. The peripheral lung parenchyma is usually fibrotic.

➤ *Descriptors:* Bronchial mucosa with preserved structure:

- atrophy
- ectatic lumen
- viscous mucus
- eosinophils
- fungus (fragments, *Aspergillus*);
- Bronchial mucosa with altered structure:
- squamous metaplasia and dysplasia;
- Lung parenchyma with altered structure:
- mononuclear inflammatory infiltrates (peribronchial)
- focal interstitial fibrosis (peribronchial)

■ *Special stains:* PAS, collagenous stains, GMS.

Hallmark of Diagnosis: Macroscopic findinngs, bronchiectasis with viscous mucus.

Differential diagnosis: Congenital bronchiectasis, immotile cilia syndrome, poststenotic bronchiectasis.

Indomethacin

Definition: Alteration of the lung parenchyma associated with intake of indomethacin, see Drug Toxicity.

Infarction, Pulmonary

Definition: Circumscribed necrosis of the lung parenchyma due to diminished arterial blood supply.

Incidence/Epidemiology: Common disorder, especially in the elderly.

Etiology/Pathophysiology: Insufficient arterial blood supply combined with increased venous pressure causes necrosis of the interstitial lung parenchyma and consequent hemorrhage and inflammatory infiltrations of neutrophils followed by lymphocytes, plasma cells, macrophages, and histiocytes. The end-stage is scarring. Acute obstruction of a lobar artery seldom induces an acute infarction due to the rapid establishment of a collateral circulation. The following disorders may cause pulmonary infarction: infection of arteries, especially aspergillosis, fusariosis, mucormycosis, pseudallescheriasis, trichosporonosis; intravascular parasites, especially nematodes; thrombembolic diseases; right heart insufficiency; atherosclerosis of the pulmonary arteries.

Clinical Presentation: Pulmonary infarctions may be asymptomatic or may cause severe chest pain and dyspnea. Acute death due to massive thromboembolism is usually not associated with massive infarction.

Prognosis: Usually good; however, bacterial superinfection can cause serious sequelae, such as abscessing pneumonia.

Radiology: Chest radiographs show subpleural, circumscribed (triangular) densities and focal pleural thickening. Pleural effusions may be present.

Pathology:

Gross: The lungs show dense, hemorrhagic, red-brown areas firm in consistency.

Histology: The interalveolar septula are necrotic. The distant air spaces are filled with blood. The texture of the lung parenchyma is preserved. Older lesions show inflammatory infiltrates with hemosiderin-laden macrophages at the boundary. Resorption of the infarction starts from the periphery. Infection with bacteria inducing purulent necrosis is not uncommon. Irregularly shaped subpleural scars may correspond to healed infarctions.

➤ *Descriptors:* Lung parenchyma with preserved structure:
- mixed inflammatory infiltrates
- macrophages (hemosiderin-laden);
- Lung parenchyma with altered structure:
- necrosis and hemorrhage
- focal interstitial fibrosis (scarring);
- Pulmonary vessels with preserved structure:
- thrombosis (pulmonary arteries)

■ *Special stains:* PAS, Collagenous stains, Prussian blue.

Hallmark of Diagnosis: Hemorrhagic necrosis with preserved lung texture.

Differential diagnosis: Pulmonary hemorrhage, idiopathic hemosiderosis, infarction due to the underlying disorder.

Infection

Definition: Alteration of the lung parenchyma associated with various infectious organisms, see Algae, Arthropods, Bacterial Infections, Fungus, Parasites, Protozoal Diseases.

Infiltrative Lung Disease

Definition: Variety of disorders with equivalent clinical (dry rales) and radiologic findings (diffuse interstitial infiltrations).

Incidence/Epidemiology: The broad spectrum of disorders includes infections (miliary tuberculosis, fungal, amebic, virus), allergic reactions, malignant neoplasms, connective tissue disorders (rheumatoid diseases, progressive systemic sclerosis), sarcoidosis, interstitial pneumonias, angiitis (Wegener's disease), pneumoconioses, congenital disorders (cystic fibrosis, pulmonary lymphangiectasis), parasites.

Etiology/Pathophysiology: A variety of agents induce similar clinical symptoms and radiological features. The details are listed under the specific headings.

Clinical Presentation: The symptoms include dyspnea, chronic cough, expectoration, loss of weight, sometimes fever, night sweats.

Prognosis: Depends upon the underlying disease.

Radiology: Chest radiographs show irregular lines, small nodules, "ground glass" nodules, patchy infiltrates, linear or irregular markings.

Pathology:

Gross: The lungs are usually heavy and wet and may have multiple, small, white nodules or large areas of necrosis. The details are listed under the particular headings.

Histology: According to the broad spectrum of disorders the light microscopic appearance varies considerably. The different components of the peripheral lung parenchyma (distant air spaces, conducting airways, arteries, veins, lymphatics) are involved with specific or nonspecific features which are listed in detail under the relevant headings.

➤ *Descriptors:* Bronchial mucosa with preserved structure:
- atrophy;
- Bronchial mucosa with altered structure:
- squamous metaplasia and dysplasia;
- Lung parenchyma with altered structure:
- caseous epithelioid granulomas
- noncaseous epithelioid granulomas
- palisading histiocytes
- mononuclear inflammatory infiltrates
- enlarged distant air spaces
- focal interstitial fibrosis
- diffuse interstitial fibrosis
- fungus
- infectious organisms (protozoans);
- Newly formed textures with metastasis potential:
- mesenchymal growth pattern
- epithelial growth pattern
- Newly formed textures without metastasis potential:

- mesenchymal growth pattern
- epithelial growth pattern

■ *Special stains:* PAS, collagenous stains, Prussian blue, see under the particular headings.

Hallmark of Diagnosis: Destruction of the lung parenchyma by inflammatory disorders or neoplasias, for details see specific headings.

Differential diagnosis: According to the underlying disease, for details see under the particular headings.

Inflammatory Pseudotumor

Definition: Benign circumscribed (postinflammatory) lesion of the lung, see Plasma Cell Tumor (synonyms histiocytoma fibrous, xanthoma fibrous, mast cell tumor solitary).

Influenzavirus Infection

Definition: Alteration of the lung parenchyma due to infection with influenzavirus.

Incidence/Epidemiology: Infection with influenzavirus has occurred in epidemics in the Western countries. Primary viral pneumonia is usually seen in elderly persons with weakened immunodefence mechanism or in infants. Infection occurs by person-to-person transmission.

Etiology/Pathophysiology: The influenzavirus belongs to the so-called group of orthomyxoviruses which contain RNA measuring 80–120 nm. The ribonucleic core of the virus can be classified by three antigens, types A, B, and C. The virus containing type A is responsible for the epidemic disease, and that with type C causes less severe infections.

Clinical Presentation: Infection is either asymptomatic or of sudden onset with shivering, headache, backache, febrile convulsions, irritation of the upper respiratory tract, and fatal outcome. Severe infection of the lower respiratory tract causes tachypnea, hypotension, dyspnea, cyanosis. Bacterial superinfection occurs in about 80% of patients.

Prognosis: Usually good; however serious sequelae and fatal outcome can occur in infants, elderly, and immunocompromised patients (approximately 10%).

Radiology: Chest radiographs show diffuse densities in both lungs, areas of consolidation, or circumscribed necrotizing nodules.

Pathology:

Gross: The lungs are heavy, wet, and red-brown. The mucosa of the conducting airways is swollen and inflammatory red in color.

Histology: The mucosa of the major bronchi show ulceration, necrosis, and dense inflammatory infiltrates. The peripheral lung parenchyma is necrotic and filled with mononuclear cells and polymorphonuclear neutrophils. Hyaline membranes are present and are apposed directly to the damaged interalveolar septula. The epithelial cells may undergo metaplastic regeneration. Mitoses can be demonstrated. Complete resolution of the infection and restitutio ad integrum may occur as well as bronchiolitis obliterans or fibrotic healing with scarring.

➤ *Descriptors:* Lung parenchyma with altered structure:

- necrosis
- mixed inflammatory infiltrates
- intrabronchiolar fibrinoid material and histiocytes
- ulceration of bronchiolar mucosa;
- Lung parenchyma with preserved structure:
- hyaline membranes
- desquamation, hypertrophy, hyperplasia and dysplasia of pneumocytes;
- Bronchial mucosa with altered structure:
- necrosis (small bronchi)
- mixed inflammatory infiltrates
- squamous metaplasia and dysplasia

■ *Special stains:* PAS, collagenous stains, isolation of the virus from bronchial washings or swabs, culture of the virus in tissue culture, embryonated eggs or monkey kidney tissue.

Hallmark of Diagnosis: Clinical history, necrotizing broncho-pneumonia, isolation of the virus.

Differential diagnosis: Bronchopneumonia due to other agents.

Inhalation of Toxic Substances

Definition: Alteration of the lung parenchyma due to inhaled toxic substances.

Incidence/Epidemiology: A variety of substances toxic to the lung are known, including oxygen, ammonia, nitrous dioxide, sulfur dioxide, gasoline, kerosene, phosgene, chlorine, cadmium, mercury, zinc, beryllium, isoproterenol, sodium cromoglycate, acetylcysterine, polymyxin B, smoke.

Etiology/Pathophysiology: Inhalation of toxic agents induces acute pulmonary edema which remains largely interstitial with minimal intraalveolar leakage. Higher concentrations induce hyaline membranes, degeneration of epithelial cells, and a subsequent proliferative phase with epithelial hypertrophy, hyperplasia and sometimes squamous metaplasia. In infants, bronchiolitis obliterans, usual interstitial pneumonia, microatelectasis, and fibrosis may occur.

Clinical Presentation: The onset of symptoms may be within minutes or hours and usually includes dyspnea, cough, malaise, hemoptysis.

Prognosis: Usually good; however, serious sequelae (bronchiolitis obliterans, usual interstitial pneumonia, honeycombing) can occur, especially in young children.

Radiology: Chest radiographs show diffuse alveolar damage and interstitial edema.

Pathology:

Gross: The lungs are heavy and wet. Areas of consolidation and bacterial superinfection may be present.

Histology: The architecture of the lung parenchyma is preserved. The interalveolar septula are thickened and display invasive mononuclear inflammatory infiltrates. Hyaline membranes, necrosis of epithelial cells, agglutinations of macrophages within the distant air spaces, and hypertrophy, hyperplasia and dysplasia of cells of the alveolar lining can be seen 24–48 h after exposure. Formation of noncaseating granulomas occurs after inhalation of beryllium fumes. Late stages involve interstitial fibrosis and honeycombing.

➤ *Descriptors:* Lung parenchyma with preserved structure:

- interstitial edema
- mononuclear inflammatory infiltrates
- hyaline membranes
- desquamation, hypertrophy, hyperplasia and dysplasia of pneumocytes
- macrophages;
- Lung parenchyma with altered structure:
- noncaseous granulomas
- intrabronchiolar fibrinoid material and histiocytes
- ulceration of bronchiolar mucosa
- focal interstitial fibrosis

■ *Special stains:* PAS, collagenous stains, X-ray diffraction or related physical techniques, endogenous lectins.

Hallmark of Diagnosis: Clinical history, acute edema, adult respiratory distress syndrome.

Differential diagnosis: Nontoxic (cardial) edema, radiation pneumonitis, allergic reaction of the lung due to drugs, usual interstitial pneumonia, pneumonitis due to obstruction, viral pneumonia.

Intrauterine Pneumonia

Definition: Primary pneumonia occurring up to 48 h after birth.

Incidence/Epidemiology: In about 25% of all neonatal and premature babies, pneumonias occur up to 48 h after birth.

Etiology/Pathophysiology: The majority of these pneumonias is induced by inhalation of infected amniotic fluid or meconium during or shortly after traversing the birth passage. Aseptic pneumonitis (lipid pneumonia) may occur due to inhalation of the fatty acids of the meconium. The infective agents include *Haemophilus influenzae, Staphylococcus aureus, Streptococcus viridans, Escherichia coli.* Advanced stages of bronchiolitis obliterans indicate the rare cases of pulmonary inflammation during the late stages of pregnancy.

Clinical Presentation: The infants present with tachypnea, cyanosis, hemoptysis.

Prognosis: Fair, depending upon the birth weight.

Radiology: Chest radiographs show dense patchy infiltrates.

Pathology:

Gross: Neonatal pneumonia is difficult to detect. The lungs may be heavy and wet.

Histology: The alveoli contain polymorphous neutrophils, inspirated amniotic fluid, necrotic interalveolar septula, and almost no fibrin.

➤ *Descriptors:* Lung parenchyma with altered structure:

- neutrophils
- intraalveolar amniotic fluid
- necrosis (interalveolar septula)

- *Special stains:* PAS, collagenous stains.

Hallmark of Diagnosis: Clinical history, polymorphous neutrophils and amniotic contents in the distant airways, necrotic interalveolar septula.

Differential diagnosis: Postdelivery pneumonia, intrauterine pneumonia due to various agents.

Iodine

Definition: Alteration of the lung parenchyma associated with intake of iodine, see Drug Toxicity.

Iodinized Oils

Definition: Alteration of the lung parenchyma associated with intake of iodinized oils (Lipiodol), see Drug Toxicity.

Iron Encrustation of Elastic Tissue

Definition: Deposits of iron in the elastic tissue of the lung, see Elastic Tissue Iron Encrustation.

Isoguanazepam

Definition: Alteration of the lung parenchyma associated with intake of isoguanazepam, see Drug Toxicity.

Isomerism Syndrome, Bronchial

Definition: Congenital malformation with bilateral right or left lung, see Congenital Abnormalities.

Isoniazid

Definition: Alteration of the lung parenchyma associated with intake of isoniazid, see Drug Toxicity.

Isoproteronol

Definition: Alteration of the lung parenchyma associated with intake of isoproteronol, see Drug Toxicity.

Isoquinazepam

Definition: Alteration of the lung parenchyma associated with intake of isoquinazepam, see Drug Toxicity.

Jaagsiekte

Definition: Alteration of the lung parenchyma in sheep due to pleuropneumonia-like organisms (PPLO).

Incidence/Epidemiology: Sheep in South Africa, Iceland, Montana (USA), Peru and Bulgaria were found to be infected by a pleuropneumonia-like organism inducing specific alterations of the lung parenchyma mimicking bronchioloalveolar carcinoma.

Etiology/Pathophysiology: The infective agent induces a transformation of cells of the alveolar lining with focal areas of proliferation.

Clinical Presentation: The animals present with progressive dyspnea with a fatal outcome.

Prognosis: The animals usually die within a year.

Radiology: Chest radiographs show multiple miliary nodules and diffuse patchy densities.

Pathology:

Gross: The lungs show multiple small, grayish-white nodules measuring a few millimeters in diameter associated with larger, diffuse, grayish-white areas firm in consistency.

Histology: The architecture of the lung is preserved. Multiple small foci of proliferating cells of the alveolar lining are seen which cluster in the distant air spaces. Inflammatory response of host tissue or invasion of the interalveolar septula is not a sign of jaagsiekte infection.

➤ *Descriptors:* Newly formed textures without metastasis potential:
  - epithelial growth pattern
  - adenoid textures
  - nests of tumor cells
  - absent or infrequent mitoses

- absent necrosis
- absent inflammatory infiltrates

■ *Special stains:* PAS, collagenous stains, Giemsa, DNA measurements.

Hallmark of Diagnosis: Proliferation of clusters of pneumocytes resembling bronchioloalveolar carcinoma.

Differential diagnosis: Bronchioloalveolar carcinoma, desquamative interstitial pneumonia.

Juvenile Cirrhosis

Definition: Alteration of the lung parenchyma associated with juvenile cirrhosis of the liver.

Incidence/Epidemiology: Infrequent involvement of the lung parenchyma has been reported in patients with chronic liver disease.

Etiology/Pathophysiology: The etiology of the disorder is unknown. The alterations of the lung parenchyma imply direct vascular connections between the pulmonary arteries and veins near the hilum, in the peripheral lung parenchyma, and attached to the pleura.

Clinical Presentation: Symptoms include dyspnea, cyanosis, and partial oxygen desaturation of arterial blood.

Prognosis: Fair, with slow progressive respiratory failure.

Radiology: The lesions are usually too small to be detected on chest radiographs.

Pathology:

Gross: The angiomas usually measure less than 1 mm in diameter.

Histology: Arteriovenous fistulae with widespread dilatation of the small pulmonary arteries and large variation in the width of the vessel walls.

➤ *Descriptors:* Lung parenchyma with altered structure:

- focal interstitial fibrosis;
- Pulmonary vessels with preserved structure:
- ectatic lumen (pulmonary arteries, small branches)
- fistula (arteriovenous)

■ *Special stains:* Collagenous stains, resin injection technique.

Hallmark of Diagnosis: Juvenile liver cirrhosis, minute angiovenous fistulae.

Differential diagnosis: Congenital angioma, capillary telangiectasis, cavernous angioma.

Kala-azar – Lymphoproliferative Diseases

Kala-azar

Definition: Alteration of the lung parenchyma associated with infection by *Leishmania donovani*. See: Leishmaniasis.

Kaolin

Definition: Alteration of the lung parenchyma associated with inhalation of hydrated aluminum silicate crystals, see also Aluminum Dust.

Incidence/Epidemiology: Persons working in mines or factories for explosives and aluminum purification are endangered.

Etiology/Pathophysiology: Interstitial fibrosis is mainly related to the amount of intermingled silica. Aluminum itself is fibrogenic in its flake type and may cause severe fibrosis.

Clinical Presentation: Characteristic symptoms are shortness of breath, dyspnea, and cough.

Prognosis: Usually good; however, progressive fibrosis can occur.

Radiology: Chest radiographs show diffuse interstitial markings and a thickened pleura.

Pathology:

Gross: Grayish-dark lungs firm in consistency. The lungs may be shrunken and present with fibrotic pleura and subpleural emphysema.

Histology: Deposits of fine gold-brown crystals with primarily peribronchiolar distribution, but alveolar proteinosis may be present in acute intoxication. Severe stages may show diffuse interstitial fibrosis and endarteritis obliterans.

➤ *Descriptors:* Lung parenchyma with preserved structure:

- dust (dark-brown particles, silica)
- intraalveolar serous fluid
- macrophages (dust-laden);
- Lung parenchyma with altered structure:
- diffuse interstitial fibrosis

■ *Special stains:* Collagenous stains, Aurine stain, X-ray diffraction or similar physical techniques for identification of aluminum.

Hallmark of Diagnosis: Clinical history, identification of aluminum deposits and silica in the lung parenchyma.

Differential diagnosis: Pneumoconiosis due to other agents, smoking, aged lung.

Kaposi's Sarcoma

Definition: Pulmonary involvement in a specific, slow-growing malignant entity.

Incidence/Epidemiology: Kaposi's sarcoma contributes to 10% of all malignant tumors in equatorial Africa. In the past it has been reported in Ashkenazi Jews and is now seen frequently in young persons suffering from acquired immunodeficiency syndrome (AIDS). Pulmonary Kaposi's sarcoma occurs in 25–75% of AIDS patients. Renal transplant patients have a 400-fold increased risk of Kaposi's sarcoma compared with the normal population.

Etiology/Pathophysiology: Three clinical forms of the malignancy have been described: (a) a nodular plaque form growing slowly and expanding in the lower extremities; (b) a more aggressive form growing in infiltrative nodules in the lower extremities; (c) a generalized form growing in multiple nodules and lymph nodes and as visceral metastases. In AIDS patients mucocutaneous manifestations of the malignancy usually precede the manifestation of pulmonary metastases.

Clinical Presentation: Patients present with fever, cough, dyspnea, episodes of respiratory compromise, and hemoptysis.

Prognosis: Poor; as most of patients with pulmonary involvement die within 2 years.

Radiology: Chest radiographs show multiple, small, circumscribed densities in the peripheral lung parenchyma and in the central parts of the lung.

Pathology:

Gross: The lungs show multiple grayish-red densities, and multiple violaceous plaques in the pleura visceralis.

Histology: The tumors are composed of spindle cells separated by slitlike vascular textures which contain red blood cells. Various amounts of mononuclear infiltrates and expanded blood and lymphatic vessels are present in the periphery of the tumor. The central parts are usually solid and show bundles of proliferating spindle cells resembling fibrosarcoma. The tumor cells may undergo erythrophagocytosis. The destruction of the interstitial lung parenchyma and of the bronchial walls is complete; inflammatory response of the host tissue is usually weak. Mitoses are rare. Early lesions contain only a small number of spindle tumor cells and can be recognized by their dilated vascular spaces and the increased number of inflammatory cells, especially lymphocytes, plasma cells, macrophages, and eosinophils.

➤ *Descriptors:* Newly formed textures with metastasis potential:
- mesenchymal growth pattern
- sarcomatous textures
- vascular textures
- plump spindle cells
- numerous capillaries
- homogeneous nuclear and cellular size
- infrequent mitoses
- mononuclear inflammatory infiltrates (scattered)

■ *Special stains:* PAS, collagenous stains, Giemsa, immunohistochemistry for vimentin, desmin, desmoplakin, neuroendocrine markers, endogenous lectins, DNA analysis.

Hallmark of Diagnosis: Clinical history, preceding skin lesions, spindle tumor cells with slitlike vascular spaces intermingled with abundant erythrocytes.

Differential diagnosis: Fibrosarcoma, inflammatory granulation, bronchiolitis obliterans, tuberous sclerosis, lymphangioleiomyomatosis, interstitial fibrosis.

Kartagener's Syndrome

Definition: Congenital disorder producing situs inversus, chronic sinusitis, and bronchiectasis, associated with a defect of the dynein arm of the cilia in nasal and bronchial epithelial cells.

Incidence/Epidemiology: Uncommon disorder with familial risk.

Etiology/Pathophysiology: The congenital abnormality of the dynein arms of ciliated cells induces dysmotility or immotility of ciliary beats. The failure of airways clearance causes recurrent infections of the upper and lower respiratory tract. Bronchiectases are frequently observed. The dynein arms are formed by ATPase-rich proteins and are attached to one central and nine peripheral doublets of microtubules. The microtubules are the main part of the cilium.

Clinical Presentation: Symptoms are related to recurrent bacterial infections of the upper and lower respiratory tract and include chronic cough, expectoration, and fever.

Prognosis: Usually good; recurrent chronic infections induce chronic bronchitis and bronchiectasis after 10–30 years.

Radiology: Chest radiographs show diffuse patchy densities and bronchiectasis.

Pathology:

Gross: The bronchi are ectatic. Severe peribronchial fibrosis is usually present.

Histology: The mucosa of the conducting airways is hyperplastic, while the submucosa shows fibrosis and rarification of submucosal glands. The surrounding lung parenchyma exhibits fibrotic changes that may reach the degree of honeycombing. The abnormal functioning of the cilia can be analyzed in wet slides using living tissue (mounted at 37° C).

➤ *Descriptors:* Bronchial mucosa with preserved structure:
- noncoordinated beats of cilia
- mononuclear inflammatory infiltrates
- ectatic lumen

■ *Special stains:* Electron microscopy, wet (37° C) mounting, PAS, collagenous stains.

Hallmark of Diagnosis: Clinical history, identification of functional abnormality of the cilia of bronchial epithelial cells.

Differential diagnosis: Chronic bacterial infections due to other causes such as congenital immunodefects, smoking, alcoholism.

Kasabach-Merritt Syndrome

Definition: Alteration of the lung parenchyma associated with the Kasabach-Merritt syndrome (congenital cavernous hemangiomas and thrombocytopenia).

Incidence/Epidemiology: Relatively uncommon disease, and involvement of the lung or pleura is extremely rare.

Etiology/Pathophysiology: The congenital disorder is characterized by giant hemangioendotheliomas which are usually localized unilaterally. Association with intravascular, disseminated, or localized coagulation is thought to be caused by abnormal sequestering sites for platelets. Patients may present with hyposomia or giantism.

Clinical Presentation: Patients present with bleeding, which can be massive.

Prognosis: Fair, if surgical excision of the hemangiomas can be performed.

Radiology: Chest radiographs may be normal or display circumscribed peripheral or subpleural densities. Angiography can confirm the hemangiomas.

Pathology:

Gross: The affected lung or pleura shows ectatic tortuous vessels measuring several centimeters in size.

Histology: The lesions are composed of numerous ectatic vessels. Adherent fresh and older thromboses and moderate mononuclear inflammatory infiltrates are usually present.

➤ *Descriptors:* Newly formed textures without metastasis potential:

- mesenchymal growth pattern
- vascular textures
- angiomatoid textures
- absent or infrequent mitoses
- homogeneous nuclear and cellular size
- hemorrhage

■ *Special stains:* PAS, collagenous stains, Giemsa.

Hallmark of Diagnosis: Clinical history, tortuous ectatic vessels with thrombosis and hemorrhage.

Differential diagnosis: "Ordinary" cavernous hemangioendothelioma, lymphangiectasis, postinflammatory cavernous lesions.

Klebsiella

Definition: Alteration of the lung parenchyma associated with infection by *Klebsiella pneumoniae.*

Incidence/Epidemiology: Infection with *Klebsiella pneumoniae* (Friedländer pneumonia) is usually a disease of adults occurring in persons with diminished immunodefence such as alcoholics and diabetics and in those with poor oral hygiene.

Etiology/Pathophysiology: The bacillus usually enters the lung by aspiration of contaminated oral secretions and induces either an acute or chronic pneumonia.

Clinical Presentation: Patients are severely ill and present with high fever, dyspnea, expectoration, and chest pain.

Prognosis: Poor in immunocompromised patients, premature babies with low birth weight and elderly persons.

Radiology: Chest radiographs usually show the involvement of several lobes and abscess formation.

Pathology:

Gross: The lungs are wet and consolidated and may display abscess formation.

Histology: The diffuse intraalveolar exudate is composed of fibrin, debris, and a large number of macrophages and neutrophilic granulocytes. The interalveolar septula are necrotic. Abscess formation and histiocytic infiltrates are seen in older lesions. The macrophages are found to contain several ingested gram-negative and methenamine-positive bacilli measuring 1.5–6.0 µm.

➤ *Descriptors:* Lung parenchyma with altered structure:

- necrosis and hemorrhage (abscess formation)
- neutrophils
- macrophages
- focal interstitial fibrosis

■ *Special stains:* PAS, Gram's, methenamine silver, collagenous stains.

Hallmark of Diagnosis: Bacterial pneumonia, identification of the organisms by microbiology.

Differential diagnosis: Bacterial pneumonia due to other organisms.

Kulchitzky Cell Tumor

Definition: Pulmonary neoplasm of neuroendocrine origin with low to moderate malignancy, see Carcinoid Tumor.

Lagochilascaris minor

Definition: Infection of the lung by the nematode *Lagochilascaris minor*.

Incidence/Epidemiology: Sporadic parasitic infections have been reported from Central and South America.

Etiology/Pathophysiology: Contamination occurs in traumatic lesions of the lung. Abscesses have been reported in the subcutaneous fatty tissue around the head and neck. Infections of the upper respiratory tract are usually seen in the nasopharynx.

Clinical Presentation: Patients complain about severe pains. Moving worms are usually seen in the subcutaneous lesions.

Prognosis: Usually good and without serious sequelae.

Radiology: No specific findings have been reported.

Pathology:

Gross: The lesions are putriform abscesses with surrounding fibrotic organization. Worms can be seen in the center of the necrosis.

Histology: The abscesses contain debris, neutrophils, macrophages, lymphocytes, and fibroblasts at their boundaries. The centers may contain worms, larvae, and eggs.

➤ *Descriptors:* Lung parenchyma with altered structure:

- necrosis and hemorrhage (abscess formation)
- mixed inflammatory infiltrates
- macrophages
- parasites (worms, larvae and eggs)
- proliferating fibroblasts

■ *Special stains:* PAS, Movat.

Hallmark of Diagnosis: Clinical history, necrotizing pneumonia with parasites, identification of the worms.

Differential diagnosis: Infections with other parasites.

Large Cell Carcinoma of the Lung

Definition: Malignant tumor of the lung with a specific histomorphological appearance.

Incidence/Epidemiology: About 10% of all primary lung carcinomas are classified as large cell undifferentiated carcinoma of the lung. The sex ratio and the age distribution are similar to that of all lung carcinomas.

Etiology/Pathophysiology: Smoking is considered to be the major risk factor in large cell anaplastic carcinoma. It is questionable whether these carcinomas are a specific entity. There is evidence that large cell undifferentiated carcinomas can be grouped into adenocarcinoma and epidermoid carcinoma in the majority of cases by electron microscopic examinations. The survival of patients with large cell anaplastic carcinoma is as poor as that of patients with small cell anaplastic carcinoma, i.e., worse than that of patients with adenocarcinoma or epidermoid carcinoma.

Clinical Presentation: Patients complain of chronic cough, chest pain, loss of weight and malaise.

Prognosis: Poor, similar to that of patients with small cell anaplastic carcinoma: about 90% of patients die within 2 years after clinical diagnosis.

Radiology: Chest radiographs show central tumor masses in 50–70% of patients, and peripherally circumscribed densities in about 30–50%.

Pathology:

Gross: The tumors are grayish-white with firm, gritty consistency. They usually show a clear-cut boundary with the surrounding lung tissue and are often of spheroid shape.

Histology: The tumors grow in solid patterns and usually preserve the interalveolar septula. They are composed of large tumor cells in which can be seen a low to moderate number of mitoses. The nuclei are large and of irregular shape and contain prominent nucleoli. Inflammatory response of the host tissue is weak or missing. Hemorrhagic areas of necrosis can be seen. They stain positively with keratin and also, frequently, vimentin.

➤ *Descriptors:* Newly formed textures with metastasis potential:

- epithelial growth patterns
- solid textures
- large tumor cells
- inhomogeneous nuclear and cellular size
- infrequent mitoses
- prominent nucleoli
- hemorrhage and necrosis
- absent or weak inflammatory infiltrates
- micrometastases

■ *Special stains:* PAS, collagenous stains, immunohistochemistry for keratin, vimentin, desmin, neuroendocrine and lymphocytic markers, DNA analysis.

Hallmark of Diagnosis: Large tumor cells, no specific growth texture, PAS-negative, prominent nucleoli, absence of keratin, expression of intercellular bridges.

Differential diagnosis: Undifferentiated adenocarcinoma or epidermoid carcinoma, metastatic hypernephroid carcinoma, amelanotic melanoma, large cell lymphocytic lymphoma.

Large Cell Lymphoma of the Lung

Definition: Involvement of the lung with large cell non-Hodgkin's lymphoma.

Incidence/Epidemiology: Primary lymphomas of the lung are rare and include a variety of non-Hodgkin's lymphomas with different degrees of malignancy. The tumors may arise in children and usually young to middle-aged adults. T-cell lymphoma and large cell lymphoma occur in a minority of the reported cases.

Etiology/Pathophysiology: The lymphomas may arise from bronchially associated lymphatic tissue (BALT) as solitary nodules or in association with extrapulmonary involvement.

Clinical Presentation: Symptoms include shortness of breath on exercise, dyspnea, and chronic cough; other patients are asymptomatic.

Prognosis: Poor, the median survival of patients with pulmonary manifestation has been estimated as 2–3 years.

Radiology: Chest radiographs show either solitary, peripherally circumscribed densities or diffuse, interstitial infiltrates, sometimes in multiple lobes. Necrosis or cavitation is rare, but does occur.

Pathology:

Gross: The lungs show solitary or multiple, grayish-tan nodules of soft consistency which may reach several centimeters in diameter.

Histology: The tumors are composed of large, atypical lymphocytes with prominent nucleoli and a relatively large amount of cytoplasm. Mitoses are frequent. The original lung texture is destroyed, and tumorous invasion of the walls of smaller vessels and bronchi occurs. The pleura is usually involved and infiltrated. Areas of hemorrhagic necrosis may be present. The lymphomas tend to proliferate in association with BALT. Invasion of the hilar lymph nodes may occur; it is, however, only observed in a minority of cases.

➤ *Descriptors:* Newly formed textures with metastasis potential:
- mesenchymal growth pattern
- lymphomatoid textures
- large tumor cells (lymphomatoid)
- homogeneous nuclear and cellular size
- prominent nucleoli
- frequent mitoses
- necrosis (focal)
- absent or weak inflammatory infiltrates

■ *Special stains:* PAS, Giemsa, collagenous stains, immunohistochemistry for lymphocytic markers, keratin, neuroendocrine markers.

Hallmark of Diagnosis: Classification of the malignant lymphoma according to light microscopic and immunohistologic features.

Differential diagnosis: Lymphomatoid granulomatosis, lymphoid hyperplasia, pseudolymphoma, interstitial lymphomatoid pneumonia, small cell anaplastic carcinoma, other forms of lymphoma.

Larva Migrans (Visceral)

Definition: Infection of the lung with visceral larva migrans (*Toxocara canis* and *cati*).

Incidence/Epidemiology: Human infection of the lung with *toxocara canis* and *cati* has been reported in various countries, especially in the southeastern and eastern parts of the USA. The infections occur most frequently in children.

Etiology/Pathophysiology: *Toxorana canis* (*toxorana cati*) are common infectious agents of dogs (cats). Infection occurs by ingesting eggs of the parasites in the feces of dogs (cats). The larvae develop in the stomach or small intestines, penetrate to the blood vessels and are swept to the liver, lung, brain, eyes, and other organs. The larvae cannot mature in man.

Prognosis: Usually good and without serious sequelae.

Clinical Presentation: Symptoms include anorexia, weakness, fever, eosinophilia, chronic cough, dyspnea, hemoptysis, and nausea.

Radiology: Chest radiographs show bilateral, diffuse, patchy infiltrates.

Pathology:

Gross: The lungs reveal multiple, small (several millimeters) grayish-white nodules with central hemorrhage.

Histology: The larvae cause a granulomatous reaction of the lung parenchyma with predominant neutrophils and eosinophils and larvae measuring 20 x 500 μm at their center. Histiocytic inflammatory reaction at the boundary of the granulomas may be present. The larvae are usually dead and have degenerated.

➤*Descriptors:* Lung parenchyma with altered structure:

- noncaseous epithelioid granulomas
- parasites (intragranulomatous, degenerated)
- palisading histiocytes
- eosinophils
- mononuclear inflammatory infiltrates

■ *Special stains:* PAS, Movat, collagenous stains, Giemsa.

Hallmark of Diagnosis: Clinical history, necrotizing pneumonia, ill defined granulomas, identification of the larvae.

Differential diagnosis: Infection with other parasites, especially *Ascaris*, *Trichuris*, and other nematodes.

Leeches

Definition: Alteration of the lung parenchyma associated with aspiration of leeches, see Hirudiniasis.

Legionnaires' Disease

Definition: Infection of the lung with *Legionella.*

Incidence/Epidemiology: Infection occurs as a sporadic disease acquired in the community and as an epidemic disease. Persons working in air-conditioned rooms are at particular risk.

Etiology/Pathophysiology: Infection of the lung precedes a bacteremia with extrapulmonary manifestations in the kidneys, gastrointestinal tract, and central nervous system.

Clinical Presentation: Patients complain of fever, malaise, and myalgia several days before the outbreak of pulmonary and extrapulmonary manifestations, which can be recognized by expectoration, diarrhea, and renal failure.

Prognosis: Fair, about 30–40% of patients will have complete resolution after one month, while others may present with progressive respiratory failure. The mortality has been estimated at 2–10%.

Radiology: Chest radiographs show dense lobar or lobular infiltrates.

Pathology:

Gross: The lungs are heavy and show multiple, grayish-white densities limited to the lobes or lobules.

Histology: The original lung texture is preserved and infiltrated by numerous neutrophilic granulocytes, lymphocytes, plasma cells, and macrophages. The inflammatory infiltrates are intermingled with excessive fibrin deposits (fibrinopurulent pneumonia). Resolution occurs by infiltration of histiocytes.

➤*Descriptors:* Lung parenchyma with preserved structure:

- mixed inflammatory infiltrates
- intraalveolar fibrinoid material
- bacteria (Warthin-Starry stain)

■ *Special stains:* PAS, Gram's (organisms are weakly positive), Warthin-Starry stain, Dieterle's stain, collagenous stains.

Hallmark of Diagnosis: Fibrinoid pneumonia, identification of *Legionella* by microbiology.

Differential diagnosis: Bacterial pneumonia due to other organisms.

Leiomyoblastoma

Definition: Malignant tumor of the lung with a specific microscopic growth pattern.

Incidence/Epidemiology: Unusual malignant tumor in the lung.

Etiology/Pathophysiology: It arises as a primary tumor of the lung or metastasizes into the lung.

Clinical Presentation: Patients are usually asymptomatic.

Prognosis: Poor.

Radiology: Chest radiographs show a solitary nodule in the peripheral lung.

Pathology:

Gross: Circumscribed, yellowish mass of firm consistency.

Histology: The tumors are composed of small spindle cells and small round cells with unsuspicious nucleoli. Mitoses can be noted infrequently. An inflammatory response of the host tissue is absent or weak. Necroses may occur. The original lung texture is completely destroyed.

➤*Descriptors:* Newly formed textures with metastasis potential:

- mesenchymal growth pattern

- sarcomatous textures
- small tumor cells (spindle)
- homogeneous nuclear and cellular size
- finely distributed nuclear chromatin
- infrequent mitoses
- necrosis and hemorrhage (small areas)
- weak or absent inflammatory infiltrates

■ *Special stains:* PAS, Giemsa, collagenous stains, immunohistochemistry for keratin, vimentin, desmin, desmoplakin, neuroendocrine markers, lysozyme.

Hallmark of Diagnosis: Spindle tumor cells intermingled with small round tumor cells.

Differential diagnosis: Glomus tumor in the lung, hemangiopericytoma, carcinoid, epithelioid leiomyosarcoma.

Leiomyoma

Definition: Benign mesenchymal tumor of the lung.

Incidence/Epidemiology: Rare tumor of the larger bronchi and trachea. About 30 cases have been reported.

Etiology/Pathophysiology: The tumors arise from smooth muscle cells of the bronchi, trachea, or vessels.

Clinical Presentation: The symptoms are due to the central location of the lesions and include chronic cough, hemoptysis, and shortness of breath during exercise.

Prognosis: Usually good and without serious sequelae.

Radiology: Chest radiographs are normal or are related to air trapping induced by the centrally located submucosal tumors.

Pathology:

Gross: The tumors are solid in consistency and grayish.

Histology: The tumors are composed of dense bundles of smooth muscle cells. They may show central hyalinization. Mitoses are very rare. The tumors grow in the submucosa of the trachea or larger bronchi and lead to obstruction of the lumen.

➤ *Descriptors:* Newly formed textures without metastasis potential:

- mesenchymal growth pattern
- fibromatous textures
- smooth muscle cells
- homogeneous nuclear and cellular size
- small nuclei
- absent or infrequent mitoses
- absent necrosis
- mononuclear inflammatory infiltrates (weak)

■ *Special stains:* PAS, Masson Goldner, collagenous stains, immunohistochemistry for vimentin, desmin, desmoplakin, lysozyme, actin, myosin, DNA analysis.

Hallmark of Diagnosis: Proliferating smooth muscle cells with central hyalinization and homogeneous nuclear pattern, distinct tumor nodules.

Differential diagnosis: Benign metastasizing leiomyoma, lymphangioleiomyomatosis, leiomyosarcoma, granular cell tumor, fibrosarcoma.

Leiomyoma, Benign Metastasizing

Definition: Intrapulmonary mesenchymal tumor with specific histomorphologic and clinical features.

Incidence/Epidemiology: Unusual tumor occurring in women with a history of hysterectomy.

Etiology/Pathophysiology: The tumors are considered to be metastases of low-grade, smooth muscle tumors. Most of these tumors have their origin in the uterus. Others have been reported to originate in the cervix, saphenous vein, gluteal region, or diaphragm. Other lesions include primary leiomyomas of the lung (arising from smooth muscle cells of the larger and smaller bronchi and arteries), fibrous hamartomas, and fibrosarcomas.

Clinical Presentation: Patients are usually asymptomatic. The lesions are considered to be benign or of only low-grade malignancy as long as they are of small size (below 2 cm in diameter).

Prognosis: Most patients survive several years; however, curative treatment is usually not possible.

Radiology: Chest radiographs show solitary nodules in the peripheral lung parenchyma.

Pathology:

Gross: The tumors are grayish-white and firm in consistency.

Histology: The tumors are composed of bundles of smooth muscle cells growing in different directions. Mitotic figures are rare and hard to detect. Entrapped air spaces with hyperplastic epithelial cells are the remains of the original lung textures. Necroses and inflammatory response of host tissue are not features of benign metastasizing leiomyomas.

➤ *Descriptors:* Newly formed textures without metastasis potential:
- mesenchymal growth pattern
- fibromatous textures
- smooth muscle cells
- homogeneous nuclear and cellular size
- absent or infrequent mitoses
- entrapped air spaces
- absent necrosis
- absent inflammatory infiltrates

■ *Special stains:* PAS, collagenous stains, Masson Goldner, immunohistochemistry for vimentin, desmin, desmoplakin, actin, myosin, DNA analysis.

Hallmark of Diagnosis: Clinical history, proliferating smooth muscle cells with entrapped distant air spaces, "benign features" of the tumor.

Differential diagnosis: Primary leiomyoma of the lung, lymphangioleiomyomatosis, leiomyosarcoma, plasma cell granuloma.

Leiomyosarcoma

Definition: Malignant mesenchymal tumor of the lung with a specific histomorphological growth pattern.

Incidence/Epidemiology: Rare tumor occurring in children and young adults.

Etiology/Pathophysiology: There is evidence that the tumors are of congenital origin. Some of the reported cases have had additional fibromatous proliferations in extrapulmonary organs.

Clinical Presentation: Symptoms include chronic cough, dyspnea, and hemoptysis. The tumors are of low- to medium-grade malignancy.

Prognosis: Fair, most patients survive 5 years or longer.

Radiology: Chest radiographs show central tumor masses in association with major bronchi.

Pathology:

Gross: The tumors are red-grayish and firm in consistency.

Histology: The tumors are composed of dense bundles of proliferating smooth muscle cells with numerous mitotic figures and large variation in cellular and nuclear size. Necrotic areas may be present. The original interstitial lung parenchyma and the submucous glands are destroyed and no longer recognizable.

➤ *Descriptors:* Newly formed textures with metastasis potential:
- mesenchymal growth pattern
- sarcomatous textures
- smooth muscle cells
- inhomogeneous nuclear and cellular size
- frequent mitoses
- necrosis and hemorrhage
- absent or weak inflammatory infiltrates

■ *Special stains:* PAS, collagenous stains, Masson Goldner, immunohistochemistry for keratin, vimentin, desmin, desmoplakin, actin, myosin, lysozyme, DNA analysis.

Hallmark of Diagnosis: Clinical history, proliferating smooth muscle cells with large variation in cellular and nuclear size, numerous mitotic figures.

Differential diagnosis: Inflammatory pseudotumor, congenital generalized fibromatosis, thoracoblastoma, neurogenous sarcoma.

Leishmaniasis

Definition: Infection of the lung with *Leishmania donovani* (synonyms Kala-azar, dumdum fever, black fever.

Incidence/Epidemiology: The disease occurs predominantly in South America, Africa, Mediterranean countries, and Asia. It is a disease of children and young adults in India, whereas in China and Brazil it is an infection of children and infants.

Etiology/Pathophysiology: The protozoan organisms are transferred to man by insects (sandflies). The amastigotes measure 1.3–3.0 µm, are of round to oval shape, and have a thin cell membrane, a large nucleus, and a rod-shaped kinetoblast. They stain positively with HE, Giemsa, and Wilder's reticulum stain. The protozoa multiply in histiocytes after inoculation into the skin. In the insect vector the protozoa change to leptomonads and multiply in the midgut of the fly.

Clinical Presentation: Patients display five cardinal conditions: (a) hepatosplenomegaly, (b) pancytopenia, (c) generalized lymphadenopathy, (d) fever, and (e) cachexia. Chronic cough indicates the rare involvement of the lung.

Prognosis: The mortality of untreated patients is 80% in children and 90% in adults. Recurrent infections within 2 years occur in 5–15% of patients.

Radiology: Chest radiographs show the displacement of the diaphragm due to the extremely large hepatosplenomegaly. Diffuse interstitial densities may be present.

Pathology:

Gross: Atelectatic lungs with excessive hepatosplenomegaly.

Histology: The protozoa are usually numerous in histiocytes of the liver and spleen, and in the subcutaneous fatty tissue. The original lung texture is preserved. The distant air spaces contain fibrin, detritus, mononuclear inflammatory infiltrates and histiocytes. The latter display in the interstitium and are laden with protozoan amastigotes.

➤ *Descriptors:* Lung parenchyma with preserved structure:

- intraalveolar fibrinoid material
- mononuclear inflammatory infiltrates
- histiocytes (amastigotes-laden)

■ *Special stains:* Giemsa, Wilder's reticulum stain.

Hallmark of Diagnosis: Clinical history, hepatosplenomegaly, identification of *Leishmania donovani*.

Differential diagnosis: Infections with other protozoan organisms.

Lentil Pneumonia

Definition: Chronic pneumonitis due to aspiration of starch grains from legumes.

Incidence/Epidemiology: Unusual disease seen in persons working in agriculture or accidentally exposed to legume preparation.

Etiology/Pathophysiology: The inhaled grains induce a granulomatous foreign-body reaction in the lung parenchyma. They are, to a certain degree, inert to digestion.

Clinical Presentation: Usually no complaints.

Prognosis: Good and without serious sequelae.

Radiology: Chest radiographs may be normal.

Pathology:

Gross: Occasional, small, granulomatous nodules may be seen.

Histology: Granulomatous foreign-body reaction of the lung parenchyma with neutrophilic granulocytes, lymphocytes, plasma cells, macrophages, and multinucleated giant cells. In the center of the granuloma, foreign-body material may resemble the eggs of helminths.

➤ *Descriptors:* Lung parenchyma with altered structure:

- noncaseous epithelioid granulomas
- mixed inflammatory infiltrates
- multinucleated giant cells
- foreign-body material (intraalveolar, resembling eggs of parasites)

■ *Special stains:* PAS, Giemsa.

Hallmark of Diagnosis: Identification of starch grains, granulomatous foreign-body reaction.

Differential diagnosis: Parasitic infections, adiaspiromycosis.

Letterer-Siwe Disease

Definition: Alteration of the lung parenchyma caused by infiltrations of histiocytes resembling Langerhans' cells in the acute stage of the disease, see Histiocytosis X.

Leukemia

Definition: Leukemic infiltrates in the lung parenchyma.

Incidence/Epidemiology: A considerable number of patients suffering from leukemia develop pulmonary leukemic infiltrates. The rates range from 25–70% in autopsies and from 5–15% while living. All kinds of lymphomas can involve the lung; however, patients with high blast counts and T-cell lymphoma are at higher risk. Patients with pseudolymphoma are at higher risk of developing pulmonary lymphoma than the general population.

Etiology/Pathophysiology: The lung and the liver belong to the group of organs with a fine capillary network and a dense reticuloendothe-

lial cellular population. Lymphocytic tumor cells usually follow the pathways along the veins and bronchi within the bronchially associated lymphatic tissue (BALT) and penetrate from the interstitial capillary network into the distant air spaces. Bacterial superinfection is frequently seen in patients with acute or recurrent leukemia.
Clinical Presentation: Patients complain about dyspnea, chronic cough, malaise, fever, and symptoms of bacterial pneumonia.

Prognosis: Fair, patients may survive for several years depending upon the malignancy grade of the underlying disease.

Radiology: Chest radiographs show diffuse interstitial densities.

Pathology:
Gross: The lungs are heavy and show multiple grayish-white densities of soft consistency measuring several centimeters in diameter. The pleura is usually involved.

Histology: Leukemic tumor infiltrates are present, depending on the leukocytic cell type. They invade the pleura and the walls of smaller vessels and of bronchi and spread along the BALT. The tumor infiltrates start from the interstitial tissue and move into the alveoli. The boundary between tumorous lung areas and healthy lung parenchyma is usually distinct and clear-cut. The larger conducting airways are often empty.

➤ *Descriptors:* Newly formed textures with metastasis potential:
- mesenchymal growth pattern
- lymphomatoid textures
- homogeneous nuclear and cellular size
- infrequent mitoses
- absent necrosis

■ *Special stains:* PAS, Giemsa, collagenous stains, immunohistochemistry for leukocytic cellular subtypes, endogenous lectins, DNA analysis.

Hallmark of Diagnosis: Clinical history, identification of lymphocytic tumor cells.

Differential diagnosis: Pseudolymphoma, inflammatory pseudotumor, small cell anaplastic carcinoma, metastatic small cell sarcoma into the lung (Ewing's sarcoma, Askin tumor, etc.).

Levodopa

Definition: Alteration of the lung parenchyma associated with intake of levodopa, see Drug Toxicity.

Librium

Definition: Alteration of the lung parenchyma associated with intake of librium, see Drug Toxicity.

Lidocaine

Definition: Alteration of the lung parenchyma associated with intake of lidocaine, see Drug Toxicity.

Limestone

Definition: Alteration of the lung parenchyma associated with inhalation of limestone dust.
Incidence/Epidemiology: Development of mild pneumoconiosis in a few workers exposed to limestone has been reported.
Etiology/Pathophysiology: Limestone is considered to be inert if storage in the lung parenchyma occurs. Development of pneumoconiosis associated with limestone is probably induced by the contamination by silica (up to 15%).
Clinical Presentation: Symptoms include chronic cough, shortness of breath during exercise, dyspnea; they are, however, usually mild and progress only a little.
Prognosis: Usually good and without progression.
Radiology: Chest radiographs may be normal or show slight, interstitial, diffuse densities.
Pathology:
Gross: The lungs are dark brown and may display small silicotic nodules.
Histology: The deposits of limestone are associated with the bronchioles and may intermingle with deposits of silica and circumferential fibrosis.
➤ *Descriptors:* Lung parenchyma with preserved structure:
- dust

- macrophages (dust-laden);
- Lung parenchyma with altered structure:
- focal interstitial fibrosis (mild)

■ *Special stains:* PAS, collagenous stains, polarization, Prussian blue, X-ray diffraction or related physical techniques.

Hallmark of Diagnosis: Clinical history, identification of deposits of limestone by X-ray diffraction or related physical techniques.

Differential diagnosis: Exposure of the lung to other external agents such as smoking, silica, hard metals, coal.

Lipid Pneumonia

Definition: Lipoid deposits in the lung parenchyma due to endogenous causes or aspiration of oil.

Incidence/Epidemiology: Aspiration of oil-containing media may occur with cooking oil, cod liver oil, fat-soluble preparations (children), oily nosedrops, or mineral oil. Iatrogenic agents include radiographic contrast media and aerosols. Endogenous causes are the compression of lymphatic drainage or hyperlipemia and diabetes mellitus.

Etiology/Pathophysiology: Some of the lipid drops are phagocytosed by macrophages, and some remain within the distant airways. In later stages, the formation of multinucleated, foreign-body giant cells, the invasion of histiocytes, and the induction of interstitial fibrosis may result in honeycombing. Mononuclear interstitial infiltration is related to the specific component of the inhaled oil.

Clinical Presentation: The symptoms of inhaled oil drops are usually mild or absent. Larger amounts of aspirated oil induce acute dyspnea, chest pain, cough, and cyanosis. Endogenous lipoid pneumonias usually have a mild onset and are of slow progression.

Prognosis: Usually good, as progression is absent or very slow.

Radiology: Chest radiographs show diffuse interstitial densities with increased markings in the basilar parts of the lower lobes.

Pathology:

Gross: The lungs are solid in consistency and grayish to yellow. Oil droplets may be seen on the cut surfaces in severe intoxication.

Histology: The lung texture is often preserved. The distant air spaces contain lipid droplets and clusters of foamy macrophages which have also ingested oil droplets. Mononuclear interstitial infiltrates are present depending upon the degree and components of the inhaled oil. Later stages show interstitial fibrosis with decomposition of the original lung texture.

➤ *Descriptors:* Lung parenchyma with preserved structure:

- lipoid material (intraalveolar droplets)
- macrophages (foamy)
- mononuclear inflammatory infiltrates (mild);
- Lung parenchyma with altered structure:
- diffuse interstitial fibrosis (mild)

■ *Special stains:* PAS, collagenous stains, oil red O stain on frozen tissue.

Hallmark of Diagnosis: Clinical history, identification of lipid droplets in the distant air spaces and in macrophages.

Differential diagnosis: Obstructive pneumonia, centroacinar emphysema, lipoma, liposarcoma.

Lipiodol

Definition: Alteration of the lung parenchyma associated with intake of lipiodol, see Drug Toxicity.

Lipoid Proteinosis of Trachea and Bronchi

Definition: Involvement of the trachea and bronchi in the heritable disease hyalinosis cutis et mucosae (Urbach-Wiethe syndrome).

Incidence/Epidemiology: Rare disease of autosomal-recessive inheritance involving the larynx, pharynx, and skin.

Etiology/Pathophysiology: The disease is characterized by deposits of small amounts of glycoproteins in the skin, pharynx, larynx, and internal viscera. The deposits are perineural and perivascular.

Clinical Presentation: The symptoms are usually manifest in adults and consist of obstructive pulmonary complaints.

Prognosis: Fair.

Radiology: Chest radiographic findings are related to the obstruction of the trachea or major bronchi.

Pathology:

Gross: The narrowed trachea or bronchi contain multiple, small, yellowish nodules in the submucosa.

Histology: Deposits of hyalinized acellular material in the submucosa of the trachea or bronchi have been mentioned. The submucosal glands are destroyed. The mucosa undergoes squamous metaplasia.

➤ *Descriptors:* Bronchial mucosa with altered structure:

- hyaline material
- destruction of submucosal glands
- squamous metaplasia and dysplasia

■ *Special stains:* PAS, oil red O stain, Congo stain.

Hallmark of Diagnosis: Identification of submucosal hyaline deposits in the trachea or major bronchi.

Differential diagnosis: Amyloidosis, hamartoma, submucosal scars due to antecedent trauma (biopsy).

Lipoma

Definition: Benign mesenchymal tumor with specific histomorphological appearance.

Incidence/Epidemiology: Unusual tumor arising in young and middle-aged adults. Sex ratio 9:1 (men:women). Specific risk factors are not known.

Etiology/Pathophysiology: The tumors are associated with mature fatty tissue. They usually originate from bronchial or peribronchial fatty tissue. Some tumors are located in the peripheral (subpleural) lung parenchyma.

Clinical Presentation: Symptoms are related to the central localization and consist of shortness of breath, asthmatic complaints, and chronic cough.

Prognosis: Good and without serious sequelae.

Radiology: Chest radiographs are usually normal or may show peripheral atelectasis.

Pathology:

Gross: The lumen of a major bronchus is narrowed by submucosal fatty tissue.

Histology: The tumors are characterized by mature fatty tissue localized in the submucosa and in the peripheral subpleural lung tissue. Necroses, inflammatory response of host tissue, and mitoses are absent.

➤ *Descriptors:* Newly formed textures without metastasis potential:

- mesenchymal growth pattern
- myxomatoid textures
- fatty tissue (mature)
- small nuclei (round)
- absent or infrequent mitoses
- absent necrosis
- absent inflammatory infiltrates

■ *Special stains:* None.

Hallmark of Diagnosis: Mature fatty tissue.

Differential diagnosis: Lipomatoid hamartoma.

Lipoproteinosis

Definition: Disease of the peripheral lung parenchyma characterized by diffuse lipid-proteinaceous material located in the alveoli, see Alveolar Proteinosis.

Liposarcoma

Definition: Malignant tumor of the lung derived from fatty tissue.

Incidence/Epidemiology: Extremely rare tumor of the lung. Only a few cases have been reported.

Etiology/Pathophysiology: The reported tumors are related to the peribronchial, periarterial, and subpleural fatty tissue.

Clinical Presentation: The symptoms arise from the central localization of the tumors and include chronic cough, dyspnea, and atelectasis.

Prognosis: Exact data are not known; however, it is suggested that patients have a poor survival.

Radiology: Chest radiographs show a centrally located, circumscribed tumor mass.

Pathology:

Gross: The lung contains a circumscribed, yellowish-white, tumor mass of soft consistency measuring 2–4 cm in diameter.

Histology: The tumors consist of immature fat cells with wide variation in nuclear and cellular size. Mitoses, areas of necrosis, and complete disturbance of the underlying texture of the lung parenchyma are present. Focal areas of spindle cells and small tumor cells resembling small cell anaplastic carcinoma may exist.

➤ *Descriptors:* Newly formed textures with metastasis potential:
- mesenchymal growth pattern
- sarcomatous textures
- fatty tissue (immature)
- large tumor cells (lipid droplets)
- inhomogeneous nuclear and cellular size
- frequent mitoses
- necrosis and hemorrhage (focal)
- absent or weak inflammatory infiltrates

■ *Special stains:* PAS, collagenous stains, oil red O fat stain, immunohistochemistry for vimentin, keratin, desmin, desmoplakin, lysozyme, actin, myosin, neuroendocrine markers, endogenous lectins, DNA analysis.

Hallmark of Diagnosis: Clinical history, histomorphological features including identification of sarcomatous origin and fatty droplets in the cytoplasm of the tumor cells.

Differential diagnosis: Metastasis of liposarcoma into the lung, sarcomas of other classification, lipoma, small cell anaplastic carcinoma, malignant histiocytoma.

Listeriosis, Congenital

Definition: Alteration of the lung parenchyma associated with infection by *Listeria monocytogenes.*

Incidence/Epidemiology: Rare infection of the lung seen in infants during the fetal, neonatal, or perinatal period and in prematures.

Etiology/Pathophysiology: The organisms spread from the infected mother through the placenta or through an infected birth canal to the infants. As in infections with *Toxoplasma gondii* or *Treponema pallidum*, sepsis will occur, with pulmonary and hepatic manifestations.

Clinical Presentation: The infants present with cutaneous pustules, respiratory distress, or meningitis. The placenta shows villitis and abscess formation. Late onset of symptoms is usually associated with meningitis.

Prognosis: Usually good, if prompt treatment is instituted.

Radiology: Chest radiographs show circumscribed areas with abscessing pneumonia.

Pathology:

Gross: The lungs show large areas of necrosis with some consolidation at the boundary.

Histology: The distant airways have necrotic areas filled with debris, neutrophilic granulocytes, lymphocytes, plasma cells, histiocytes, macrophages, and gram-positive organisms.

➤ *Descriptors:* Lung parenchyma with altered structure:
- necrosis and hemorrhage
- fibrinoid material
- mixed inflammatory infiltrates
- infectious organisms (*Listeria*, Dieterle's stain)

■ *Special stains:* PAS, Gram's, collagenous stains, Dieterle's stain, immunohistochemistry for *Listeria*.

Hallmark of Diagnosis: Clinical history, identification of the rods.

Differential diagnosis: Toxoplasmosis, congenital syphilis, pulmonary abscess due to other infectious agents.

Lithiasis

Definition: Deposits of calcified material in the proximal and/or distant air spaces, see Alveolar Microlithiasis, Broncholithiasis, Calcification.

Lobar Pneumonia

Definition: Homogeneous infection of one or more lobes.

Incidence/Epidemiology: Lobar pneumonia is less common than lobular pneumonia (bronchopneumonia). However, it is not infrequently seen in immunocompromised patients or those with chronic pulmonary disease, alcoholism, liver cirrhosis, malignancies, and congenital pulmonary abnormalities.

Etiology/Pathophysiology: In principle, any organism which is able to spread rapidly from one single focus into the surrounding lung parenchyma can produce a lobar pneumonia. Among the bacterial infections, lobar pneumonia is most frequently seen in association with *Streptococcus pneumoniae*.

Clinical Presentation: The patients present with high fever, chest pain, cough, and dyspnea and are usually quite sick.

Prognosis: Usually good; however, depending upon the infective organisms and general condition of the patients fatal courses occur.

Radiology: Chest radiographs show homogeneous densities occupying one or several complete lobes.

Pathology:

Gross: The infected lobes are heavy and either red-brown and wet or grayish-white, ribby, and consolidated depending upon the stage of the bacterial infection.

Histology: The histomorphological changes depend upon the stage of the disease and can be classified into four different levels (see bacterial pneumonia): (a) initial response of the lung (edema); (b) red hepatization (extravasation of red blood cells and invasion of neutrophils); (c) gray hepatization (deposits of fibrin, an enormous number of granulocytes and macrophages); (d) yellow hepatization (resolution stage, restoration of tissue texture).

➤ *Descriptors:* Lung parenchyma with preserved structure:

- intraalveolar serous fluid
- hemorrhage
- neutrophils
- intraalveolar fibrinoid material
- mixed inflammatory infiltrates
- macrophages;
- Lung parenchyma with altered structure:
- proliferating fibroblasts
- focal interstitial fibrosis

■ *Special stains:* PAS, Gram's, collagenous stains, immunofluorescence for identification of the organisms.

Hallmark of Diagnosis: Clinical history, radiology, homogeneous infection of one or several lobes.

Differential diagnosis: Lobular pneumonia, lobar pneumonia due to the underlying organisms.

Löffler's Syndrome

Definition: Alteration of the lung parenchyma in acute eosinophilic pneumonia.

Incidence/Epidemiology: The disease is seen fairly frequently due to the broad variety of underlying agents.

Etiology/Pathophysiology: In developed countries the causative agent most frequently seen is related to intake of drugs. These include virtually all kinds of drugs such as antibiotics (penicillin, sulfa, streptomycin, isoniazid, etc.), cytostatics (bleomycin, azathioprine, procarbazine, etc.), antiinflammatory drugs (aspirin, naproxine, etc.), antihyperglycemics (chlorpropamide, etc.), antihypertensives (hydralazine, etc), anticonvulsives (chlorpromazine, carbamazepine, etc.). In developing countries the causative agent is most frequently related to infections (fungi, parasites, especially *Ascaris lumbricoides, Wuchereria bancrofti, Brugia malayi*, bacteria (*Brucella, Proteus, Staphylococcus*, viruses). Additional agents are fumes of metals (nickel, beryllium, zinc)and organic and inorganic allergens (pollen, beeswax, mineral oil, cooking oil, etc.). The disease is now understood to be an acute usually mild and self-healing reaction of the lung to a broad variety of exogenous agents (limited hypersensitivity reaction).

Clinical Presentation: The symptoms are absent or mild (shortness of breath during exercise, mild fever, cough). Blood eosinophil count is elevated.

Prognosis: Usually good and without serious sequelae.

Radiology: Chest radiographs show small to massive diffuse shadows which shift from one location to another within a couple of days and which disappear without treatment after 20–30 days.

Pathology:

Gross: The lungs display ill-defined, red-tan areas with somewhat increased consistency.

Histology: The texture of the lung parenchyma is preserved. The distant airways and the interalveolar septula contain an enormous number of eosinophilic granulocytes which can also be detected in the sputum or with bronchoalveolar lavage. An increased number of lymphocytes, macrophages, and histiocytes indicates a shift of acute eosinophilic pneumonia to chronic eosinophilic pneumonia.

➤ *Descriptors:* Lung parenchyma with preserved structure:

- eosinophils
- mixed inflammatory infiltrates

■ *Special stains:* PAS, Giemsa.

Hallmark of Diagnosis: Clinical history, radiologic findings, increased number of eosinophilic infiltrates.

Differential diagnosis: Chronic eosinophilic pneumonia, hypersensitivity reaction of the lung, histiocytosis X.

Löfgren's Syndrome

Definition: Manifestation of sarcoidosis with bilateral hilar lymphadenopathy and erythema nodosum and, infrequently, uveitis, parotitis, fever.

Incidence/Epidemiology: Löfgren's syndrome can be seen in about 10% of all patients suffering from sarcoidosis.

Etiology/Pathophysiology: The etiology of sarcoidosis is not known.

Clinical Presentation: The majority of patients are asymptomatic. Symptoms include chronic cough, shortness of breath during exercise, and dyspnea.

Prognosis: Worse than with common sarcoidosis, the mortality rate related to Löfgren's syndrome can be estimated 15–25%.

Radiology: Chest radiographs show bilateral hilar lymphadenopathy. In addition, diffuse interstitial infiltrates may be present.

Pathology:

Gross: The hilar lymph nodes are enlarged and of grayish-white color, often with increased consistency.

Histology: The lymphatic tissue reveals multiple, noncaseating, epithelioid granulomas with multinucleated giant cells. A fibrotic ring usually surrounds the granulomas. The number of lymphocytes and plasma cells is less than that found in intrapulmonary sarcoid granulomas. For details, see Sarcoidosis.

➤ *Descriptors:* Lung parenchyma with altered structure:

- noncaseous epithelioid granulomas
- mononuclear inflammatory infiltrates
- multinucleated giant cells
- focal interstitial fibrosis (circumferential, scarring);
- Lung parenchyma with preserved structure:
- mononuclear inflammatory infiltrates (focal)
- unsuspicious pneumocytes

■ *Special stains:* PAS, collagenous stains, Giemsa, Ziehl-Neelsen, endogenous lectins.

Hallmark of Diagnosis: Clinical history, radiologic findings, noncaseating epithelioid granulomas with peripheral fibrosis, and multinucleated giant cells.

Differential diagnosis: Tuberculosis, fungal infections, sarcoid-like lesions (in patients with malignancies).

Lupus Erythematosus, Systemic

Definition: Alterations of the lung parenchyma associated with systemic lupus erythematosus (SLE).

Incidence/Epidemiology: Pulmonary manifestation is seen in 40–60% of all diseased patients.

Etiology/Pathophysiology: SLE is an autoimmune disorder with development of autoimmune antibodies against antigens of the nuclear membranes, erythrocytes, and/or connective tissue. The circulating autoimmune complexes may deposit on any basal membrane and thus lead to an inflammatory response of the involved textures (vessels, glomeruli, interalveolar septula, etc.). Intrapulmonary manifestation may involve pulmonary hemorrhage, acute interstitial pneumonitis (lupus pneumonitis), acute vasculitis, lymphomatoid interstitial pneumonia, interstitial fibrosis, pulmonary hypertension, or bronchiolitis obliterans.

Clinical Presentation: Symptoms include acute respiratory distress, chest pain (painful pleuritis with pleural effusions), dyspnea, chronic cough, and hemoptysis.

Prognosis: About 77% of patients will survive 5 years or longer. Cause of death is most frequently related to cardiac or renal failure.

Radiology: Chest radiographs show diffuse interstitial densities, atelectasis and pleural effusions.

Pathology:

Gross: The lungs show fibrinoid deposits on the pleural surface, pleural thickening, and increased consistency of the lung parenchyma.

Histology: The histomorphologic image varies and may show: (a) infiltration of polymorphonuclear cells in the capillaries of the interalveolar septula, fibrin deposits on the basal membranes, hyperplasia and hypertrophy of pneumocytes, intraalveolar hemorrhage; (b) broad hyalinized basal membranes and fibrotic denaturation of the submucosal glands; (c) diffuse, lymphocytic interstitial infiltrates with marked desquamative reaction in the distant air spaces; (d) dense mononuclear and polymorphous infiltrates in the walls of smaller and medium-sized arteries; (e) granulomatous erosion of small bronchi and bronchioles; (f) thickening and dense polymorphous infiltrates in the pleura with fibrinoid deposits on the pleural surfaces.

➤ *Descriptors:* Lung parenchyma with preserved structure:
- mixed inflammatory infiltrates (intracapillary)
- intraalveolar fibrinoid material
- hemorrhage
- desquamation, hypertrophy, hyperplasia and dysplasia of pneumocytes
- hyaline material (basal membranes)
- mononuclear inflammatory infiltrates;
- Pleura with preserved structure:
- hyalinosis
- mixed inflammatory infiltrates
- fibrinoid material;
- Pulmonary vessels with preserved structure:
- mixed inflammatory infiltrates
- mononuclear inflammatory infiltrates;
- Bronchial mucosa with altered structure:
- fibrinoid material
- histiocytes
- ulceration
- destruction of submucosal glands
- lymphomatoid granulomas

■ *Special stains:* PAS, Giemsa, collagenous stains, immunohistochemistry for IgG, DNA analysis, endogenous lectins.

Hallmark of Diagnosis: Clinical history, identification of LE cells, lymphomatoid interstitial pneumonia, vasculitis, pleuritis, hyalinization of basal membranes, capillaritis.

Differential diagnosis: Usual interstitial pneumonia, lymphoid interstitial pneumonia, acute respiratory distress syndrome, organizing pneumonia, vasculitis, and granulomatosis.

Lycoperdonosis

Definition: Alteration of the lung parenchyma associated with inhalation of puffball spores.

Incidence/Epidemiology: Rare disorder seen in mushroom collectors.

Etiology/Pathophysiology: Inhalation of puffball spores (*Basidiomycele* fungus) causes an extrinsic allergic reaction of the lung parenchyma.

Clinical Presentation: Usually acute or subacute onset of symptoms with chills, dyspnea, and dry cough.

Prognosis: Usually good and without serious sequelae.

Radiology: Chest radiographs show diffuse interstitial infiltrates.

Pathology:

Gross: The lungs are wet and of grayish-tan color.

Histology: The lungs show interstitial mononuclear and eosinophilic inflammatory infiltrates such as are usually seen in allergic extrinsic alveolitis.

➤ *Descriptors:* Lung parenchyma with altered structure:
- noncaseous epithelioid granulomas
- eosinophils
- multinucleated giant cells
- intrabronchiolar fibrinoid material and histiocytes
- ulceration of bronchiolar mucosa;
- Lung parenchyma with preserved structure:
- macrophages
- desquamation, hypertrophy, hyperplasia and dysplasia of pneumocytes
- mononuclear inflammatory infiltrates
- intraalveolar serous fluid

■ *Special stains:* PAS, collagenous stains, Giemsa, endogenous lectins.

Hallmark of Diagnosis: Clinical history, histopathologic changes such as are seen in allergic extrinsic alveolitis.

Differential diagnosis: Adult respiratory distress syndrome, usual interstitial pneumonia, lymphocytic interstitial pneumonia, desquamative interstitial pneumonia, sarcoidosis.

Lymphadenopathy

Definition: Unusual enlargement of the hilar and mediastinal lymph nodes as evidenced by radiologic techniques.

Incidence/Epidemiology: Frequent disorder seen in a wide variety of patients.

Etiology/Pathophysiology: Enlargement of the hilar and mediastinal lymph nodes is caused by a variety of disorders such as metastatic carcinoma (from lung, kidney, gastrointestinal tract), sarcoidosis, fungal infections, tuberculosis, pneumoconiosis (silicosis, hematite miner's, kaolin), lymphoma, angioimmunoblastic lymphadenopathy.

Clinical Presentation: Patients may be asymptomatic or present with dyspnea, chest pain, and/or chronic cough.

Prognosis: Depends upon the underlying disease.

Radiology: Chest radiographs show enlargement and broadening of the mediastinal and hilar structures.

Pathology:

Gross: The lymph nodes are enlarged and evince changes associated with the underlying disease. In a small percentage of cases no morphologic equivalent to the radiologic changes can be detected. Angioimmunoblastic lymphadenopathy is usually associated with generalized lymphadenopathy, hepatosplenomegaly, hemolytic anemia, skin rash, or polyclonal hypergammaglobulinemia.

Histology: The characteristic changes are described under the particular chapters. Angioimmunoblastic lymphadenopathy involves proliferating immunoblasts, plasma cells, histiocytes, prominent vascularity, "burned out" germinal centers, and eosinophilic intercellular deposits.

➤ *Descriptors:* Lymphatic tissue with preserved structure:

- mixed inflammatory infiltrates
- mononuclear inflammatory infiltrates
- dust;
- Lymphatic tissue with altered structure:
- caseous epithelioid granulomas
- noncaseous epithelioid granulomas
- focal interstitial fibrosis (scarring)
- dust;
- Newly formed textures without metastasis potential:
- angiomatoid textures
- lymphomatoid textures
- mononuclear inflammatory infiltrates
- hyaline material;
- Newly formed textures with metastasis potential:
- mesenchymal growth pattern
- lymphomatoid textures
- sarcomatous textures
- epithelial textures

▪ *Special stains:* PAS, collagenous stains, Giemsa, and, depending upon the underlying disorder, immunohistochemistry, endogenous lectins, Ziehl-Neelsen, DNA analysis.

Hallmark of Diagnosis: Radiologic findings.

Differential diagnosis: Due to the underlying disorder.

Lymphadenopathy, Angioimmunoblastic

Definition: Alteration of the lung parenchyma associated with angioimmunoblastic lymphadenopathy, see Angioimmunoblastic Lymphadenopathy.

Lymphangiectasis

Definition: Congenital disorder characterized by dilated and increased number of (subpleural) lymphatic vessels.

Incidence/Epidemiology: The incidence of the disorder has been estimated to be 5–15% of all premature infants with a sex ratio of 1.5:1 (males:females). Additional abnormalities are frequent and include asplenia syndrome, cardiovascular abnormalities (septal defects, atrioventricular communication), renal abnormalities, ichthyosis congenita.

Etiology/Pathophysiology: Familial occurrence and increased occurrence with maternal polyhydramnios have been reported. Additional cardiovascular abnormalities suggest lymphomatoid malformation secondary to obstruction of lymphatic drainage. Complications include chylothorax, pleural effusions, pneumothorax, and interstitial pulmonary emphysema. It can be classified into three general categories: (a) primary disorder, (b) secondary disorder associated with cardiovascular abnormalities, and (c) generalized disorder associated with visceral lymphangiomas and hemangiomas.

Clinical Presentation: Infants present with a severe disorder, usually with obstructive cardiovascular lesions.

Prognosis: Primary lymphangiectasis is usually fatal; patients with secondary or generalized lymphangiectasis may survive without serious sequelae.

Radiology: Chest radiographs show dense subpleural areas and prominent interstitial and subpleural lymphatic vessels (Kerley's B lines), a diffuse hyperlucency of the lung parenchyma, and depression of the diaphragm.

Pathology:

Gross: The lungs are overinflated and display a fibrous network of grayish-white vessels of subpleural and peribronchial origin.

Histology: Beneath the pleura, multiple, ectatic, lymphatic vessels are present. The lymphatic vessels are separated from each other by fibrous connective tissue or just by small layers of endothelial cells. Inflammation is weak, and the surrounding lung parenchyma may be immature.

➤ *Descriptors:* Pulmonary vessels with preserved structure:

- ectatic lumen (lymphatic vessels, beneath the pleura)
- tortuous vessels
- fibrosis (between the ectatic lymphatic spaces)

■ *Special stains:* PAS, collagenous stains.

Hallmark of Diagnosis: Multiple, dilated, lymphatic vessels lying beneath the pleura and partly separated by fibrous connective tissue.

Differential diagnosis: Interstitial pulmonary emphysema, infantile lobar emphysema, adenomatoid cystic malformation, angioma.

Lymphangiographic Dyes

Definition: Alteration of the lung parenchyma associated with exposure to lymphangiographic dyes, see Drug Toxicity.

Lymphangioleiomyomatosis

Definition: Uncontrolled proliferation of smooth muscle cells in the lung parenchyma.

Incidence/Epidemiology: Rare disorder seen in young and middle aged women (18–48 years old). Renal angiopathy is seen in 10–20% of patients. All reported cases were women in their reproductive years.

Etiology/Pathophysiology: The etiology is not known. It is considered to be a form of tuberous sclerosis. The lymph nodes are involved in 50–70% of reported cases. The angiomyomatous lesions are found in the central lymph nodes, the thoracic duct, or peripheral lung parenchyma and remain limited to these organ systems. Estrogen receptors in the proliferating smooth muscle cells and elevated estrogen levels in the serum have been reported. (There is evidence that estrogen stimulates the growth of smooth muscle cells).

Clinical Presentation: The symptoms include chylothorax, pneumothorax, increasing shortness of breath, and hemoptysis.

Prognosis: Poor, as progressive pulmonary failure usually causes death after a few years, although prolonged course without progression have been described.

Radiology: Chest radiographs show linear, diffuse, basilar densities, often in bihilar symmetry. In later stages signs of honeycombing with large cysts, overexpanded lungs, flattening of the diaphragm, and fibrotic changes occur.

Pathology:

Gross: The original lung texture is replaced by large cysts of varying size separated by small amounts of healthy lung parenchyma. The pleura is fibrotic, and chylous pleural effusions may be present.

Histology: Numerous, plump, spindle-shaped, smooth muscle cells proliferate around the terminal bronchioles and other centroacinar structures causing complete dissolution of the original lung texture.The lymphatic vessels and the veins are obstructed. The proliferating smooth muscle cells run in bundles and cause cystic dilatation of the lung parenchyma. The nuclei are broadly varied in size and shape. Mitoses are infrequent. Additional infiltrates of histiocytes and fibroblasts may be seen. Within the lymph nodes the proliferating smooth muscle cells derive from the subcapsular sinus and the lymphatic wall and extend from the periphery to the center.

➤ *Descriptors:* Newly formed textures without metastasis potential:

- mesenchymal growth pattern
- fibromatous textures
- smooth muscle cells (proliferating)
- plump spindle cells
- inhomogeneous nuclear and cellular size
- absent or infrequent mitoses
- entrapped air spaces
- mononuclear inflammatory cells
- hemorrhage

■ *Special stains:* PAS, collagenous stains, Masson Goldner, Giemsa, immunohistochemistry for actin, myosin, vimentin, estrogen, progesterone, endogenous lectins, DNA analysis.

Hallmark of Diagnosis: Age and sex of the patient, proliferating smooth muscle cells forming large, irregularly sized cysts.

Differential diagnosis: Interstitial pulmonary fibrosis, adult generalized myofibromatosis, Kaposi's sarcoma, benign metastasizing leiomyoma, leiomyosarcoma.

Lymphangioma

Definition: Benign vascular lesion of the lymphatic vessels.

Incidence/Epidemiology: Rare disorder seen in infants, children, and young to middle-aged adults.

Etiology/Pathophysiology: Neoplastic process of the lymphatic vessels closely associated with hemangioma.

Clinical Presentation: Patients may be asymptomatic or present with chylothorax.

Prognosis: Usually good and without serious sequelae.

Radiology: Chest radiographs show small, peripheral, ill-defined lesions.

Pathology:
Gross: Small, grayish-white, subpleural lesions.

Histology: Beneath the pleura several ectatic lymphatic vessels of highly variable diameter can be seen. The surrounding lung parenchyma may be fibrotic.

➤ *Descriptors:* Newly formed textures without metastasis potential:
- vascular textures (ectatic lymphatic vessels)
- homogeneous nuclear and cellular size
- fibrosis

■ *Special stains:* Collagenous stains, immunohistochemistry for endothelial cells, DNA analysis.

Hallmark of Diagnosis: Cluster of ectatic lymphatic vessels.

Differential diagnosis: Hemangioma, arteriovenous malformation, lymphangioleiomyomatosis.

Lymphangitis Carcinomatosa

Definition: Spread of primary lung carcinoma into the lymphatic vessels of the bronchial submucosa.

Incidence/Epidemiology: The disorder is seen in about 10–20% of primary adenocarcinoma patients and those with small cell anaplastic carcinomas of the lung. Patients with adenoid-cystic carcinoma are at higher risk, and those with epidermoid carcinoma and large cell anaplastic carcinoma are at lower risk.

Etiology/Pathophysiology: Spread of carcinoma cells is seen toward the lymphatic drainage to the central hilar and mediastinal lymph nodes. Lymphangiosis carcinomatosa is of special importance in lung surgery (boundaries of the resected bronchi and arteries).

Clinical Presentation: The bronchial mucosa is often unsuspicious.

Prognosis: Very poor; patients with lymphangiosis carcinomatosa usually suffer from generalized malignancies.

Radiology: Chest radiographs show no specific findings.

Pathology:
Gross: The bronchi may be normal or evidence a thickened submucosa.
Histology: Proliferating carcinoma cells in the submucosal lymphatic and venous vessels.

➤ *Descriptors:* Newly formed textures with metastasis potential:
- epithelial growth pattern
- vascular and pleural invasion

■ *Special stains:* PAS, collagenous stains, immunohistochemistry depending upon the cell type of the carcinoma, DNA analysis.

Hallmark of Diagnosis: Proliferating carcinoma cells in the submucosal lymphatic and venous vessels.

Differential diagnosis: According to the underlying neoplasm, hyperplasia of endothelial cells, crush artifacts of glandular epithelial cells.

Lymphocytic Angiitis and Granulomatosis, Benign

Definition: Benign lymphocytic vasculitis with formation of granulomas.

Incidence/Epidemiology: Unusual disease occurring in young to middle-aged adults with an estimated prevalence of 20–40% of other granulomatous disorders (Wegener's disease, lymphomatoid granulomatosis).

Etiology/Pathophysiology: The etiology is not known. Association with chronic relapsing panniculitis (Weber-Christian disease) has been suggested.

Clinical Presentation: Symptoms include shortness of breath, dyspnea, and malaise.

Prognosis: Usually good, about 60–70% of patients survive for 10–20 years without serious sequelae or recurrence.

Radiology: Chest radiographs show multiple well-defined nodules (80%) or single, circumscribed densities (20%).

Pathology:

Gross: The lungs show dense grayish-white infiltrates of soft consistency.

Histology: The lung parenchyma is erased by dense lymphocytic infiltrates which invade the walls of small and medium-sized arteries and veins. Poorly defined granulomas with giant cells may be present. Coagulative necrosis is associated with the arteries at the center of the lesion. Reed-Sternberg cells, marked cellular atypia, mitoses, necrosis, and the formation of germinal centers are not signs of benign lymphocytic angiitis and granulomatosis.

➤ *Descriptors:* Newly formed textures without metastasis potential:

- mesenchymal growth pattern
- lymphomatoid textures
- vascular and pleural invasion
- lymphoid granulomas (ill-defined)
- multinucleated giant cells (scattered)
- necrosis (coagulative, small areas);
- Bronchial mucosa with altered structure:
- intrabronchiolar fibrinoid material and histiocytes
- ulceration of bronchiolar mucosa

■ *Special stains:* PAS, collagenous stains, Giemsa, immunohistochemistry for lymphocytic subpopulations and immunoglobulins, endogenous lectins, DNA analysis.

Hallmark of Diagnosis: Homogeneous lymphocytic infiltrates with angiitis and formation of poorly defined granulomas.

Differential diagnosis: Wegener's granulomatosis, lymphomatoid granulomatosis, well-differentiated lymphoma, pseudolymphoma, lymphoid interstitial pneumonia, Churg-Strauss syndrome.

Lymphocytic Interstitial Pneumonia

Definition: Chronic interstitial pneumonia with mononuclear inflammatory infiltrates (predominantly lymphocytes).

Incidence/Epidemiology: The disorder is more common in women than in men and is associated with a broad variety of clinical features such as Sjögren's syndrome, nodular lymphoid hyperplasia of the intestines, amyloidosis, drug intake, chronic active hepatitis, agammaglobulinemia, systemic lupus erythematosus, Hashimoto's thyroiditis.

Etiology/Pathophysiology: The etiology is not known. Some authors consider lymphocytic interstitial pneumonia to be a premalignant stage prior to lymphoma.

Clinical Presentation: Symptoms include chronic cough, dyspnea, fever, chest pain and loss of weight.

Prognosis: Fair, about 30% of patients remain stable, but others show progressive respiratory failure with honeycomb lung in the end stage.

Radiology: Chest radiographs show coarse, bibasilar, reticulonodular densities or soft, fluffy infiltrates.

Pathology:

Gross: The lungs show ill-defined, yellowish-tan densities with increased consistency. Honeycombing may be present.

Histology: The interstitial lung parenchyma is densely infiltrated with small lymphocytes, plasma cells, and histiocytes. Occasionally multinucleated giant cells and ill-defined granulomas may be seen. The boundary with healthy lung parenchyma is clear. Older lesions evidence invading fibroblasts and collagen deposits.

➤ *Descriptors:* Lung parenchyma with altered structure:

- mononuclear inflammatory infiltrates
- atypical lymphoid cells
- germinal centers
- unsuspicious pneumocytes

■ *Special stains:* PAS, collagenous stains, Giemsa, immunohistochemistry for lymphocytic subpopulations and immunoglobulins (lymphoid interstitial pneumonia is of polymorphous composition), endogenous lectins, DNA analysis.

Hallmark of Diagnosis: Dense interstitial inflammatory infiltrates composed of lymphocytes, plasma cells, and histiocytes.

Differential diagnosis: Lymphocytic lymphoma, allergic alveolitis, pseudolymphoma, follicular bronchiolitis, angioimmunoblastic lymphadenopathy, lymphoid hyperplasia.

Lymphoid Hyperplasia

Definition: Hyperplasia of lymphatic tissue in the lung.

Incidence/Epidemiology: Frequently seen in association with a broad variety of disorders such as chronic infections, bronchiectasis, cystic fibrosis, pneumoconiosis, and rheumatoid lesions, especially rheumatoid arthritis.

Etiology/Pathophysiology: Chronic infection or inflammation of the lung parenchyma and conducting airways induces follicular hyperplasia, most prominently along the airways and beneath the pleura.

Clinical Presentation: The lesions are asymptomatic.

Prognosis: Good and without known serious sequelae.

Radiology: Chest radiographs show central or (most frequently) peripheral, well-defined densities often resembling primary carcinoma or metastases.

Pathology:

Gross: Grayish-black nodules of soft to firm consistency.

Histology: Well defined nodules consisting of mature lymphocytes, often intermingled with dust-laden macrophages. Fibrosis may be present.

➤ *Descriptors:* Newly formed textures without metastasis potential:

- mesenchymal growth pattern
- lymphomatoid textures
- lymphocytes (mature)
- dust
- macrophages (scattered)
- germinal centers (few)

■ *Special stains:* Giemsa, immunohistochemistry for lymphocytic subpopulations, DNA analysis.

Hallmark of Diagnosis: Well defined lymphocytic infiltrates with germinal centers resembling lymph nodes.

Differential diagnosis: Lymphocytic interstitial pneumonia, pseudolymphoma, angioimmunoblastic lymphadenopathy, lymphoma.

Lymphoma, Angiocentric, Large Cell

Definition: Pulmonary involvement of highly malignant non-Hodgkin's lymphoma associated with angiocentric necrosis, see Angiocentric Large Cell Lymphoma.

Lymphoma of the Lung

Definition: Malignant neoplasm of the lung with characteristic cell type.

Incidence/Epidemiology: About 10% of patients with malignant lymphoma may present with involvement of the lung clinically. They include children and young to middle-aged adults with an equal sex ratio. Risk factors for pulmonary involvement are not known.

Etiology/Pathophysiology: The lymphomas either arise from intrapulmonary lymphatic tissue or are manifest as metastatic intrapulmonary tumor infiltrates.

Clinical Presentation: Most patients are asymptomatic, but some present with malaise, cough, dyspnea, and pulmonary infections.

Prognosis: Depends upon the malignancy grade of the lymphomas, but usually poor. Patients with plasmacytoid differentiation tend to have a prolonged survival and less recurrences.

Radiology: Chest radiographs show diffuse dense infiltrates.

Pathology:

Gross: The lungs are heavy and show areas of grayish-white color and soft consistency.

Histology: The lymphomas may be subclassified as follows: (a) Hodgkin's disease; (b) non-Hodgkin's disease which includes well-differentiated (small cell) lymphoma; mixed cell lymphoma; and large cell lymphoma. Immunohistochemistry subclassifies the above into T-cell and B-cell lymphomas.

➤ *Descriptors:* Newly formed textures with metastasis potential:

- mesenchymal growth pattern

- lymphomatoid textures
- small tumor cells
- large tumor cells
- homogeneous nuclear and cellular size
- inhomogeneous nuclear and cellular size

■ *Special stains:* PAS, collagenous stains, Giemsa, immunohistochemistry for lymphocytic subclassification, immunoglobulins, endogenous lectins, DNA analysis.

Hallmark of Diagnosis: Classification of the lymphoma according to the cell type.

Differential diagnosis: Pseudolymphoma, small cell anaplastic carcinoma, lymphocytic interstitial pneumonia, lymphomatoid granulomatosis.

Lymphomatoid Granulomatosis

Definition: Lymphoproliferative disease belonging to the category of pulmonary angiitis and granulomatosis.

Incidence/Epidemiology: Unusual disease seen more frequently in young to middle-aged adults with a slight predominance in men. Specific risk factors are not known.

Etiology/Pathophysiology: The etiology is not known. The involvement of extrapulmonary organs such as the kidneys, skin, or nervous system suggests association of the disease with malignant reticulosis.

Clinical Presentation: Symptoms include chest pain, chronic cough, shortness of breath, fever, malaise, and loss of weight.

Prognosis: Poor, about 70% of patients die within 2 years after clinical diagnosis.

Radiology: Chest radiographs show multiple, bilateral, well-defined nodules measuring up to several centimeters in diameter.

Pathology:

Gross: The lungs contain multiple, grayish-yellowish, firm, circumscribed masses which may show massive, central, hemorrhagic necrosis.

Histology: The original texture of the lung parenchyma is destroyed by a dense infiltrate consisting of lymphocytes, plasma cells, histiocytes, and atypical lymphoreticular cells resembling immunoblasts. Mixed inflammatory infiltrates can be seen in the walls of smaller arteries and veins. Prominent necrosis may be present. Multinucleated giant cells, epithelioid histiocytes, and eosinophilic granulocytes are not features of lymphomatoid granulomatosis.

➤ *Descriptors:* Lung parenchyma with altered structure:

- mononuclear inflammatory infiltrates
- atypical cells (lymphoid, resembling immunoblasts)
- necrosis and hemorrhage (focal, prominent);
- Pulmonary vessels with preserved structure:
- mixed inflammatory infiltrates (arteries and veins)

■ *Special stains:* PAS, collagenous stains, Giemsa, immunohistochemistry for lymphocytic subpopulations and immunoglobulins, endogenous lectins, DNA analysis.

Hallmark of Diagnosis: Interstitial polymorphous inflammatory infiltrates, atypical lymphoreticular cells (immunoblasts), fibrotic changes.

Differential diagnosis: Malignant lymphoma, necrotizing sarcoid granulomatosis, Wegener's disease, Churg-Strauss syndrome.

Lymphoproliferative Diseases

Definition: Benign and malignant disorders of the lung characterized by abnormal processes of lymphoid tissue.

Incidence/Epidemiology: Unusual diseases seen predominantly in young to middle-aged adults of both sexes.

Etiology/Pathophysiology: The diseases are made up of benign hyperplastic processes of lymphoid tissue (lymphoid hyperplasia, angioimmunoblastic lymphadenopathy, lymphoid interstitial pneumonia, pseudolymphoma, hypersensitivity reaction), malignant neoplasms (Hodgkin's disease, non-Hodgkin's lymphoma, malignant histiocytosis, plasma cell tumor, mycosis fungoides – Sezary's syndrome), and disorders of unknown etiology (lymphomatoid granulomatosis, angiitis, and granulomatous diseases).

Clinical Presentation: Patients are either asymptomatic or present with cough, fever, chest pain, shortness of breath, and dyspnea.

Prognosis: Usually good for hyperplastic disorders, poor for true neoplastic disorders or those with unknown etiology.

Radiology: Most often chest radiographs show multiple, circumscribed densities, and less frequently diffuse, fluffy infiltrates are seen.

Pathology:

Gross: The lungs show multiple, well-defined, grayish-yellowish nodules with varying degrees of honeycombing.

Histology: The lesions are characterized by interstitial inflammatory infiltrates with partial or complete destruction of the original lung texture and with infiltrates destroying the walls of small and medium-sized arteries and veins. Specific alterations of the lung parenchyma are described under their particular headings.

➤ *Descriptors:* Lung parenchyma with altered structure:
- mononuclear inflammatory infiltrates (lymphomatoid)
- necrosis and hemorrhage;
- Pulmonary vessels with preserved structure:
- mixed inflammatory infiltrates
- mononuclear inflammatory infiltrates;
- Newly formed textures without metastasis potential:
- mesenchymal growth pattern
- lymphomatoid textures
- absent or infrequent mitoses
- germinal centers
- absent necrosis;
- Newly formed textures with metastasis potential:
- epithelial growth pattern
- mesenchymal growth pattern
- lymphomatoid textures
- adenoid textures
- epidermoid textures
- solid textures
- frequent mitoses
- necrosis (focal)

■ *Special stains:* PAS, collagenous stains, Giemsa, immunohistochemistry for lymphocytic subpopulations, immunoglobulins, endogenous lectins, DNA analysis.

Hallmark of Diagnosis: Dense interstitial mononuclear infiltrates, morphologic changes such as are described under the particular headings.

Differential diagnosis: Benign and malignant lymphoreticular infiltrates such as are described under the particular headings.

MacLeod Syndrome – Myxoma

MacLeod Syndrome

Definition: Unilateral hyperlucent lung, see Swyer-James Syndrome.

Macroglobulinemia of Waldenström

Definition: Alteration of the lung parenchyma associated with macroglobulinemia of Waldenström.

Incidence/Epidemiology: Patients with macroglobulinemia and pulmonary involvement are between 20 and 75 years old. The sexes are equally involved.

Etiology/Pathophysiology: Pulmonary involvement may occur without metastasis into the hilar or mediastinal lymph nodes. Patients usually present with IgM monoclonal gammopathy or cryoglobulinemia.

Clinical Presentation: The majority of patients are asymptomatic, but some present with cough, dyspnea, loss of weight, and chest pain.

Prognosis: The disease may be slowly progressive or rapidly fatal.

Radiology: Chest radiographs show single or multiple, dense nodules, diffuse interstitial or intraalveolar infiltrates. Cavitation and hilar lymphadenopathy are rare.

Pathology:

Gross: The lungs display single or multiple yellowish-white nodules of soft consistency.

Histology: The lung parenchyma is destroyed by dense homogeneous lymphoplasmacytoid infiltrates spreading from the interalveolar septula into the distant air spaces. Mitoses are rare. Small sclerotic areas and some necrosis may be present.

➤ *Descriptors:* Newly formed textures with metastasis potential:

- mesenchymal growth pattern
- lymphomatoid textures
- small tumor cells (lympho-plasmacytoid)
- homogeneous nuclear and cellular size
- infrequent mitoses
- necrosis (focal)

■ *Special stains:* PAS, collagenous stains, Giemsa, immunohistochemistry for immunoglobulins, lymphocytic subpopulations, endogenous lectins, DNA analysis.

Hallmark of Diagnosis: Clinical history, well-differentiated lymphocytic lymphoma with plasmacytoid differentiation.

Differential diagnosis: Lymphoid interstitial pneumonia, pseudolymphoma, other groups of lymphomas.

Malacoplakia

Definition: Disorder with incomplete function of macrophages.

Incidence/Epidemiology: Unusual disease, most common in the bladder mucosa. Only a few cases with pulmonary involvement have been described.

Etiology/Pathophysiology: Macrophages show a decrease in the ability to digest bacteria, most frequently *Escherichia coli*. However, other gram-positive or gram-negative bacteria or mycobacteria may be involved. The disorder is most frequently seen in immunocompromised patients.

Clinical Presentation: Patients are usually asymptomatic but may present with cough, chest pain, or shortness of breath during exercise.

Prognosis: Usually fair, depending upon the underlying disorder.

Radiology: Chest radiographs show either single or multiple dense nodules in the peripheral lung parenchyma.

Pathology:

Gross: The nodules are yellowish in color and soft in consistency and may show necrosis.

Histology: The original lung texture is preserved. The distant air spaces and interstitial tissue are filled with foamy macrophages. Some of them contain Michaelis-Gutmann bodies which are intracytoplasmic round to oval inclusion bodies measuring 3–20 μm. They stain positively with Prussian blue and calcium stains and often display a halo.

➤ *Descriptors:* Lung parenchyma with preserved structure:

- macrophages (foamy, inclusion bodies)

■ *Special stains:* PAS, collagenous stains, Prussian blue, calcium stains, Gram's (for intracytoplasmic bacteria), endogenous lectins, electron microscopy.

Hallmark of Diagnosis: Foamy, granular macrophages with Michaelis-Gutmann bodies, bacteria ingested by histiocytes, and preserved texture of the lung parenchyma.

Differential diagnosis: Endogenous lipid pneumonia, Whipple's disease, infection with *Mycobacterium avium intracellulare*, Niemann-Pick disease, Gaucher's disease, other storage disorders.

Malaria

Definition: Alteration of the lung parenchyma associated with infection by *Plasmodium falciparum, vivax, ovale*, and *malariae*.

Incidence/Epidemiology: Falciparum malaria is limited to tropical countries whereas vivax malaria has a worldwide distribution. Plasmodium malariae was once common in Europe (Italy). Ovale malaria has been reported from Africa and Vietnam. The number of infected persons amounts to 1–2 millions.

Etiology/Pathophysiology: Malaria is transmitted from person to person by female *Anopheles* mosquitoes. The mosquito becomes infected by sucking blood containing the sexual forms of the parasites (micro- and macrogametocytes). The sexual life cycle within the mosquito produces ookinetes and motile sporozoites living near and in the salivary glands of the mosquito. In man the sporozoites enter the liver and change into merozoites which then multiply in the erythrocytes. Approximately 5–10% of patients infected with *Plasmodium falciparum* develop an acute (severe) respiratory distress syndrome.

Clinical Presentation: The disorder starts abruptly with shortness of breath and circumoral cyanosis 2–3 days after onset of malarial chills and fever. The disorder usually displays dramatic deterioration involving dyspnea and cyanosis, leading to death within a couple of days.

Prognosis: Usually fatal within a few days.

Radiology: Chest radiographs show patchy, diffuse densities in the lower lobes and interstitial markings in the upper lobes suggesting severe edema.

Pathology:

Gross: The lungs are wet, edematous and heavy and may show focal, intrapulmonary hemorrhage and pleural and pericardial effusions.

Histology: The interalveolar septula are thickened and edematous and contain trophozoites. The distant air spaces are filled with macrophages containing malarial pigment and an edematous transudate. Hyaline membranes and multinucleated giant cells may be seen.

➤ *Descriptors:* Lung parenchyma with preserved structure:

- interstitial edema
- infectious organisms (trophozoites)
- macrophages (malarial pigment)
- hyaline membranes
- multinucleated giant cells

■ *Special stains:* PAS, collagenous stains, Prussian blue.

Hallmark of Diagnosis: Clinical history, severe pulmonary edema, identification of trophozoites in the interalveolar septula.

Differential diagnosis: Adult respiratory distress syndrome due to other reasons (drug reaction).

Malformation

Definition: Congenital abnormalities of the lung parenchyma, see Congenital Abnormalities.

Malt Worker's Lung

Definition: Alteration of the lung parenchyma associated with exposure to malt dust.

Incidence/Epidemiology: Rare disorder most frequently seen in persons susceptible to a hypersensitivity reaction.

Etiology/Pathophysiology: Dust of malt products may induce a hypersensitivity reaction of the lung.

Clinical Presentation: Symptoms are related either to acute or chronic onset of a hypersensitivity reaction and include cough, shortness of breath, dyspnea, and malaise.

Prognosis: Usually good and without serious sequelae.

Radiology: Chest radiographs show diffuse bilateral densities or may be normal.

Pathology:

Gross: The lungs are wet and heavy and may show edematous and fibrinoid areas.

Histology: The histomorphological changes include intraalveolar and interstitial edema, hyperplasia and hypertrophy of cells of the alveolar lining and formation of granulomas as described under the heading Allergic (Extrinsic) Alveolitis.

➤ *Descriptors:* Lung parenchyma with altered structure:
- noncaseous epithelioid granulomas
- eosinophils
- multinucleated giant cells
- intrabronchiolar fibrinoid material and histiocytes
- ulceration of bronchiolar mucosa;
- Lung parenchyma with preserved structure:
- macrophages
- desquamation, hypertrophy, hyperplasia and dysplasia of pneumocytes
- mononuclear inflammatory infiltrates
- intraalveolar serous fluid

■ *Special stains:* PAS, collagenous stains, Giemsa, endogenous lectins.

Hallmark of Diagnosis: Clinical history, histomorphological findings of allergic extrinsic alveolitis.

Differential diagnosis: Acute respiratory distress syndrome, bronchioloalveolar carcinoma, desquamative interstitial pneumonia, usual interstitial pneumonia, allergic alveolitis due to the underlying agent.

Mammomonogamiasis

Definition: Alteration of the lung parenchyma associated with infection by *Mammomonogamus laryngeus.*

Incidence/Epidemiology*:* The disease is endemic in the Caribbean Islands, Guyana, Brazil, and the Philippines. About 100 human infections have been reported.

Etiology/Pathophysiology: Humans are infected through an unknown association with cattle, probably by eating infected food. The worms are in male/female pairs located within the throat. Their eggs may be recognized in the sputum.

Clinical Presentation: The worms provoke violent symptoms including cough, asthmatic complaints, and malaise.

Prognosis: Usually good.

Radiology: Chest radiographs are usually normal or may reflect dysatelectatic signs.

Pathology:

Gross: The worms, measuring 3 mm in length by 0.5 mm in width or up to 10 mm in length by 0.7 mm in width, can be identified in the throat.

Histology: The worms lie in pairs and may be accompanied by severe inflammation involving lymphocytes, plasma cells, and eosinophilic granulocytes.

➤ *Descriptors:* Lung parenchyma with altered structure:
- parasites (pairs, in the throat)
- mixed inflammatory infiltrates
- eosinophils

■ *Special stains:* PAS, Giemsa, Movat.

Hallmark of Diagnosis: Clinical history, parasites in the throat (pairs), identification of the worms.

Differential diagnosis: Infections by other parasites, especially hookworms.

Manganese Fumes

Definition: Alteration of the lung parenchyma associated with inhalation of manganese fumes.

Incidence/Epidemiology*:* Manganese is used in steel hardening processes and is incorporated into bronze. Manganese oxide, which is mined in various countries, is used as a bleaching agent and oxidizing salt. Persons working in mines and manganese mills may be exposed to poisoning concentrations of manganese oxide or permanganate. Acute intoxications are rare.

Etiology/Pathophysiology: Inhaled manganese particles will reach the distant air spaces and induce a mild to moderate interstitial pneumonitis. They will be ingested by macrophages, and the inflammatory reaction usually disappears after several weeks. Interstitial fibrosis is absent or mild. Manganese has – if at all – a low fibrinogenic potency.

Clinical Presentation: The symptoms include shortness of breath, cough, dyspnea, and fever.

Prognosis: Usually good, but mild fibrotic changes of the lung can remain.

Radiology: Chest radiographs show diffuse interstitial densities or are normal.

Pathology:

Gross: The lungs are heavy, wet and brownish-red in acute intoxications.

Histology: The distant air spaces contain numerous mononuclear inflammatory infiltrates and dust-laden macrophages. The cells of the alveolar lining display hyperplasia and hypertrophy.

➤ *Descriptors:* Lung parenchyma with preserved structure:

- mononuclear inflammatory infiltrates
- macrophages (dust laden)

■ *Special stains:* PAS, Prussian blue, collagenous stains, X-ray diffraction or related techniques for identification of manganese.

Hallmark of Diagnosis: Clinical history, (desquamative) interstitial pneumonitis, identification of manganese.

Differential diagnosis: Acute intoxication of the lung due to other agents, desquamative interstitial pneumonia, allergic (extrinsic) alveolitis.

Mansonellosis

Definition: Infection of the lung with the filarial nematode *Mansonella ozzardi*.

Incidence/Epidemiology*:* Infection of humans with *Mansonella ozzardi* is endemic in Guyana, northern Argentina, the Amazon region, and Central America.

Etiology/Pathophysiology: The parasite is well adapted to man and lives in the thoracic and peritoneal region and within the lymphatics. It is transferred by insect vectors (species of *Culicoides* and *Simulium*).

Clinical Presentation: The parasite seldom causes symptoms which, when they do appear, may include itchy, cutaneous plaques, mild fever, eosinophilia, headache, slight vertigo, or pleural effusions.

Prognosis: Usually good and without serious sequelae.

Radiology: Chest radiographs are usually normal or may show pleural effusions.

Pathology:

Gross: The parasites measure about 70 mm in length by 0.2 mm in width and are rarely encountered.

Histology: The microfilariae may be seen in peripheral blood capillaries which usually show a granulomatous inflammatory infiltrate.

➤ *Descriptors:* Lung parenchyma with altered structure:

- noncaseous epithelioid granulomas
- necrosis and hemorrhage (focal)
- mixed inflammatory infiltrates
- eosinophils;
- Pulmonary vessels with altered structure:
- noncaseous epithelioid granulomas
- parasites (capillaries, small arteries, and veins)
- mixed inflammatory infiltrates

■ *Special stains:* PAS, collagenous stains, Movat, Giemsa.

Hallmark of Diagnosis: Clinical history, identification of microfilariae in the peripheral capillaries.

Differential diagnosis: Infection with other nematodes, granulomatous inflammation due to other agents.

Maple Bark Stripper's Lung

Definition: Alteration of the lung parenchyma associated with exposure to maple bark.

Incidence/Epidemiology*:* Unusual disorder seen in some persons working with maple bark.

Etiology/Pathophysiology: Exposure to maple bark may induce a hypersensitivity reaction of the lung. The specific etiologic agent has been identified as spores of *Cryptostroma corticale*.

Clinical Presentation: Symptoms are related either to an acute or chronic form of the disease and include high fever, cough, chest pain, and dyspnea.

Prognosis: Usually good; however, prolonged courses may occur.

Radiology: Chest radiographs show diffuse, soft, interstitial infiltrates in both lungs.

Pathology:

Gross: The lungs are heavy and of increased consistency.

Histology: The causative organisms can be identified in the cytoplasm of histiocytes and macrophages, which contains 3–5 μm brown, ovoid, thick-walled, intracytoplasmic inclusions. Formation of epithelioid granulomas and bronchiolitis obliterans is frequent.

➤ *Descriptors:* Lung parenchyma with altered structure:
- noncaseous epithelioid granulomas
- eosinophils
- multinucleated giant cells
- intrabronchiolar fibrinoid material and histiocytes
- ulceration of bronchiolar mucosa;
- Lung parenchyma with preserved structure:
- macrophages
- desquamation, hypertrophy, hyperplasia and dysplasia of pneumocytes
- mononuclear inflammatory infiltrates
- intraalveolar serous fluid

■ *Special stains:* PAS, collagenous stains, Giemsa.

Hallmark of Diagnosis: Clinical history, allergic extrinsic alveolitis with intracytoplasmic inclusions of spores of *Cryptostroma corticale*.
Differential diagnosis: Usual interstitial pneumonia, sarcoidosis, bronchiolitis obliterans, allergic extrinsic alveolitis due to other agents.

Mazzotti Reaction

Definition: Sensitive diagnostic test in onchocerciasis and streptocerciasis (filariasis). Intake of 50 mg diethylcarbamazine (DEC) by mouth produces erythema and pruritus within a few hours (positive test), see Filariasis.

Measles

Definition: Alteration of the lung parenchyma associated with infection by the measles virus.
Incidence/Epidemiology: Pneumonic changes of the lung parenchyma associated with measles virus infection is a rare disorder seen in young children and infants with damaged lung parenchyma (mucoviscidosis) and in immunocompromised children and adults (kwashiorkor, acute leukemia, renal transplants, etc.). A skin rash can usually be seen prior to onset of the viral pneumonia.
Etiology/Pathophysiology: The virus invades respiratory epithelial cells and induces necrosis and desquamation.
Clinical Presentation: The viral pneumonia can be severe, with dyspnea, high fever, malaise, and cough.
Prognosis: Progressive measles syndrome arising in immunocompromised patients is often fatal.
Radiology: Chest radiographs show diffuse, bilateral, interstitial infiltrates with some areas of consolidation.

Pathology:
Gross: The lungs are heavy and red-brown or may contain consolidated areas with red-grayish color and small foci of hemorrhage and increased, meaty consistency.

Histology: The histomorphologic changes result in necrosis of epithelial bronchoalveolar cells and interalveolar septula, dense infiltrates of lymphocytes and plasma cells into the interalveolar and interlobar septula, formation of hyaline membranes in the distant airways, and the presence of multinucleated giant cells. The giant cells also contain eosinophilic, Feulgen-negative, intranuclear and intracytoplasmic inclusions. Healing areas contain infiltrates of histiocytes and macrophages and a resolution of hyaline membranes.

➤ *Descriptors:* Lung parenchyma with preserved structure:
- hemorrhage
- degeneration of pneumocytes
- hyaline membranes
- mononuclear inflammatory infiltrates
- multinucleated giant cells
- inclusion bodies (intracytoplasmic)

■ *Special stains:* PAS, collagenous stains, Giemsa and immunofluorescence for demonstration of the measles virus.

Hallmark of Diagnosis: Clinical history, necrotizing lymphocytic pneumonia with multinucleated giant cells.

Differential diagnosis: Pneumonia caused by other viruses, desquamative interstitial pneumonia, giant cell interstitial pneumonia, usual interstitial pneumonia, lymphoid interstitial pneumonia.

Mecamylamine

Definition: Alteration of the lung parenchyma associated with intake of mecamylamine, see Drug Toxicity.

Meconium Aspiration

Definition: Alteration of the lung parenchyma due to aspiration of meconium.

Incidence/Epidemiology: Unusual disease seen in infants with perinatal stress.

Etiology/Pathophysiology: The infant passes meconium into the amniotic fluid and aspirates it with respiratory movements. Meconium aspiration is usually seen in full-term infants.

Clinical Presentation: The skin, larynx, trachea, and the main bronchi of the infants are covered with green mucoid meconium which causes severe respiratory distress syndrome, pneumothorax and quite high mortality.

Prognosis: Depending upon the amount of aspirated meconium, the mortality may be 50% or more.

Radiology: Chest radiographs show patchy, diffuse densities, air trapping, and signs of pneumothorax.

Pathology:

Gross: The lungs are soft in consistency and silver-green. The major bronchi are obliterated by green meconium.

Histology: The proximal and distant airways are obliterated by green meconium and viscous mucus containing desquamated epithelial cells. Additional bacterial superinfection may be present.

➤ *Descriptors:* Bronchial mucosa with preserved structure:

- meconium
- ulceration
- desquamation, hypertrophy, hyperplasia and dysplasia of epithelial cells
- mixed inflammatory infiltrates

■ *Special stains:* PAS, collagenous stains, Giemsa.

Hallmark of Diagnosis: Clinical history, macroscopic findings, obliteration of the conducting airways by mucus and meconium.

Differential diagnosis: Bronchopulmonary dysplasia, bacterial pneumonia, mucoviscidosis.

Mediastinitis, Sclerosing

Definition: Chronic aggressive fibrosis of mediastinal structures.

Incidence/Epidemiology: Rare disease affecting more women than men.

Etiology/Pathophysiology: The etiology of the disease is not known.

Clinical Presentation: Symptoms include shortness of breath, progressive dyspnea, and obstruction of the upper cephalic arteries and veins.

Prognosis: Poor, as most patients present with progressive respiratory failure and progressive obstruction of the upper cephalic arteries and veins.

Radiology: Chest radiographs show an enlargement and broadening of the mediastinum.

Pathology:

Gross: The mediastinal structures are gray and firm to hard in consistency.

Histology: The mediastinal structures are destroyed by proliferating fibroblasts, histiocytes, and deposits of collagen fibers. Scattered mononuclear inflammatory infiltrates are present.

➤ *Descriptors:* Lung parenchyma (mediastinum) with altered structure:

- diffuse interstitial fibrosis
- proliferating fibroblasts
- mononuclear inflammatory infiltrates
- absent necrosis

■ *Special stains:* PAS, Giemsa, collagenous stains, immunohistochemistry for lymphocytic subpopulations and immunoglobulins.

Hallmark of Diagnosis: Clinical history, severe fibrous inflammation of the mediastinum.

Differential diagnosis: Hodgkin's disease of sclerosing type, histiocytic lymphoma.

Mefenamic Acid

Definition: Alteration of the lung parenchyma associated with intake of mefenamic acid, see Drug Toxicity.

Meglumine Diatrizoate

Definition: Alteration of the lung parenchyma associated with intake of diatrizoate meglumine, see Drug Toxicity.

Melanoma

Definition: Malignant tumor in the lung with characteristic histomorphological appearance.

Incidence/Epidemiology: Primary pulmonary melanoma is a rare malignancy. The majority of intrapulmonary melanomas are metastases, and a detailed confirmation of the primary localization is often an impossible task.

Etiology/Pathophysiology: Melanomas of the main bronchi may arise from neuroendocrine cells of the mucosa.

Clinical Presentation: Symptoms are related to the localization of the melanoma and include cough, dyspnea, hemoptysis, or nonspecific findings.

Prognosis: Poor, similar to that of patients with bronchial carcinomas.

Radiology: Chest radiographs show either peripherally localized, circumscribed densities or centrally located tumor masses.

Pathology:

Gross: The tumors are firm in consistency and either grayish-white or dark brown.

Histology: The majority of centrally localized melanomas contain heavily pigmented, atypical melanocytes which may show numerous mitoses. Peripheral melanomas are usually composed of large, amelanotic tumor cells with irregularly formed nuclei. Prominent nucleoli and diffuse tumor spread with complete destruction of the interstitial lung parenchyma are usually present.

➤ *Descriptors:* Newly formed textures with metastasis potential:
- mesenchymal growth pattern
- solid textures
- large tumor cells (melanin pigment)
- prominent nucleoli
- frequent mitoses
- inhomogeneous nuclear and cellular size
- micrometastases
- absent or weak inflammatory infiltrates

■ *Special stains:* PAS, collagenous stains, Giemsa, Prussian blue, Fontana Masson's stain for melanin, immunohistochemistry for neuroendocrine and melanoma markers, S-100 protein, DNA analysis.

Hallmark of Diagnosis: Clinical history, poorly differentiated or anaplastic malignoma, demonstration of melanin pigment in tumor cells.

Differential diagnosis: Undifferentiated large cell carcinoma, large cell lymphoma, undifferentiated sarcoma.

Melioidosis

Definition: Infection of the lung with *Pseudomonas pseudomallei*.

Incidence/Epidemiology: Chronic infections of the lung have been reported in persons living in or visiting southeast Asia, including the Philippines, Vietnam, and Malaysia, where the disease is endemic.

Etiology/Pathophysiology: The bacteria are present in endemic areas and infection does only limited damage in healthy persons. A long latent period before clinical onset of the disease is characteristic.

Clinical Presentation: Symptoms include those of either acute septicemia with dyspnea, high fever, and chest pain or a chronic disorder with progressive shortness of breath and abscesses of the skin and visceral organs (liver, lung, kidneys).

Prognosis: Usually good if no septicemia occurs. About 50% of patients with melioidosis septicemia have a fatal outcome.

Radiology: Chest radiographs show multiple, small densities in the upper lobes suggesting microabscesses.

Pathology:

Gross: The lungs display multiple small grayish-red nodules in the upper lobes measuring a few millimeters in diameter.

Histology: The original lung texture is destroyed and replaced by neutrophilic and eosinophilic granulocytes, lymphocytes, plasma cells, macrophages, fibrin, debris, and hemorrhage. The bacteria which stain positively with Giemsa and Gram's stain may be seen in macrophages.

➤ *Descriptors:* Lung parenchyma with altered structure:
- necrosis and hemorrhage
- mixed inflammatory infiltrates
- bacteria (gram-positive)
- macrophages (gram-positive bacteria)

■ *Special stains:* PAS, collagenous stains, Giemsa, Gram's stain, immunofluorescence.

Hallmark of Diagnosis: Clinical history, hemorrhagic microabscesses in the upper lobes, identification of the bacteria.
Differential diagnosis: Abscessing pneumonia due to other infectious agents.

Melphalan

Definition: Alteration of the lung parenchyma associated with intake of melphalan, see Drug Toxicity.

Mendelson's Syndrome

Definition: Clinical findings (cough, cyanosis, shock, hypoxemia, etc.) in patients with gastric acid aspiration, see Acid Gastric Aspiration.

Mephenesin

Definition: Alteration of the lung parenchyma associated with intake of mephenesin, see Drug Toxicity.

Mephenytoin

Definition: Alteration of the lung parenchyma associated with intake of mephenytoin, see Drug Toxicity.

Mercaptopurine

Definition: Alteration of the lung parenchyma associated with intake of mercaptopurine, see Drug Toxicity.

Mercury Fumes

Definition: Alteration of the lung parenchyma due to inhalation of mercury fumes.
Incidence/Epidemiology: Rare disease seen in persons working with metallic mercury and in persons working with organic compounds of mercury.
Etiology/Pathophysiology: Inhalation of sufficient amounts of mercury induces severe pulmonary damage affecting the conducting and distant airways.
Clinical Presentation: Symptoms develop after a few hours of intoxication and include dyspnea, cough, and fever.
Prognosis: Fair, as slow progressive respiratory failure is seen after survival of severe acute intoxications.
Radiology: Chest radiographs show diffuse patchy densities, interstitial emphysema, and pneumothorax. Later stages show consolidated areas and signs of interstitial fibrosis.
Pathology:
Gross: The lungs are edematous, heavy, and soft in consistency.
Histology: Early lesions show a marked intraalveolar and interstitial edema, necrosis of the bronchioles and cells of the alveolar lining, and desquamated pneumocytes. Later stages show agglutination of fibroblasts, histiocytes, macrophages, formation of hyaline membranes, deposits of collagen, and interstitial fibrosis. The end stage may be partial resolution and honeycombing.

➤ *Descriptors:* Lung parenchyma with preserved structure:
- interstitial edema
- degeneration of pneumocytes
- desquamation, hypertrophy, hyperplasia and dysplasia of pneumocytes
- mononuclear inflammatory infiltrates
- hyaline membranes;
- Lung parenchyma with altered structure:
- necrosis (bronchioles)
- proliferating fibroblasts
- diffuse interstitial fibrosis
- honeycombing

■ *Special stains:* PAS, collagenous stains, Giemsa, endogenous lectins, X-ray diffraction and related physical techniques.

Hallmark of Diagnosis: Clinical history, adult respiratory distress syndrome, identification of mercury in the distant airways.
Differential diagnosis: Adult respiratory distress syndrome due to other agents.

Mesenchymal Tumors

Definition: Benign and malignant tumors of the lung of mesenchymal origin.

Incidence/Epidemiology: Malignant mesenchymal tumors of the lung are rare, and metastatic tumor growth must be excluded. Malignant mesenchymal tumors can be classified into various forms of sarcomas (fibro-, leiomyo-, rhabdomyo-, neuro-, osteo-, chondro-, lipo-, angio-, epithelioid hemangio-), fibrous histiocytoma, Kaposi's sarcoma. They usually occur in children or in young to middle aged adults. Associated risk factors (except AIDS for Kaposi's sarcoma) have not been identified.
Benign mesenchymal tumors of the lung are more common and include hamartomas, leiomyomas, fibromas, fibromyxomas, myxomas, lipomas, neurofibromas (nerve sheath tumors), hemangiopericytomas.

Etiology/Pathophysiology: The tumors are related to the corresponding intrapulmonary structures. Hamartomas are considered to be a tumorlike malformation and are the most common benign tumor of the lung.

Clinical Presentation: Symptoms are related to the localization of the tumors. Patients may be asymptomatic cr present with cough, dyspnea and chest pain.

Prognosis: Patients with benign mesenchymal tumors usually have a good prognosis without serious sequelae, but those with malignant mesenchymal tumors have a poor prognosis, usually worse than that of patients with bronchial carcinomas.

Radiology: Chest radiographs show circumscribed dense nodules.

Pathology:

Gross: The lungs display dense, circumscribed, grayish-white nodules which are soft in consistency in malignant tumors (and may reveal hemorrhage) or solid and bony in consistency in benign tumors (especially hamartomas).

Histology: The tumors are classified according to their tumor cell population which is described under their particular headings. Differentiation between benign and malignant lesions may be difficult. Features indicating malignant tumor growth are tumor size (greater than 3 cm in maximum diameter), the presence of necrotic areas, marked inflammatory response of host tissue, and numerous mitoses.

➤ *Descriptors:* Newly formed textures without metastasis potential:

- mesenchymal growth pattern
- solid textures
- homogeneous nuclear and cellular size
- absent or infrequent mitoses
- absent necrosis;
- Newly formed textures with metastasis potential:
- mesenchymal growth pattern
- sarcomatous textures
- frequent mitoses
- inhomogeneous nuclear and cellular size
- necrosis and hemorrhage

■ *Special stains:* PAS, collagenous stains, Giemsa, immunohistochemistry for mesenchymal markers such as vimentin, desmin, desmoplakin, actin, myoglobulin, neurofilaments, S-100 protein, DNA analysis, endogenous lectins (especially heparin).

Hallmark of Diagnosis: Proliferating mesenchymal cells.

Differential diagnosis: As described under the particular headings.

Mesenchymoma

Definition: Neoplasms of the lung with various degrees of malignancy derived from the mesenchyma, see Mesenchymal Tumors.

Mesothelioma

Definition: Benign or malignant neoplasm derived from the serosa cells of the pleura, pericardium, and peritoneal cavity.

Incidence/Epidemiology: Rare tumor accounting for less than 1% of all cancer deaths in the Western hemisphere. It has an increasing incidence in the Western countries due to its close association with exposure of patients to asbestos. The incidence is estimated to be 2–4/100 000 in men and 0.5–1.5/100 000 in women. It occurs most frequently in middle-aged men and women (40–60 years old). However, it has also been reported in children. The neoplasms arise 15–25 years after exposure to asbestos. In addition, other agents and occupations have been associated with an increased risk for the development of mesothelioma, including mineral fibers (erionite), nickel, beryllium, radiation, organic chemicals (silicone, ethylene oxide, stilbestrol, mineral oil, liquid paraffin), viruses, chronic inflammation (tuberculous pleuritis, familial Mediterranean fever, recurrent lung infections), workers in the ship, petrochemical, stone cutting, fiberglass, nickel, copper, rubber, leather, textile, and glass industries.

Etiology/Pathophysiology: The etiology of mesothelioma is not known. The association with exposure to asbestos has been confirmed by various studies. However, a close dose-response relationship could not be derived. The asbestos bodies and asbestos fibers are usually found within the distant airways of the lung parenchyma and not within the pleural tissue. The majority of mesotheliomas arise from the parietal pleura and not from the visceral pleura. It has been suggested that the physical properties of asbestos fibers (length-to-width ratio) are of importance for the development of mesotheliomas and that the commercial amphiboles, crocidolite and amosite, are more carcinogenic than chrysotile. In addition, a familial risk of developing mesothelioma has been suggested. About 20% of patients with mesothelioma have no history of associated risk factors.

Clinical Presentation: The neoplasms occur either as a single, solid nodule or as diffuse, pleural tumor growth. Symptoms include chest pain, dyspnea, pleural effusion, cough, and loss of weight.

Prognosis: Poor for patients with diffuse mesotheliomas, the median survival after clinical manifestation is less than 1 year. Curative resections are extremely rare. Patients with benign localized mesotheliomas have a good prognosis without known sequelae or recurrent tumors.

Radiology: Chest radiographs show either a solid tumor mass within the pleural cavity or a diffuse thickening of the pleura with effusion. Solid mesotheliomas usually appear in the middle parts of the pleura whereas the diffuse mesotheliomas are most often seen in the lower parts.

Pathology:

Gross: The neoplasms can be classified into solid and diffuse tumors according to their macroscopic features. Diffuse mesotheliomas are always malignant. Localized mesotheliomas may be malignant or benign. The tumors have a grayish-yellowish color, are solid or soft in consistency, and spread along the pleural cavity. The lung parenchyma is usually atelectatic and meaty in consistency. Solid mesotheliomas resemble fibromas or histiocytomas.

Histology: The histomorphologic structures of mesothelioma range widely. The tumors can be classified into epithelial or mixed mesothelioma and fibrous or sarcomatous mesothelioma. Epithelial mesotheliomas grow in adenoid patterns forming tubular and papillar structures surrounded by a single layer of large to medium-sized tumor cells. Solid growth patterns are present in addition. Mitoses are found infrequently, and a relation to small lymphatic or venous vessels is not found. In addition, various numbers of spindle tumor cells resembling fibroblasts or histiocytes are present. The nuclei contain prominent nucleoli. Fibrous mesotheliomas are composed of large polygonal to plump spindle cells growing in sarcomatous textures. Bundles of anisotropic tumor cell clusters are usually observed. The inflammatory response of host tissue may be impressive in both types of mesothelioma. Small necrotic areas are present.

➤ *Descriptors:* Newly formed textures without metastasis potential:
- mesenchymal growth pattern
- fibromatous textures
- plump spindle cells
- absent or infrequent mitoses
- homogeneous nuclear and cellular size
- absent necrosis;
- Newly formed textures with metastasis potential:
- mesenchymal growth pattern
- epithelial growth pattern
- sarcomatous textures
- adenoid textures (tubuli and papillae)
- solid textures
- large tumor cells
- plump spindle cells
- lining of tumor cells (epithelial tumor cells)
- homogeneous nuclear and cellular size
- prominent nucleoli
- infrequent mitoses
- necrosis (small areas)

■ *Special stains:* PAS (with and without digestion; mesotheliomas are usually negative to PAS or contain digestible glycogen which is, however, also present in metastatic adenocarcinoma of the lung), Hale's colloidal iron stain or alcian blue (for demonstration of hyaluronic acid, for which about 20% of mesotheliomas are positive), Giemsa, collagenous stains, electron microscopy for demonstration of microvilli, immunohistochemistry for vimentin, cytokeratin, epithelial membrane antigen (EMA), S-100 protein, carcinoembryonic antigen (CEA), human epithelium-specific antigen (HEA-125), DNA analysis, syntactic structure analysis, endogenous lectins (GlcNAc).

Hallmark of Diagnosis: Clinical history, macroscopic findings, histological features of sarcomatous structures or of adenomatoid patterns with tubular and papillar textures, monolayers of tumor cells, immunohistochemistry (negative for CEA, EMA), syntactic structure analysis, electron microscopy.

Differential diagnosis: Metastatic adenocarcinoma into the pleura, metastatic sarcoma into the pleura.

Metal Fumes

Definition: Alteration of the lung parenchyma associated with exposure to metal fumes.

Incidence/Epidemiology: Chronic exposure has been reported in a few cases. Industrial accidents are the common cause of exposure.

Etiology/Pathophysiology: Inhalation of compounds containing fumes of heavy metals such as cadmium, mercury, or zinc induce acute damage of the lung parenchyma which may become chronic inflammation and interstitial fibrosis in survivors. Inhalation of welding fumes, aluminum fumes, or metal fumes associated with silica from sandblasting may induce acute pulmonary alveolar proteinosis.

Clinical Presentation: Symptoms include dyspnea, chest pain, and cough.

Prognosis: Fair, as slow progressive respiratory failure is the usual course.

Radiology: Chest radiographs show diffuse, bilateral, patchy densities.

Pathology:

Gross: The lungs are edematous, heavy, and reddish-gray. Late stages show honeycombing and centrilobular emphysema.

Histology: Acute stages show interstitial and intraalveolar edema, hyaline membranes, desquamation and necrosis of cells of the alveolar lining, and interstitial inflammation. Late stages reveal interstitial fibrosis, centrilobular emphysema, and destruction of the original lung texture with honeycombing.

➤ *Descriptors:* Lung parenchyma with preserved structure:

- intraalveolar serous fluid
- interstitial edema
- degeneration of pneumocytes
- desquamation, hypertrophy, hyperplasia and dysplasia of pneumocytes
- mononuclear inflammatory infiltrates
- hyaline membranes;
- Lung parenchyma with altered structure:
- necrosis (bronchioles)
- proliferating fibroblasts
- diffuse interstitial fibrosis
- honeycombing

■ *Special stains:* PAS, collagenous stains, Giemsa, X-ray diffraction and related physical techniques, endogenous lectins.

Hallmark of Diagnosis: Clinical history, acute alveolar damage, interstitial fibrosis, identification of metal deposits.

Differential diagnosis: Acute alveolar damage or diffuse interstitial fibrosis due to other agents.

Metaraminol

Definition: Alteration of the lung parenchyma associated with intake of metaraminol, see Drug Toxicity.

Metastases into the Lung

Definition: Growth of intrapulmonary neoplasms arising from extrapulmonary organs.

Incidence/Epidemiology: About 20–80% of all malignant neoplasms metastasize into the lung in the terminal stage of the disease. Surgical treatment of intrapulmonary metastases can be performed in 20–60% of young and middle-aged adults, inducing partial or complete remission. The risk of developing intrapulmonary metastases increases with increasing size of the primary tumor (TNM-stage). Intrapulmonary metastases of various malignancies (including colorectal carcinomas) can develop without or prior to intrahepatic metastases.

Etiology/Pathophysiology: Metastases into the lung arise from tumor spread via the lymphatic, venous, and arterial vessels. The majority of patients with metastatic tumor growth present with a solitary or only a few isolated tumor nodules. Diffuse intrapulmonary metastatic tumor spread has been noted in 20–40% of tumor patients. Metastases arising from renal carcinomas, bladder carcinomas, uterine carcinomas, and colon carcinomas are frequently seen in hilar and proximal intrapulmonary lymph nodes associated with major bronchi. These tumors may simulate primary bronchial carcinomas.

Clinical Presentation: Pulmonary symptoms depend upon the localization of the metastases. Patients may be asymptomatic or present with cough, malaise, dyspnea, and/or hemoptysis.

Prognosis: Poor; the median survival is 1–3 years after clinical manifestation.

Radiology: Chest radiographs show solitary or multiple densities within the lung parenchyma. A notable number of metastases are located in the subpleural lung parenchyma.

Pathology:

Gross: The lungs contain a solitary nodule or multiple, circumscribed, grayish-white densities, often with central hemorrhagic necrosis and soft in consistency.

Histology: The intrapulmonary metastases of sarcomas frequently differ in their microscopic appearance from the primary. They grow in undifferentiated structures and are composed of plump spindle cells. Metastases of carcinomas may be indistinguishable from primary lung carcinoma. They are frequently highly differentiated tumors, especially metastases from the colon and uterus. Intrapulmonary metastases usually grow without detectable inflammatory response of host tissue, as opposed to primary lung carcinomas.

➤ *Descriptors:* Newly formed textures with metastasis potential:

- sarcomatous growth pattern
- epithelial growth pattern
- inhomogeneous nuclear and cellular size
- micrometastases
- absent inflammatory infiltrates

■ *Special stains:* PAS, Giemsa, immunohistochemistry depending upon the cell type, DNA analysis, syntactic structure analysis, endogenous lectins (metastases usually possess binding capacity to heparin, in contrast to primary bronchial carcinomas).

Hallmark of Diagnosis: Clinical history, cell type of the primary and the metastasis, similarities in DNA patterns, and syntactic structure analysis.

Differential diagnosis: Primary lung neoplasm of similar cell type.

Methacholine

Definition: Alteration of the lung parenchyma associated with intake of methacholine, see Drug Toxicity.

Methadone

Definition: Alteration of the lung parenchyma associated with intake of methadone, see Drug Toxicity.

Methotrexate

Definition: Alteration of the lung parenchyma associated with intake of methotrexate, see Drug Toxicity.

Methyl dopa

Definition: Alteration of the lung parenchyma associated with intake of methyl dopa, see Drug Toxicity.

Methylphenidate

Definition: Alteration of the lung parenchyma associated with intake of methylphenidate, see Drug Toxicity.

Methylthiouracil

Definition: Alteration of the lung parenchyma associated with intake of methylthiouracil, see Drug Toxicity.

Methysergide

Definition: Alteration of the lung parenchyma associated with intake of methysergide, see Drug Toxicity.

Meyers-Kouwenaar Syndrome

Definition: Clinical symptoms (cough, wheezing, peripheral eosinophilia, diffuse densities on chest X-radiographs) seen in tropical pulmonary eosinophilia, see Eosinophilia, Tropical Pulmonary.

Michaelis-Gutmann Bodies

Definition: Intracytoplasmic inclusion bodies seen in macrophages with incomplete cellular function, see Malacoplakia.

Microlithiasis

Definition: Disease of the peripheral lung parenchyma characterized by intraalveolar deposits of calcospherites, see Alveolar Microlithiasis.

Microliths

Definition: Deposits of calcified material in the lung parenchyma, see Chronic Airflow Obstruction.

Micronemiasis

Definition: Infection of the lung with the nematode *Micronema deletrix*.

Incidence/Epidemiology: Unusual infection of humans. A few cases have been reported in Canada and the USA. The nematode infects horses and is usually not pathogenic in man.

Etiology/Pathophysiology: *M. deletrix* is a free-living parasite and infects humans probably by invasion through traumatized skin. It spreads throughout the body via the venous blood stream and invades the brain and the lung most frequently.

Clinical Presentation: Symptoms are related to infection of the central nervous system (meningoencephalitis).

Prognosis: The reported patients died due to meningoencephalitis.

Radiology: Chest radiographs have been normal.

Pathology:

Gross: Small areas of hemorrhagic necrosis may be seen. The parasites measure 0.3×0.02 mm and the eggs 40×12 µm.

Histology: The parasites can be seen in the capillaries and in the alveolar walls and are usually surrounded by dense granulomatous inflammatory infiltrates.

➤ *Descriptors:* Lung parenchyma with altered structure:

- noncaseous epithelioid granulomas
- necrosis and hemorrhage
- mixed inflammatory infiltrates
- eosinophils;
- Pulmonary vessels with altered structure:
- parasites (capillaries)
- noncaseous epithelioid granulomas
- mixed inflammatory infiltrates
- eosinophils

■ *Special stains:* PAS, collagenous stains, Giemsa, Movat.

Hallmark of Diagnosis: Clinical history, identification of the parasites within the central nervous system and within the small vessels of the lung.

Differential diagnosis: Infection of the lung by other parasites, granulomatous inflammation of the lung due to other agents.

Middle Lobe Syndrome

Definition: Chronic or recurrent atelectasis of the right middle lobe seen on chest X-radiographs, see Atelectasis, Bronchiectasis, Obstructive Pulmonary Disease.

Miller's Lung

Definition: Alteration of the lung parenchyma associated with inhalation of proteins derived from the wheat weevil.

Incidence/Epidemiology: Rare disorder observed in persons working with dust-contaminated grain.

Etiology/Pathophysiology: The insect proteins induce an allergic reaction of the lung parenchyma (allergic extrinsic pneumonitis).

Clinical Presentation: Symptoms may be acute or subacute and include cough, chills, dyspnea, fever, and malaise.

Prognosis: Usually good without serious sequelae.

Radiology: Chest radiographs show diffuse, bilateral, patchy densities.

Pathology:
Gross: Wet, heavy, red-grayish lung.

Histology: All histomorphological features as described under the heading Allergic (Extrinsic) Alveolitis can be seen.

➤ *Descriptors:* Lung parenchyma with altered structure:
- noncaseous epithelioid granulomas
- eosinophils
- multinucleated giant cells
- intrabronchiolar fibrinoid material and histiocytes
- ulceration of bronchiolar mucosa;
- Lung parenchyma with preserved structure:
- macrophages
- desquamation, hypertrophy, hyperplasia and dysplasia of pneumocytes
- mononuclear inflammatory infiltrates
- intraalveolar serous fluid

■ *Special stains:* PAS, collagenous stains, Giemsa, immunohistochemistry for immunoglobulins, lymphocytic subpopulations, HLA-DR.

Hallmark of Diagnosis: Clinical history, features of allergic extrinsic pneumonitis.

Differential diagnosis: Due to other extrinsic agents, sarcoidosis, berylliosis, lymphoid interstitial pneumonia, usual interstitial pneumonia, desquamative interstitial pneumonia.

Mineral Oil

Definition: Alteration of the lung parenchyma associated with exposure to Mineral Oil, see Drug Toxicity.

Mineral Pneumoconiosis

Definition: Alteration of the lung parenchyma due to deposits of abnormal amounts of dust.

Incidence/Epidemiology: Abnormal amounts of dust in the peripheral lung parenchyma are frequently seen in miners and persons exposed to various sources of silica, metal fumes, or fly ash or working in the manufacture of ceramics, paints, cosmetics, silverware, rubber, etc. The details are described under the particular headings.

Etiology/Pathophysiology: The deposition of mineral particles in the terminal air spaces is closely related to the size of the particles, the number of inhaled particles, and their clearance rate. Particles have to be in the size range of 1–5 μm in order to reach the distant airways. Particles measuring below 0.5 μm move by diffusion and Brownian motion. Particles greater than 10 μm are to a large extent removed by the proximal conducting airways. Deposits of particles in the terminal airways may remain inert and biologically inactive or may induce a progressive inflammatory response of host tissue and subsequently generate fibrosis. Minerals considered to be of minor fibrogenic activity include coal, talc, kaolin, bentonite, cement, limestone, titanium, iron, zirconium, tin, antimony, barium, and cerium. Mineral fibers of high fibrinogenic potential include silica, asbestos, shale, nepheline, nickel, aluminum, and chromium. Additional factors such as tuberculosis, chronic infection, familial predisposition, and admixture of a small amount of silica can induce severe fibrosis or complicated pneumoconiosis in persons exposed to primarily inert mineral fibers.

Clinical Presentation: Symptoms include progressive shortness of breath, dry cough, pulmonary hypertension, and dyspnea.

Prognosis: Fair, but slow progressive respiratory failure is the usual outcome.

Radiology: Chest radiographs show a wide range of morphological features that should be graded according to the ILO classification which is based upon diffuse, granular and nodular densities being graded separately.

Pathology:
Gross: The lungs show multiple, usually black to grayish-brown densities of firm consistency. Central necrosis may be seen in coal pneumo-

coniosis. Silicosis is characterized by concentric fibrous nodules measuring a few millimeters to several centimeters in diameter. The hilar lymph nodes are commonly involved in pneumoconiosis.

Histology: The deposits of dust are composed of agglutinations of commonly birefringent crystals and black amorphous material. Fibrosis, if present, may obscure the dust particles which are concentrated at the periphery of the fibrotic nodule. Asbestos induces a diffuse, ill-defined fibrosis, as opposed to silica and related minerals. Smoking without additional exposure to mineral fibers seldom induces fibrosis. However, it may enhance the fibrotic potential in mineral-exposed persons.

➤ *Descriptors:* Lung parenchyma with preserved structure:

- dust (birefringent crystals)
- macrophages (dust-laden)
- mononuclear inflammatory infiltrates;
- Lung parenchyma with altered structure:
- proliferating fibroblasts
- diffuse interstitial fibrosis
- focal interstitial fibrosis (with dust particles)

■ *Special stains:* PAS, collagenous stains, Prussian blue, Giemsa, X-ray diffraction method or related physical techniques, electron microscopy (including scanning electron microscopy).

Hallmark of Diagnosis: Clinical history, deposits of dust in the terminal air spaces, identification of the dust particles by physical techniques.

Differential diagnosis: Dust deposits of various mineral particles, smoking.

Mites

Definition: Alteration of the lung parenchyma due to inhalation of mites.

Incidence/Epidemiology*:* Rare disorder. An allergic reaction of the lung parenchyma to inhaled dust containing mites or their products is more prevalent.

Etiology/Pathophysiology: Mites and products of mites in dust are allergens and may induce a mild to moderate allergic reaction.

Clinical Presentation: Symptoms include asthmatic complaints, cough, and shortness of breath.

Prognosis: Usually good and without serious sequelae

Radiology: Chest radiographs are usually normal.

Pathology:

Gross: The lungs appear normal.

Histology: Very infrequently, mites can be demonstrated in the smaller bronchi.

➤ *Descriptors:* Bronchial mucosa with preserved structure:

- mites (in the lumen of small bronchi)
- mixed inflammatory infiltrates
- eosinophils

■ *Special stains:* None.

Hallmark of Diagnosis: Demonstration of mites in the lung.

Differential diagnosis: Allergic reaction of the lung parenchyma to other agents.

Mitomycin

Definition: Alteration of the lung parenchyma associated with intake of mitomycin, see Drug Toxicity.

Monocrotaline

Definition: Alteration of the lung parenchyma associated with intake of monocrotaline, see Drug Toxicity.

Monod's Sign

Definition: Particular findings on chest X-radiographs (large round densities surrounded by crescents of air). See: Aspergillosis.

Mononucleosis

Definition: Infection of the lung with Cytomegalovirus, see Cytomegalovirus, Viral Infection.

Mounier-Kuhn Syndrome

Definition: Chronic sinusitis and tracheitis with descending bronchitis.

Incidence/Epidemiology: Infrequent disorder usually seen in young to middle-aged men (20–40 years old) and sometimes in young children. Familial occurrence has been reported.

Etiology/Pathophysiology: Chronic infection of the nasal and ethmoidal sinus induces chronic infections of the trachea and the major bronchi with resultant tracheobronchiomegaly. An autosomal recessive type of inheritance has been suggested.

Clinical Presentation: Symptoms include recurrent bacterial infection of the upper and lower respiratory tract, chronic cough with expectoration, mild fever, and recurrent bronchopneumonias.

Prognosis: Fair, as slow progressive respiratory failure is the usual outcome.

Radiology: Chest radiographs may be normal or show ectatic bronchi and peribronchiolar infiltrates.

Pathology:

Gross: The trachea and the major bronchi show an ectatic lumen and a swollen, reddish mucosa.

Histology: The submucosa is infiltrated by mononuclear inflammatory infiltrates and displays fibrotic changes with rarefaction of the glands and muscular fibers. The mucosa may be atrophic or may show squamous metaplasia.

➤ *Descriptors:* Bronchial mucosa with altered structure:

- fibrosis (submucosa)
- atrophic mucosa
- destruction of submucosal glands
- erosion of cartilage
- mononuclear inflammatory infiltrates

■ *Special stains:* PAS, Giemsa.

Hallmark of Diagnosis: Clinical history, ectasia of the trachea and major bronchi.

Differential diagnosis: Tracheomalacia, congenital or postinflammatory bronchiectasis.

Mountain Sickness

Definition: Acute pulmonary edema due to high altitude.

Incidence/Epidemiology: Several cases have been reported among those climbing to altitudes above 3 000 m; they developed a fatal acute pulmonary edema.

Etiology/Pathophysiology: The disorder affects persons who have not yet adapted to longer stays at high altitudes, i.e., most frequently young healthy persons or soldiers transported to high altitudes without acclimatization. The main cause is seen in pulmonary venous vasoconstriction and redistribution of blood from systemic to pulmonary blood flow.

Clinical Presentation: Symptoms include progressive dyspnea, dry cough, vomiting, headache, and insomnia. Death may occur after 1–7 days.

Prognosis: Fair, mortality rate of patients with acute edema may be 20% or more. Chronic damage of lung may be seen in survivors.

Radiology: Chest radiographs show diffuse, dense, bilateral infiltrates.

Pathology:

Gross: The lungs are heavy, edematous, and enlarged.

Histology: The distant airways and the interstitium are filled with edematous fluid. The formation of hyaline membranes is seen. The alveoli contain macrophages and clusters of erythrocytes. The capillaries are occluded by thrombotic lesions. Bacterial superinfection may be present in extended disease courses.

➤ *Descriptors:* Lung parenchyma with preserved structure:

- intraalveolar serous fluid
- macrophages
- hemorrhage
- hyaline membranes;
- Lung parenchyma with altered structure:
- focal interstitial fibrosis;
- Pulmonary vessels with preserved structure:
- thrombosis (in the capillaries)

■ *Special stains:* PAS, collagenous stains, Giemsa.

Hallmark of Diagnosis: Clinical history, acute pulmonary edema, hyaline membranes.

Differential diagnosis: Adult respiratory distress syndrome due to other causes, acute bacterial pneumonia.

Mucinous Cystadenoma

Definition: Low-grade tumor of the lung with specific histomorphological features.

Incidence/Epidemiology: Extremely rare tumor, only a few cases have been reported.

Etiology/Pathophysiology: The tumors may arise from peripheral epithelial cells with mucinous hypertrophy, hyperplasia and dysplasia.

Clinical Presentation: Patients are usually asymptomatic.

Prognosis: Good and without known serious sequelae.

Radiology: Chest radiographs show circumscribed densities several centimeters in diameter.

Pathology:

Gross: The tumors appear as large, semitranslucent, solitary, gelatinous masses.

Histology: The tumor is surrounded by hyperplastic and slightly atypical mucinous lining cells (goblet cells) which produce enormous amounts of mucus. The original lung parenchyma is destroyed. An inflammatory response of the host tissue with multinucleated foreign-body giant cells may be present.

➤ *Descriptors:* Newly formed textures without metastasis potential:

- epithelial growth pattern
- adenoid textures
- cysts (large, mucinous)
- large tumor cells (polar oriented nuclei)
- absent or infrequent mitoses
- homogeneous nuclear and cellular size
- absent necrosis
- mononuclear inflammatory infiltrates
- multinucleated giant cells

■ *Special stains:* PAS, collagenous stains, Giemsa, DNA analysis.

Hallmark of Diagnosis: Adenomatoid tumor with extraordinary mucus production and hyperplastic lining cells in the boundary.

Differential diagnosis: Adenocarcinoma, mucus gland adenoma, metastasis of ovary carcinoma into the lung.

Mucocele

Definition: Cystic formation in the lung filled with viscous mucus, see Cyst.

Mucoepidermoid Carcinoma

Definition: Carcinoma arising from the bronchial submucosal glands with different grades of malignancy.

Incidence/Epidemiology: Unusual tumor most frequently seen in young to middle-aged adults with equal frequency in both sexes. It may also occur in children and aged persons. No associated risk factors are known.

Etiology/Pathophysiology: The carcinoma arises from the submucosal glands of the major bronchi and trachea. Low-grade mucoepidermoid carcinomas are of benign behavior; high-grade mucoepidermoid carcinomas metastasize and have a poor prognosis.

Clinical Presentation: Symptoms are related to the proximal localization of the tumors and include chronic cough, shortness of breath, asthmatic irritation of the bronchi, and obstructive atelectasis.

Prognosis: Patients with low-grade mucoepidermoid carcinomas have a good prognosis without serious sequelae; those with high-grade mucoepidermoid carcinomas have a poor prognosis similar to those with bronchial carcinomas.

Radiology: Chest radiographs may be normal or reveal signs associated with bronchial obstruction.

Pathology:

Gross: The conducting airways display a firm, grayish tumor mass with polypoid growth into the bronchial lumen. The size varies from several millimeters to a few centimeters in maximum diameter.

Histology: The carcinoma contains two different textures, (a) the development of glandular patterns and (b) the presence of epidermoid areas with solid growth patterns. The glandular areas contain multiple separated glands with atypical, epithelial, mucus-producing cells. The epidermoid areas are composed of large, atypical cells growing in solid sheets. However, keratinization is usually absent. According to the differentiation of growth textures and of the degree of cellular abnormality, low-grade and high-grade mucoepidermoid carcinomas can be distinguished. Low-grade mucoepidermoid carcinomas show well-differentiated glandular and solid textures, a small number of mitoses, no inflammatory response of the host tissue, and no necrotic areas. High-grade ones have marked nuclear atypias in the glandular areas, numerous tubular glands, moderate inflammatory response of the host tissue, and multiple areas of hemorrhagic necrosis.

➤ *Descriptors:* Newly formed textures with metastasis potential:
- epithelial growth pattern
- epidermoid textures
- adenoid textures
- solid textures
- mucus production
- intercellular bridges
- infrequent mitoses
- homogeneous nuclear and cellular size
- absent necrosis
- inhomogeneous nuclear and cellular size
- necrosis and hemorrhage
- absent or weak inflammatory infiltrates

■ *Special stains:* PAS, Giemsa, immunohistochemistry for CEA, keratin, EMA; endogenous lectins, DNA analysis.

Hallmark of Diagnosis: Simultaneous glandular and epidermoid textures with various degrees of differentiation.

Differential diagnosis: Mixed adeno-epidermoid carcinoma, adenocarcinoma with various degrees of differentiation, acinus cell tumor, carcinoid, bronchial gland adenoma.

Mucoid Impaction

Definition: Bronchiectasis with intrabronchial viscous mucus, see Bronchiectasis.

Mucormycosis

Definition: Infection of the lung with fungi of the order Mucorales.

Incidence/Epidemiology: Opportunistic infection seen in immunocompromised patients such as those with leukemia, diabetes mellitus, lymphomas, or severe burns. It has been estimated to be the third most common opportunistic infection in patients under cytostatic therapy.

Etiology/Pathophysiology: The infection may occur as a localized, nonopportunistic infection of the skin, as a fulminant infection of the paranasal sinus and the central nervous system, or as an invasive pulmonary and disseminated infection. The fungi usually spread from the bronchial tree through the bronchial walls into the adjacent distant airways and blood vessels. Infective genera include *Rhizopus, Absidia, Mucor, Rhizomurum, Saksenaea, Cunninghamella, Mortierella, Syncephalastrum*, and *Apophysomyces*.

Clinical Presentation: Symptoms include fever, cough, chest pain, and hemoptysis.

Prognosis: Fair, depending upon the general condition of the patient.

Radiology: Chest radiographs show centrally localized, ovoid densities, signs of hemorrhagic infarcts, or a miliary and nodular pattern.

Pathology:

Gross: The lung has a centrally localized, hemorrhagic mass with necrosis and consolidation at the periphery.

Histology: The infected parts show areas of hemorrhagic necrosis intermingled with neutrophilic and eosinophilic granulocytes, lymphocytes, and plasma cells. Broad pleomorphic hyphae with perpendicular branching can be seen with HE stain. They are often cut in different directions and may display oval to round transections. They measure 10–15 μm in diameter and are wider than those associated with the *Aspergillus*. In contrast to *Aspergillus* the hyphae of mucor are less uniform, irregularly septated, and less anisotropic in orientation.

➤ *Descriptors:* Lung parenchyma with altered structure:
- necrosis and hemorrhage
- fungus (hyphae and spores)
- mixed inflammatory infiltrates
- eosinophils

■ *Special stains:* PAS, GMS, methenamine silver stain, immunofluorescence.

Hallmark of Diagnosis: Identification of the fungal hyphae in sputum, bronchial washings, or biopsies.

Differential diagnosis: Infections by other species, especially *Aspergillus.*

Mucoviscidosis

Definition: Alteration of the lung parenchyma associated with cystic fibrosis, see Cystic Fibrosis.

Mullite Fibers

Definition: Alteration of the lung parenchyma associated with inhalation of (nonasbestos) mullite fibers, see Nonasbestos Fibers.

Mushroom Worker's Lung

Definition: Alteration of the lung parenchyma seen in mushroom workers.

Incidence/Epidemiology: Rare disorder seen in workers exposed to mushrooms growing in humidified rooms or to moldy mushroom compost.

Etiology/Pathophysiology: The disorder is considered to be a hypersensitivity reaction of the lung caused by inhalation of spores of *Thermoactinomyces sacchari*.

Clinical Presentation: Symptoms are subacute or of acute onset and include fever, malaise, chest pain, dyspnea, and cough.

Prognosis: Usually good and without serious sequelae.

Radiology: Chest radiographs may be normal or show diffuse ground-glass infiltrates or miliary densities.

Pathology:

Gross: The lungs may be normal or show areas of reddish-gray consolidations.

Histology: The interstitial lung texture is preserved and may show acute interstitial infiltrates, intraalveolar edema with hypertrophy, hyperplasia and dysplasia of cells of the alveolar lining, noncaseating granulomas, and features of desquamative interstitial pneumonia (DIP), usual interstitial pneumonia (UIP), or lymphocytic interstitial pneumonia (LIP). The details are described under the heading Allergic (Extrinsic) Alveolitis.

➤ *Descriptors:* Lung parenchyma with altered structure:
- noncaseous epithelioid granulomas
- eosinophils
- multinucleated giant cells
- intrabronchiolar fibrinoid material and histiocytes
- ulceration of bronchiolar mucosa;
- Lung parenchyma with preserved structure:
- macrophages
- desquamation, hypertrophy, hyperplasia and dysplasia of pneumocytes
- mononuclear inflammatory infiltrates
- intraalveolar serous fluid

■ *Special stains:* PAS, collagenous stains, Giemsa, endogenous lectins.

Hallmark of Diagnosis: Clinical history, histomorphologic findings of allergic extrinsic alveolitis.

Differential diagnosis: Infectious and noninfectious granulomatous diseases, usual interstitial pneumonia, desquamative interstitial pneumonia. For details, see Allergic (Extrinsic) Alveolitis.

Mustard Gas

Definition: Alteration of the lung parenchyma associated with inhalation of mustard gas (increased risk of lung cancer). See: Cancer of the Lung, Toxic Injury.

Mycetoma

Definition: Circumscribed densities seen on chest X-radiographs of patients with fungal infections, see Fungus.

Mycobacteria, Atypical

Definition: Infection of the lung with atypical mycobacteria.

Incidence/Epidemiology: Formerly a rare disease, infection by atypical mycobacteria has become more common in immunocompromised patients, especially those suffering from AIDS.

Etiology/Pathophysiology: Atypical mycobacteria are found in water, soil, and dust, and are usually acquired from the environment. The most important strains include *Mycobacterium avium-intercellulare* and *kansasii*. Infections of various organs such as the lungs, kidneys, and liver and bacteremia are common.

Clinical Presentation: Symptoms include cough, fever, and malaise. Patients may be severely ill.

Prognosis: Usually good; however, prolonged courses and poor response to antituberculous chemotherapy may induce slow progressive respiratory failure.

Radiology: Chest radiographs show diffuse granular (miliary) densities or larger areas of consolidation and patchy infiltrates.

Pathology:

Gross: The lungs show multiple, grayish nodules of firm consistency or larger, grayish-white areas with consolidation.

Histology: Atypical mycobacteria seldom form caseating granulomas. Diffuse inflammatory infiltrates made up of neutrophilic and eosinophilic granulocytes, lymphocytes, plasma cells, and predominantly histiocytes and macrophages can be seen in the distant airways and in the interalveolar walls.

➤ *Descriptors:* Lung parenchyma with altered structure:
- necrosis (small areas)
- mixed inflammatory infiltrates
- macrophages
- multinucleated giant cells
- caseous epithelioid granulomas (ill-defined);
- Pulmonary vessels with preserved structure:
- mononuclear inflammatory infiltrates

■ *Special stains:* Ziehl-Neelsen, PAS, rhodamin fluorescence, auramine, Wright's stain.

Hallmark of Diagnosis: Clinical history, ill-defined epithelioid granulomas, identification of bacteria.

Differential diagnosis: Pneumonia due to other bacteria.

Mycoplasma pneumonia

Definition: Infection of the lung with *Mycoplasma pneumoniae*.

Incidence/Epidemiology*:* Community acquired infectious disorder not infrequently seen on military and college campuses.

Etiology/Pathophysiology: The infective agent is of low viral capacity and usually induces a self-healing pneumonia. Diagnosis is based upon the clinical picture and a positive complement fixation titer (positive cold agglutination assay).

Clinical Presentation: Symptoms include fever, chest pain, chills, malaise, headache, and/or myalgia. Fatal cases may develop septicemia and neurologic symptoms.

Prognosis: Usually good, even in untreated patients who often present with prolonged courses.

Radiology: Chest radiographs show diffuse, dense, patchy, interstitial infiltrates.

Pathology:

Gross: The lungs are heavy and show edematous changes or consolidated yellowish-white areas.

Histology: The small bronchi and bronchioles are heavily infiltrated by lymphocytes, macrophages, and plasma cells, which are also present in the interalveolar walls. The epithelial cells are desquamated, necrotic, or hyperplastic. A fibrinous exudate can be seen in later stages.

➤ *Descriptors:* Lung parenchyma with preserved structure:
- degeneration of pneumocytes
- mononuclear inflammatory infiltrates
- desquamation, hypertrophy, hyperplasia and dysplasia of pneumocytes;
- Bronchial mucosa with preserved structure:
- mononuclear inflammatory infiltrates
- desquamation, hypertrophy, hyperplasia and dysplasia of epithelial cells

■ *Special stains:* PAS, collagenous stains, Giemsa, Gram's, DNA hybridization.

Hallmark of Diagnosis: Clinical history, positive complement fixation titer (binding assay), dense interstitial mononuclear infiltrate in the bronchioles and distant airways.

Differential diagnosis: Pneumonia due to infection with virus, *Legionella, Chlamydia*, or *Rickettsia*.

Mycosis Fungoides

Definition: Infiltration of mycosis fungoides into the lung parenchyma.

Incidence/Epidemiology*:* Mycosis fungoides is a T-cell lymphoma of the skin. The extracutaneous manifestation is most frequently seen in the lymph nodes and in the lung. The Sezary syndrome includes erythrodermia, lymphadenopathia, and leukemia.

Etiology/Pathophysiology: The disorder is considered to be a neoplasm arising from T-helper cells (seldom from T-suppressor cells) of the skin. The disorder may disseminate into the lymph nodes and next most frequently into the peripheral lung parenchyma.

Clinical Presentation: Symptoms include shortness of breath on exercise, chest pain, and cough.

Prognosis: Median survival of patients with pulmonary involvement is less than 5 years.

Radiology: Chest radiographs show diffuse, patchy infiltrates.

Pathology:

Gross: The lungs show small areas of grayish-white infiltrates propagating along the smaller and major bronchi.

Histology: The tumorous infiltrates propagate along the intrapulmonary lymphatic vessels and are composed of atypical lymphocytoid cells with polymorphous and convoluted nuclei. Large mycosis cells are present.

➤ *Descriptors:* Newly formed textures with metastasis potential:
- mesenchymal growth pattern
- lymphomatoid textures
- large tumor cells (myçosis cells)
- small nuclei (polymorphous and convoluted)
- infrequent mitoses

■ *Special stains:* PAS, collagenous stains, Giemsa, immunohistochemistry for lymphocytic subpopulations, DNA analysis.

Hallmark of Diagnosis: Clinical history, tumor infiltrates in the peripheral lung consistent with mycosis fungoides.

Differential diagnosis: Other type of lymphoma, lymphomatoid granulomatosis, lymphoid interstitial pneumonia.

Myeloblastoma, Granular Cell

Definition: Benign tumor of the lung derived from Schwann cells.

Incidence/Epidemiology: Unusual tumor most frequently found in young to middle-aged adults and of equal sex distribution. No associated risk factors are known.

Etiology/Pathophysiology: The tumor is thought to arise from Schwann cells. It is located in the major bronchi and in the trachea with obstructive growth pattern.

Clinical Presentation: Symptoms are related to the proximal location of the tumors and include cough, obstructive pneumonitis, dyspnea and blood tinged sputum.

Prognosis: Usually good and without serious sequelae.

Radiology: Chest radiographs show either no abnormalities or findings related to obstruction of a major bronchus.

Pathology:

Gross: The tumors appear as solitary or multiple, small, grayish-white endobronchial polypoid tumor masses within the lower trachea or major bronchi.

Histology: The tumors are composed of large, plump spindle cells with abundant granular cytoplasm and small, round nuclei. Mitotic figures, necrosis, or an inflammatory response of host tissue is absent or rare. The bronchial epithelial cells usually show squamous metaplasia, sometimes with severe atypia.

➤ *Descriptors:* Newly formed textures without metastasis potential:
- mesenchymal growth pattern
- fibromatous textures
- plump spindle cells
- large tumor cells
- small nuclei (round)
- homogeneous nuclear and cellular size
- abundant cytoplasm (granular)
- absent or infrequent mitoses
- absent necrosis

■ *Special stains:* PAS, Congo, collagenous stains, Giemsa, Prussian blue, immunohistochemistry for neuroendocrine markers, S-100 protein, DNA analysis, endogenous lectins.

Hallmark of Diagnosis: Localization, solid textures composed of granular cells.

Differential diagnosis: Malacoplakia, Whipple's disease, oncocytoma, carcinoid.

Myeloma, Multiple

Definition: Involvement of the lung in patients with multiple myeloma.

Incidence/Epidemiology: Rare disease, but one observed more frequently than primary plasma cell tumors of the lung.

Etiology/Pathophysiology: Low grade, malignant, non-Hodgkin's lymphoma arising from reticular plasma cells.

Clinical Presentation: Patients may be asymptomatic or present with cough, chest pain, dyspnea, and pleural effusions.

Prognosis: Survival of patients may last for 5–20 years.

Radiology: Chest radiographs show diffuse, interstitial densities or multiple, circumscribed nodules measuring a few centimeters in maximum diameter.

Pathology:

Gross: The lungs show several grayish-white nodules of soft consistency. Necrotic areas are usually not present.

Histology: The texture of the lung parenchyma is usually preserved. The interalveolar walls and the distant airways contain densely packed, uniform, plasmacytoid tumor cells. Mitotic figures are present, but necrotic areas are usually missing.

➤ *Descriptors:* Newly formed textures with metastasis potential:
- mesenchymal growth pattern
- lymphomatoid textures
- small tumor cells (plasmacytoid cells)
- homogeneous nuclear and cellular size
- infrequent mitoses
- absent necrosis

■ *Special stains:* PAS, Giemsa, immunohistochemistry for lymphocytic subpopulations, DNA analysis.

Hallmark of Diagnosis: Clinical history, plasmacytoid tumor cells within the distant airways.

Differential diagnosis: Primary plasmacytoma of the lung, LIP, plasma-cell granuloma, lymphomatoid granulomatosis.

Myiasis

Definition: Infection of the lung with larvae dipterans.

Incidence/Epidemiology: Unusual disorder seen in tropical countries. Infection of the lung has been reported only in a few (less than 10) cases.

Etiology/Pathophysiology: The arthropod larvae dipterans invades the skin of humans after a bite from an infected mosquito. The organisms invade the skin, eyes, brain, ear, gastro-intestinal tract, kidneys, nasopharynx, and lung. Due to its poor adaptation to man, a severe inflammatory reaction is seen in the involved organs.

Clinical Presentation: Patients may be asymptomatic or complain about cough, hemoptysis, chest pain, and dyspnea.

Prognosis: Usually good; however, fatal cases have been reported.

Radiology: Chest radiographs show coin lesions or small granular densities in the peripheral lung.

Pathology:

Gross: The lungs show multiple, grayish-white, small nodules with consolidation.

Histology: The parasites are surrounded by dense inflammatory infiltrates composed of lymphocytes, plasma cells, granulocytes, histiocytes, and macrophages. Granulomatous reaction, hemorrhage, and necrosis may be seen.

➤ *Descriptors:* Lung parenchyma with altered structure:
- mixed inflammatory infiltrates (dense)
- parasites (maggots)
- necrosis and hemorrhage
- noncaseous epithelioid granulomas (poorly defined)

■ *Special stains:* PAS, collagenous stains, Giemsa, Movat.

Hallmark of Diagnosis: Clinical history, identification of the parasites in host tissue showing an inflammatory reaction.

Differential diagnosis: Infection of the lung with other parasites, bacterial bronchopneumonia.

Myofibromatosis, Generalized

Definition: Proliferation of diffuse spindle cells of low-grade malignancy in the lung.

Incidence/Epidemiology: Rare disorder most frequently seen in the newborns and infants (congenital generalized fibromatosis). However, a few cases have been reported in middle-aged and elderly adults.

Etiology/Pathophysiology: The etiology of the disorder is not known. The diffuse proliferation of smooth muscle cells may derive from a chronic inflammatory stimulus with the progressive behavior of a true neoplasm.

Clinical Presentation: Symptoms include progressive shortness of breath, dyspnea, and cyanosis.

Prognosis: The prognosis is poor, but more favorable if only one lung is affected.

Radiology: Chest radiographs show diffuse interstitial densities, sometimes with miliary appearance.

Pathology:

Gross: The lungs are of stiff consistency and of grayish-white color. The pleura may be fibrotic.

Histology: The interalveolar septula contain clusters of proliferating smooth muscle cells which concentrate around the bronchioles and small vessels. Cells of the alveolar lining are normal. Within the distant airways, agglutinations of macrophages and fibrinoid deposits may be seen.

➤ *Descriptors:* Lung parenchyma with altered structure:

- focal interstitial fibrosis
- proliferating smooth muscle cells;
- Lung parenchyma with preserved structure:
- intraalveolar fibrinoid material
- macrophages

■ *Special stains:* PAS, collagenous stains, Congo, Giemsa, immunohistochemistry for immunoglobulins, actin, myosin, desmin, desmoplakin, vimentin, neurofilaments, endogenous lectins, DNA analysis.

Hallmark of Diagnosis: Clinical history, clusters of proliferating smooth muscle fibers without major chronic inflammation in the lung.

Differential diagnosis: Progressive interstitial fibrosis, lymphangioleiomyomatosis, metastatic leiomyosarcoma.

Myxedema

Definition: Alteration of the lung parenchyma associated with severe untreated hypothyroidism.

Incidence/Epidemiology*:* Extremely rare disorder described only in a few patients (autopsy study).

Etiology/Pathophysiology: Long-term hypothyroidism induces edematous changes in the interstitial tissue with hyalin deposits of proteins, fibrinoid material, and glycoproteins.

Clinical Presentation: Symptoms include dyspnea, restrictive lung function, and chronic cough.

Prognosis: Usually good; however, long-lasting myxedema may induce slow progressive respiratory failure.

Radiology: Chest radiographs show diffuse interstitial infiltrates in both lungs.

Histology: The interalveolar septula are widened and contain a pale hyaline substance. Inflammatory cells are absent. Hyperplasia and hypertrophy of cells of the alveolar lining are absent. The alterations are marked around the small arteries and bronchi.

➤ *Descriptors:* Lung parenchyma with preserved structure:

- interstitial edema
- hyaline material
- absent inflammatory infiltrates

■ *Special stains:* PAS, collagenous stains, Giemsa, Congo, endogenous lectins.

Hallmark of Diagnosis: Clinical history, diffuse hyaline deposits in the interalveolar septula and around the small arteries and bronchi.

Differential diagnosis: Interstitial fibrosis, amyloidosis, chronic interstitial edema due to other causes.

Myxoma

Definition: Metastatic (continuous) spread of myxoma of the heart into the lung.

Incidence/Epidemiology*:* Rare disorder usually seen in young adults.

Etiology/Pathophysiology: Myxomas derive from the endocardium and are primarily benign. They may, however, show malignant behavior after reaching a certain age or size. They usually reach the lung via the pulmonary arteries and may spread into the adjacent lung parenchyma per continuum.

Clinical Presentation: Patients present with symptoms related to the endocardial and endovascular growth of the tumors.

Prognosis: Poor, most of patients die within 1 year if the tumor has already infiltrated the pulmonary vessels or lung parenchyma.

Radiology: Chest radiographs are usually normal or may show widened pulmonary arteries.

Pathology:

Gross: Yellowish, mucinous tumors within the proximal pulmonary arteries.

Histology: The tumors are composed of spindle cells with enclosed myxomatoid gelatinous material. Mitoses are infrequent. Necrotic areas are usually not present.

➤ *Descriptors:* Newly formed textures without metastasis potential:
- mesenchymal growth pattern
- fibromatous textures
- myxomatoid textures
- plump spindle cells
- hyaline material (myxomatoid, gelatinous)
- homogeneous nuclear and cellular size
- absent or infrequent mitoses
- absent necrosis

■ *Special stains:* PAS, collagenous stains, Prussian blue, Giemsa, immunohistochemistry for vimentin, desmin, desmoplakin, actin, myosin, DNA analysis, endogenous lectins.

Hallmark of Diagnosis: Clinical history, myxomatoid tumors in the proximal pulmonary arteries.

Differential diagnosis: Myxosarcoma, organized thromboemboli, metastatic sarcomas of various origins.

Naloxone – Rutile Fibers

Naloxone

Definition: Alteration of the lung parenchyma associated with intake of naloxone, see Drug Toxicity.

Narcotics

Definition: Alteration of the lung parenchyma associated with intake of narcotics, see Drug Toxicity.

Necrosis

Definition: Complete destruction of the lung parenchyma caused by various agents, see Abscess.

Nematodes

Definition: Infection of the lung with nematode species.
Incidence/Epidemiology: The percentage of infected persons amounts to 20–25% of the world population. The most successful nematodes are *Ascaris lumbricoides* and *Strongyloides stercoralis*. Several nematodes are well adapted to humans and seldom cause severe symptoms.
Etiology/Pathophysiology: The following disorders of the lung caused by nematodes have been described: angiostrongyliasis, anisakiasis, baylisascariasis, capillariasis, dirofilariasis, enterobiasis, filariasis, gnathostomiasis, lagochilascariasis, visceral larva migrans, mammomonogamiasis, mansonellosis, metastrongyliasis, strongyliasis, trichinosis. The majority of nematodes need a transient host in order to be able to infect man. The life cycle and the special features of infection are described under the particular headings.
Clinical Presentation: Well adapted nematodes seldom cause severe symptoms. Others like *Capillaria, Trichinella spiralis, Metastrongylus elongatus, Lagochilascaris minor*, or *Baylisascaris procyonis* are more adapted to lower mammals and are not considered to be natural parasites of man. Infection of the central nervous system usually determines the major clinical symptoms; infection of the lower respiratory tract may be of minor clinical importance.
Prognosis: Usually good and without serious sequelae. The clinical course is, in general, determined by the occurrence of infections of the central nervous system.
Radiology: The parasites may appear on chest radiographs as circumscribed peripheral densities; however, a nontrivial percentage of chest radiographs are normal.
Pathology:
Gross: The parasites may be recognized macroscopically within larger areas of the lung parenchyma that show dense inflammatory infiltrations. In other cases only serial sections can identify the nematodes which are often killed by the inflammatory response of the host tissue.
Histology: Identification of the parasites or eggs may be difficult due to a severe granulomatous inflammatory response of the host tissue. In special cases only shadows of former parasites can be identified, but others may show immature worms or eggs. The details are described under the particular headings.

➤ *Descriptors:* Lung parenchyma with altered structure:
- noncaseous epithelioid granulomas
- parasites (intragranulomatous, "shadows")
- mixed inflammatory infiltrates
- eosinophils

■ *Special stains:* PAS, collagenous stains, Giemsa, Movat, immunofluorescence.

Hallmark of Diagnosis: Clinical history, identification of the parasites.
Differential diagnosis: According to the species, other infection by parasites, nonspecific bacterial infection.

Neocarcinostatin

Definition: Alteration of the lung parenchyma associated with intake of neocarcinostatin, see Drug Toxicity.

Neonatal and Pediatric Disorders

Definition: Congenital and acquired diseases of the lung in newborns, infants, and children.

Incidence/Epidemiology: The lung is involved in nearly all acquired (infectious) and congenital disorders of major clinical importance. In addition, treatment of pulmonary disorders during early childhood may lead to chronic alterations of the lung parenchyma, resulting in interstitial fibrosis or chronic asthmatic complaints.

Etiology/Pathophysiology: The lung is one of the most vulnerable organs in newborns and the target of several traumatic lesions during birth. The possibly insufficient function of the lung during the early days after birth has to be overcome by artificial ventilation which may lead to characteristic damage to the lung. The following congenital disorders have been described: abnormalities in development of the lung, malformation of the trachea and major bronchi, agenesis and hypoplasia of the lung parenchyma, herniation of the lung, abnormal vascular supply (Scimitar syndrome), infantile emphysema, pulmonary lymphangiectasis, cystic adenoid malformation, abnormalities of the diaphragm, and involvement of the lung in genetically inherited systemic disorders. The acquired neonatal and pediatric disorders include: interstitial pneumonitis, hyaline membrane disease, bronchopulmonary dysplasia, interstitial pulmonary emphysema, pulmonary hemosiderosis, pulmonary hemorrhage, Goodpasture's syndrome, bacterial and viral infections, intralobar sequestration, infections with *Rickettsia*, *Mycoplasma*, *Chlamydia* and fungus, and benign and malignant tumors.

Clinical Presentation: Clinical characteristics and symptoms are described under the particular headings and usually include dyspnea, fever, and cyanosis.

Prognosis: Usually serious disorders whose outcome strongly depends upon the birth weight.

Radiology: The radiologic findings are described under the particular headings.

Pathology:

Gross: The findings are described under the particular headings.

Histology: The findings are described under the particular headings.

➤ *Descriptors:* Lung parenchyma with preserved structure:

- mixed inflammatory infiltrates
- desquamation, hypertrophy, hyperplasia and dysplasia of pneumocytes;
- Lung parenchyma with altered structure:
- necrosis and hemorrhage
- caseous epithelioid granulomas
- noncaseous epithelioid granulomas
- diffuse interstitial fibrosis
- focal interstitial fibrosis;
- Newly deformed textures without metastasis potential:
- epithelial growth pattern
- mesenchymal growth pattern
- homogeneous nuclear and cellular size;
- Newly formed textures with metastasis potential:
- epithelial growth pattern
- mesenchymal growth pattern
- inhomogeneous nuclear and cellular size
- necrosis and hemorrhage
- frequent mitoses

■ *Special stains:* Usually PAS, collagenous stains, Giemsa.

Hallmark of Diagnosis: Variable inflammatory infiltrates, benign and malignant neoplasms. For details, see under the particular headings.

Differential diagnosis: As described under the particular headings.

Neoplasia

Definition: Benign or malignant tumor of the lung, see Cancer of the Lung, Hamartoma, Mesenchymal Tumors.

Neostigmine

Definition: Alteration of the lung parenchyma associated with intake of neostigmine, see Drug Toxicity.

Neuroblastoma

Definition: Metastasis of neuroblastoma into the lung, see Metastasis into the Lung.

Neuroendocrine Tumors of the Lung

Definition: Benign and malignant neoplasms of the lung derived from dispersed neuroendocrine cells.

Incidence/Epidemiology: About 20–30% of all primary neoplasms of the lung are thought to be of neuroendocrine origin. The majority of these tumors are comprised of small cell anaplastic carcinomas followed by tumorlets and carcinoids. About 10% of all non-small cell carcinomas express binding capacities to neuroendocrine markers. There is no difference in age and sex distribution compared with patients with carcinomas of nonneuroendocrine origin.

Etiology/Pathophysiology: The dispersed neuroendocrine system refers to cells within various organs and within the lung; the latter are most frequently localized in the bronchial mucosa, which are able to take up and decarboxylate amine precursors. These cells can be identified by immunohistochemical markers which are specific for neuron-specific enolase (γ enolase), gastrin-releasing peptide (bombesin), synaptophysin, and chromogranins. Neoplasms expressing antigens to these markers are classified as neuroendocrine neoplasms and include: tumorlets, mature and atypical carcinoids, small cell anaplastic carcinomas, and a minority of non-small cell carcinomas.

Clinical Presentation: The neoplasms show a broad variety of biological behavior ranging from benign tumors to high-grade malignancies with poor prognosis. Symptoms are usually related to the localization of the tumors, and only a small percentage (10–20%) of patients with neuroendocrine tumors present with symptoms related to hormonal activity of the neoplasms. The prognosis of patients is independent of immunohistochemical staining behavior.

Prognosis: Very poor in most cases, the major exception being carcinoid, which usually show a good prognosis without serious sequelae.

Radiology: About 70–80% of the neoplasms arise from central parts of the lower respiratory tract. Chest radiographs usually show central tumor masses with obstructive changes of the peripheral lung parenchyma. Tumorlets are normally not seen on chest radiographs.

Pathology:
Gross: The tumors are yellowish, and soft in consistency and generally have a good blood supply.
Histology: The light microscopic findings are discussed under the specific headings. Particular light microscopic findings related to expression of neuroendocrine binding capacities are not known. About 30–50% of small cell anaplastic carcinomas are negative to neuroendocrine markers in immunohistochemistry analysis.

➤ *Descriptors:* Newly formed textures with metastasis potential:

- epithelial growth pattern
- solid textures
- endocrine textures
- inhomogeneous nuclear and cellular size
- finely distributed nuclear chromatin
- frequent mitoses
- necrosis and hemorrhage;
- Newly formed textures without metastasis potential:
- epithelial growth pattern
- solid textures
- endocrine textures
- homogeneous nuclear and cellular size
- absent or infrequent mitoses
- absent necrosis
- hemorrhage (focal)

■ *Special stains:* Immunohistochemistry for neuroendocrine markers such as NSE, bombesin, synaptophysin, chromogranin A, chromogranin B, electron microscopy.

Hallmark of Diagnosis: Positive staining with neuroendocrine markers.

Differential diagnosis: Neoplasms of nonneuroendocrine origin according to immunohistochemical and electron microscopic features.

Neurofibromatosis

Definition: Involvement of the lung in neurofibromatosis.

Incidence/Epidemiology: Involvement of the lung in neurofibromatosis occurs in about 10–30% of these patients.

Etiology/Pathophysiology: Neurofibromatosis (von Recklinghausen's disease) is a phakomatosis, a congenital disease with dominant inheritance. It is characterized by multiple, soft neurofibromas in the central, peripheral, and vegetative nervous system. Involvement of the lung may be caused by primary changes (phakomatosis) and by secondary factors such as increased risk of chronic infections.

Clinical Presentation: Symptoms include chronic progressive shortness of breath during exercise, cough. Decreased lung function occurs.

Prognosis: Fair, but slow progressive respiratory failure is common.

Radiology: Chest radiographs show diffuse interstitial densities, increased transparency in the upper parts of the lung (bullous emphysema), and very occasionally circumscribed nodules.

Pathology:

Gross: The upper lobes display large bullous cysts, while the lower lobes have fibrotic areas and changes seen with honeycombing.

Histology: The lung parenchyma of the upper lobes is destroyed and replaced by large air spaces (bullous emphysema). The lower parts of the lung show mononuclear interstitial infiltrates with deposits of fibrinoid material in the distant airways resembling usual interstitial pneumonia (UIP). Other chronic interstitial changes may be more related to desquamative interstitial pneumonia (DIP). Interstitial fibrosis is usually present.

➤ *Descriptors:* Lung parenchyma with altered structure:
- mononuclear inflammatory infiltrates
- macrophages
- enlarged distant air spaces
- proliferating fibroblasts
- diffuse interstitial fibrosis
- honeycombing

■ *Special stains:* PAS, collagenous stains, Giemsa, Congo, immunohistochemistry for immunoglobulins, endogenous lectins.

Hallmark of Diagnosis: Clinical history, bullous emphysematous changes in the upper lobes, UIP or DIP in the lower lobes.

Differential diagnosis: Idiopathic emphysema, idiopathic UIP, DIP or similar changes related to various agents.

Neurogenic Neoplasms

Definition: Neoplasms of the lung arising from nervous tissue in the lung.

Incidence/Epidemiology: Extremely rare tumors of the lung seen in children and young to middle-aged adults.

Etiology/Pathophysiology: Small nerve fibers and scattered peripheral neurogenic cells may enter into uncontrolled growth with benign or malignant behavior. The tumors are most frequently described as schwannomas and granular cell blastomas. Extremely rare are multiple circumscribed nodules resembling aggressive neurofibromatosis.

Clinical Presentation: Symptoms are related to the localization of the tumors and are usually obstructive complaints.

Prognosis: Usually good and without serious sequelae.

Radiology: Chest radiographs usually show centrally localized tumors and suggest findings related to central obstruction of a major bronchus.

Pathology:

Gross: Firm, grayish-white tumor masses usually localized in association with a major bronchus.

Histology: The tumors are composed of atypical, spindle-shaped cells growing in anisotropic textures (sheets), often with so-called palisading. The specific findings are discussed under the particular headings.

➤ *Descriptors:* Newly formed textures without metastasis potential:
- mesenchymal growth pattern
- fibromatous textures
- plump spindle cells
- absent or infrequent mitoses
- hemorrhage (focal)

■ *Special stains:* PAS, collagenous stains, immunohistochemistry for neurofilaments, vimentin, S-100 protein, desmin, desmoplakin.

Hallmark of Diagnosis: Mesenchymal growth pattern, myxomatoid textures, spindle-shaped cells with palisading. For details, see under the particular headings.

Differential diagnosis: As described under the particular headings, especially fibromatous neoplasms, chronic inflammatory lesions, and atypical tuberculosis.

Neurosarcoma

Definition: Malignant neoplasm of the lung derived from intrapulmonary nerve cells.

Incidence/Epidemiology: Extremely rare neoplasm with equal sex distribution.

Etiology/Pathophysiology: Neoplasm derived from intrapulmonary neural elements.

Clinical Presentation: Symptoms are related to the location. Some tumors may be associated primarily with benign neurofibromas which have become malignant growths.

Prognosis: Poor, as most patients die within 2 years after clinical manifestation of the tumors.

Radiology: Chest radiographs usually show centrally localized tumor masses and suggest findings related to obstruction of a major bronchus.

Pathology:

Gross: Yellowish, soft tumor masses with some necrotic areas and hemorrhage.

Histology: The tumors are composed of plump spindle cells which may show palisading textures. The features of the nuclei and tumor cells show wide variation and may suggest benign tumors in about 20–30% of cases. Necrotic areas, hemorrhage, and myxomatoid changes occur in the more undifferentiated tumors.

➤ *Descriptors:* Newly formed textures with metastasis potential:
- mesenchymal growth pattern
- sarcomatous textures
- plump spindle cells
- palisading tumor cells
- necrosis and hemorrhage
- infrequent mitoses

■ *Special stains:* PAS, collagenous stains, Giemsa, immunohistochemistry for S-100 protein, neurofilaments, desmin, vimentin, desmoplakin.

Hallmark of Diagnosis: Sarcomatous growth pattern, positive neurogenic markers.

Differential diagnosis: Neurofibroma, fibrosarcoma, other types of sarcoma.

Nickel

Definition: Alteration of the lung parenchyma associated with exposure to nickel.

Incidence/Epidemiology: Nickel is mined in the USA, USSR, Cuba and Norway. Alterations of the lung parenchyma associated with exposure to nickel have also been reported in persons working in nickel refineries (UK, particular Wales, and Norway).

Etiology/Pathophysiology: Nickel is a hard metal widely used in the chemical industry and in metallurgy. It is suspected of inducing precancerous lesions and cancer of the upper and lower respiratory tract especially carcinoma of the nasal epithelium. Posing special risk are the nickel compound Ni_3S_2 and additional contaminating arsenic and cobalt. Nickel is also fibrogenic to the lung parenchyma, probably by inhibiting normal defence mechanisms of macrophages which are rendered unable to ingest and kill certain bacteria (*Staphylococcus pyogenes*) by exposure to nickel.

Clinical Presentation: The majority of patients are asymptomatic until the development of lung cancer or cancer of the nose.

Prognosis: Fair, patients have a high risk of lung cancer and cancer of the nose occurring 10–20 years after exposure to nickel.

Radiology: Chest radiographs show a circumscribed density related to lung cancer and mild interstitial fibrotic changes.

Pathology:

Gross: The lungs are normal or slightly fibrotic and in addition show a solid grayish-white tumor.

Histology: Mild interstitial and usually diffuse fibrosis is present in addition to the carcinoma which is usually epidermoid carcinoma and less frequently adenocarcinoma. The nasal epithelium may evidence squamous metaplasia with different grades of dysplasia.

➤ *Descriptors:* Lung parenchyma with altered structure:
- diffuse interstitial fibrosis (mild);
- Bronchial mucosa with altered structure:
- squamous metaplasia and dysplasia;
- Newly formed textures with metastasis potential:
- epithelial growth pattern
- epidermoid textures
- adenoid textures
- keratin production
- mucus production
- homogeneous nuclear and cellular size
- inhomogeneous nuclear and cellular size

- frequent mitoses
- infrequent mitoses
- necrosis

■ *Special stains:* PAS, collagenous stains, Giemsa, X-ray diffraction method or related physical techniques, immunohistochemistry for immunoglobulins and lymphocytic subpopulations, endogenous lectins, DNA analysis (for carcinoma).

Hallmark of Diagnosis: Clinical history, identification and quantification of nickel deposits in the lung parenchyma.

Differential diagnosis: Alteration of the lung parenchyma (fibrosis, lung cancer) due to other causes.

Nicotine

Definition: Alteration of the lung parenchyma associated with exposure to nicotine, see Smoking.

Niemann-Pick Disease

Definition: Involvement of the lung in Niemann-Pick disease.

Incidence/Epidemiology: Involvement of the lung with the infantile form of Niemann-Pick disease can be seen in 50–70% of patients. It is less common in patients suffering from the adult form.

Etiology/Pathophysiology: Niemann-Pick disease is a storage disorder of autosomal recessive inheritance involving abnormal deposits of sphingomyelin in reticuloendothelial cells. Four different forms are distinguishable: (a) an infantile form with fatal outcome during childhood; (b) a prolonged form with onset during childhood, characterized by hepatosplenomegaly and interstitial fibrosis of the lung; (c) an adult form with predominantly neurological symptoms; (d) a mild adult form with slowly progressive hepatosplenomegaly.

Clinical Presentation: The symptoms include progressive shortness of breath with subsequent dyspnea, cyanosis, and severely restricted lung function.

Prognosis: Poor in infantile forms, fair in prolonged forms and in adult forms, which usually present with slow progressive respiratory failure.

Radiology: Chest radiographs show diffuse patchy densities, nodular infiltrates, and honeycombing in late stages.

Pathology:

Gross: The lungs are fibrotic, show honeycombing, and are pale yellow.

Histology: The distant airways show dense agglutinations of large foamy macrophages (Niemann-Pick cells) associated with lymphocytes and plasma cells. Interstitial fibrosis and honeycombing are present in late stages.

➤ *Descriptors:* Lung parenchyma with preserved structure:

- macrophages (foamy)
- mononuclear inflammatory infiltrates;
- Lung parenchyma with altered structure:
- proliferating fibroblasts
- diffuse interstitial fibrosis
- honeycombing

■ *Special stains:* PAS, collagenous stains, Giemsa, Prussian blue, electron microscopy, endogenous lectins.

Hallmark of Diagnosis: Clinical history, demonstration of Niemann-Pick cells by use of electron microscopy.

Differential diagnosis: Involvement of the lung in other storage disorders, atypical tuberculosis, granular cell myoblastoma.

Niridazole

Definition: Alteration of the lung parenchyma associated with intake of niridazole, see Drug Toxicity.

Nitrofurantoin

Definition: Alteration of the lung parenchyma associated with intake of nitrofurantoin, see Drug Toxicity.

Nitrogen Dioxide

Definition: Alteration of the lung parenchyma associated with inhalation of Nitrogen Dioxide, see Drug Toxicity.

Nitrogen Mustards

Definition: Alteration of the lung parenchyma associated with intake of nitrogen mustards, see Drug Toxicity.

Nocardiosis

Definition: Infection of the lung with *Nocardia asteroides*.

Incidence/Epidemiology: *N. asteroides* is an aerobic bacterium, order Actinomycetaceae, with worldwide distribution. It is an opportunistic, gram-positive organism growing in immunocompromised patients such as those receiving steroid therapy, transplants, cytostatic drug regimes, or with AIDS.

Etiology/Pathophysiology: *N. asteroides* is usually inhaled from environmental sources and causes chronic abscessing pneumonia with surrounding fibrotic changes of the necrotic areas. *N. brasiliensis* and *caviae* seldom induce lung infections and are more frequently seen in cutaneous infections. Pulmonary and cerebral infection with *N. asteroides* may be associated with pulmonary alveolar proteinosis, i.e., alveolar proteinosis increases the risk of infection with *N. asteroides*.

Clinical Presentation: The symptoms include cough, dyspnea, expectoration, fever, and chills.

Prognosis: Usually fatal after several months or even years.

Radiology: Chest radiographs show a solitary or multiple, circumscribed densities with central necrosis.

Pathology:

Gross: The lungs show a solitary or multiple, yellowish-reddish nodules with central necrosis and surrounding fibrosis.

Histology: The necrotic areas contain numerous neutrophilic granulocytes, plasma cells, and lymphocytes. The organisms consist of elongated filaments with irregular branches forming rods of various lengths. They may appear similar to ice crystals or chinese characters and stain positively with Gram's stain and methenamine silver stain and negative with Ziehl-Neelsen stain.

➤ *Descriptors:* Lung parenchyma with altered structure:

- necrosis and hemorrhage
- mixed inflammatory infiltrates
- infectious organisms (gram-positive, filamentous)

■ *Special stains:* PAS, collagenous stains, Giemsa, Gram's stain, methenamine silver stain.

Hallmark of Diagnosis: Abscessing opportunistic pneumonia with gram-positive, adhesive ("ice crystals") branching organisms.

Differential diagnosis: Abscessing pneumonias due to other infective organisms such as *Actinomyces* or melioidosis.

Nonasbestos Mineral Fibers

Definition: Alteration of the lung parenchyma associated with inhalation of nonasbestos mineral fibers.

Incidence/Epidemiology: Exposure of persons to nonasbestos mineral fibers is steadily increasing, especially to those mineral fibers replacing asbestos.

Etiology/Pathophysiology: The etiology of fibrosis of the lung parenchyma induced by certain asbestos and nonasbestos fibers is still unknown. Of undoubted importance are the physical properties and the "surface conditions" of the inhaled fibers. The lung defence mechanisms such as incorporation of the fibers by macrophages, oxygen radicals, and nonspecific activation of fibroblasts are probably involved.

Clinical Presentation: The patients may be asymptomatic or present with chronic cough, shortness of breath during physical exercise, dyspnea, etc.

Prognosis: Prognosis depends upon the nature and the amount of inhaled mineral fibers.

Radiology: Chest radiographs may be normal or show diffuse interstitial densities, circumscribed nodules, pleural effusions, and focal scarring. Classification of the radiologic findings according to the ILO scheme (see under Pneumoconiosis) results in three categories depending on the size and profusion of the lesions.

Pathology:

Gross: The lungs may be normal or show diffuse grayish-white densities and a firm consistency. They can display focal, brownish-black nodules as well as pleural thickening and honeycombing.

Histology:
The mineral fibers can be seen in the distant air spaces and may be ingested by macrophages. Diffuse interstitial fibrosis of various degrees or focal scarring and subpleural emphysematous changes are usually associated with clustered mineral fibers. The histomorphological findings may resemble alterations induced by asbestos fibers, silica or hard metal fumes. Sequelae are diffuse interstitial fibrosis, honeycombing, bronchial carcinomas, and probably mesotheliomas.

➤ *Descriptors:* Lung parenchyma with preserved structure:

- ferruginous bodies
- dust (intraalveolar, amorphous, birefringent)
- macrophages (mineral fibers, dust);
- Lung parenchyma with altered structure:
- diffuse interstitial fibrosis
- focal interstitial fibrosis
- mononuclear inflammatory infiltrates
- honeycombing;
- Pleura with altered structure:
- hyaline material
- acellular collagen (basket-weave appearance);
- Newly formed structures with metastasis potential:
- epithelial growth pattern
- mesenchymal growth pattern
- epidermoid textures
- solid textures
- adenoid textures
- sarcomatous textures

■ *Special stains:* PAS, collagenous stains, Prussian blue, X-ray diffraction methods or related physical techniques.

Hallmark of Diagnosis: Clinical history, intraalveolar mineral fibers, focal or diffuse interstitial fibrosis, identification of the mineral fibers.

Differential diagnosis: Lung damage induced by other extrinsic or intrinsic agents, smoking, asbestos fibers, or metal fumes.

Obstructive Pulmonary Disease

Definition: Alteration of the lung parenchyma due to complete or partial obstruction of the conducting airways.

Incidence/Epidemiology: Frequent disorder seen in patients at any age. The most frequent causes in newborns and infants are congenital malformations and aspiration and in adults centrally located tumors.

Etiology/Pathophysiology: Complete or partial obstruction of the larger bronchi may be acute or chronic. Acute complete obstruction causes atelectasis and usually induces subsequent bacterial infections, if it is not resolved. Acute partial obstruction may persist over a long period of time and induces chronic deformation of the distant conducting airways and chronic pneumonitis, often with bacterial superinfection. The related obstructive disorders are bronchiectasis, bronchopneumonia, interstitial pneumonitis with associated fibrosis, scarring, and honeycombing.

Clinical Presentation: Symptoms include cough, expectoration, asthmatic complaints, chest pain and dyspnea.

Prognosis: Depends upon the underlying disease, slow progression of the pulmonary dysfunction is frequently observed.

Radiology: Chest radiographs show peripheral diffuse densities, often related to anatomical segments.

Pathology:

Gross: The major bronchi usually show a central narrowing of the lumen caused by foreign bodies, tumors, scarring, lymph nodes, etc.

Histology: The peripheral lung parenchyma contains agglutinations of macrophages, often with foamy cytoplasm, ectatic bronchi, additional mononuclear inflammatory infiltrates, exudation of fibrin, and granulocytic infiltrates if a bacterial superinfection has occurred.

➤ *Descriptors:* Bronchial mucosa with preserved structure:

- ectatic lumen
- mononuclear inflammatory infiltrates
- eosinophils
- increased number of goblet cells;
- Lung parenchyma with preserved structure:
- macrophages
- mononuclear inflammatory infiltrates
- intraalveolar fibrinoid material;
- Lung parenchyma with altered structure:
- focal interstitial fibrosis
- honeycombing

■ *Special stains:* PAS, collagenous stains, Giemsa.

Hallmark of Diagnosis: Clinical history, narrowing of the bronchial lumen, desquamative changes of the distant airways, bronchiectasis.
Differential diagnosis: Asthmatic bronchitis, desquamative interstitial pneumonia (DIP), opportunistic infection, interstitial lung diseases due to other agents.

Oil Aspiration

Definition: Alteration of the lung parenchyma due to aspiration of oil.
Incidence/Epidemiology: Aspiration of oil has been most frequently described under infants and children or in elderly persons receiving nosedrops, oily vitamin preparations, or cod liver oil. Adults may aspirate mineral oil or oil-based contrast media. Chronic oil aspiration may be seen in drug-dependent persons (sniffing).
Etiology/Pathophysiology: Oil is relatively inert to phagocytosis and to biochemical digestion in the lung parenchyma. However, differences exist between different oils according to their proportion of unsaturated fatty acids. Mineral oils and vegetable oils are usually inert or may produce a mild to moderate inflammatory reaction of host tissue, as opposed to animal oils, which elicit a very intense inflammatory reaction.
Clinical Presentation: Patients may be asymptomatic or may present with chest pain, dyspnea, and cough.
Prognosis: Depending upon the amounts of inhaled oil and the compartments involved, slow recovery from the symptoms or slow progression to respiratory failure may occur.
Radiology: Chest radiographs show diffuse interstitial and intraalveolar densities with marked propagation in the lower parts of the lung.
Pathology:
Gross: The lungs are firm in consistency and of grayish to yellow color. Oil droplets may arise from the cut surface in severe intoxication.
Histology: The distant airways are filled with oil droplets and macrophages digesting oil droplets. Mononuclear infiltrates are usually present. However, the degree of inflammatory infiltration varies to a large extent. Fibrotic changes may be seen in late phases.

➤ *Descriptors:* Lung parenchyma with preserved structure:
- lipoid material (intraalveolar oil droplets)
- macrophages (foamy, oil-laden)
- mononuclear inflammatory infiltrates;
- Lung parenchyma with altered structure:
- focal interstitial fibrosis
- proliferating fibroblasts
- honeycombing

■ *Special stains:* PAS, collagenous stains, Giemsa, Oil red O stain, endogenous lectins.
Hallmark of Diagnosis: Clinical history, identification of oil droplets in the distant airways.
Differential diagnosis: Endogenous lipid pneumonia, lipoma, liposarcoma.

Oncocytoma

Definition: Benign neoplasms of the lung derived from cells of the mucus glands of the bronchial submucosa.
Incidence/Epidemiology: Rare neoplasm usually seen in elderly patients.
Etiology/Pathophysiology: Oncocytic change of glandular cells is associated with an increased number of mitochondria in these cells. Oncocytomas are tumors with an increased number of mitochondria and negative binding capacities to neurosecretory markers.
Clinical Presentation: Symptoms are related to the central location of the tumors and include chronic cough, asthmatic complaints and dyspnea.
Prognosis: Usually good and without serious sequelae.
Radiology: Chest radiographs may be normal or may show findings related to obstructive changes of the peripheral lung parenchyma.
Pathology:
Gross: The tumors measure 2–4 cm in maximum diameter at time of clinical symptomatology and are grayish with a firm consistency.
Histology: The neoplasms are composed of large, homogeneous cells with abundant granular cytoplasm. Adenoid growth textures are usually present. Mitotic figures, necrosis, or inflammatory response of the host tissue are usually not detectable.

➤ *Descriptors:* Newly formed textures without metastasis potential:

- epithelial growth pattern
- adenoid textures
- large tumor cells (abundant cytoplasm)
- homogeneous nuclear and cellular size
- absent or infrequent mitoses
- absent necrosis
- absent inflammatory infiltrates

■ *Special stains:* PAS, Giemsa, immunohistochemistry for neuroendocrine markers (to exclude carcinoids), DNA analysis (to exclude adenocarcinoma), endogenous lectins.

Hallmark of Diagnosis: Oncocytic appearance of tumor cells with adenoid growth pattern. Absent mitotic figures, necrosis, or inflammatory infiltrations.

Differential diagnosis: Carcinoid, adenocarcinoma, acinic cell tumor, mucoepidermoid carcinoma, mucus gland adenoma.

Opisthorchosis

Definition: Infection of the lung with *Opisthorchis viverrini.*

Incidence/Epidemiology: *Opisthorchis viverrini* is endemic in the northeastern part of Thailand, in Poland, USSR, Vietnam, India, Japan, and Korea. In contrast to infections of the liver (about 25% of the population) infections of the lung are very rare and usually seen in farmers.

Etiology/Pathophysiology: The eggs of the trematode pass through the bile duct of man and are ingested by snails from the feces. Within the snail cercariae develop and enter fresh water as free-swimming parasites, where they are ingested by a wide variety of fish and crayfish. Upon eating raw or undercooked fish man ingests the parasites which penetrate into the liver. They form large cysts in the liver which may rupture, and the parasites may invade the diaphragm and the right lung. Patients have an increased risk of developing cholangiocarcinoma.

Clinical Presentation: The infection usually does not produce symptoms early on, but they may develop later and comprise anorexia, diarrhea, eosinophilia, and dyspnea if the lung is involved.

Prognosis: Usually good; however, heavy worm burdens can cause serious sequelae including liver abscess, pancreatitis, hepatobronchial fistula, and cholangiocarcinoma.

Radiology: Chest radiographs show a dense circumscribed mass in the lower right lung with continuation to the diaphragm and liver.

Pathology:

Gross: The right lung displays grayish-white areas of necrosis and cystic alterations in the lower lobe.

Histology: The parasites measure approximately 7 × 1 mm, the eggs 20–30 µm. Infection can be identified by finding the eggs in the feces. The parasites usually do not invade the liver and lie within the bile ducts which can become obstructed and may rupture. Infection of the lung is accompanied by severe inflammatory infiltrates and biliary-bronchial fistula.

➤ *Descriptors:* Lung parenchyma with altered structure:

- mixed inflammatory infiltrates
- necrosis
- parasites (eggs)
- eosinophils

■ *Special stains:* PAS, collagenous stains, Giemsa, Movat.

Hallmark of Diagnosis: Clinical history, hepato-bronchial fistula, identification of the parasites.

Differential diagnosis: Infection of the lung with other species of parasites, especially *Echinococcus, Schistosoma, Fasciola.*

Opportunistic Infections

Definition: Alteration of the lung parenchyma associated with opportunistic infections, see Bacterial Infections.

Ornithosis

Definition: Infection of the lung by *Chlamydia psittaci*, see Psittacosis.

Orthomyxovirus

Definition: Infection of the lung by orthomyxovirus, see Influenzavirus Infection.

Ossification of the Lung

Definition: Development of osteoid tissue in the lung parenchyma.

Incidence/Epidemiology: An unusual disorder most frequently seen either in middle-aged men (nodular form) or in older men (racemose form).

Etiology/Pathophysiology: Two different types of ossification can be distinguished: (a) a nodular form with nodules measuring 2–8 mm and (b) a racemose form with linear deposits. Both forms are related to chronic inflammation of the lung, chronic pulmonary venous hypertension, and chronic renal disease (renal failure).

Clinical Presentation: Patients are usually asymptomatic.

Prognosis: Usually good; however, slow progression into respiratory failure has been reported.

Radiology: Chest radiographs show multiple, nodular densities, predominantly in the lower lobes.

Pathology:

Gross: The lungs exhibit multiple, hard, white nodules.

Histology: The ossified nodules lie in the distant airways and are of various sizes. They contain a matrix of mature lamellar bone, sometimes with bone marrow. Fibrotic changes surrounding the nodules are present and are related to the size of the nodules. Larger nodules are surrounded by fibrous tissue, in contrast to smaller bony nodules. Severe interstitial inflammation is usually absent.

➤ *Descriptors:* Lung parenchyma with altered structure:

- bony nodules (intraalveolar, mature)
- focal interstitial fibrosis (perinodular)
- mononuclear inflammatory infiltrates

■ *Special stains:* PAS, collagenous stains, Giemsa, endogenous lectins.

Hallmark of Diagnosis: Deposits of mature bony nodules within the distant airways.

Differential diagnosis: Metastatic osteosarcoma, calcification of the lung.

Osteosarcoma

Definition: Malignant neoplasm of the lung with osteoid differentiation.

Incidence/Epidemiology: Primary osteosarcomas of the lung are extremely rare, and only a few cases have been reported. Metastases of osteosarcoma into the lung are more frequent and are usually seen in young to middle-aged adults several months to some years after development of the primary.

Etiology/Pathophysiology: The neoplasms derive from cartilaginous or osteous tissue of the lung.

Clinical Presentation: The few cases of primary lung osteosarcomas observed were centrally localized, and symptoms were related to the central location of the tumors.

Prognosis: Poor and similar to that of patients with bronchial carcinoma.

Radiology: Chest radiographs show dense tumor masses in the central areas of the lung.

Pathology:

Gross: The tumors measure 2–4 cm in maximum diameter at the time of detection and are of solid, firm, pearly consistency and white in color.

Histology: The neoplasms show characteristic differentiation into osteoid formations with trabecules, atypical multinucleated giant cells, and small spindle-shaped tumor cells. Mitotic figures are present, and necrotic and cystic areas are small.

➤ *Descriptors:* Newly formed textures with metastasis potential:

- mesenchymal growth pattern
- sarcomatous textures
- osteoid textures
- large tumor cells
- multinucleated giant cells (atypical)
- inhomogeneous nuclear and cellular size
- plump spindle cells
- frequent mitoses
- necrosis and hemorrhage

■ *Special stains:* PAS, collagenous stains, Giemsa, immunohistochemistry for vimentin, desmin, desmoplakin, endogenous lectins, DNA analysis.

Hallmark of Diagnosis: Clinical history, osteoid growth pattern of the neoplasms.

Differential diagnosis: Metastatic osteosarcoma, sarcomas of other tissue.

Ovarian Carcinoma

Definition: Metastasis of ovarian carcinoma into the lung, see Metastasis into the Lung.

Oxygen

Definition: Alteration of the lung parenchyma due to inhalation of pure oxygen.
Incidence/Epidemiology: Inhalation of pure oxygen and of ozone is of practical importance in therapeutic regimes of newborns and of patients at any age presenting with reduction of blood oxygen levels. Inhalation of air with small but detectable concentrations of ozone now occurs in air-polluted areas, especially during summertime.
Etiology/Pathophysiology: Excessive oxygen is harmful to the lung and causes severe damage, especially in lungs with preexisting lesions. Oxygen disturbs the air-interstitial fluid barrier and consequently induces the formation of hyaline membranes, desquamation of epithelial cells, degeneration of endothelial cells and interstitial edema. Damage may be seen as soon as 8–12 h after exposure.
Clinical Presentation: Symptoms include progressive dyspnea and acute respiratory distress.
Radiology: Chest radiographs show diffuse bilateral densities.
Prognosis: Fair, but slow progressive respiratory failure is often observed.
Pathology:
Gross: The lungs are edematous, heavy, and red-pink.
Histology: The normal texture of the lung parenchyma is preserved. The distant airways contain hyaline membranes, fragments of pneumocytes, and a moderate inflammatory infiltrate consisting of neutrophilic and eosinophilic granulocytes, plasma cells,and macrophages. The interalveolar septula are widened by protein-rich fluid. Fibroblasts and organized fibrinoid deposits are seen in later stages. Bronchiolitis obliterans is frequently present in later stages, especially in infants. Scarring and honeycombing may be the outcome of the intoxication.

➤ *Descriptors:* Lung parenchyma with preserved structure:

- mixed inflammatory infiltrates
- hyaline membranes
- intraalveolar serous fluid;
- Lung parenchyma with altered structure:
- intraalveolar fibrinoid material
- macrophages
- proliferating fibroblasts
- focal interstitial fibrosis
- intrabronchiolar fibrinoid material and histiocytes
- ulceration of bronchiolar mucosa
- honeycombing

■ *Special stains:* PAS, collagenous stains, Giemsa, endogenous lectins.

Hallmark of Diagnosis: Clinical history, interstitial edema, hyaline membranes, bronchiolitis obliterans, organizing pneumonia.
Differential diagnosis: Acute alveolar damage due to other agents, pulmonary edema, bacterial pneumonia.

Oxyphenisatin

Definition: Alteration of the lung parenchyma associated with intake of oxyphenisatin, see Drug Toxicity.

Oxyprenolol

Definition: Alteration of the lung parenchyma associated with intake of oxyprenolol, see Drug Toxicity.

Ozon

Definition: Alteration of the lung parenchyma associated with inhalation of ozon, see Oxygen.

Pancoast's Tumor

Definition: Malignant neoplasm of the lung arising in the superior sulcus.
Incidence/Epidemiology: About 10% of all malignancies are located within the superior sulcus. The age distribution and the sex ratio of patients are similar to those of all lung carcinomas.
Etiology/Pathophysiology: Patients with Pancoast's tumors present with the same risk fac-

tors as the population of all patients with bronchial carcinomas.

Clinical Presentation: Symptoms are usually late in appearing and include chest pain, Horner's syndrome and subcutaneous masses.

Prognosis: Poor; however, patients with Pancoast's tumors have a better prognosis than patients with tumors which are also graded pT3 due to other reasons.

Radiology: Chest radiographs show a peripheral density with continuation into the upper chest wall.

Pathology:

Gross: The tumors are firm in consistency, and white and infiltrate the pleura parietalis and adjacent tissue.

Histology: Surgical specimens usually show poorly differentiated carcinomas with dense inflammatory infiltrates due to radiation treatment prior to excision. All cell types of the lung carcinoma can develop in the upper sulcus region, but epidermoid carcinoma and adenocarcinoma are most frequent.

➤ *Descriptors:* Newly formed textures with metastasis potential:

- epithelial growth pattern
- adenoid textures
- epidermoid textures
- inhomogeneous nuclear and cellular size
- prominent nucleoli
- frequent mitoses
- micrometastases
- dense inflammatory infiltrates

■ *Special stains:* PAS, collagenous stains, Giemsa, immunohistochemistry for various tumor markers, DNA analysis, endogenous lectins.

Hallmark of Diagnosis: Localization of the carcinoma.

Differential diagnosis: Due to the specific cell type.

Pancreatin

Definition: Alteration of the lung parenchyma associated with intake of pancreatin, see Drug Toxicity.

Papillary Adenoma

Definition: Benign neoplasm of the lower respiratory tract, see Adenoma.

Papilloma

Definition: Benign tumor of the glandular and bronchial surfaces of the lung.

Incidence/Epidemiology: Unusual tumor arising in children and young to middle-aged adults. Squamous papillomas often occur as multiple lesions. Adult patients with papillomas are usually heavy cigarette smokers.

Etiology/Pathophysiology: Papillomas are thought to arise from papillomavirus-infected epithelial cells. However, none of the common papillomavirus types seen in the cervix has been identified in bronchial papillomatous lesions.

Clinical Presentation: Symptoms are related to endobronchial and endotracheal growth and, hence, to asthmatic complaints and to obstructive changes of the distant lung parenchyma. Spread of papillomatous lesions from the larynx to the trachea and major bronchi occurs in 2–5% of cases.

Prognosis: Children younger than 5 years old, usually have a poor prognosis and present with multiple recurrences. Malignant transformation can occur even after 10–30 years. The mortality rate related to multiple squamous papillomas has been estimated to be 30–40%.

Radiology: Chest radiographs are normal or show lesions associated with obstruction of a major conduction airway.

Pathology:

Gross: Exophytic lesions soft in consistency and grayish-white. Continuous growth into subcartilaginous tissue may occur.

Histology: The bronchial or tracheal epithelial cells undergo squamous metaplasia with bland acanthosis. Dysplasia of the epithelial cells is usually present and may proceed in severity to carcinoma in situ or invasive carcinoma. The stromal reaction is moderate to severe and includes numerous mononuclear inflammatory infiltrates. The distant lung parenchyma may show obstructive pneumonitis with additional bacterial superinfection. Inverted papillomas may show transitional cell layers with glandular appearance.

➤*Descriptors:* Newly formed textures without metastasis potential:

- epithelial growth pattern
- epidermoid textures
- polypoid endobronchial textures
- absent or infrequent mitoses
- homogeneous nuclear and cellular size
- preserved bronchial mucosa;
- Bronchial mucosa with altered structure:
- squamous metaplasia and dysplasia
- mononuclear inflammatory infiltrates

▪ *Special stains:* PAS, Giemsa, immunohistochemistry or in situ hybridization for papillomavirus infection, DNA analysis, and syntactic structure analysis for grading of dysplasia.

Hallmark of Diagnosis: Exophytic growth of benign epithelial tumor comprising squamous metaplasia, papillomatosis, and acanthosis.

Differential diagnosis: Epidermoid carcinoma, squamous metaplasia, carcinoid, bronchial adenoma, mucoepidermoid carcinoma.

Papillomatosis

Definition: Multiple, benign exophytic lesions arising in the larynx or in the trachea.

Incidence/Epidemiology: Unusual disorder usually seen in infants or in children.

Etiology/Pathophysiology: About 50% of children with laryngeal papillomatosis have a history of infection of the genital tract of the mother with papillomavirus type 6. Continuous extension of the papillomas into the trachea and major bronchi rarely occurs.

Clinical Presentation: Symptoms include cough, hoarseness, and complaint associated with obstruction of the conducting airways.

Prognosis: Usually poor, children present with multiple recurrencies.

Radiology: Chest radiographs are usually normal.

Pathology:

Gross: The tumors are grayish-white and soft in consistency and seldom exceed 1 cm in maximum diameter.

Histology: The neoplasms show sheets of epidermoid cells with various degrees of dysplasia. Mitotic figures may be present as well as koilocytic features and moderate stromal reaction. Nests of small papillomas may be present even in the distant conducting airways.

➤*Descriptors:* Newly formed textures without metastasis potential:

- epithelial growth pattern
- epidermoid textures
- polypoid endobronchial textures
- absent or infrequent mitoses
- prominent nucleoli
- preserved bronchial mucosa;
- Bronchial mucosa with altered structure:
- squamous metaplasia and dysplasia
- koilocytosis
- mononuclear inflammatory infiltrates

▪ *Special stains:* PAS, Giemsa, immunohistochemistry and in situ hybridization for papillomavirus (type 6), DNA analysis and syntactic structure analysis for grading of dysplasia.

Hallmark of Diagnosis: Exophytic papillomatous growth of epidermoid (transitional cell) structures with various degrees of dysplasia and koilocytosis.

Differential diagnosis: Squamous metaplasia, chronic inflammation, epidermoid carcinoma, mucoepidermoid carcinoma.

Papillomavirus

Definition: Infection of the lower respiratory tract with papillomavirus, see Papillomatosis, Viral Infection.

Paprika Slicer's Lung

Definition: Alteration of the lung parenchyma associated with inhalation of paprika dust.

Incidence/Epidemiology: The disorder has been described under Yugoslavian workers exposed to moldy paprika pods. Poor workhouse conditions induce the growth of the fungus *Mucor stolonifer*.

Etiology/Pathophysiology: Inhalation of fungal spores induces an allergic reaction of the lung parenchyma.

Clinical Presentation: Symptoms may be acute or subacute and include cough, chest pain, shortness of breath on exercise, dyspnea, and fever.

Radiology: Chest radiographs show diffuse, interstitial densities or a fine granular pattern.

Prognosis: Usually good and without known sequelae.

Pathology:

Gross: The lungs are edematous and reddish-pink.

Histology: The histomorphological findings include interstitial edema, exudation of fibrin, interstitial mononuclear infiltrates, eosinophilic infiltrates, formation of noncaseating epithelioid granulomas. Fibromatous changes may occur in advanced phases.

➤ *Descriptors:* Lung parenchyma with altered structure:

- noncaseous epithelioid granulomas
- eosinophils
- multinucleated giant cells
- intrabronchiolar fibrinoid material and histiocytes
- ulceration of bronchiolar mucosa;
- Lung parenchyma with preserved structure:
- macrophages
- desquamation, hypertrophy, hyperplasia and dysplasia of pneumocytes
- mononuclear inflammatory infiltrates
- intraalveolar serous fluid

■ *Special stains:* PAS, collagenous stains, Giemsa, immunohistochemistry for immunoglobulins, endogenous lectins.

Hallmark of Diagnosis: Clinical history, histomorphological findings as described under the heading Allergic (Extrinsic) Alveolitis.

Differential diagnosis: Infectious and noninfectious granulomatous diseases, lymphocytic interstitial pneumonia, desquamative interstitial pneumonia. For details, see Allergic (Extrinsic) Alveolitis.

Paraaminosalicylic Acid

Definition: Alteration of the lung parenchyma associated with intake of paraaminosalicylic acid, see Drug Toxicity.

Paracoccidioidomycosis

Definition: Infection of the lung by *Paracoccidioides brasiliensis.*

Incidence/Epidemiology: The disease is endemic in South America, especially in the tropical and subtropical areas of Brazil, Columbia, and Venezuela. The diagnosis of pulmonary infection may be delayed as long as 20–30 years after the infective contact. At specific risk are persons with intensive contact with the soil (rural inhabitants).

Etiology/Pathophysiology: *P. brasiliensis* is a dimorphic fungus growing as a white mold at lower temperatures and in cerebri forms at higher temperatures. It forms oval, yeast-like organisms measuring 5–40 μm in maximum diameter with a characteristic adherence of large and small cells.

Clinical Presentation: The infection occurs in two different clinical forms: (a) an acute progressive (disseminated) course (10% of patients, usually young persons) with fungemia and septical metastases into the liver, spleen, and lymph nodes after initial infection of the lung; (b) a chronic progressive form (90% of patients, usually older persons) which has a latent period of several years before clinical detection. The progression is limited to the lung in about 50–70% of patients, whereas 30–50% of patients present with a limited or disseminated spread of the fungus. Symptoms include chest pain, fever, dyspnea, cough, and hemoptysis.

Prognosis: Fair, as it is a self-limited infection in 50–70% of patients. Acute, progressive, life-threatening forms occur in 10% of patients. The mortality rate is less than 5%.

Radiology: Chest radiographs show bilateral, diffuse, nodular infiltrates often with parahilar markings. Cavities are observed in 10–40% of patients.

Pathology:

Gross: The lungs are fibrotic and the structure is dissolved into honeycombing. Caseating, yellowish-white, crumbling nodules and parahilar fibrosis are present.

Histology: The organisms can be seen in a suppurative alveolar exudate which is usually surrounded by irregularly formed fibrous bundles destroying the adjacent lung parenchyma. Multinucleated giant cells, macrophages, and histiocytes may be present.

➤ *Descriptors:* Lung parenchyma with preserved structure:

- intraalveolar fibrinoid material
- mixed inflammatory infiltrates
- fungus (yeast);
- Lung parenchyma with altered structure:

- caseous epithelioid granulomas (ill-defined)
- multinucleated giant cells
- fungus (yeast)
- mixed inflammatory infiltrates
- focal interstitial fibrosis

■ *Special stains:* PAS, collagenous stains, Giemsa, methenamine silver stain.

Hallmark of Diagnosis: Clinical history, intraalveolar fibrinoid material with mixed inflammatory infiltrates, identification of the fungus.

Differential diagnosis: Histoplasmosis, cryptococcosis, blastomycosis.

Paraffinoma

Definition: Granulomatous alteration of the lung parenchyma after aspiration of oil.

Incidence/Epidemiology: Rare disease seen months to years after initial aspiration.

Etiology/Pathophysiology: The reaction of the lung parenchyma to aspirated oil depends upon the amount of unsaturated fatty acids and chemical admixtures. Oil droplets can be ingested by macrophages and be inert to the host tissue or may induce a chronic, progressive, granulomatous, inflammatory reaction.

Clinical Presentation: Patients are usually asymptomatic.

Prognosis: Usually good; however, slow progressive respiratory failure can occur in patients with extensive intoxication.

Radiology: Chest radiographs show solitary densities, usually in the lower lobes.

Pathology:

Gross: The lungs exhibit solitary, yellowish nodules and are firm in consistency.

Histology: The granulomas consist of foamy macrophages, histiocytes, lymphocytes, plasma cells, multinucleated foreign-body giant cells, and lipoid droplets in the adjacent distant air spaces.

➤ *Descriptors:* Lung parenchyma with altered structure:

- lipoid material (lipid droplets)
- noncaseous epithelioid granulomas
- multinucleated giant cells
- macrophages (foamy)
- mononuclear inflammatory infiltrates

■ *Special stains:* PAS, collagenous stains, Giemsa, Oil red O stain.

Hallmark of Diagnosis: Clinical history, noncaseating granulomas with foamy macrophages and lipoid droplets.

Differential diagnosis: Desquamative interstitial pneumonia, atypical tuberculosis, sarcoidosis, allergic extrinsic alveolitis.

Paraganglioma

Definition: Metastasis of paraganglioma into the lung parenchyma, see Metastasis into the Lung.

Paragonimiasis

Definition: Infection of the lung by species of the genus *Paragonimus*, especially *P. westermani*.

Incidence/Epidemiology: The *genus Paragonimus* is endemic in Asia, Africa, and South America. Several species are known to live in specific endemic areas. The parasite is acquired by eating raw or undercooked infected crabs or crayfish.

Etiology/Pathophysiology: *P. westermani* and related species are the only true human pulmonary parasites and thus well adapted to the pulmonary environment and able to mature and settle in the lung. The parasite eggs, which are produced in the lungs, are coughed up, swallowed, and passed with the feces. The eggs are taken in by snails and develop to free-swimming cercariae which infect crabs and crayfish by penetrating the gills and becoming metacercariae. After being eaten by man the metacercariae penetrate the wall of the stomach and settle into the lung after passing the diaphragm. The ovoid eggs measure 90×50 µm, and the adult worms 10×5 mm.

Clinical Presentation: Patients may be asymptomatic or complain about the insidious onset of chest pain, cough and hemoptysis. Pleural effusions have been reported in 40–50% of patients.

Prognosis: Usually good; however, a fatal outcome has been reported if cerebral infections exist.

Radiology: Chest radiographs show normal lungs.

Pathology:
Gross: The lungs contain one or more cysts measuring 1–2 cm in diameter. The cysts and possible inflammatory reaction can be seen adjacent to small bronchi and bronchioles.
Histology: The mature parasites usually lie in clusters and are surrounded by an eosinophilic and granulocytic inflammatory exudate. Other lesions are small scars or granulomatous areas with embedded eggs. The worms may be covered by fibrous walls which form cysts up to 15 mm in maximum diameter.

➤ *Descriptors:* Lung parenchyma with altered structure:
- parasites (eggs and larvae)
- focal interstitial fibrosis (at boundary)
- cysts (pseudocysts, fibrous walls)
- noncaseous epithelioid granulomas
- mixed inflammatory infiltrates
- eosinophils

■ *Special stains:* PAS, collagenous stains, Giemsa, Movat.

Hallmark of Diagnosis: Clinical history and triad: cough, hemoptysis, and identification of eggs in sputum or in feces.
Differential diagnosis: Infection of the lung with other parasites, especially alariasis or schistosomiasis.

Parainfluenza

Definition: Infection of the lung by parainfluenzavirus.
Incidence/Epidemiology: Infection of the upper and lower respiratory tract with parainfluenza virus accounts for 5–10% of all acute respiratory diseases in hospitalized children. It is less common in adults.
Etiology/Pathophysiology: Transmission of the virus is due to person-to-person contact or droplets. The infection usually manifests in the nasal epithelium with an incubation time of 4–8 days. The virus spreads from the nasal epithelium to the trachea and to the lower respiratory tract as far as the terminal airways. Four different types of parainfluenzavirus can be distinguished according to their antigenicity. The disorder has a self-healing tendency, and death seldom occurs. However, patients with immunologic deficiency (T-cell abnormalities) are at specific risk.
Clinical Presentation: Symptoms include rhinorrhea, hoarseness, cough, rhonchi, stridor, wheezing, fever, and chest pain.
Prognosis: Usually good; however, immunocompromised patients often present with bacterial superinfections and serious sequelae.

Radiology: Chest radiographs are usually normal or may show mild signs of bronchitis and peribronchiolar infiltrates.

Pathology:
Gross: The trachea and the bronchi are red, and the mucosa is edematous and swollen.

Histology: The epithelial cells of the small bronchi and bronchioles are damaged and desquamated. A moderate mononuclear infiltration is present in the submucosa. Infection of the terminal airways causes an intraalveolar edema, fibrin exudation, hyperplasia and hypertrophy of the cells of the alveolar lining and formation of multinucleated giant cells. Interstitial fibrosis may develop in late stages or in immunocompromised patients. The giant cells show cytoplasmic inclusion bodies, and the epithelial cells often show koilocytosis.

➤ *Descriptors:* Bronchial mucosa with preserved structure:
- desquamation, hypertrophy, hyperplasia and dysplasia of epithelial cells
- mononuclear inflammatory infiltrates;
- Lung parenchyma with preserved structure:
- intraalveolar serous fluid
- desquamation, hypertrophy, hyperplasia and dysplasia of pneumocytes
- koilocytosis
- multinucleated giant cells;
- Lung parenchyma with altered structure:
- focal interstitial fibrosis

■ *Special stains:* PAS, Giemsa, collagenous stains, immunohistochemistry and in situ hybridization.

Hallmark of Diagnosis: Clinical history, identification of virus infection by serum antibodies in hemagglutination tests, complement fixation, neutralization tests.

Differential diagnosis: Infection of the respiratory tract with other viruses (especially respiratory syncytial virus), bronchopneumonia due to other agents, allergic reaction of bronchial epithelium.

Paraquat

Definition: Alteration of the lung parenchyma associated with inhalation of paraquat.

Incidence/Epidemiology: Paraquat is a potent herbicide and has been used in Mexico for spraying marihuana plants. It is also sold in solid, liquid and aerosol forms as a grass killer. Intoxications have been reported in the USA.

Etiology/Pathophysiology: Paraquat probably induces its severe damage to lung parenchyma by the release of free oxygen radicals. Intoxication occurs as severe acute alveolar damage and most frequently has a fatal outcome.

Clinical Presentation: The intoxication starts with burning in the throat and mouth and proceeds to progressive dyspnea, hypoxemia and cyanosis after a few days. Death is usually unavoidable.

Prognosis: Poor, a mortality rate of 80–100% has been reported.

Radiology: Chest radiographs show bilateral, diffuse infiltrates.

Pathology:

Gross: The lungs are edematous, heavy, and pink.

Histology: The lung texture is preserved. The interalveolar walls have diffuse, mononuclear, inflammatory infiltrates. The distant airways contain fibrin deposits, macrophages, lymphocytes, and plasma cells. Formation of hyaline membranes, hypertrophy, hyperplasia, dysplasia, and desquamation of the cells of the alveolar lining indicate the diffuse alveolar damage. Bronchiolitis obliterans is common. Interstitial fibrosis with honeycombing may occur in the end-stage.

➤ *Descriptors:* Lung parenchyma with preserved structure:

- intraalveolar fibrinoid material
- mononuclear inflammatory infiltrates
- hyaline membranes
- desquamation, hypertrophy, hyperplasia and dysplasia of pneumocytes;
- Lung parenchyma with altered structure:
- intrabronchiolar fibrinoid material and histiocytes
- ulceration of bronchiolar mucosa
- focal interstitial fibrosis
- honeycombing

■ *Special stains:* PAS, collagenous stains, Giemsa, endogenous lectins.

Hallmark of Diagnosis: Clinical history, diffuse alveolar damage.

Differential diagnosis: Diffuse alveolar damage due to other agents, usual interstitial pneumonia, desquamative interstitial pneumonia, bronchiolitis obliterans due to other agents, bronchioloalveolar carcinoma.

Parasitelike Structures

Definition: Alteration of the lung parenchyma associated with aspiration of vegetal material, see Lentil Pneumonia.

Parasites

Definition: Infection of the lung by more highly organized organisms.

Incidence/Epidemiology: Parasites such as protozoa, nematodes, and trematodes are a severe public health problem, especially in the tropics, and kill several million people each year. Invasion of parasites into the lung is quite rare and often an aberrancy. However, individual patients may present with severe clinical problems. In addition, the spectrum of parasitic invasion of the lung in Western countries has changed due to the problem of immunocompromised patients such as those with AIDS or undergoing organ transplantation who are highly susceptible to infection by protozoa.

Etiology/Pathophysiology: The lungs may be the host of arthopods (acariasis: inhalation of mites; myiasis: larva dipterans; pentastomiasis: *Pentastoma armilifer, linguatula*; hirundiasis: leeches); cestodes (cysticercosis, echinococcosis, sparganosis); nematodes (anisakiasis, ascariasis, dilofilariasis, filariasis, which include the so-called tropical pulmonary eosinophilia, capillariasis, strongyloidiasis, mammomonogamiasis, toxocariasis, trichinosis, visceral larva migrans, and rare infections with baylisascariasis, *Lagochilascaris, Gnathostoma, Enterobius vermicularis, Micronea, Metastrongylus, Angiostrongylus, Mansonella*); protozoa (acanthamebiasis, amebiasis, Chagas' disease, cryptosporidiasis, kala-azar, malaria, *Pneumocystis carinii*, toxoplasmosis, trichomoniasis); trematodes (alariasis, opistorchiasis, paragonimiasis, schistosomiasis, and rare infections with *Clinostomum, Fasciola*). The details are discussed under the particular headings.

Clinical Presentation: The severity of pulmonary symptoms depends upon the severity of infection and upon the species. Well-adapted species seldom cause severe symptoms and may remain virtually undetected until the death of the host. Nonadapted parasites usually induce marked symptoms which include chest pain, cough, eosinophilia, hemoptysis and dyspnea.

Prognosis: Usually good; however, fatal courses occur and are often related to cerebral infections.

Radiology: Chest radiographs are usually normal.

Pathology:

Gross: Only cestodes, nematodes, trematodes and leeches can be seen macroscopically.

Histology: The histomorphological diagnosis may be difficult due to the severe inflammatory response of host tissue and degeneration of the parasite. Severe infections can be identified by the presence of eggs in the sputum and feces.

➤ *Descriptors:* Lung parenchyma with altered structure:

- noncaseous epithelioid granulomas
- parasites (intraalveolar, larvae, eggs, "shadows")
- mixed inflammatory infiltrates
- eosinophils
- focal interstitial fibrosis (scarring);
- Pulmonary vessels with altered structure:
- parasites
- noncaseous epithelioid granulomas
- mixed inflammatory infiltrates
- eosinophils

■ *Special stains:* PAS, collagenous stains, Movat, complement-binding assay, immunofluorescence.

Hallmark of Diagnosis: Clinical history, identification and classification of the parasite.

Differential diagnosis: Due to the infective agent, bacterial infections, infarction.

Penicillamine

Definition: Alteration of the lung parenchyma associated with intake of penicillamine, see Drug Toxicity.

Penicillin

Definition: Alteration of the lung parenchyma associated with intake of penicillin, see Drug Toxicity.

Penicilliosis

Definition: Infection of the lung by *Penicillium marnefei.*

Incidence/Epidemiology: The pulmonary infection has been described in about 20 patients, half of them with decreased immunity. All patients were visitors or residents of Southeast Asia (including Vietnam).

Etiology/Pathophysiology: The source of infection and the incubation period are not known. The organisms are probably inhaled and settle in the peripheral lung parenchyma. However, cases due to accidental trauma of the skin have also been reported.

Clinical Presentation: Patients may be asymptomatic or present with a history of intermittent moderate fever, chest pain, loss of weight, expectoration and hepatosplenomegaly.

Prognosis: Fair, but fatal cases have been reported, who developed progressive respiratory failure ranging from 2 months to 3 years.

Radiology: Chest radiographs show solitary peripheral nodules or diffuse patchy densities in the lower lobes, and pleural effusions.

Pathology:

Gross: The lungs show multiple small to medium-sized, necrotic, yellowish to grayish areas of crumble consistency.

Histology: The organisms appear as yeastlike, oval cells lying in clusters or in separate lines. Suppurative exudation and numerous histiocytes indicate the reaction of host tissue. Older lesions may show surrounding fibrosis, cavitation, and honeycombing. In contrast to *Histoplasma capsulatum*, the organisms have no buds.

➤ *Descriptors:* Lung parenchyma with altered structure:

- necrosis (abscess formation)
- fungus (yeastlike cells)
- mixed inflammatory infiltrates
- palisading histiocytes
- necrosis and hemorrhage (cavitation)
- focal interstitial fibrosis

- honeycombing;
- Lung parenchyma with preserved structure:
- fungus (yeastlike cells)
- intraalveolar fibrinoid material
- mixed inflammatory infiltrates

■ *Special stains:* PAS, collagenous stains, Giemsa, GMS, methenamine silver stain.

Hallmark of Diagnosis: Clinical history, identification of the fungus.

Differential diagnosis: Infection with other species of fungus, especially *Histoplasma capsulatum.*

Pentastomiasis

Definition: Infection of the lung by pentastomes of the orders *Armillifer* and *Linguatula*.

Incidence/Epidemiology: Human infection by pentastomes is common in endemic areas of central Africa and Malaysia, and has been reported in southeast Europe, southeast Asia, south and central America. The percentage of human infection ranges between 20% and 40% in autopsy series from Africa.

Etiology/Pathophysiology: The organisms are bloodsucking endoparasites of reptiles, birds, and mammals. The species are not definitely classified and may be included under the arthropods, the annelids, or as the specific order Pentastomida. The life cycle of the parasites varies considerably. Reptiles usually serve as specific hosts and carry the parasites within their lungs. The embryonated eggs are deposited into water or on leaves with the feces or bronchial secretions and are ingested by intermediate hosts which are usually rodents. Larvae at various developmental stages penetrate the walls of the intestines and attach themselves to the peritoneal wall of the rodents. The reptiles become infected by eating contaminated rodents, and the life cycle is completed. Man may serve as an intermediate host (in this case the infective larvae will not survive), as temporary specific host (by eating raw or undercooked meat of goats, sheep or rodents contaminated with mature larvae), or as specific host by eating the meat of snakes with living parasites. The infective larvae usually settle in the nasopharyngeal tissues, and the adult worms in the peritoneal tissues and diaphragm.

Clinical Presentation: Infection with mature worms is usually asymptomatic, and the patients seldom complain about cough, chest pain, or dyspnea due to pneumothorax. Infective larvae commonly induce the halzoun syndrome (discomfort in the throat, cough, sneezing, and occasionally dysphagia, and vomiting).

Prognosis: Usually good; however, a few fatal cases with cerebral infections have been reported.

Radiology: Chest radiographs may show calcified nodules attached to the diaphragm and the so called C-shape in the right lower lobe.

Pathology:

Gross: The adult worms measure 1–10 cm in length and 0.2–0.6 cm in diameter and have a long annulate abdomen. They are usually attached to the diaphragm. The larvae measure a few millimeters in length and diameter.

Histology: The worms usually induce no or only a weak inflammatory reaction of host tissue whereas the infective larvae may provoke dense inflammatory mononuclear infiltrates. The larvae have a chitinous cuticle 5–10 µm in diameter and prominent acidophilic glands. The worms have two pairs of anterior hooks and a mouth of similar histomorphologic appearance.

➤ *Descriptors:* Lung parenchyma with preserved structure:

- parasites (encysted larvae)
- absent inflammatory infiltrates;
- Lung parenchyma with altered structure:
- parasites (larvae, dead)
- mixed inflammatory infiltrates
- eosinophils
- focal interstitial fibrosis

■ *Special stains:* PAS, collagenous stains, Movat.

Hallmark of Diagnosis: Clinical history, identification of the parasite.

Differential diagnosis: Infection with other parasites.

Pentazocine

Definition: Alteration of the lung parenchyma associated with intake of pentazocine, see Drug Toxicity.

Pentolinium

Definition: Alteration of the lung parenchyma associated with intake of pentolinium, see Drug Toxicity.

Phaeocopulariopsis

Definition: Allergic (extrinsic) pneumonitis associated with inhalation of *Phaeocopulariopsis brunghii*.

Incidence/Epidemiology: The fungus lives in soil and wood. Allergic reaction of the lung parenchyma has been reported of Vietnam soldiers.

Etiology/Pathophysiology: The organisms induce an allergic reaction of the lung parenchyma.

Clinical Presentation: Acute and chronic stages of the pneumonitis can occur. For details, see Allergic (Extrinsic) Pneumonitis.

Prognosis: Usually good and without serious sequelae.

Radiology: Chest radiographs are normal or show diffuse bilateral densities.

Pathology:

Gross: The lungs are normal or heavy, wet and reddish, or of firm and rubbery in consistency.

Histology: The findings include interstitial, noncaseous epithelioid granulomas, bronchiolitis obliterans, desquamative interstitial pneumonia or organizing pneumonia. For details, see Allergic (Extrinsic) Pneumonitis.

➤ *Descriptors:* Lung parenchyma with altered structure:

- noncaseous epithelioid granulomas
- eosinophils
- multinucleated giant cells
- intrabronchiolar fibrinoid material and histiocytes
- ulceration of bronchiolar mucosa;
- Lung parenchyma with preserved structure:
- macrophages
- desquamation, hypertrophy, hyperplasia and dysplasia of pneumocytes
- mononuclear inflammatory infiltrates
- intraalveolar serous fluid

■ *Special stains:* PAS, collagenous stains, methenamine silver stain, immunohistochemistry, endogenous lectins.

Hallmark of Diagnosis: Clinical history, histomorphological findings consistent with allergic extrinsic pneumonitis.

Differential diagnosis: Sarcoidosis, berylliosis, granulomatous infections, usual interstitial pneumonia, desquamative interstitial pneumonia, lymphocytic interstitial pneumonia. For details, see Allergic (Extrinsic) Pneumonitis.

Phaeohyphomycosis

Definition: Opportunistic infection of the lung by various species of dematiacious fungi.

Incidence/Epidemiology: The fungi live as soil and wood saprophytes in all parts of the world and may grow in subcutaneous nodules in immunocompromised (seldom in healthy) persons. Infection usually occurs following traumatic lesions of the skin.

Etiology/Pathophysiology: Injury by wood splinters or other infective traumatic lesions enable the fungi to enter the subcutaneous fatty tissue where they form subcutaneous abscesses measuring several centimeters in diameter. The most common species are *Phialophora parasitica, jeanselmi, richardsiae*, and *Wangiella dermatidis*. Some patients develop systemic infection including that of the brain (especially the cerebral hemispheres) and the lung. Other organs are seldom involved.

Clinical Presentation: Symptoms include headache, nausea, vomiting, fever, chest pain, dyspnea, and hemoptysis.

Prognosis: Usually good and without serious sequelae; however, cerebral infections can be of fatal outcome.

Radiology: Chest radiographs show circumscribed, usually multiple nodules measuring several centimeters in diameter.

Pathology:

Gross: The lungs show multiple grayish-white, necrotic nodules, sometimes with surrounding granulomatous tissue.

Histology: The organisms can be identified by yeastlike cells comprising hyphae and spores. A granulomatous epithelioid reaction of host tissue may be present as well as suppurative alveolar exudate. The septated and branched hyphae measure 2–6 μm in diameter and are intermingled with numerous spores.

➤ *Descriptors:* Lung parenchyma with altered structure:
- caseous epithelioid granulomas
- mixed inflammatory infiltrates
- eosinophils
- fungus (yeastlike cells)
- necrosis and hemorrhage (abscess formation)

■ *Special stains:* PAS, collagenous stains, GMS, methenamine silver stain.

Hallmark of Diagnosis: Clinical history, epithelioid granuloma or suppurative pulmonary infection by fungal hyphae and spores.

Differential diagnosis: Infection of the lung by other fungal species, especially *Chlamydium*, *Aspergillus*.

Phenylbutazone

Definition: Alteration of the lung parenchyma associated with intake of phenylbutazone, see Drug Toxicity.

Phosgene

Definition: Alteration of the lung parenchyma associated with inhalation of phosgene, see Toxic injury.

Phosphorus

Definition: Alteration of the lung parenchyma associated with intake of phosphorus, see Drug Toxicity.

Phycomycosis

Definition: Acute fungal infection of the lung (synonym mucormycosis), see Mucormycosis.

Pickwickian Syndrome

Definition: Alteration of the lung parenchyma associated with impaired respiration due to adiposis.

Incidence/Epidemiology: Pickwickian syndrome is frequent in persons with severe adiposis.

Etiology/Pathophysiology: Adiposis may induce impaired respiration, recurrent prolonged duration of sleep, polyglobulia, and pulmonary hypertension. The detailed etiology is not known. Symptoms are reversible after reduction of weight.

Clinical Presentation: Symptoms include dyspnea, cough, attacks of sleep, and prolonged duration of sleep.

Prognosis: Usually good; however, slow progressive respiratory failure may occur.

Radiology: Chest radiographs are usually normal.

Pathology:

Gross: The lungs are normal or may show a mild interstitial edema.

Histology: The changes of the lung parenchyma are associated with pulmonary hypertension. The arterial walls are thickened and the smooth muscle cells are hypertrophied. The arterioles show distinct muscularization. The intima is usually not altered.

➤ *Descriptors:* Lung parenchyma with preserved structure:
- intraalveolar serous fluid;
- Pulmonary vessels with altered structure:
- hyaline material (media of arterial walls)
- proliferating smooth muscle cells (arteries)

■ *Special stains:* Collagenous stains.

Hallmark of Diagnosis: Clinical history, mild features of pulmonary hypertension.

Differential diagnosis: Pulmonary hypertension due to other causes.

Pigeon Breeders Lung

Definition: Alteration of the lung parenchyma seen in pigeon breeders, see Psittacosis.

Pindolol

Definition: Alteration of the lung parenchyma associated with intake of pindolol, see Drug Toxicity.

Pink Buffer

Definition: Syndrome seen in patients with chronic airflow obstruction and maintained blood gases (thin patients with increased minute ventilation), see Chronic Airflow Obstruction.

Piperazine

Definition: Alteration of the lung parenchyma associated with intake of piperazine, see Drug Toxicity.

Pituitary Snuff Taker's Lung

Definition: Alteration of the lung parenchyma associated with inhalation of pituitary snuff.
Incidence/Epidemiology: Not infrequently seen in young patients living in a poor social environment or unstable family relationships.
Etiology/Pathophysiology: Allergic reaction of the lung parenchyma associated with mammalian proteins.
Clinical Presentation: Acute and chronic hypersensitivity reactions have been described.
Prognosis: Usually good and without serious sequelae.
Radiology: Chest radiographs may be normal or show diffuse bilateral densities.
Pathology:
Gross: The lung may be normal or show firm, consolidated areas. For details, see Allergic (Extrinsic) Alveolitis.
Histology: The findings include noncaseous epithelioid granulomas, mononuclear inflammatory infiltrates, bronchiolitis obliterans and hyperplasia and dysplasia of the cells of the alveolar lining. For details, see Allergic (Extrinsic) Alveolitis.

➤ *Descriptors:* Lung parenchyma with altered structure:
- noncaseous epithelioid granulomas
- eosinophils
- multinucleated giant cells
- intrabronchiolar fibrinoid material and histiocytes
- ulceration of bronchiolar mucosa;
- Lung parenchyma with preserved structure:
- macrophages
- desquamation, hypertrophy, hyperplasia and dysplasia of pneumocytes
- mononuclear inflammatory infiltrates
- intraalveolar serous fluid

■ *Special stains:* PAS, collagenous stains, methenamine silver stain, immunohistochemistry, endogenous lectins.
Hallmark of Diagnosis: Clinical history, histomorphologic findings consistent with allergic (extrinsic) alveolitis.
Differential diagnosis: Sarcoidosis, berylliosis, granulomatous infections, desquamative interstitial pneumonia, usual interstitial pneumonia. For details, see Allergic (Extrinsic) Alveolitis.

Plague

Definition: Infection of the lung by *Yersinia pestis*.
Incidence/Epidemiology: Whereas the disorder was common during the Middle Ages (black death), it is nowadays an extremely rare disorder.
Etiology/Pathophysiology: Infections with the gram-negative bacterium *Y. pestis* may induce a bubonic or a pneumonic form. The lung is involved in a similar way in both courses. *Y. pestis* has its reservoir in rodents (rats) and is transmitted to man by flea bites. The bacteria can also be accidentally inhaled in laboratories and induce severe infections by direct pulmonary infection.
Clinical Presentation: The regional lymph nodes are swollen and enlarged with painful fluctuant buboes. Symptoms include high fever, progressive dyspnea, hemoptysis, and chest pain.
Prognosis: Due to modern chemotherapy the mortality rate has decreased from 90% in earlier days to 5–10%.
Radiology: Chest radiographs show bilateral confluent densities.
Pathology:
Gross: The lungs are necrotic and brownish-red.
Histology: The lung texture is destroyed and replaced by a hemorrhagic necrosis with moderate granulomatous infiltrates and macrophages in the periphery of the lesions. The necrotic areas comprise complete lobes. The

peribronchial and mediastinal lymph nodes are usually involved. The bacteria measure 1–2 μm in length and are usually numerous in the necrotic areas.

➤ *Descriptors:* Lung parenchyma with altered structure:
- necrosis and hemorrhage
- mixed inflammatory infiltrates
- bacteria (numerous)

■ *Special stains:* PAS, collagenous stains, Brown and Hopps, Warthin Starrey, direct immunofluorescence.

Hallmark of Diagnosis: Clinical history, necrotizing pneumonia, identification of *Y. pestis*.

Differential diagnosis: Abscessing pneumonia due to other agents.

Plaque, Pleural

Definition: Fibrotic nodules of the pleura, often calcified.

Incidence/Epidemiology: Frequent disorder associated with various agents.

Etiology/Pathophysiology: Pleural plaques may develop in association with chronic inflammation of the subpleural lung parenchyma or after exposure of the lung parenchyma to exogenous agents. Inhalation of small amounts of asbestos fibers induces pleural plaques in 40–60% of persons after a latent period of 10–20 years.

Clinical Presentation: Patients are usually asymptomatic.

Prognosis: Usually good and without serious sequelae.

Radiology: Chest radiographs show a thickening of the pleura, usually laterally over the lower lobes following the extensions between the ribs.

Pathology:

Gross: The thickening appears like "sugar icing" (Zuckerguss). The surface may be either smooth or granular. The consistency is hard and partly stony. Impressions of the ribs are present.

Histology: The plaques consist of thick, avascular, and acellular bundles of collagen with basket-weave patterns and scattered mononuclear inflammatory infiltrates near the boundary of the subpleural fatty tissue. The boundary of the lesions is abrupt. Asbestos fibers or bodies are usually not demonstrable in the collagenous network.

➤ *Descriptors:* Pleura with altered structure:
- acellular collagen (basket-weave pattern)
- hyaline material
- absent inflammatory infiltrates

■ *Special stains:* PAS, collagenous stains, Prussian blue (for demonstration of asbestos bodies).

Hallmark of Diagnosis: Solitary or multiple nodules of acellular and avascular collagenous bundles at the pleural surface.

Differential diagnosis: Mesothelioma of the pleura.

Plasma Cell Granuloma

Definition: Benign, circumscribed (postinflammatory?) lesion of the lung parenchyma with peculiar histomorphology, see Pseudotumor, Inflammatory.

Plasmacytoma

Definition: Malignant, low-grade non-Hodgkin's lymphoma of the lung derived from lymphoplasmacytoid cells.

Incidence/Epidemiology: Rare disorder usually seen in young to middle-aged adults or in elderly persons.

Etiology/Pathophysiology: The tumors derive from lymphoplasmacytoid cells. Secondary metastases of multiple myeloma into the lung are more frequent than primary plasmacytoma of the lung.

Clinical Presentation: Patients are asymptomatic or may have chronic cough, shortness of breath, and chest pain.

Prognosis: Fair, but the reported number of primary plasmacytomas is too small to estimate their degree of malignancy.

Radiology: Chest radiographs show a solitary or multiple densities.

Pathology:

Gross: The lungs show a solitary, yellowish-white nodule soft in consistency.

Histology: The lung parenchyma is destroyed and replaced by dense infiltrations of plasmacytoid lymphocytes intermingled with plump spindle cells which may show mitotic figures and invasion of the walls of small vessels, usually in the pleura.

➤ *Descriptors:* Newly formed textures without metastasis potential:

- mesenchymal growth pattern
- lymphomatoid textures
- small tumor cells (plasmacytoid lymphocytes)
- homogeneous nuclear and cellular size
- absent or infrequent mitoses
- plump spindle cells
- vascular and pleural invasion

■ *Special stains:* PAS, collagenous stains, Giemsa, immunohistochemistry for lymphocytic subpopulations, endogenous lectins, DNA analysis.

Hallmark of Diagnosis: Malignancy consisting of plasmacytoid lymphocytes, no evidence of metastases into the lung.

Differential diagnosis: Multiple myeloma, lymphoma of other origin, small cell anaplastic carcinoma.

Plastics Workers

Definition: Alteration of the lung parenchyma seen in plastics workers.

Incidence/Epidemiology: Acute damage of the lung parenchyma has been reported in plasties workers involved in accidents or in silo fillers. Workers involved in the production of sulfuric, chromic, or picric acid or nitrocellulose are at specific risk of developing adult respiratory distress syndrome (ARDS).

Etiology/Pathophysiology: The toxic agents are nitric acid (HNO_3) and nitrogen dioxide (NO_2, N_2O_4). The gases are easily absorbed in the fluid of the peripheral lung parenchyma and induce acute alveolar damage with bronchiolitis obliterans. The safety levels are about 10 ppm.

Clinical Presentation: Symptoms include burning in the upper and lower respiratory tract, chest pain, cough, and dyspnea.

Prognosis: Usually good; however, slow progressive respiratory failure can occur in patients with severe intoxication.

Radiology: Chest radiographs show diffuse edema and at a later stage consolidating areas.

Pathology:
Gross: The lungs are edematous and reddish-pink.
Histology: Severe intoxication provokes massive intraalveolar and interstitial edema with infiltration of neutrophilic granulocytes, desquamation of epithelial cells and fibrin exudation. At later stages bronchiolitis obliterans occurs as well as invasion of histiocytes and macrophages. Fibrosis and honeycombing may be the end-stage.

➤ *Descriptors:* Lung parenchyma with preserved structure:

- intraalveolar serous fluid
- desquamation, hypertrophy, hyperplasia and dysplasia of pneumocytes
- hyaline membranes
- mixed inflammatory infiltrates;
- Lung parenchyma with altered structure:
- necrosis (bronchiolar walls)
- intrabronchiolar fibrinoid material and histiocytes
- ulceration of bronchiolar mucosa
- focal interstitial fibrosis
- mononuclear inflammatory infiltrates
- proliferating fibroblasts
- honeycombing

■ *Special stains:* PAS, collagenous stains, Giemsa, endogenous lectins.

Hallmark of Diagnosis: Clinical history, acute alveolar damage.

Differential diagnosis: Adult respiratory distress syndrome due to other causes, usual interstitial pneumonia, desquamative interstitial pneumonia, organizing bacterial pneumonia.

Pleural Effusion

Definition: Transudation or exudation into the pleural cavity.

Incidence/Epidemiology: A variety of disorders can induce pleural effusions which may be transudative, chylous, suppurative, or carcinomatous. Pleural effusions are most frequently seen in the elderly.

Etiology/Pathophysiology: Pleural effusions are induced either by increased production of pleural fluid, by diminished absorption, or both. Congestive heart failure and hepatic and renal disorders induce decreased absorption of pleural fluid, which is also seen in obstruction by metastatic tumors of lymphatic drainage into the lymph nodes. Increased production and/or abnormal chemical composition of pleural fluid are observed in primary or metastatic malignancies of the pleura, infectious diseases such as tuberculosis, and inflammatory diseases, for example, rheumatic disorders. Peripheral lung infarctions induce hemorrhagic pleural effusions. Asbestos induces pleural effusions a long time after exposure. Pleural effusions are also seen in chronic pulmonary infections such as actinomycosis, or in lymphangioleiomyomatosis. Any alteration of the fluid dynamics, chemical composition of the fluid, or capillary permeability induces pleural effusions.

Clinical Presentation: Patients may be asymptomatic if the amount of pleural effusion is limited to 100–200 cm^3. Symptoms include dyspnea, shortness of breath on exercise and chest pain.

Prognosis: Fair; depending upon the underlying disease pleural effusions may be difficult to treat, and recurrences may be frequently observed.

Radiology: Chest radiographs show densities in the pleural cavities which vary according to the position of the patient.

Pathology:

Gross: Pleural effusions may be clear and amber-yellowish, suppurative, or milky in color.

Histology: The histology of pleural biopsies usually shows a marked proliferation of mesothelial cells which tend to desquamate and hypertrophy. Mitoses and marked atypias may be present. The changes are more severe and mimic a malignancy if therapeutic or repeated diagnostic treatments have been performed such as puncture, installation of antibiotics, etc. The cytologic criteria for malignancy should be based upon the findings in small cellular agglutinations which show unusual atypical changes in reactive hyperplasia.

➤ *Descriptors:* Pleura with preserved structure:

- mononuclear inflammatory infiltrates
- mixed inflammatory infiltrates
- hyperplasia and dysplasia of mesothelial cells;
- Pleura with altered structure:
- caseous epithelioid granulomas
- noncaseous epithelioid granulomas
- hyperplasia and dysplasia of mesothelial cells;
- Newly formed textures without metastasis potential:
- mesenchymal growth pattern;
- Newly formed textures with metastasis potential:
- epithelial growth pattern
- mesenchymal growth pattern
- adenoid textures
- sarcomatous textures
- lymphomatoid textures
- infrequent mitoses
- homogeneous nuclear and cellular size
- prominent nucleoli

■ *Special stains:* PAS, Giemsa, Prussian blue, immunocytology.

Hallmark of Diagnosis: Clinical history, cytologic findings.

Differential diagnosis: According to the underlying disorder, metastatic neoplasms, mesothelioma, infectious and inflammatory disorders.

Pleuritis

Definition: Inflammation or infection of the pleura.

Incidence/Epidemiology: Acute or chronic inflammation or infection of the pleura is a frequent disorder in middle-aged and older persons. Inflammation of the pleura is usually a reaction due to disorders of peripheral lung parenchyma and is seldom caused by penetrative disorders of the liver or stomach.

Etiology/Pathophysiology: Inflammation of the pleura is common (20–40%) in connective tissue disorders such as rheumatoid diseases, chronic interstitial pneumonitis, and metabolic abnormalities and is less frequent in sarcoidosis (5–10%) or vasculitides and angiocentric lymphoproliferative diseases. Any infection of the lower respiratory tract can involve the pleura. Examples are tuberculosis, abscessing bacterial pneumonias such as actinomycosis, and fungal infections such as penicilliosis. Parasitic infections are rare and may be seen in *Echinococcus* or in pentastomiasis. Inhalation of toxic agents such as asbestos, hard metals, fumes, nitrogen oxide, ozone, etc. can also induce pleuritis.

Clinical Presentation: Symptoms include chest pain, dyspnea, and fever.

Prognosis: Usually good, depending upon the underlying disease.

Radiology: Chest radiographs may be normal or may show pleural effusions or pleural fibrosis.

Pathology:

Gross: The lung surface is thickened and blunt, often grayish. Fibrinoid deposits may be seen.

Histology: The mesothelial cells are hypertrophic and hyperplastic and have a tendency toward desquamation and local growth. Inflammatory infiltrates are circumscribed and consist of clusters of mononuclear cells. Eosinophilic infiltrates are present in chronic pneumothorax in about 20–50% of cases, indicating an exogenous allergic reaction of the pleura to the air content in the pleural cavity. Multinucleated giant cells are often intermingled with eosinophils. Well-defined tuberculous granulomas are formed only in a minority of patients with proven bacterial pleuritis tuberculosa. Dense inflammatory infiltrates of lymphocytes and plasma cells in the pleura indicate tuberculous pleuritis as long as no other infective or inflammatory agent has been proven.

➤ *Descriptors:* Pleura with preserved structure:
- mononuclear inflammatory infiltrates
- mixed inflammatory infiltrates
- eosinophils
- hyperplasia and dysplasia of mesothelial cells;
- Pleura with altered structure:
- caseous epithelioid granulomas
- noncaseous epithelioid granulomas
- lymphomatoid granulomas
- hyperplasia and dysplasia of mesothelial cells

■ *Special stains:* PAS, collagenous stains, Giemsa, Prussian blue, Ziehl-Neelsen.

Hallmark of Diagnosis: Clinical history, inflammatory infiltrates of various types and degrees.

Differential diagnosis: According to the underlying disorder, mesothelioma.

Pneumococcal Pneumonia

Definition: Infection of the lung with *Staphylococcus pneumoniae*.

Incidence/Epidemiology: Infection with *S. pneumoniae* is one of the most frequent community-acquired bacterial pulmonary disorders.

Etiology/Pathophysiology: Infection with *S. pneumoniae* occurs by inhalation of the bacteria, is usually severe, and has a significant mortality. Superinfection may occur in patients with adult respiratory distress syndrome.

Clinical Presentation: Symptoms include high fever, dyspnea, and chest pain.

Prognosis: Fair; the mortality rate in patients between 12–50 years old is 15–20%; in patients of other ages or with underlying chronic diseases, it is significantly higher.

Radiology: Chest radiographs show either solid densities of one complete lobe or diffuse, patchy densities distributed over several parts of the lungs.

Pathology:

Gross: The macroscopic features of the lungs are related to the stage of the pneumonia and may show large, pink-reddish areas soft in consistency or grayish-white with a firm consistency.

Histology: The histomorphologic findings include dense infiltrates of neutrophilic granulocytes, lymphocytes, and plasma cells in the stage of gray hepatization, presenting diffuse nodular consolidation. Earlier stages show severe edema and hyperemia of the lungs, or extravasation of erythrocytes and fibrin into the distant airways.

➤ *Descriptors:* Lung parenchyma with preserved structure:
- intraalveolar serous fluid
- intraalveolar fibrinoid material
- mixed inflammatory infiltrates
- bacteria;
- Lung parenchyma with altered structure:
- necrosis and hemorrhage
- mixed inflammatory infiltrates
- bacteria
- proliferating fibroblasts
- focal interstitial fibrosis

■ *Special stains:* PAS, collagenous stains, Giemsa, Gram's (*S. pneumoniae* is positive).

Hallmark of Diagnosis: Clinical history, severe bacterial pneumonia, identification of *S. pneumoniae*.

Differential diagnosis: Bacterial infections with other organisms.

Pneumoconiosis

Definition: Alteration of the lung parenchyma associated with inhalation of dust.

Incidence/Epidemiology: Inhalation of dust and related material such as mineral fibers and granules, metal fumes, or coal is still frequently observed in persons working in mines, in production plants, and in customers. Due to the long interval between exposure and development of clinically relevant symptoms, the incidence of certain pneumoconioses is still rising, especially changes of the lung parenchyma associated with exposure to asbestos.

Etiology/Pathophysiology: Dust particles of a certain size (0.5–5 μm) may reach the terminal airways and are usually deposited close to the terminal bronchioles. Deposits of particles or crystals with certain physical and chemical properties induce activation of macrophages and of immunodefence mechanisms and subsequently fibrotic changes of the lung parenchyma. Other particles are inert and seldom cause severe damage of the lung. Deposits of silica, asbestos or coal are usually associated with fibrosis and those of talc and beryllium with noncaseating granulomas, whereas those of kaolin, titanium, or tin seldom give rise to severe fibrotic changes.

Clinical Presentation: Patients are usually asymptomatic; however, slowly progressive dyspnea, chronic cough, and recurrent infections may indicate the fibrogenic potential of inhaled substances.

Prognosis: Fair, depending upon the nature of the inhaled substances; slow progressive respiratory failure is the most frequently observed course.

Radiology: Chest radiographs are classfied according to the rules of the International Labor Office (ILO), and include the following:

(a) Small opacities, grouped according to their maximum diameter r (round nodules p: $r < 1.5$ mm; q: $1.5 < r < 3.0$ mm; r: $3.0 < r < 10.0$ mm; irregular opacities s: $r < 1.5$ mm; t: $1.5 < r < 3.0$ mm; u: $3.0 < r < 10.0$ mm).

(b) Larger opacities are classified according to the sum of the greatest parameters present and grouped into A (sum < 5 cm), and B (single or sum > 5 cm, and a total less than the area of the right upper zone), and C (others).

(c) The additional category "profusion" is based upon the comparison of the densities of opacities in comparision with standard radiographs and grouped into four categories (0: absent opacities or < category 1; 1, 2, 3 according to the standard radiographs with increasing density). Pleural thickening is noted separately.

Pathology:

Gross: The lungs usually show circumscribed, black densities of firm, fibrous consistency. Diffuse fibrosis and honeycombing are present in advanced stages, or in cases with chronic superinfection.

Histology: The deposits are most frequently birefringent and can be demonstrated in the distant airways. Fibrous nodules contain only a few crystals or particles. Asbestos fibers may be covered with a protein shell (asbestos bodies). Silica induces nodular fibrosis, asbestos fibers a diffuse interstitial fibrosis.

The details are discussed under the particular headings.

➤ *Descriptors:* Lung parenchyma with preserved structure:

- dust (birefringent fibers, crystals)
- macrophages (dust-laden);
- Lung parenchyma with altered structure:
- diffuse interstitial fibrosis
- focal interstitial fibrosis
- mononuclear inflammatory infiltrates

■ *Special stains:* PAS, collagenous stains, Giemsa, Prussian blue, endogenous lectins, X-ray diffraction method or related techniques.

Hallmark of Diagnosis: Clinical history, identification of the crystals or dust, grading of fibrotic changes.

Differential diagnosis: Smoking, due to the chemistry of the dust deposits (crystallography).

Pneumocystis Carinii

Definition: Infection of the lung with *Pneumocystis carinii.*

Incidence/Epidemiology: Infection of the lung with the protozoan *P. carinii* is common in immunocompromised patients regardless of the underlying disorder. Patients with AIDS are at special risk, and about 50% of them develop *P. carinii* infections. Other populations at risk are infants and children with acute lymphocytic leukemia, patients with kidney, bone marrow, or liver transplants, patients with advanced cancer.

Etiology/Pathophysiology: *P. carinii* is an ubiquitous organism, probably of protozoan order. It also infects different species of mammals, especially rats, and it has not been proven whether the organism is specific for different species. Its life cycle involves first maturing trophozoites, then cysts with merozoites, and finally collapsed cysts. It is suggested that asymptomatic human carriers exist.

Clinical Presentation: Patients may be asymptomatic or present with only mild pulmonary symptoms such as cough or shortness of breath during exercise. Others are severely ill and present with dyspnea, hypoxemia, and fever.

Prognosis: The mortality rate ranges between 40–60%.

Radiology: Chest radiographs show patchy densities in both lungs.

Pathology:

Gross: The lungs are edematous and have pale grayish to pale tan areas firm in consistency. The areas may occupy a whole lobe or be confluent and patchy.

Histology: The lung texture is preserved, and the interalveolar septula slightly thickened and invaded by a mild mononuclear infiltrate. The distant air spaces contain a foamy exudate of hyaline color with HE stain. The exudate resembles alveolar proteinosis with intermingled erythrocytes. Other histomorphologic changes are the formation of noncaseating histiocytic granulomas, exudation of fibrin and formation of hyaline membranes and agglutination of macrophages within the distant air spaces. Interstitial fibrosis, abscess formation, and granulomatous inflammatory reaction of the lung are not features of infection with *P. carinii* but may occur in rare cases. The organisms appear in precysts and cysts measuring 3–6 µm in maximum diameter. They usually contain one or several (up to 8) intracystic bodies and comma-shaped thickening of the cystic wall.

➤ *Descriptors:* Lung parenchyma with preserved structure:

- intraalveolar serous fluid
- mononuclear inflammatory infiltrates
- macrophages (precysts)
- infectious organisms (cysts and precysts)

■ *Special stains:* PAS, collagenous stains, Giemsa, Grocott's stain or other methenamine silver stains, immunofluorescence. The organisms do not stain with HE.

Hallmark of Diagnosis: Clinical history of immunocompromise, foamy intraalveolar exudate, and demonstration of the organisms with Grocott's stain or direct immunofluorescence.

Differential diagnosis: Infection with other organisms such as *Coccidioides immitis, Candida* species, *Histoplasma capsulatum.*

Pneumonia

Definition: Alteration of the lung parenchyma associated with infection by various organisms.

Incidence/Epidemiology: Infection of the lung is one of the most common disorders in man. Mild bronchopneumonic infections are closely associated with cold seasons. Severe pneumonias are frequently seen in terminal stages of several diseases such as cancer, heart infarction, collagenous disorders, congenital malformations, and neurological diseases.

Etiology/Pathophysiology: Infection of the terminal air spaces may occur with organisms descending from the upper respiratory tract, rapid growth of inhaled agents, septicemia, or contiguous spread from adjacent organs such as the liver or stomach. Bacterial infections usually induce changes which show a close time-morphology relationship (edematous stage, red hepatization, gray hepatization, lysis; see bacterial pneumonia). Viral infections induce hypertrophy, hyperplasia and dysplasia of cells of the alveolar lining, and may be cytologically indistinguishable from adenocarcinoma. Bacterial superinfection by viral pneumonias and vice versa is common and often of specific clinical importance. Fungal infections of the lung are usually transmitted through the conducting airways and may be limited to endobronchial growth over a long period of time. Parasites settle most frequently in the vascular system, and several species develop large cysts. Protozoan infections induce changes in pulmonary macrophages and in histiocytes, usually accompanied by intraalveolar exudate.

Clinical Presentation: Patients show high fever, cough, expectoration, hemoptysis and dyspnea.

Prognosis: Usually good and without serious sequelae; however, high mortality rates exist for specific infectious organisms or for patients with severe underlying disorders.

Radiology: Chest radiographs show multiple, patchy or circumscribed densities which may occupy a complete lobe.

Pathology:

Gross: The lungs are usually edematous, heavy, and of increased consistency. Firm, yellowish-white nodules or areas of consolidation may be present.

Histology: The texture of the lung parenchyma is necrotic and replaced by a granulocytic or lymphocytic infiltrate which characteristically comprises plasma cells and macrophages. Eosinophilic granulocytes indicate parasitic infections, absence of granulocytes viral infections, and marked intraalveolar exudation protozoan infection. Cellular atypias with abnormal size and shape of nuclei and koilocytosis are seen in viral infections. Formation of granulomas indicates tuberculosis or fungal infection. The details are discussed under the particular headings.

➤ *Descriptors:* Lung parenchyma with preserved structure:

- intraalveolar serous fluid
- hemorrhage
- intraalveolar fibrinoid material
- macrophages
- desquamation, hypertrophy, hyperplasia and dysplasia of pneumocytes
- koilocytosis
- hyaline membranes;
- Lung parenchyma with altered structure:
- caseous epithelioid granulomas
- necrosis and hemorrhage
- mixed inflammatory infiltrates
- intrabronchiolar fibrinoid material and histiocytes
- ulceration of bronchiolar mucosa
- proliferating fibroblasts
- focal interstitial fibrosis
- diffuse interstitial fibrosis
- honeycombing

■ *Special stains:* PAS, collagenous stains, Giemsa, GMS, methenamine silver stains, Ziehl-Neelsen, Movat, Warthin-Starry.

Hallmark of Diagnosis: Clinical history, necrosis of the lung parenchyma, marked inflammatory infiltrates, and identification of the organisms.

Differential diagnosis: Due to the organisms, vasculitides and granulomatous disorders, infarction, necrotic lung cancer.

Pneumonitis

Definition: Acute or chronic inflammation of the lung parenchyma (synonym alveolitis).

Incidence/Epidemiology: Acute or chronic, noninfectious inflammation of the lung parenchyma is associated with a broad variety of agents, such as drug intake, radiation, inhalation of toxic gases, or alterations of the immune system. The incidence of pneumonitis can be estimated at 5/100 000–10/100 000 per year in the European population.

Etiology/Pathophysiology: The terms alveolitis, pneumonia, and pneumonitis are widely used synonymously. Toxic agents can reach the lung via the conducting airways, the capillary system or the lymphatics. The reaction pattern of the lung parenchyma is related to the enormous surface of cells of the alveolar lining and of the capillary system. In the majority of cases both systems are involved. Damage of the cells of the alveolar lining induces desquamation, proliferation, and cellular atypia. Involvement of the immune system and of the capillaries induces exudation of fibrin and the formation of hyaline membranes. Invasion of lymphocytes may be predominant in the interstitial tissue whereas some cases show dense agglutinations of macrophages and the formation of giant cells. Bacterial superinfection may be seen in some cases. Any lung injury can proceed to fibrosis and honeycombing.

Clinical Presentation: Symptoms include acute dyspnea, fever, and cough or unsuspicious onset of dyspnea, cough, and malaise.

Prognosis: Acute pneumonitis has a variable clinical course, development of chronic stages with progressive respiratory failure is not infrequently seen. Patients with chronic interstitial pneumonitis seldom survive 5 years after clinical manifestation of the disease. Those with DIP or GIP have a better prognosis and may respond to therapeutic regimes.

Radiology: Chest radiographs show diffuse, bilateral densities and ground glass appearance, usually predominant in the lower zones.

Pathology:

Gross: The lung are edematous, red-tan or grayish, and increased in consistency.

Histology: The histomorphological image of acute pneumonitis is characterized by intraalveolar edema, desquamation, hypertrophy, hyperplasia and dysplasia of the pneumocytes, mild interstitial polymorphous inflammatory infiltrates, and by fibrin deposits, hyaline membranes, and intraalveolar histiocytes at later stages. The histomorphological changes of (chronic) interstitial pneumonitis can be grouped into the following categories: (a) usual interstitial pneumonia (UIP); (b) desquamative interstitial pneumonia (DIP); (c) lymphocytic interstitial pneumonia (LIP); (d) giant cell interstitial pneumonia (GIP). According to the underlying course or agent the following diseases can be identified: radiation pneumonitis, allergic extrinsic alveolitis (pneumonitis) and eosinophilic pneumonitis. The histomorphological details are described under the particular headings.

➤ *Descriptors:* Lung parenchyma with preserved structure:

- intraalveolar serous fluid
- mixed inflammatory infiltrates
- desquamation, hypertrophy, hyperplasia and dysplasia of pneumocytes
- hyaline membranes
- intraalveolar fibrinoid material
- mononuclear inflammatory infiltrates
- macrophages
- multinucleated giant cells
- eosinophils;
- Lung parenchyma with altered structure:
- mononuclear inflammatory infiltrates
- proliferating fibroblasts
- multinucleated giant cells
- diffuse interstitial fibrosis
- enlarged distant air spaces
- honeycombing

■ *Special stains:* PAS, collagenous stains, Giemsa, endogenous lectins.

Hallmark of Diagnosis: Clinical history, desquamation of pneumocytes, interstitial mononuclear infiltrates, cellular atypias of pneumocytes, intraalveolar macrophages.

Differential diagnosis: Infectious pneumonia, bronchioloalveolar carcinoma, congenital disorders, collagenous tissue diseases, lymphangioleiomyomatosis.

Pneumopericardium

Definition: Alteration of the pericardium in interstitial pulmonary emphysema.

Incidence/Epidemiology: About 40–70% of all infants with interstitial pulmonary emphysema develop a pneumopericardium.

Etiology/Pathophysiology: Presence of air in the interstitial tissue tends to induce a pneumothorax and to proceed along the interlobar septa, along the vessels, and into the adjacent tissues such as the pericardium and mediastinum.

Clinical Presentation: Infants present with severe pulmonary and cardiac problems that are difficult to handle and are associated with high mortality.

Prognosis: The mortality rate is between 40–60% and closely related to the birth weight.

Radiology: Chest radiographs show lucent linear lines and cystic spaces in the lung parenchyma associated with dense markings. The mediastinum is widened.

Pathology:

Gross: The pericardium shows edematous changes and fibrinoid deposits.

Histology: Small layers of fibrin are present on the mesothelial cells accompanied by scattered mononuclear infiltrates. Eosinophilic granulocytes and multinucleated giant cells may be seen in late stages.

➤ *Descriptors:* Pericardium with preserved structure:

- fibrinoid material
- mononuclear inflammatory infiltrates
- multinucleated giant cells
- eosinophils
- effusion (serous fluid)

■ *Special stains:* PAS, collagenous stains, Giemsa.

Hallmark of Diagnosis: Clinical history, presence of interstitial pulmonary emphysema and of nonspecific inflammatory reaction of the pericardium.

Differential diagnosis: Pericarditis due to other agents.

Pneumothorax

Definition: Presence of air in the thoracic cavity.

Incidence/Epidemiology: Spontaneous pneumothorax is frequently seen in patients with chronic asthmatic bronchitis, emphysema, tuberculosis, bronchiectasis, connective tissue disorders, lymphangioleiomyomatosis, and less frequently bronchial carcinoma, pulmonary infarction, *Pneumocystis carinii*, or pneumoconiosis. It may also occur in young asthenic adults without preceding clinical symptoms.

Etiology/Pathophysiology: Pneumothorax develops as a result of a leak, either of the pleura visceralis or of the pleura parietalis (chest trauma). The peripheral lung parenchyma is usually characterized by emphysematous cysts of various sizes. The pleura show fibrotic and atrophic changes.

Clinical Presentation: Symptoms include acute dyspnea and chest pain.

Prognosis: Usually good and without serious sequelae.

Radiology: Chest radiographs reveal a collapse of the lung with a distinct boundary at the pleura visceralis.

Pathology:

Gross: The pleura is thickened, and subpleural fibrous areas are usually present adjacent to emphysematous cysts which are covered by thin, atrophic areas of the pleura.

Histology: The lung parenchyma contains enlarged distant airways with rarefaction of the interalveolar septula and usually interstitial fibrosis in the periphery. The pleura shows fibrosis and atrophy in closely related areas and infiltration of mononuclear inflammatory cells (lymphocytes, plasma cells). Eosinophilic leukocytes and multinucleated giant cells can be seen in persistent pneumothorax or in recurrent courses. The walls of the small bronchi and bronchioles are infiltrated with mononuclear cells and may be hyperplastic.

➤ *Descriptors:* Lung parenchyma with altered structure:

- enlarged distant air spaces
- mononuclear inflammatory infiltrates
- focal interstitial fibrosis;
- Pleura with altered structure:
- fibrosis (focal)
- mononuclear inflammatory infiltrates (scattered)
- eosinophils
- multinucleated giant cells
- atrophy (focal)

■ *Special stains:* PAS, collagenous stains, Giemsa.

Hallmark of Diagnosis: Clinical history, subpleural emphysema, fibrosis and atrophy of the pleura visceralis.

Differential diagnosis: Chronic pleuritis due to other agents.

Polyalveolar Lobe

Definition: Congenital malformation of the lung with increased number of alveoli.

Incidence/Epidemiology: Unusual disorder, only a few cases have been reported.

Etiology/Pathophysiology: The size of the lobe is increased due to an abnormal number of alveoli which are, however, of normal volume. The increased volume of the lobe induces a shift of the mediastinum and atelectatic compression of other lobes.

Clinical Presentation: The disorder mimics infantile lobar emphysema with respiratory distress and dyspnea.

Prognosis: Fair, but a fatal outcome has been reported.

Radiology: Chest radiographs show a shift of the mediastinum and increased density of adjacent lobes.

Pathology:

Gross: The lobe is two to three times as large as normal.

Histology: The lung texture is maintained. The size of the alveoli is normal. The adjacent lobes show atelectasis.

➤ *Descriptors:* Lung parenchyma with preserved structure:

- no morphological abnormalities

■ *Special stains:* None.

Hallmark of Diagnosis: Clinical history, increased size of a lobe due to increased number of normal alveoli.

Differential diagnosis: Infantile lobar emphysema.

Polyarteritis Nodosa

Definition: Alteration of the lung parenchyma associated with polyarteritis nodosa.

Incidence/Epidemiology: Involvement of the lung in patients with classic polyarteritis nodosa is estimated to occur in 5–10% of cases.

Etiology/Pathophysiology: Polyarteritis nodosa is a disorder affecting many organs, characterized by necrosis, thrombosis, and chronic inflammation of small and medium-sized arteries. The disorder induces ischemic or hemorrhagic infarctions of the tissue areas supplied by the affected arteries. High incidence of hepatitis B antigenemia (HBsAg) and of circulating HBsAg-anti-HBs immune complexes in sera of drug-addicted patients with polyarteritis nodosa suggest involvement of viral infection and atypical immunoresponse in the etiology of the disorder.

Clinical Presentation: Patients complain about chest pain, dyspnea,and hemoptysis or blood-tinged sputum.

Prognosis: Poor, the 5-year survival rate is between 10–25% after clinical manifestation.

Radiology: Chest radiographs show multiple, ill-defined, peripheral densities in both lungs.

Pathology:

Gross: The small and medium-sized arteries are occluded by thromboses which cannot be seen macroscopically. The peripheral lungs are usually normal or may infrequently show multiple hemorrhagic infarction of various sizes and stages of organization and is red-brown or pink and firm in consistency.

Histology: The walls of medium-sized and small arteries are invaded by neutrophilic granulocytes, lymphocytes, and plasma cells. The lumen is occluded by older thromboembolic lesions, and the lamina elastica interna and externa are destroyed and show fragments of collagenous fibers. Areas of hemorrhagic infarctions may be present if larger arteries are involved.

➤ *Descriptors:* Pulmonary vessels with altered structure:
- fragmentation of elastic fibers
- mixed inflammatory infiltrates
- stenosis
- thrombosis (old, in the smaller arteries);
- Lung parenchyma with preserved structure:
- mixed inflammatory infiltrates
- hemorrhage;
- Lung parenchyma with altered structure:
- necrosis and hemorrhage
- mononuclear inflammatory infiltrates
- focal interstitial fibrosis

■ *Special stains:* PAS, collagenous stains, Giemsa, methenamine silver stain, immunohistochemistry for hepatitis B antigens, endogenous lectins.

Hallmark of Diagnosis: Clinical history, vasculitis of small and medium-sized arteries with necrosis and thrombosis.

Differential diagnosis: Vasculitides of other origin, necrotizing pneumonia, Hodgkin's disease, lymphomatoid granulomatosis.

Polymer Fume Fever

Definition: Alteration of the lung parenchyma associated with inhalation of polymer fumes.

Incidence/Epidemiology: Unusual disorder seen in accidents, in workers exposed to fumes arising from the production of Teflon or Fluon (polytetrafluoroethylene), or in persons smoking contaminated cigarettes.

Etiology/Pathophysiology: The reaction of the lung tissue to the fumes is probably related to damage of type 1 pneumocytes.

Clinical Presentation: High fever, chills, and cough develop a few hours after intoxication.

Prognosis: Usually good and without serious sequelae.

Radiology: Chest radiographs are usually normal or may show mild, diffuse, patchy densities.

Pathology:

Gross: The lungs are normal or may be edematous.

Histology: The terminal alveoli may be filled with fibrinoid exudate, macrophages, and erythrocytes. The lung parenchyma alterations are completely reversible. Detailed data are not known due to the complete remission of the disorder.

➤ *Descriptors:* Lung parenchyma with preserved structure:
- intraalveolar serous fluid
- macrophages
- mononuclear inflammatory infiltrates
- hemorrhage

■ *Special stains:* PAS, collagenous stains, Giemsa, Movat pentachrome, endogenous lectins.

Hallmark of Diagnosis: Clinical history, findings consistent with (mild) acute alveolar damage, hemorrhage.
Differential diagnosis: Acute alveolar damage due to other agents.

Polymyositis-Dermatomyositis

Definition: Alteration of the lung parenchyma associated with polymyositis-dermatomyositis.
Incidence/Epidemiology: About 5–10% of all patients suffering from polymyositis-dermatomyositis present with primary involvement of the lung.
Etiology/Pathophysiology: A high percentage of patients with polymyositis-dermatomyositis have antibodies against antimyoglobin, nuclear-specific antibodies, and high titers against hepatitis B and coxsackievirus B. The skeletal muscles are swollen and atrophic. Perivascular mononuclear infiltrates and fibrosis indicate the involvement of small arteries.
Clinical Presentation: Symptoms include progressive dyspnea, chest pain, and cough. The course may be rapid or prolonged with recurrent episodes.
Prognosis: Fair; a few patients will recover completely, most patients will present with relapses occurring after 1–15 years, and only a few patients will die due to pulmonary, renal, or cardiac failure.
Radiology: Chest radiographs show multiple, patchy densities or diffuse interstitial infiltrates.
Pathology:
Gross: The lungs are usually of normal appearance.
Histology: The interalveolar septula are infiltrated by mononuclear cells comprising lymphocytes and plasma cells and less frequently histiocytes. Formation of ill-defined granulomas may occur. Interstitial fibrosis is rare and restricted to perivascular collagenous fibers. Bronchiolitis obliterans may occur.

➤ *Descriptors:* Lung parenchyma with preserved structure:
- mononuclear inflammatory infiltrates
- hyaline material (basal membranes);
- Pulmonary vessels with preserved structure:
- mononuclear inflammatory infiltrates;
- Lung parenchyma with altered structure:
- focal interstitial fibrosis (perivascular)
- noncaseous epithelioid granulomas (ill-defined)
- intrabronchiolar fibrinoid material and histiocytes
- ulceration of bronchiolar mucosa

■ *Special stains:* PAS, collagenous stains, Giemsa, immunohistochemistry for hepatitis B or coxsackie-virus B, endogenous lectins.
Hallmark of Diagnosis: Clinical history, diffuse lymphocytic interstitial infiltrates.
Differential diagnosis: Usual interstitial pneumonia, involvement of the lung in other systemic disorders.

Polyp, Fibroblastic

Definition: Fibromatous endobronchiolar mass seen in bronchiolitis obliterans.
Incidence/Epidemiology: Organizing fibroblastic polyps are the histomorphological characteristic finding in bronchiolitis obliterans which is associated with (a) virus, mycoplasma, rickettsia, fungus, and mycobacteria infection; (b) toxic fumes (nitrogen dioxide, tin, ammonia, acid fumes); (c) obstructive lesions; (d) aspiration; (e) collagen vascular disorders; (f) side effects of drugs; (g) transplants; (h) idiopathic disorders.
Etiology/Pathophysiology: The fibroblastic polyps usually occlude the terminal bronchioles and adhere to about half of the bronchiolar wall. They have the appearance of organizing fibrinoid deposits which cannot completely resolve or transform into collagenous tissue. They are probably induced by partial necrosis and desquamation of bronchiolar epithelial cells.
Clinical Presentation: Symptoms have an ill-defined onset and include cough and flu-like complaints.
Prognosis: Depends upon the underlying disease.
Radiology: Chest radiographs show patchy, ground-glass densities in both lungs with a preference for the upper right lobe.
Pathology:
Gross: The lungs show multiple, grayish-white nodules measuring 1–2 mm in maximum diameter, especially in the upper right lobe.
Histology: The polyps consist of collagenous fibers attached to one side of the bronchioles. The epithelial cells are destroyed on the adher-

ent side and well-preserved at the opposite side. Entrapped plasma cells and lymphocytes are usually present in the polyps.

➤ *Descriptors:* Lung parenchyma with altered structure:
- intrabronchiolar fibrinoid material and histiocytes
- ulceration of bronchiolar mucosa

■ *Special stains:* PAS, collagenous stains, Giemsa, Movat pentachrome stain, endogenous lectins.

Hallmark of Diagnosis: Collagenous fibers attached to one side of the bronchioles with preserved epithelial cells of the opposite side.

Differential diagnosis: Patchy organizing (bacterial) pneumonia.

Pompe's Disease

Definition: Alteration of the lung parenchyma associated with Pompe's disease, see Acid Maltase Deficiency.

Pontiac Fever

Definition: Acute febrile illness with high fever induced by infection with *Legionella pneumophila*.

Incidence/Epidemiology: The specific response to infection with *L. pneumophila* is not uncommon.

Etiology/Pathophysiology: The sudden onset of the febrile reaction to infection with *Legionella* and its benign course suggest a potent and fast developing immunity reaction of host tissue.

Clinical Presentation: Symptoms include high fever, chills, and dyspnea after an incubation time of 2–4 days. Resolution occurs after several days.

Prognosis: Usually good and without serious sequelae.

Radiology: Chest radiographs show multiple patchy bilateral densities.

Pathology:

Gross: No specific findings have been reported due to the benign course.

Histology: The lung texture is preserved. The distant airways are filled with a fibrinoid exudate of neutrophilic granulocytes, lymphocytes, plasma cells, and macrophages. The bacteria are mainly demonstrable within the histiocytes and macrophages.

➤ *Descriptors:* Lung parenchyma with preserved structure:
- intraalveolar fibrinoid material
- mixed inflammatory infiltrates
- macrophages

■ *Special stains:* PAS, collagenous stains, Giemsa, Dieterle's stain, immunofluorescence.

Hallmark of Diagnosis: Clinical history, identification of the bacteria.

Differential diagnosis: Legionnaire's disease, pneumonia due to other infective organisms.

Practolol

Definition: Alteration of the lung parenchyma associated with intake of practolol, see Drug Toxicity.

Prematurity

Definition: Alteration of the lung parenchyma associated with prematurity.

Incidence/Epidemiology: The incidence of premature infants is estimated to 0.5–2% in larger series. Prematurity is nearly always associated with dysfunction of the lung to various degrees.

Etiology/Pathophysiology: Immaturity of the lung is associated with disturbances in production and resorption of surfactant. Mature surfactant is a necessary precondition for accurate expansion of the lung. Inadequate amounts of physiologically active surfactant induce incomplete expansion of the lung and respiratory distress syndrome. Therapeutic regimes include artificial respiration in severe stages, which can cause secondary lung parenchyma alterations such as bronchopulmonary dysplasia or interstitial pulmonary emphysema.

Clinical Presentation: Infants present with respiratory distress syndrome of various degrees.

Prognosis: The prognosis is closely related to the birth weight.

Radiology: Chest radiographs show diffuse interstitial densities and opacities.

Pathology:

Gross: The bulky lungs show areas of overexpansion and atelectasis and usually consolidated areas of infection.

Histology: The histomorphological lesions include formation of hyaline membranes (hyaline membrane disease) or of interstitial emphysema, morphologic changes as described under bronchopulmonary dysplasia, focal narrowing of the trachea, and seldom massive hemorrhage.

➤ *Descriptors:* Lung parenchyma with preserved structure:

- hyaline membranes
- mononuclear inflammatory infiltrates
- macrophages
- intraalveolar fibrinoid material
- desquamation, hypertrophy, hyperplasia and dysplasia of pneumocytes;
- Lung parenchyma with altered structure:
- macrophages
- mononuclear inflammatory infiltrates
- necrosis
- diffuse interstitial fibrosis;
- Bronchial mucosa with altered structure:
- necrosis
- mixed inflammatory infiltrates
- squamous metaplasia and dysplasia

■ *Special stains:* PAS, collagenous stains, Giemsa, endogenous lectins.

Hallmark of Diagnosis: Clinical history, hyaline membranes, interstitial emphysema, organizing pneumonia.

Differential diagnosis: Depends on the underlying disorder, acquired infection of the lung.

Preneoplasia

Definition: Alteration of the bronchial mucosa and lung parenchyma associated with subsequent malignant growth.

Incidence/Epidemiology: Preneoplastic changes of the bronchial mucosa have frequently been observed with exposure to potential carcinogenic substances. They include basal cell hyperplasia, goblet cell hyperplasia, squamous metaplasia, dysplasia, and micropapillomatosis, or hyperplasia and dysplasia of the cells of the alveolar lining. The reported frequency in autopsy cases lies between 10–40% in heavy smokers. Patients with bronchial carcinomas reveal preneoplastic changes of the bronchial mucosa in 30–50% of cases. The preneoplastic changes are closely related to the cell type of the carcinomas (basal cell hyperplasia and small cell carcinoma, goblet cell hyperplasia and adenocarcinoma, and squamous metaplasia and epidermoid carcinoma). The frequency of preneoplastic changes decreases with increasing distance from the malignancies.

Etiology/Pathophysiology: The development of malignant growth is now understood to be the final state of recurrent (toxic) damages of the affected tissue (multiple hit theory). Repair mechanisms try to push back the altered tissue into its former normal state, inducing stable cellular and structural abnormalities of the tissue. Tissue with these abnormalities is at higher risk of changing into uncontrolled cellular proliferation than that with a normal appearance. However, preneoplastic changes of the bronchial mucosa or peripheral lung parenchyma are not essential for development of bronchial carcinomas. Preneoplastic changes reveal altered cytoskeletons and altered endogenous lectins.

Clinical Presentation: Preneoplastic changes are accidental findings in surgical specimens, autopsy cases, or biopsy specimens taken at bronchoscopy. They usually do not cause symptoms.

Prognosis: It has been estimated that preneoplastic changes may transform into malignant growth after 5–15 years. Exact data are not known.

Radiology: The lesions are not detectable on chest radiographs.

Pathology:

Gross: The bronchial mucosa is thick and has a rough surface.

Histology: The basal cells of the bronchial mucosa lie in several (4–12) unordered layers (basal cell hyperplasia) and reveal signs of increased proliferation. The number of goblet cells is increased and the number of ciliated cells reduced (goblet cell hyperplasia). Ciliated and goblet cells are absent and replaced by squamous epithelium with various degrees of dysplasia (squamous metaplasia). Several small, vascularized, papilliform vaultings covered with hyperplastic or metaplastic epithelial cells define the micropapillomatosis. Mononuclear inflammatory infiltrates are usually present.

➤ *Descriptors:* Bronchial mucosa with preserved structure:

- desquamation, hypertrophy, hyperplasia and dysplasia of epithelial cells
- mononuclear inflammatory infiltrates
- increased number of basal cells
- increased number of goblet cells;
- Bronchial mucosa with altered structure:
- squamous metaplasia and dysplasia

■ *Special stains:* PAS, collagenous stains, Giemsa, immunohistochemistry (cytokeratins), endogenous lectins.

Hallmark of Diagnosis: Increased number of basal cells, goblet cells, or squamous metaplasia and various degrees of dysplasia.

Differential diagnosis: Viral infection.

Primidone

Definition: Alteration of the lung parenchyma associated with intake of primidone, see Drug Toxicity.

Procainamide

Definition: Alteration of the lung parenchyma associated with intake of procainamide, see Drug Toxicity.

Procarbazine

Definition: Alteration of the lung parenchyma associated with intake of procarbazine, see Drug Toxicity.

Propoxur

Definition: Alteration of the lung parenchyma associated with intake of propoxur, see Drug Toxicity.

Propoxyphene

Definition: Alteration of the lung parenchyma associated with intake of propoxyphene, see Drug Toxicity.

Propranolol

Definition: Alteration of the lung parenchyma associated with intake of propranolol, see Drug Toxicity.

Propylthiouracil

Definition: Alteration of the lung parenchyma associated with intake of propylthiouracil, see Drug Toxicity.

Prostaglandin F_{3a}

Definition: Alteration of the lung parenchyma associated with intake of prostaglandin F_{3a}, see Drug Toxicity.

Proteinosis

Definition: Disease of the peripheral lung parenchyma characterized by diffuse intraalveolar lipid proteinaceous material, see Alveolar Proteinosis.

Protothecosis

Definition: Infection of the lung with achlorophyllus algae of genus *Prototheca.*

Incidence/Epidemiology: Unusual disorder seen in man and in mammals. About 30 cases have been reported, most frequently in the USA.

Etiology/Pathophysiology: Two different species, *P. wickerhamii* and *zopfii* are known to infect humans. The prototheca species are ubiquitous and live in soil, stream water, and sewage. Infections occur most frequently in patients with decreased immune defences. The organisms usually become virulent via skin lesions with subsequent, progressive, papular or eczematous dermatitis and spread of the organisms into the regional lymph nodes. Hematogenous dissemination induces infection of the lung.

Clinical Presentation: Symptoms include a preceding cutaneous infection which is followed by recurrent pneumonia with fever, chest pain, dyspnea, and cough.

Prognosis: Usually good and without serious sequelae.

Radiology: Chest radiographs show multiple, patchy, and ill-defined densities.

Pathology:

Gross: The lungs may show areas of consolidation or suppurative pneumonia. No specific findings have been reported.

Histology: The organisms induce a necrotic lesion with lymphocytes, plasma cells, and multinucleated giant cells. Invasion of histiocytes may mimic rheumatoid nodules. The organisms are composed of ovoid cells (sporangia, measuring 5–15 μm) and of molded endospores which appear in clusters of 4–15 units.

➤ *Descriptors:* Lung parenchyma with altered structure:

- necrosis
- mononuclear inflammatory infiltrates
- multinucleated giant cells
- infectious organisms (ovoid sporangia, molded endospores)
- caseous epithelioid granulomas (ill-defined)

■ *Special stains:* PAS, collagenous stains, GMS, Gridley's, Giemsa, immunofluorescence.

Hallmark of Diagnosis: Clinical history, identification of prototheca in skin lesions and transbronchial biopsies.

Differential diagnosis: Infection of the lung with other organisms, especially *Cryptococcus*, *Cryosporium*, fungus of phaeohyphomycosis, geotrichosis.

Protozoal Infections

Definition: Infection of the lung parenchyma by protozoal organisms.

Incidence/Epidemiology: The most frequent protozoal infection of the lung seen in the Western hemisphere is caused by *Pneumocystis carinii*. Other infectious organisms are: *Trypanosoma* (Chagas' disease), *Leishmania* (leishmaniasis), *Plasmodium* (malaria), *Toxoplasma* (toxoplasmosis), *Entamoeba* (amebiasis), *Acanthamoeba* (acanthamebiasis), *Cryptosporidium* (cryptosporidiosis) and *Trichomonas* (trichomoniasis). The details are described under the particular headings.

Etiology/Pathophysiology: The majority of the organisms are transmitted by blood-sucking mosquitoes and occur in healthy persons. *Pneumocystis carinii* infections are, however, most frequently seen in immunocompromised persons. Rodents usually serve as natural reservoirs. The details are described under the particular headings.

Clinical Presentation: Symptoms are described under the particular headings.

Prognosis: Usually good. For details, see under the particular headings.

Radiology: Chest radiographs usually show diffuse or patchy densities. For details, see under the particular headings.

Pathology:

Gross: The lungs are usually heavy, wet and firm in consistency. For details, see under the particular headings.

Histology: The specific findings are described under the corresponding headings.

➤ *Descriptors:* Lung parenchyma with altered structure:

- infectious organisms
- macrophages
- necrosis and hemorrhage;
- Lung parenchyma with preserved structure:
- intraalveolar fibrinoid material
- intraalveolar serous fluid
- mononuclear inflammatory infiltrates
- histiocytes (ingested organisms)

■ *Special stains:* PAS, collagenous stains, Movat, Grocott's stain.

Hallmark of Diagnosis: Clinical history, identification of the infectious organisms.

Differential diagnosis: Infection with other organisms, alveolar proteinosis. For details see under the particular headings.

Pseudallescheriasis

Definition: Infection of the lung by the asexual fungus *Scedosporium (Monosporium) apiospermum* or the sexual form *Pseudallescheria (Allescheria boydii)*. See also Allescheriasis.

Incidence/Epidemiology: The fungus has a worldwide distribution and occurs in soil, sewage, and polluted water. Those infected are frequently farmers or rural dwellers.

Etiology/Pathophysiology: The infection occurs either as saprophytic growth in preformed cavities such as tuberculous cavities, bronchiectasis, bronchogenic cysts, and infarction or as invasive pulmonary infection in immunocompromised patients. Infection of the skin, eyes, and meninges has been reported.

Clinical Presentation: Patients present with cough, dyspnea, and hemoptysis.

Prognosis: Patients with saphrophytic infection have a good prognosis, whereas those with invasive pulmonary infection often die with septicemia.

Radiology: Chest radiographs show either cavities with intracavitary densities suggesting mycetoma or diffuse, patchy infiltrates.

Pathology:

Gross: The lungs show abscess formation with central brown-red masses or diffuse areas of consolidation, often with small areas of necrosis.

Histology: The fungus grows in small hyphae 2–5 μm wide. Multiple branches, often perpendicular to the main stem, can be seen. Additional inflammatory infiltrates comprise neutrophilic and eosinophilic granulocytes, lymphocytes, plasma cells, and histiocytes. Formation of epithelioid granulomas may occur.

➤ *Descriptors:* Bronchial mucosa with preserved structure:

- ectatic lumen
- fibrinoid material
- fungus (hyphae)
- mixed inflammatory infiltrates
- eosinophils;
- Lung parenchyma with altered structure:
- necrosis and hemorrhage
- caseous epithelioid granulomas
- fungus (intragranulomatous, hyphae)
- eosinophils
- mixed inflammatory infiltrates

■ *Special stains:* PAS, collagenous stains, Gridley's, GMS, Grocott, Gram's, immunofluorescence.

Hallmark of Diagnosis: Caseous epithelioid granulomas, identification of the fungus.

Differential diagnosis: Infection by other species of fungus such as *Aspergillus, Botryomyces, Actinomyces, Candida, Fusarium.*

Pseudoasbestos Bodies

Definition: Intraalveolar mineral fibers of nonasbestos origin coated with iron-protein mucopolysaccharide substances, see Ferruginous Bodies, Titanium, Arc Welder's Lung.

Pseudolymphoma

Definition: Localized lymphoid proliferation in the lung parenchyma resembling lymphocytic interstitial pneumonia (LIP).

Incidence/Epidemiology: Unusual disorder seen most frequently in young to middle-aged adults. No specific risk factors have been evaluated.

Etiology/Pathophysiology: The circumscribed lesion is considered to be similar to LIP. The majority of authors agree that the pseudolymphoma is a preneoplastic lymphomatoid lesion; patients have an increased risk of developing pulmonary lymphoma.

Clinical Presentation: Patients often have no complaints.

Prognosis: Usually good; however, patients have an increased risk for the development of malignant pulmonary lymphoma.

Radiology: Chest radiographs show a circumscribed, well-defined homogeneous density in the central or peripheral part of the lung.

Pathology:

Gross: The lungs show a well-defined, grayish-white, homogeneous mass of soft consistency measuring a few centimeters in maximum diameter.

Histology: The lesion is composed of mixed cellular inflammatory infiltrates comprising mature lymphocytes and plasma cells. A few histiocytes and the formation of germinal centers may be seen. No invasion of the small vascular walls, the bronchial walls, or pleura can be detected. Multinucleated giant cells and central fibrosis are occasional findings. The noninvolved areas of the lung parenchyma are unsuspicious.

➤ *Descriptors:* Newly formed textures without metastasis potential:
- mesenchymal growth pattern
- lymphomatoid textures
- absent or infrequent mitoses
- homogeneous nuclear and cellular size
- multinucleated giant cells
- germinal centers
- mononuclear inflammatory infiltrates (lymphocytes and plasma cells, mature)

■ *Special stains:* PAS, collagenous stains, Giemsa, immunohistochemistry for lymphocytic subpopulations and for immunoglobulins, endogenous lectins, DNA analysis.

Hallmark of Diagnosis: Circumscribed lymphomatoid proliferation without features of an invasive lymphoma.

Differential diagnosis: Lymphocytic interstitial pneumonia, malignant (low-grade) lymphoma, lymphomatoid hyperplasia.

Pseudomonas

Definition: Infection of the lung by *Pseudomonas* (*P. aeruginosa*).

Incidence/Epidemiology: *P. aeruginosa* is an opportunistic, aerobic, gram-negative bacterium. Patients with severe burns or under immunosuppressive therapy are susceptible to pneumonia and bacteremia with *Pseudomonas*, whereas patients with congestive heart disease or chronic lung disorders often suffer from *Pseudomonas* pneumonia without bacteremia. *Pseudomonas* pneumonia often occurs in terminal stages of various diseases and is frequently seen in autopsies. Infection is endemic in areas of southeast Asia, see Melioidosis.

Etiology/Pathophysiology: The gram-negative organisms reach the lung by inhalation or by infection of traumatized skin and hematogenous dissemination. They grow rapidly in pulmonary tissue and induce acute progressive pneumonia.

Clinical Presentation: Usually acute onset of symptoms which include high fever, chest pain, progressive dyspnea, chills, septicemia.

Prognosis: The mortality rate in patients with septicemia ranges between 70–80%, but is considerably lower if it is still a localized infection.

Radiology: Chest radiographs show patchy, bilateral densities with marked involvement of the lower lobes and usually pleural effusions.

Pathology:

Gross: The lungs are heavy and congested and show red-tan or grayish-white areas in the lower parts. The apices are usually not or only mildly involved.

Histology: The lung texture is destroyed. The necrotic areas contain an outer border with hemorrhage, a medial zone invaded by neutrophilic granulocytes, lymphocytes, and plasma cells, and an inner core containing a suppurative exudate intermingled with multinucleated histiocytes (2–3 nuclei). The severely and less severely involved parts show acute necrosis of the arterial and venous walls with agglutinated granulocytic infiltrates. The vessels contain numerous bacilli which are also present within the distant airways. Abscess formation may occur in late stages.

➤ *Descriptors:* Lung parenchyma with altered structure:
- necrosis and hemorrhage (abscess formation)
- mixed inflammatory infiltrates
- multinucleated giant cells (histiocytes, 2–3 nuclei)
- bacteria (gram-negative)

■ *Special stains:* PAS, collagenous stains, Gram's, GMS, methenamine silver stain.

Hallmark of Diagnosis: Clinical history, abscessing suppurative pneumonia with necrotic angiitis, numerous bacteria which measure 0.6×2 μm, multinucleated histiocytes.

Differential diagnosis: Abscessing pneumonia due to other infective organisms.

Pseudotumor, Inflammatory

Definition: Circumscribed mass of proliferating mixed inflammatory cells in lung (synonyms plasma cell granuloma, myofibroblastic tumor).

Incidence/Epidemiology: Unusual disorder. However, it accounts for 40–60% of all benign tumorous lesions in children and young adults, most frequently in the age group 5–10 years. It can, however, be seen in any age group.

Etiology/Pathophysiology: The etiology of the lesion is unknown. Alteration of defence mechanisms in the lung such as dysfunction of interleukin production has been suggested to be involved in the development of inflammatory pseudotumors.

Clinical Presentation: Patients are usually asymptomatic.

Prognosis: Usually good; however, patients have an increased risk of developing malignant pulmonary lymphomas.

Radiology: Chest radiographs show a well-circumscribed, homogeneous density in the peripheral lung parenchyma.

Pathology:

Gross: The lung presents with a circumscribed, firm mass of grayish-white color. The maximum diameter measures 1–8 cm.

Histology: The tumors are composed of lymphocytes, plasma cells, histiocytes, and proliferating fibroblasts and myofibroblasts. The texture of the lung parenchyma is destroyed. Dystrophic calcification may occur. Areas of necrosis are absent.

➤ *Descriptors:* Newly formed textures without metastasis potential:

- mesenchymal growth pattern
- lymphomatoid textures
- fibroblasts and myofibroblasts
- homogeneous nuclear and cellular size
- absent or infrequent mitoses
- multinucleated giant cells
- germinal centers
- mononuclear inflammatory cells (lymphocytes and plasma cells, mature)

■ *Special stains:* PAS, collagenous stains, Giemsa, electron microscopy, immunohistochemistry for lymphocytic subpopulations, immunoglobulins, vimentin, desmin, myosin, actin, desmoplakin, endogenous lectins, DNA analysis.

Hallmark of Diagnosis: Proliferation of fibroblasts, myofibroblasts, mixed inflammatory infiltrates.

Differential diagnosis: Leiomyoma, fibroma, leiomyosarcoma, pseudolymphoma, organizing pneumonia.

Psittacosis

Definition: Infection of the lung by *Chlamydia psittaci* (synonym ornithosis).

Incidence/Epidemiology: Infection in man occurs via infected birds or asymptomatic carriers. The majority of infected persons have close contact with birds, most frequently parrots. However, other species of birds can also act as infectious sources.

Etiology/Pathophysiology: The chlamydial organism consists of a cell wall containing both DNA and RNA. The organisms have different intracellular and extracellular appearances, and they depend on their host cells for ATP and other metabolites.

Clinical Presentation: Symptoms include "flu-like" illness, cough, fever, and headache and arise after an incubation time of 1–2 weeks.

Prognosis: Usually good and without serious sequelae.

Radiology: Chest radiographs show unilateral or bilateral diffuse densities, usually in the lower lobes. Areas of consolidation may be present.

Pathology:

Gross: The lungs are heavy and edematous and show areas of firm consistency.

Histology: The distant airways are filled with mononuclear infiltrates mainly comprising lymphocytes and plasma cells. Early stages show an intraalveolar edema, interstitial granulocytic infiltrates, and desquamated macrophages in the alveoli. The epithelial cells of the bronchial mucosa are desquamated. The findings resemble those of viral infections.

➤ *Descriptors:* Lung parenchyma with preserved structure:

- mononuclear inflammatory infiltrates
- intraalveolar serous fluid
- desquamation, hypertrophy, hyperplasia and dysplasia of pneumocytes
- mixed inflammatory infiltrates

■ *Special stains:* PAS, collagenous stains, Giemsa, immunofluorescence, endogenous lectins.

Hallmark of Diagnosis: Clinical history, intraalveolar edema, macrophages, interstitial and intraalveolar mononuclear inflammatory infiltrates.

Differential diagnosis: Viral infection, infection of the lung by *Chlamydia trachomatis.*

Pulmonary Adenomatosis

Definition: Benign form of pulmonary neoplasm resembling bronchioloalveolar carcinoma.

Incidence/Epidemiology: Extremely rare disorder which is still being disputed. It should not be confused with focal cellular hypertrophy or hyperplasia and dysplasia of cells lining the bronchioles.

Etiology/Pathophysiology: The etiology is not known. Viral infection similar to that in sheep and goats (Jaagsiekte) is still under discussion.

Clinical Presentation: Symptoms include cough, chest pain, expectoration and dyspnea.

Prognosis: Poor, as slow progressive respiratory failure causes death after 2–4 years.

Radiology: Chest radiographs show multiple, diffuse densities.

Pathology:

Gross: The lungs are tan, edematous, and of increased consistency.

Histology: The interstitial texture of the lung parenchyma is preserved. The cells of the alveolar lining show a tendency toward proliferation with marked cellular atypias, hypertrophy, and hyperplasia. The interalveolar septula may be fibrotic.

➤ *Descriptors:* Newly formed textures with metastasis potential:
- epithelial growth pattern
- adenoid textures (papillae, tubuli)
- islands of tumor cells
- lining of tumor cells
- homogeneous nuclear and cellular size
- absent or infrequent mitoses
- focal interstitial fibrosis
- absent or weak inflammatory infiltrates
- micrometastases (intrapulmonary)

■ *Special stains:* PAS, Giemsa, immunohistochemistry for chromosome abnormalities, DNA analysis, endogenous lectins.

Hallmark of Diagnosis: Intraalveolar neoplasm resembling bronchioloalveolar carcinoma.

Differential diagnosis: Bronchioloalveolar carcinoma, desquamative interstitial pneumonia, obstructive pneumonitis, focal scarring pneumonia, viral pneumonia.

Pulmonary Renal Syndrome

Definition: Disorders of immunologic or infectious nature affecting both the lung and the kidney.

Incidence/Epidemiology: Rare disorders, most frequently occurring in young to middle-aged adults.

Etiology/Pathophysiology: The capillary systems (basement membranes) of the lung and kidney have certain similarities in respect to antigenic potency and, thus, may react concordantly if alterations of serum immunoglobulins occur. In addition, certain classes of organisms may show the same adhesive tendency to the capillary network in the lung and in the kidneys. The pulmonary-renal syndromes include: (a) hemorrhage with glomerular basement-specific antibodies (Goodpasture's syndrome); (b) infections (Legionnaires'disease); (c) immune-complex diseases (Wegener's granulomatosis, lupus erythematosus, systemic vasculitis).

Clinical Presentation: The pulmonary symptoms often precede the renal symptoms.

Prognosis: Usually good (Goodpasture's, Legionnaires' diseases, Wegener's granulomatosis) or fair (lupus erythematosus, systemic vasculitis).

Radiology: Chest radiographs may show either diffuse, patchy densities or circumscribed, ill-defined masses with central necrosis.

Pathology:

Gross: The lung and kidney show similar alterations including grayish-white firm nodules, areas of hemorrhage, and necrosis.

Histology: The histomorphological changes are similar and include large areas of hemorrhage, ill-defined epithelioid granulomas with necrosis, formation of abscesses, etc. The details are described under the particular headings.

➤ *Descriptors:* Lung parenchyma with altered structure:
- necrosis and hemorrhage
- caseous epithelioid granulomas (ill-defined)
- mononuclear inflammatory infiltrates
- necrosis (abscess formation);
- Pulmonary vessels with preserved structure:
- mixed inflammatory infiltrates
- mononuclear inflammatory infiltrates

■ *Special stains:* PAS, collagenous stains, Prussian blue. For details, see under the particular headings.

Hallmark of Diagnosis: Clinical history, similarity of histomorphological alterations in both pulmonary and renal parenchyma.

Differential diagnosis: See under the particular headings, involvement of the lung without involvement of the kidney (for example, limited Wegener's granulomatosis).

Pyrrolizidine alkaloids

Definition: Alteration of the lung parenchyma associated with intake of pyrrolizidine alkaloids, see Drug Toxicity.

Q Fever

Definition: Infection of the lung by *Coxiella burnetii*.

Incidence/Epidemiology: The organisms have a worldwide distribution and usually infect mammals such as sheep, goats and cattle. Those infected are usually farmers or persons working in medical health care. Endemic infection of 25 physicians present during an autopsy has been reported (Freiburg, FRG).

Etiology/Pathophysiology: The organisms belong to the order of rickettsial agents and are usually transmitted by person-to-person contact. Mosquito bites may be an additional infectious source.

Clinical Presentation: Symptoms include headache, fever, malaise, and myalgia and show an abrupt onset after an incubation period of approximately 2–3 weeks.

Prognosis: The infection is only seldom fatal, and its course is usually benign and without serious sequelae.

Radiology: Chest radiographs may show diffuse lobar densities in severe infections.

Pathology:

Gross: The lungs are heavy, edematous, and red or grayish-white depending upon the stage of the pneumonia.

Histology: The alveoli are filled with a fibrinous exudate which includes lymphocytes, macrophages, plasma cells, and only a few neutrophilic granulocytes. The inflammatory cells are located within the distant airways and in the interstitial walls. The lung texture is preserved.

➤ *Descriptors:* Lung parenchyma with preserved structure:

- intraalveolar fibrinoid material
- mononuclear inflammatory infiltrates
- neutrophils (scattered)

■ *Special stains:* PAS, collagenous stains, Giemsa, immunofluorescence.

Hallmark of Diagnosis: Clinical history, identification of rickettsia, interstitial mononuclear and intraalveolar fibrinous exudative pneumonia.

Differential diagnosis: Bacterial pneumonia due to other agents.

Quinicrine Talc

Definition: Alteration of the lung parenchyma associated with intake of quinicrine talc, see Drug Toxicity.

Quinidine

Definition: Alteration of the lung parenchyma associated with intake of quinidine, see Drug Toxicity.

Radiation

Definition: Alteration of the lung parenchyma associated with radiation of the lung.

Incidence/Epidemiology: The lung may be included in concepts of radiation therapy for various malignancies, especially Pancoast's tumors or tumors of the mediastinum. Radiation of axillary lymph nodes in patients with breast carcinoma often induces changes in the lung parenchyma due to scattered X-rays. Other sources of radiation are exposure to radioactive particles especially after accidents at nuclear power plants.

Etiology/Pathophysiology: Radiation of the lung induces interstitial pneumonitis of various degrees depending upon the intensity of the radiation. Damaged tissue includes the capillary system, the bronchioles, and epithelial cells. The late stage is characterized by progressive fibrosis, which may develop as late as years after exposure. Several drugs can "trigger" the occurrence of radiation pneumonitis several years after exposure to radiation (radium recall). Other drugs can potentiate the radiation damage (bleomycin, cyclophosphamide, methotrexate).

Clinical Presentation: Patients may be asymptomatic or may complain of progressive dyspnea and cough, but seldom of chest pain.

Prognosis: Fair, virtually every radiation exposure induces lung damage which may proceed to slow progressive respiratory failure after years.

Radiology: Chest radiographs show diffuse interstitial densities often with unclear boundaries between the lung and adjacent structures (mediastinum) and marked shrinkage of the lung.

Pathology:
Gross: The lungs are of stiff consistency and pale in color. Honeycombing can be seen in late stages.

Histology: The radiation induces a marked proliferation of the endothelial and epithelial cells in combination with extravasation of fibrinous fluid. The capillaries and small arterial and venous vessels are occluded by microthrombi and proliferated endothelial cells. The cells of the alveolar lining show marked hyperplasia and hypertrophy. Cellular atypias are frequent and may mimic carcinomatous changes. Bronchiolitis obliterans may occur. Hyaline membranes are seen in early stages, whereas in late stages marked interstitial fibrosis often with proliferating smooth muscle cells in the fibrotic bundles can be seen.

➤ *Descriptors:* Lung parenchyma with preserved structure:
- intraalveolar serous fluid
- hyaline membranes
- desquamation, hypertrophy, hyperplasia and dysplasia of pneumocytes
- mixed inflammatory infiltrates;
- Lung parenchyma with altered structure:
- proliferating smooth muscle cells
- intrabronchiolar fibrinoid material and histiocytes
- ulceration of bronchiolar mucosa
- proliferating fibroblasts
- diffuse interstitial fibrosis
- honeycombing;
- Bronchial mucosa with altered structure:
- squamous metaplasia and dysplasia

▪ *Special stains:* PAS, collagenous stains, endogenous lectins, immunohistochemistry for immunoglobulins and lymphocytic subpopulations, DNA analysis.

Hallmark of Diagnosis: Clinical history, diffuse alveolar damage and marked alteration of the capillaries and small vessels, prominent cellular hyperplasia and hypertrophy associated with cellular atypias.

Differential diagnosis: Interstitial pneumonitis due to other agents (especially drug toxicity), adenocarcinoma of the lung.

Radon

Definition: Patients exposed to radon have an increased risk of lung cancer, see Cancer of the Lung.

Reid Index

Definition: Ratio of the transverse thickness of the bronchial mucus glands divided by the bronchial wall thickness. It measures in nonbronchitics 0.25–0.40, and in bronchitics and miners 0.40–0.59, see Chronic Airflow Obstruction.

Rendu-Osler-Weber Disease

Definition: Alteration of the lung parenchyma associated with familial telangiectasis.

Incidence/Epidemiology: Rare disorder with dominant inheritance. Pulmonary involvement may be seen.

Etiology/Pathophysiology: The disorder is characterized by multiple angiomatous telangiectases of the skin, mucus membranes, and visceral organs such as liver, lung, or spleen.

Clinical Presentation: Patients may be asymptomatic or may present with a clinically relevant shunt volume.

Prognosis: Usually good and without serious sequelae.

Radiology: Chest radiographs may show multiple arteriovenous fistulae.

Pathology:
Gross: Multiple, usually small plexuses of tortuous vessels with ectatic lumen and thin walls can be seen in the peripheral lung parenchyma.
Histology: The walls of the vessels are of small diameter and usually show arterial characteristics with abrupt transformation to venous structures. The interposed capillary bed is absent.

➤ *Descriptors:* Pulmonary vessels with preserved structure:
- tortuous vessels (veins, lymphatics)
- ectatic lumen
- atrophy of media

■ *Special stains:* Collagenous stains.

Hallmark of Diagnosis: Clinical history, multiple arteriovenous fistulae.

Differential diagnosis: Lymphangiectasis, cavernous hemangioma.

Reserpine

Definition: Alteration of the lung parenchyma associated with intake of reserpine, see Drug Toxicity.

Respiratory Distress

Definition: Clinical syndrome related to damage of the alveolar capillary membrane representing a heterogeneous group of disorders, see Adult Respiratory Distress Syndrome, Bronchopulmonary Dysplasia, Hyaline Membrane Disease.

Respiratory Syncytial Virus Infection

Definition: Infection of the lung by respiratory syncytial virus.
Incidence/Epidemiology: Infection of the lower respiratory tract with this virus is common in children and may reach an infection rate of 100–200/1 000 children during the first year of life. Usually adults are repeatedly infected until old age in community epidemics.

Etiology/Pathophysiology: The RNA virus is usually transmitted by direct contact with the mucosa of the nose (fingers). After an incubation period of a week, infection of the upper respiratory tract (rhinorrhea, anorexia) develops, spreading along the airways to the lower respiratory tract. The virus replicates in the cytoplasm of the epithelial cells. Immunity to the virus is incomplete and is partially lost after several months. The virus has been identified in children with sudden infant death syndrome. Virus specific IgE and a depressed number of suppressor T lymphocytes could be identified in patients suffering from infectious bronchiolitis.

Clinical Presentation: Patients develop symptoms of infection of the upper respiratory tract followed by cough, tachypnea, low-grade fever, and signs of bronchiolar obstruction. Cyanosis and high-grade fever indicate severe pulmonary infections. The mortality rate may reach 1% in normal children and may rise to 30% in the elderly or in children with additional damage of the lung (bronchopulmonary dysplasia) or with underlying heart diseases.

Prognosis: Usually good and without serious sequelae; however, immunocompromised patients, aged persons, or children with preexisting lung damage have a mortality rate reaching 30%.

Radiology: Chest radiographs may be normal or may reveal signs of air trapping, diffuse patchy infiltrates, or multiple, ill-defined densities in both lungs.

Pathology:
Gross: The lungs are overexpanded, heavy, and reddish-brown.

Histology: The epithelial cells of the distant airways and of the small bronchi are desquamated and necrotic. The distant airways are filled with proteinaceous fluid, erythrocytes, and mononuclear inflammatory cells to various degrees. Multinucleated giant cells containing intracytoplasmic inclusion bodies may be present. The interalveolar septula are widened and contain inflammatory infiltrates. Hyaline membranes and debris invaded by macrophages and by fibroblasts indicate more severe infections.

➤ *Descriptors:* Lung parenchyma with preserved structure:
- intraalveolar fibrinoid material
- mononuclear inflammatory infiltrates
- multinucleated giant cells
- inclusion bodies (intracytoplasmic)
- hyaline membranes

- desquamation, hypertrophy, hyperplasia and dysplasia of pneumocytes;
- Bronchial mucosa with preserved structure:
- desquamation, hypertrophy, hyperplasia and dysplasia of epithelial cells
- mononuclear inflammatory infiltrates;
- Bronchial mucosa with altered structure:
- necrosis
- mixed inflammatory infiltrates

■ *Special stains:* PAS, collagenous stains, Giemsa, immunofluorescence.

Hallmark of Diagnosis: Clinical history, infectious bronchiolitis associated with interstitial pneumonia, hyaline membranes. Identification of the virus by circulating RSV antigen and other serologic diagnostic techniques (complement fixation, enzyme immuno assay, etc).

Differential diagnosis: Bronchopneumonia due to other organisms, especially adenovirus, rhinovirus, influenzavirus, mumps virus, *Mycoplasma pneumoniae*, rickettsial infections.

Rhabdomyosarcoma

Definition: Malignant tumor of the lung with characteristic histology.

Incidence/Epidemiology: Extremely rare tumor occurring in the peripheral lung parenchyma and in association with the larger bronchi and trachea. About 20 cases, mostly adult males, have been published.

Etiology/Pathophysiology: The tumor, with solely rhabdomyoblastic differentiation, may arise from the muscular layer of the bronchi, trachea, or vessels.

Clinical Presentation: Patients may be asymptomatic or present with symptoms related to the proximal localization of the tumor.

Prognosis: Usually poor and similar to that of patients with ordinary bronchial carcinomas.

Radiology: Chest radiographs show either centrally or peripherally localized circumscribed densities.

Pathology:

Gross: The tumors are firm in consistency and yellowish-white.

Histology: The tumors are composed of plump spindle cells which show characteristic cross-striations in the cytoplasm. Inflammatory response of the host tissue is weak. Necrotic areas may be present in larger tumors. Calcification and numerous mitotic figures are not a sign of rhabdomyosarcoma. Rhabdomyoblastic differentiation may be seen in certain areas of other lesions such as teratomas, blastomas, carcinosarcomas, or congenital cystic adenomatoid malformations.

➤ *Descriptors:* Newly formed textures with metastasis potential:

- mesenchymal growth pattern
- sarcomatous textures
- plump spindle cells
- inhomogeneous nuclear and cellular size
- abundant cytoplasm (cytoplasmic cross-striations)
- infrequent mitoses
- necrosis and hemorrhage
- absent or weak inflammatory infiltrates

■ *Special stains:* PAS, collagenous stains, Giemsa, electron microscopy, immunohistochemistry for myosin, actin, vimentin, desmin, desmoplakin, DNA analysis, endogenous lectins.

Hallmark of Diagnosis: Identification of rhabdomyoblastic differentiation by immunohistochemistry or electron microscopy.

Differential diagnosis: Teratoma, blastoma, carcinosarcoma, metastatic rhabdomyosarcoma.

Rheumatic Fever

Definition: Alteration of the lung parenchyma in patients suffering from rheumatic fever.

Incidence/Epidemiology: Only a few cases suffering from rheumatic fever with pulmonary involvement have been reported.

Etiology/Pathophysiology: Rheumatic fever is considered to be an abnormal reaction of the immune system associated with toxins of β-hemolytic streptococci. Patients suffer from recurrent attacks of fever with arthritis and endocarditis.

Clinical Presentation: The clinical course of the reported cases with pulmonary involvement is characterized by progressive dyspnea, cyanosis, and death occurring within a few months after onset of the disorder.

Prognosis: Poor, as patients with pulmonary symptoms usually die within a few months after clinical manifestation.

Radiology: Chest radiographs show diffuse bilateral densities.

Pathology:

Gross: The lungs are heavy, red-grayish and rubbery in consistency.

Histology: The distant airways are filled with proteinaceous material, mononuclear inflammatory infiltrates comprising macrophages, lymphocytes, and plasma cells. The interalveolar septula are widened, and edematous and contain similar inflammatory cells. The small vessels are involved in the inflammatory process.

➤ *Descriptors:* Lung parenchyma with preserved structure:

- intraalveolar fibrinoid material
- mononuclear inflammatory infiltrates
- interstitial edema;
- Pulmonary vessels with preserved structure:
- mononuclear inflammatory infiltrates

■ *Special stains:* PAS, collagenous stains, Giemsa, immunohistochemistry for immunoglobulins, lymphocytic subpopulations, endogenous lectins.

Hallmark of Diagnosis: Clinical history, diffuse alveolar damage consistent with usual interstitial pneumonia.

Differential diagnosis: Usual interstitial pneumonia due to other agents, especially drug reaction; organizing bacterial pneumonia.

Rheumatoid Disease

Definition: Alteration of the lung parenchyma associated with rheumatoid disorders.

Incidence/Epidemiology: About 40–50% of patients with rheumatoid disorders have histomorphological and functional evidence of pleuropulmonary involvement. Pulmonary involvement of rheumatoid disorders is seen more frequently in men than in women. Rheumatoid pleuritis is more frequent than pulmonary parenchymal disease.

Etiology/Pathophysiology: The etiology of the disease is not known. There is evidence that immune-complex-mediated injury, cell-mediated immunoregulation, and hereditary factors participate in pleuropulmonary involvement of rheumatoid disease.

Clinical Presentation: Symptoms related to arthritis usually precede pleuropulmonary symptoms. However, uncommonly, the opposite may occur. Pulmonary symptoms are usually related to pleuritis with pleural effusions. Lung function tests show evidence of restrictive pulmonary function abnormalities.

Prognosis: Usually good; slow progressive respiratory failure or development of honeycombing may occur but are extremely rare.

Radiology: Chest radiographs show findings related to pleural effusions and in addition, diffuse patchy densities, scarring, ill-defined nodules a few millimeters to 1–2 cm in size.

Pathology:

Gross: The lungs are firm in consistency and may show scarring with fibrotic nodules measuring a few millimeters or centimeters in maximum diameter.

Histology: The histomorphologic findings include the usual interstitial pneumonia (UIP, usually associated with fibrosis), bronchiolitis obliterans, formation of rheumatoid (seldom centrally necrotizing) nodules, fibrinoid obliteration of small vessels, and constrictive bronchiolitis. The UIP-related changes usually include advanced interstitial fibrosis with destruction of the normal lung texture, an intensive lymphocytic interstitial infiltrate, moderate hyperplasia and hypertrophy of cells of the alveolar lining, and weak exudation of proteinaceous fluid. The rheumatoid nodules are composed of epithelioid histiocytes which may show palisading, scattered lymphocytes, and rarely multinucleated Langhans' giant cells. Central necrotic areas consist of amorphous eosinophilic material. In addition, the walls of small vessels and of larger bronchi may be involved. Rheumatic nodules located within the pleura are usually ill-defined.

➤ *Descriptors:* Lung parenchyma with preserved structure:

- intraalveolar fibrinoid material
- mononuclear inflammatory infiltrates
- multinucleated giant cells;
- Pulmonary vessels with preserved structure:
- mononuclear inflammatory infiltrates;
- Lung parenchyma with altered structure:
- intrabronchiolar fibrinoid material and histiocytes
- ulceration of bronchiolar mucosa
- lymphomatoid granulomas
- proliferating fibroblasts
- diffuse interstitial fibrosis

- honeycombing;
- Pleura with altered structure:
- lymphomatoid granulomas
- hypertrophy and hyperplasia of mesothelial cells

■ *Special stains:* PAS, collagenous stains, Giemsa, immunohistochemistry for immunoglobulins (deposits of IgM) and lymphocytic subpopulations, endogenous lectins.

Hallmark of Diagnosis: Clinical history, nonspecific pleuritis with pleural effusions, histomorphological findings related to usual interstitial pneumonia, rheumatoid nodules, bronchiolitis obliterans.

Differential diagnosis: Usual interstitial pneumonia, reaction of the lung parenchyma due to toxic agents, tuberculosis, sarcoidosis, bacterial (organizing) pneumonia, Hodgkin's disease.

Rhinosporidiosis

Definition: Infection of the lung by *Rhinosporidium seeberi.*

Incidence/Epidemiology: The disorder occurs sporadically in India and Sri Lanka.

Etiology/Pathophysiology: The organisms are considered to be a fungus and cannot be cultured or transmitted to animals. Man becomes infected by contact with water or dust. Infected persons are predominantly men.

Clinical Presentation: The primary site of infection is most frequently the nose, followed by the eyes. Other sites include the skin, the genitals, or rectum. Dissemination to the viscera is uncommon. The lesions resemble allergic polyps or papilloma lesions and may last for 20–30 years.

Prognosis: Usually good and without serious sequelae.

Radiology: Chest radiographs are usually normal or may show multiple granular densities.

Pathology:

Gross: The lungs display multiple, firm, miliary, grayish-yellow nodules.

Histology: The organisms grow from small trophic cysts to large sporangia which contain multiple spores. The cysts measure 10–200 μm in maximum diameter and may be surrounded by granulomatous or fibrotic tissue.

➤ *Descriptors:* Lung parenchyma with altered structure:

- caseous epithelioid granulomas
- fungus (intragranulomatous, sporangia)
- mononuclear inflammatory infiltrates
- eosinophils

■ *Special stains:* PAS, GMS, Gridley's stain.

Hallmark of Diagnosis: Caseous epithelioid granulomas, identification of the cysts and sporangia.

Differential diagnosis: Infection with other fungal species such as *Prototheca, Chrysosporium parvum, Coccidioides immitis.*

Rhinovirus

Definition: Infection of the lung by rhinovirus.

Incidence/Epidemiology: Infection of the lower respiratory tract with rhinovirus rarely occurs despite its frequent involvement of the upper respiratory tract.

Etiology/Pathophysiology: The rhinovirus belongs to the order of picornavirus (RNA virus) and is transmitted by droplets.

Clinical Presentation: The virus causes the "common cold". Pulmonary infection may be difficult to document with absolute certainty. "Superinfective" bacterial pneumonia is the usual finding.

Prognosis: Usually good; however, immunocompromised patients or persons with preexisting lung damage may develop serious bacterial superinfection with fatal outcome.

Radiology: Chest radiographs are usually normal or may show diffuse densities.

Pathology:

Gross: No specific findings have been reported.

Histology: The histomorphologic findings include nonspecific pulmonary damage, debris, and hyaline material within the distant airways, desquamation of cells of the alveolar lining, and mononuclear interstitial infiltrates.

➤ *Descriptors:* Lung parenchyma with preserved structure:

- intraalveolar fibrinoid material
- mononuclear inflammatory infiltrates
- desquamation, hypertrophy, hyperplasia and dysplasia of pneumocytes

■ *Special stains:* PAS, collagenous stains, Giemsa, in situ hybridization.

Hallmark of Diagnosis: Identification of the virus within the lower respiratory tract.

Differential diagnosis: Bacterial pneumonia, infection with other viruses.

Rickettsial Infections

Definition: Infection of the lung by rickettsiae.

Incidence/Epidemiology: Rickettsial infection in man includes the following five groups: (a) typhus (worldwide); (b) spotted fever (Rocky Mountain spotted fever, America; north Asian tick-borne rickettsiosis, USSR; African tick typhus, Africa, India; Queensland tick typhus, Australia; rickettsial pox, USA, USSR, Korea); (c) tsutsugamushi disease (south Asia, Western Pacific); (d) Q fever (worldwide); (e) trench fever (Europe, USSR, Mexico).

Etiology/Pathophysiology: Rickettsiae usually live in arthopods (lice, ticks, mites) and are transmitted to man accidentally. They are gram-negative, bacterium-like, obligate intracellular (except the trench fever) microorganisms which grow in coccoid, diplobacillary, and chain form. They are considered to be bacteria containing DNA and RNA but lack enzymes enabling them to grow outside of a cellular environment.

Clinical Presentation: The clinical picture is usually characterized by an acute onset of high fever, skin rash, headache, malaise, muscle pain, etc. after an incubation period of 1–3 weeks. The details are described under the particular headings.

Prognosis: Usually good; however, fatal courses still occur in severe infections or with decreased immunity.

Radiology: Chest radiographs show diffuse, ill-defined densities.

Pathology:

Gross: The changes of the lung parenchyma resemble lobar pneumonia.

Histology: The peripheral lung parenchyma shows multifocal interstitial inflammation with intraalveolar exudation of fibrin, and additional alterations such as vasculitis and small foci of necrosis.

➤ *Descriptors:* Lung parenchyma with preserved structure:
- intraalveolar fibrinoid material
- mononuclear inflammatory infiltrates;
- Pulmonary vessels with preserved structure:
- mononuclear inflammatory infiltrates;
- Lung parenchyma with altered structure:
- necrosis (focal)
- mixed inflammatory infiltrates

■ *Special stains:* PAS, collagenous stains, Giemsa, immunofluorescence.

Hallmark of Diagnosis: Clinical history, identification of the organisms by immunofluorescence in lung or skin biopsy specimens, serologic tests.

Differential diagnosis: Infections with other rickettsial organisms, bacterial pneumonia.

Rock Wool Fibers

Definition: Alteration of the lung parenchyma associated with inhalation of rock wool fibers.

Incidence/Epidemiology: Exposure to rock wool occurs among persons working in rock wool factories which melt naturally occurring rock and draw out mineral fibers.

Etiology/Pathophysiology: The formed fibers may reach the distant airways depending upon their size. They are considered to be nonfibrogenic and usually do not produce chronic respiratory disease. A slightly increased risk for mesothelioma exists.

Clinical Presentation: The symptoms depend upon the amount of inhaled fibers and are usually mild.

Prognosis: Usually good; however, an increased risk for the development of malignant mesotheliomas exists.

Radiology: Chest radiographs are usually normal.

Pathology:

Gross: No specific alterations have been reported.

Histology: The birefringent fibers can be seen in the distant airways especially close to the bronchioles. Inflammatory reaction of the lung parenchyma is rare and usually weak.

➤ *Descriptors:* Lung parenchyma with preserved structure:
- dust (birefringent fibers)
- macrophages (birefringent fibers)
- mononuclear inflammatory infiltrates
- ferruginous bodies (pseudoferruginous)

■ *Special stains:* PAS, collagenous stains, polarization, X-ray diffraction method and related physical techniques.

Hallmark of Diagnosis: Clinical history, identification of the fibers.

Differential diagnosis: Inhalation of other nonasbestos or asbestos mineral fibers.

Rocky Mountain Spotted Fever

Definition: Infection of the lung with *Rickettsia rickettsii.*

Incidence/Epidemiology: Rocky Mountain spotted fever is endemic in North and South America. Most cases have been reported from the eastern States along the Atlantic seashore and occur from late spring until early autumn.

Etiology/Pathophysiology: The organisms live in the salivary glands of ticks and have their reservoir in different species of mammals. Infection of man occurs during the ticks' feeding on blood.

Clinical Presentation: The clinical picture which develops after an incubation period of 1–2 weeks is characterized by acute onset of symptoms and rash. The rash starts from the peripheral wrists and ankles, moving up the arms and legs to the abdomen, and consists of sharply defined purpuric macules. Cough, dyspnea, or even cyanosis are present if pulmonary involvement occurs.

Prognosis: Usually good with abating disease after 2 weeks; however, death may occur after 10 days as a result of toxemia in severe infections.

Radiology: Chest radiographs show bilateral, diffuse, occasionally widespread densities.

Pathology:

Gross: The lungs are heavy and of red-tan color.

Histology: The organisms induce an acute interstitial pneumonitis comprising interstitial edema, intraalveolar exudation of proteinaceous material, intraalveolar hemorrhage, and mononuclear inflammatory infiltrates in the walls of the small arteries (vasculitis). Formation of hyaline membranes may occur. The organisms can be demonstrated by direct immunofluorescence techniques on paraffin-embedded sections.

➤ *Descriptors:* Lung parenchyma with preserved structure:
- intraalveolar fibrinoid material
- mononuclear inflammatory infiltrates
- hyaline membranes
- hemorrhage

■ *Special stains:* PAS, collagenous stains, Giemsa, immunofluorescence.

Hallmark of Diagnosis: Clinical history, interstitial pneumonia, intraalveolar fibrinous exudation, vasculitis, identification of the organisms.

Differential diagnosis: Infection of the lung by other rickettsiae, viral pneumonia, usual interstitial pneumonia.

Rubella

Definition: Alteration of the lung parenchyma associated with rubella embryopathy.

Incidence/Epidemiology: About 4/100 000 pregnancies in a nonepidemic period result in rubella embryopathy, if the mother is seronegative.

Etiology/Pathophysiology: The rubella syndrome is the result of a diaplacentary infection of the fetus with the rubellavirus during the first two trimesters. The classic rubella embryopathy comprises cataracts, deafness and congenital heart disease; in addition, the expanded disorder may result in thrombocytopenia purpura, neonatal hepatitis, encephalitis, and pneumonitis.

Clinical Presentation: The infants present with respiratory distress soon after birth.

Prognosis: Fair without sequelae; resolution of the disease needs several weeks or months.

Radiology: Chest radiographs show diffuse bilateral densities.

Pathology:

Gross: The lungs are heavy and dark-red.

Histology: The lung parenchyma shows evidence of diffuse interstitial pneumonitis, either of the usual or of the desquamative type. Fibrosis does not develop in rubella pneumonitis.

➤ *Descriptors:* Lung parenchyma with preserved structure:
- intraalveolar fibrinoid material
- mononuclear inflammatory infiltrates
- desquamation, hypertrophy, hyperplasia and dysplasia of pneumocytes
- macrophages

■ *Special stains:* PAS, collagenous stains, Giemsa, immunofluorescence, electron microscopy.

Hallmark of Diagnosis: Clinical history, interstitial pneumonitis, identification of the virus by use of immunofluorescence techniques.

Differential diagnosis: Superimposed bacterial infection, infection of the lung by other viruses, usual interstitial pneumonia, desquamative interstitial pneumonia.

Rutile Fibers

Definition: Alteration of the lung parenchyma associated with inhalation of rutile fibers.

Incidence/Epidemiology: Inhalation of rutile fibers may occur in the dye industry when titanium dioxide is used.

Etiology/Pathophysiology: Rutile fibers are a form of titanium dioxide usually associated with silica. They are found in the distant airways and may be coated with iron. Animal experiments have not shown fibrogenic activity of titanium dioxide.

Clinical Presentation: Patients are usually asymptomatic.

Prognosis: Usually good and without serious sequelae.

Radiology: Chest radiographs are usually normal or may show mild diffuse densities.

Pathology:

Gross: The lungs may be of pale color.

Histology: Rutile fibers are usually located within the bronchioles and nearby lung parenchyma zones.They may be coated with iron (rutile bodies) and contain a dark central core. Inflammatory reaction of the lung parenchyma and fibrosis are not characteristic findings associated with inhaled rutile fibers.

➤ *Descriptors:* Lung parenchyma with preserved structure:

- dust (fibers)
- macrophages (dust particles)
- ferruginous bodies (iron-coated rutile bodies)

■ *Special stains:* Collagenous stains, Prussian blue, X-ray diffraction techniques or related physical methods.

Hallmark of Diagnosis: Clinical history, identification of the rutile fibers.

Differential diagnosis: Asbestos fibers, other nonasbestos mineral fibers.

Salicylates – Zygomycosis

Salicylates

Definition: Alteration of the lung parenchyma associated with intake of salicylates, see Drug Toxicity.

Salicylazosulfapyridine

Definition: Alteration of the lung parenchyma associated with intake of salicylazosulfapyridine, see Drug Toxicity.

Saline (Hypertonic)

Definition: Alteration of the lung parenchyma associated with intake of hypertonic saline, see Drug Toxicity.

Samustine

Definition: Alteration of the lung parenchyma associated with intake of samustine, see Drug Toxicity.

Sarcoid Granulomatosis, Necrotizing

Definition: Disorder of the lung characterized by noncaseating granulomatous inflammation, vasculitis, and foci of parenchymal necrosis.

Incidence/Epidemiology: Unusual disorder seen more frequently in females (sex ratio 3–5:10, men:women). Nearly all reported patients are over 20 years old (mean age 49 years). Associated risk factors are not known.

Etiology/Pathophysiology: The etiology of the disease is not known. Its association with sarcoidosis, Wegener's granulomatosis, and hypersensitivity reaction of the lung remains unclear.

Clinical Presentation: Most patients present with cough, fever, chest pain, and shortness of breath, while a few may be asymptomatic. The prognosis is excellent.

Prognosis: Usually good and without serious sequelae.

Radiology: Chest radiographs show multiple nodular densities in one or both lungs. The hilar lymph nodes are usually of normal size. Pleural effusions and cavitation occur.

Pathology:

Gross: The lungs show firm, grayish-white, well-defined nodules measuring a few centimeters in diameter.

Histology: The microscopic features are: (a) extensive, confluent, sarcoid-like, epithelioid granulomas comprising histiocytes, lymphocytes, plasma cells, multinucleated giant cells, usually surrounded by bundles of fibrous tissue; (b) irregularly shaped, fibrinous, necrotic areas which are located within the sarcoid granulomas; (c) vascular involvement seen in three distinct forms, compression of small arteries and veins by dense agglutinations of granulomas, granulomatous angiitis with multinucleated giant cells and histiocytes, and mononuclear angiitis including lymphocytes, plasma cells, and macrophages. The alterations of the lung parenchyma destroy the underlying texture, including small bronchi and vessels. The granulomatous process may destroy the pleura.

➤ *Descriptors:* Lung parenchyma with altered structure:

- caseous epithelioid granulomas
- mononuclear inflammatory infiltrates
- multinucleated giant cells
- necrosis (fibrinous)
- focal interstitial fibrosis;
- Pulmonary vessels with altered structure:
- caseous epithelioid granulomas
- multinucleated giant cells
- mononuclear inflammatory infiltrates;
- Pleura with altered structure:
- caseous epithelioid granulomas
- mononuclear inflammatory infiltrates
- multinucleated giant cells
- fibrinoid material

■ *Special stains:* PAS, collagenous stains, Giemsa, Ziehl-Neelsen, GMS, immunohistochemistry for immunoglobulins and lymphocytic subpopulations, endogenous lectins.

Hallmark of Diagnosis: Clinical history, sarcoid granulomas, fibrinous necrosis, vasculitis, and exclusion of infectious diseases.

Differential diagnosis: Infectious granulomatous diseases, abscess, necrotizing lung cancer, Wegener's granulomatosis, hypersensitivity pneumonitis, rheumatoid nodules, sarcoidosis, bronchocentric granulomatosis.

Sarcoidosis

Definition: Multisystem disorder with characteristic histomorphological appearance involving the lung in almost all cases.

Incidence/Epidemiology: The disease most frequently affects young adults. However, it may be seen at any age. Young black women are predominantly affected in the USA, whereas in Europe it is most frequently seen in the Northern countries (north of the Alps). The estimated incidence is approximately 40/100 000 per year. It is more frequently seen in persons from rural areas than in those living in large cities.

Etiology/Pathophysiology: The etiology of the disorder is not known despite an enormous amount of research. Two theories are under discussion: (a) sarcoidosis is a specific disease caused by one or several agents, probably of exogenous environmental origin; (b) sarcoidosis is a syndrome representing an abnormal immunologic response to a broad variety of (inhaled?) agents. The formation of granulomas is now understood to result from activation of the cell-mediated immune system, especially associated with the presence of activated T lymphocytes and activated mononuclear phagocytes. Monocytes, tissue macrophages, inflammatory macrophages, and epithelioid cells belong to the mononuclear phagocyte system and are attracted by various chemotactic influences. They secrete angiotensin-converting enzyme (ACE) which is found in the serum and the broncholavage fluid in patients with active sarcoidosis. T lymphocytes require interactions with macrophages in order to express certain immunologic responses. The formation of epithelioid granulomas is caused by agglutinations of mature macrophages which undergo transformation into epithelioid cells and may fuse to giant cells. The giant cells are originally of the foreign-body type and undergo reorganization into Langhans-type cells. Depending on the turnover time of the macrophages granulomas of either a "high turnover type" or a "low turnover type" can be distinguished. Sarcoid granulomas are those of a "high turnover type". The formation of granulomas starts with an agglutination of T lymphocytes (ratio T-helper:T-suppressor cells 10:1; normal 1.8:1) which are activated and release various mediators such as lymphokines, mononuclear chemotactic factor, migration inhibition factor, macrophage-activation factor, leucocytic inhibitory factor, and interleukin 2. The corresponding histomorphologic feature is a focal mononuclear interstitial pneumonitis comprising small foci of inflammatory interstitial infiltrates. Later stages yield well-developed granulomas and fibrotic changes characteristically induced in the outer layer of the granulomatous formations. "High turnover granulomas" may change into "low turnover granulomas" if the inciting agent is degraded or destroyed, and subsequently the granulomas may resolve and disappear. Depending upon the amount of type 1 collagen present within the granulomas, scars of various size may remain. Central necrosis of the granulomas is not a characteristic finding in sarcoidosis. It may, however, be noted in about 10–30% of the granulomas. The necrotic areas are of fibrinous, granular, or coagulative appearance. Presence of necrosis is probably related to the size of the formed granulomas and to the rapidity of their development.

Clinical Presentation: Patients may be asymptomatic or may present with chest pain, shortness of breath, cough, or, less commonly, hemoptysis, high fever, and arthralgias. Extrathoracic manifestations are an indicator of a relatively poor prognosis and include peripheral lymph nodes (60%), eyes (30%), liver (30%), skin (25%); spleen (25%), salivary glands (10%), bone (10%), heart (5%), kidneys (5%). The hilar lymph nodes are nearly always involved in sarcoidosis, i.e., a mediastinoscopy should be performed if the transbronchial biopsies are negative for sarcoidosis.

Prognosis: Usually good and without serious sequelae; most patients have spontaneous remissions with little or no evidence of residual disease. However, the percentage of fatal cases is 5–10%. Involvement of several organs usually indicates a poor prognosis.

Radiology: Chest radiographs are used for staging as follows: stage 0, normal appearance of the lung; stage 1, mediastinal lymphadenopathy only; stage 2, mediastinal lymphadenopathy and lung infiltrates; stage 3, lung infiltrates only; stage 4, chronic fibrotic lung disease (honeycombing). Pulmonary infiltrates may be reticular, reticulonodular, alveolar, circumscribed nodules, of ground-glass appearance, or resemble honeycombing.

Pathology:

Gross: The lungs have increased in consistency and present with multiple, firm, grayish-white nodules of various sizes. The hilar lymph nodes are enlarged and firm. Late stages evidence honeycombing.

Histology: The histomorphologic findings depend upon the stage of the disease: Early lesions exhibit focal interstitial agglutinations of lymphocytes (90%) with some additional plasma cells and macrophages. The cells of the alveolar lining are unsuspicious and usually do not show any reactive hyperplasia or hypertrophy. Intraalveolar exudation or agglutinations of macrophages are absent. The lesions have a maximum diameter of 100–300 μm and are distributed randomly within the distant airways. They are usually seen in combination with "adult" granulomas which comprise small, round lesions and larger, confluent, centrally noncaseous lesions with various amounts of surrounding connective tissue. They are made up of macrophages, epithelioid cells, multinucleated giant cells, lymphocytes, and plasma cells. They are usually located in association with bronchioles and small bronchi or small vessels, i.e., the BALT. The giant cells may contain three different types of inclusion bodies: (a) Schaumann's or conchoidal bodies which are concentrically lamellar mucopolysaccharides intermingled with calcium salts and iron deposits and which may have a crystalline component; (b) asteroid bodies which are "starlike" structures composed of microfilaments, microtubules, and centrioles; (c) Hamazaki-Wesenberg bodies which are spindle-shaped, brown, pleomorphic deposits seen intracellularly and extracellularly and which are actually giant lysosomes with light-microscopic characteristics of lipofuscin. In almost all cases the granulomas are seen within the hilar lymph nodes, and, in addition, frequently within the walls of major bronchi, small and large arteries and veins, and lobar septula and pleura visceralis. The granulomas may undergo fibrosis and may only be present in the form of large, onion-shaped fibrotic areas still containing some macrophages and giant cells. Depending upon the amount of scarring granulomas, the end stage of the scars may be a honeycomb lung with bullous emphysema and complete destruction of the original texture of the lung parenchyma.

➤ *Descriptors:* Lung parenchyma with altered structure:

- noncaseous epithelioid granulomas (confluent)
- mononuclear inflammatory infiltrates
- multinucleated giant cells
- focal interstitial fibrosis
- proliferating fibroblasts
- honeycombing;
- Lung parenchyma with preserved structure:
- mononuclear inflammatory infiltrates (focal)
- unsuspicious pneumocytes;
- Bronchial mucosa with altered structure:
- noncaseous epithelioid granulomas
- multinucleated giant cells
- mononuclear inflammatory infiltrates;
- Pleura with altered structure:
- noncaseous epithelioid granulomas
- mononuclear inflammatory infiltrates
- multinucleated giant cells

■ *Special stains:* PAS, collagenous stains, Giemsa, Ziehl-Neelsen, endogenous lectins, morphometry, syntactic structure analysis.

Hallmark of Diagnosis: Clinical history, noncaseating epithelioid granulomas, sarcoid pneumonitis.

Differential diagnosis: Tuberculosis, berylliosis, fungal infections, allergic extrinsic alveolitis, necrotizing sarcoid granulomatosis.

Sarcoma

Definition: Primary malignancy of the lung arising from mesenchymal tissue.

Incidence/Epidemiology: Uncommon malignancies which comprise about 1% of all malignant lung tumors. They occur in both sexes with similar frequency and at any age. Associated risk factors are not known.

Etiology/Pathophysiology: Sarcomas arise from mesenchymal tissue of the structures within the lung and may be classified according to their differentiation into: sarcomas of the larger vessels (pulmonary artery), chondrosarcoma, osteosarcoma, rhabdomyosarcoma, hemangiopericytoma, Kaposi's sarcoma, fibrosarcoma, malignant fibrous histiocytoma, neurogenic sarcoma, angiosarcoma, liposarcoma. In addition, carcinosarcoma (usually epidermoid/adenocarcinoma combined with fibrosarcoma) has been described.

Clinical Presentation: Patients may be asymptomatic or may present with chest pain, hemoptysis, shortness of breath, dyspnea, and loss of weight.

Prognosis: Usually poor; patients have a similar prognosis to those with bronchial carcinomas.

Radiology: Chest radiographs show either a single, circumscribed (usually very large), peripheral mass or centrally localized tumors.

Pathology:

Gross: Sarcomas are usually of larger size than their epithelial counterparts at the time of excision and may reach 10–15 cm in maximum diameter. They are soft in consistency and tan to white, usually with areas of hemorrhagic necrosis.

Histology: The histomorphologic features are described under the particular headings. In general, the malignancies show bundles of plump proliferating tumor cells with scattered areas of hemorrhage and infarctlike necrosis. Inflammatory response of host tissue is rare and weak. The original lung texture is completely destroyed.

➤ *Descriptors:* Newly formed textures with metastasis potential:

- mesenchymal growth pattern
- sarcomatous textures
- plump spindle cells
- inhomogeneous nuclear and cellular size
- necrosis and hemorrhage
- absent or weak inflammatory infiltrates

■ *Special stains:* PAS, collagenous stains, Giemsa, immunohistochemistry according to the specific appearance, DNA analysis, endogenous lectins.

Hallmark of Diagnosis: Size of the tumors, presence of necrosis, mitotic figures, specific microscopic growth pattern, DNA analysis, immunohistochemistry.

Differential diagnosis: Benign counterparts of the tumors, subclassification of sarcomas, intrapulmonary metastases.

Sauna Taker's Lung

Definition: Alteration of the lung parenchyma observed in sauna takers.

Incidence/Epidemiology: Uncommon disorder seen in adult persons regularly taking sauna.

Etiology/Pathophysiology: Extrinsic hypersensitivity reaction of the lung parenchyma due to contaminated sauna water. The underlying antigen is not known.

Clinical Presentation: Acute or chronic onset of cough, shortness of breath, dyspnea, or fever may occur. For details, see Allergic (Extrinsic) Alveolitis.

Prognosis: Usually good and without serious sequelae.

Radiology: Chest radiographs show diffuse, usually mild densities.

Pathology:

Gross: No specific findings have been reported.

Histology: The histomorphologic findings are in agreement with those described under the heading Allergic (Extrinsic) Alveolitis.

➤ *Descriptors:* Lung parenchyma with altered structure:

- noncaseous epithelioid granulomas
- eosinophils
- multinucleated giant cells
- intrabronchiolar fibrinoid material and histiocytes
- ulceration of bronchiolar mucosa;
- Lung parenchyma with preserved structure:
- macrophages
- desquamation, hypertrophy, hyperplasia and dysplasia of pneumocytes
- mononuclear inflammatory infiltrates
- intraalveolar serous fluid

■ *Special stains:* PAS, collagenous stains, Giemsa, immunohistochemistry for immunoglobulins, lymphocytic subpopulations, HLA-DR.

Hallmark of Diagnosis: Clinical history, findings of allergic extrinsic alveolitis.

Differential diagnosis: Sarcoidosis, beryl-liosis, allergic extrinsic alveolitis due to other agents.

Scar

Definition: Circumscribed lesion of inert collagenous tissue within the lung parenchyma.

Incidence/Epidemiology: Frequent finding in adult persons. Any inflammatory lesion may result in a scar.

Etiology/Pathophysiology: Scars are the result of fibrotic changes of inflammatory lesions independent of their underlying cause. They are usually located in the peripheral lung parenchyma with connection to the pleura. Scars of the apical lung zones are usually associated with bullous emphysema and are considered to be the sequel of atypical pneumonia.

Clinical Presentation: Patients are usually asymptomatic.

Prognosis: Usually good and without serious sequelae; however, peripherally localized bronchial carcinomas are often found in the lung parenchyma adjacent to the scars.

Radiology: Chest radiographs are normal or may show findings associated with bullous emphysema.

Pathology:

Gross: Usually small (a few millimeters in maximum diameter) lesions firm in consistency and grayish-white or black.

Histology: Agglutinations of collagen fibers intermingled with scattered lymphocytes and plasma cells. The surrounding lung parenchyma may be emphysematously altered.

➤ *Descriptors:* Lung parenchyma with altered structure:

- mononuclear inflammatory infiltrates
- focal interstitial fibrosis
- enlarged distant air spaces

■ *Special stains:* Collagenous stains.

Hallmark of Diagnosis: Agglutination of collagen fibers.

Differential diagnosis: Fibroma, histiocytoma.

Schaumann's Bodies

Definition: Intracytoplasmic inclusion bodies, seen in macrophages and multinucleated giant cells, see Sarcoidosis, Berylliosis.

Schistosomiasis

Definition: Infection of the lung by the genus *Schistosoma.*

Incidence/Epidemiology: There is evidence that about 10% of the world's population has been infected with *Schistosoma* parasites. The parasites are endemic in Africa (Egypt, southern countries), South America (Brazil), and in Asia (China, Japan, Philippines). Persons living in rural areas of the endemic countries are at specific risk.

Etiology/Pathophysiology: The three species of schistosoma called *S. haematobium, mansoni*, and *japonicum* are highly infective in man. Additional infective species are *S. intercalatum, mattheei, bovis,* and *spindale*. *Schistosoma* organisms are flukes which live in the blood vessels of man. They live in separate sexual forms, have nonoperculated eggs, and develop without an encysted metacercarial stage. They measure 5–20 mm in length and 0.2–1 mm in width. Man is the definite host of the schistosoma species mentioned above. The adult worms live in the portal and pelvic veins and pass their eggs in feces or urine outside the body where the eggs develop into larvae. The larvae penetrate into various species of fresh water snails where they develop into cercariae (last larval stage) which are able to swim by use of their forked tail. The cercariae return to fresh water and infect man by penetrating through the skin. The parasites drop off their tails and are carried into the lung via the blood stream. They finally settle down in the hepatic, portal, or pelvic veins and form pairs of male and female worms.

Clinical Presentation: The majority of patients remain asymptomatic due to the adaptation of the parasites to man. Late findings include arthritis and especially pulmonary hypertension and cor pulmonale. Acute schistosomiasis causes fever, cough, asthma, and dysentery. The parasites are usually diagnosed by identification of their eggs in feces or urine.

Prognosis: Usually good for patients with infections of *S. mansoni* and *haematobium*, poor for those with infection of *S. japonicum.*

Radiology: Chest radiographs are usually normal or may show findings related to cor pulmonale.

Pathology:

Gross: The lungs are of normal appearance. The most characteristic finding in the cardiopulmonary system is the cor pulmonale.

Histology: The pulmonary arterioles contain eggs measuring 50–100 μm in maximum diameter. They are usually associated with granulomatous endarteritis comprising epithelioid cells, lymphocytes, plasma cells and multinucleated giant cells. The texture of the lung parenchyma remains intact. The histomorphologic findings within the lung are usually not of diagnostic importance due to the more severe involvement of other organs such as the liver, intestines, and urogenital system.

➤ *Descriptors:* Lung parenchyma with altered structure:
- parasites (eggs, in pulmonary arterioles)
- noncaseous epithelioid granulomas
- multinucleated giant cells
- eosinophils;
- Pulmonary vessels with altered structure:
- parasites (eggs, in pulmonary arterioles)
- noncaseous epithelioid granulomas
- multinucleated giant cells
- mononuclear inflammatory infiltrates
- eosinophils

■ *Special stains:* PAS, Giemsa, Ziehl-Neelsen (the eggs stain positively), Movat.

Hallmark of Diagnosis: Clinical history, pulmonary hypertension, identification of eggs in the lung parenchyma.

Differential diagnosis: Infection of the lung by other parasites, pulmonary hypertension due to other agents.

Schwannoma

Definition: Usually benign neoplasm of neuronal origin (Schwann's cells, neurinoma), see Neurogenic Neoplasms.

Scimitar Syndrome

Definition: Abnormal right pulmonary venous drainage into the inferior vena cava combined with dextroposition of the heart and hypoplasia and systemic arterial supply of the right lung.

Incidence/Epidemiology: Rare disorder which has been reported to be of familial occurrence and autosomal dominant inheritance pattern.

Etiology/Pathophysiology: Abnormal venous drainage does not incapacitate patients unless it exceeds 50% of total drainage. The right lung may be more susceptible to recurrent infections due to its hypoplasia and possibly disturbed ventilation.

Clinical Presentation: Symptoms include dyspnea and recurrent infections of the lower respiratory tract.

Prognosis: Usually good, if the abnormal venous drainage does not exceed 50% of the total drainage of one lung.

Radiology: Chest radiographs show an enlarged left pulmonary artery and a bandlike shadow of the abnormal vein parallel to the right boundary of the heart. The shadow reaches from the hilus to the heart-diaphragm angle and in its configuration resembles a curved Turkish saber called a scimitar.

Pathology:

Gross: The right lung may exhibit hypoplasia or absence of the main upper lobe bronchus. The abnormal vein usually enters the vena cava inferior close to the diaphragm.

Histology: The structure of the lung parenchyma and of the wall of the abnormal veins (and possibly arteries) is normal.

➤ *Descriptors:* Pulmonary vessels with preserved structure:
- additional veins (normal)

■ *Special stains:* None.

Hallmark of Diagnosis: Radiologic and macroscopic findings.

Differential diagnosis: Intralobular sequestration, horseshoe lung.

Scleroderma

Definition: Alteration of the lung parenchyma associated with scleroderma (progressive systemic sclerosis).

Incidence/Epidemiology: Involvement of the lung parenchyma in scleroderma is frequent and has been reported to reach a rate of 100 % in various autopsy series. Patients with scleroderma have an increased (approximately 15-fold) risk of developing lung carcinoma, especially adenocarcinoma. Lung carcinomas have been reported in about 15% of patients with scleroderma.

Etiology/Pathophysiology: Scleroderma, a connective tissue disease with still unsettled etiology (autoimmune disorder? metabolic disease? disturbance of neurovascular regulation?) induces two different alterations in the peripheral lung parenchyma: (a) chronic interstitial pneumonitis, and (b) primary chronic vasculitis.

Neither type of involvement is related to the other. The vasculitis may induce severe pulmonary hypertension. The chronic interstitial pneumonitis is of progressive nature and causes severe diffuse interstitial fibrosis.

Clinical Presentation: The onset of the lung involvement is usually insidious. Symptoms include cough, progressive dyspnea over a period of years, cyanosis, pulmonary hypertension, and death due to respiratory failure. Patients presenting with CREST (calcinosis, Raynaud's phenomenon, esophageal involvement, sclerodactyly, telangiectasia) usually present with a less intensive involvement of the lung.

Prognosis: Fair, about 80% of patients are still alive 2 years after clinical manifestation of the disease and 10% of patients survive for 10 years or longer. Older men have the worst prognosis.

Radiology: Chest radiographs show diffuse, interstitial, reticulonodular densities which are most predominant in the lower lobes. Findings related to cor pulmonale may be present. Pleural thickening and fibrosis including pleural adhesions are common.

Pathology:

Gross: The lungs are stiff and tan colored. Honeycombing may be present, as well as pleural fibrosis and pleural adhesions.

Histology: The histomorphologic findings are those of the usual interstitial pneumonia (UIP) with various degrees of interstitial fibrosis, usually already honeycombed to a moderate degree. The basement membranes along the distant airways are thickened and may contain hyaline material which is also found in the intima of involved vessels. Angiitis manifests itself by thickening of the media and a marked proliferation of the intima, which may occlude the lumen of the vessel. Plexiform lesions and fibrinoid necrosis are not characteristic findings in sclerodermal lung. Additional changes of the lung parenchyma include bronchiolitis obliterans and bronchiolectasis.

➤ *Descriptors:* Lung parenchyma with preserved structure:
- intraalveolar fibrinoid material
- macrophages
- mononuclear inflammatory infiltrates
- hyaline membranes;
- Lung parenchyma with altered structure:
- intrabronchiolar fibrinoid material and histiocytes
- ulceration of bronchiolar mucosa
- enlarged distant air spaces
- mononuclear inflammatory infiltrates
- proliferating fibroblasts
- diffuse interstitial fibrosis
- honeycombing;
- Pulmonary vessels with altered structure:
- hyaline material (arterial intima)
- mononuclear inflammatory infiltrates
- proliferating smooth muscle cells

■ *Special stains:* PAS, collagenous stains, Giemsa, immunohistochemistry for immunoglobulins and lymphocytic subpopulations, endogenous lectins.

Hallmark of Diagnosis: Clinical history, histomorphologic findings of usual interstitial pneumonia, hyalinosis of small and medium-sized arteries, and mononuclear vasculitis.

Differential diagnosis: Usual interstitial pneumonia, vasculitis, bronchiolitis obliterans associated with other agents.

Sclerosing Hemangioma

Definition: Benign neoplasm of the lung of various histomorphology, see Hemangioma, Sclerosing.

Semustine

Definition: Alteration of the lung parenchyma associated with intake of semustine, see Drug Toxicity.

Sequestration

Definition: A mass of pulmonary parenchyma not connected to the tracheobronchial tree. Intralobar sequestration defines lung parenchyma within the right or left lung as invested with visceral pleura; extralobar sequestration defines lung parenchyma lying outside the visceral pleura of the normal lung parenchyma.

Incidence/Epidemiology: Extralobar sequestration is a rare disorder seen most frequently in infants aged 1–6 months. Intralobar sequestration is also a rare disorder seen most frequently in children aged 1–10 years. It can be detected at any age. However, it is rarely seen in infants.

Extralobar sequestration is predominant in males (sex ratio 3:1, males:females), and intralobar sequestration is slightly predominant in females (sex ratio 1:1.1; males:females). Associated anomalies are frequent in patients with extralobar sequestration and include diaphragmatic hernia, pulmonary hypoplasia, bronchogenic cysts, and cardiovascular malformations.

Etiology/Pathophysiology: In extralobar sequestration the ectopic lung parenchyma is usually located within the thoracic cavity, most frequently between the lower lobe and the diaphragm. The arterial supply and venous drainage are provided by the systemic vessels in 80–95% of cases with extralobar sequestration, as opposed to patients with intralobar sequestration, where the venous drainage is usually provided by the pulmonary veins. Chronic inflammation and infections are not infrequently observed in both extralobar and intralobar sequestrated lung masses. The extralobar sequestration is believed to be induced by an outpouching of the foregut which becomes separated from its source during the later development of the lung. Intralobar sequestration has two origins (a) acquired such as bronchial occlusion due to inflammation, aspiration, or as result of recurrent pneumonia and (b) a congenital malformation.

Clinical Presentation: Patients with extralobar sequestration present with cyanosis, dyspnea, and difficulties in feeding, and those with intralobar sequestration chronic cough, mild fever, and recurrent pulmonary infections.

Prognosis: Usually good; however, additional congenital defects or recurrent infections may cause serious problems.

Radiology: Chest radiographs show variable findings in both disorders, which may range from normal lung to cystic areas or small linear densities.

Pathology:

Gross: The lung shows a thickened pleura. The lung parenchyma is firm in consistency and may contain cystic areas in intralobar sequestration.

Histology: The lung parenchyma is of normal texture in both disorders. Cases with intralobar sequestration, however, are usually altered by chronic inflammatory processes and may display cystic areas, fibrosis, and honeycombing. Extralobar sequestrated lesions may also be altered by superimposed inflammatory processes. They usually show uniformly dilated bronchioles, alveolar ducts and alveoli separated by thick alveolar septa of immature appearance.

➤ *Descriptors:* Lung parenchyma with preserved structure:
- viscous mucus
- desquamation, hypertrophy, hyperplasia and dysplasia of pneumocytes;
- Lung parenchyma with altered structure:
- cysts (multilocular)
- mononuclear inflammatory infiltrates
- proliferating fibroblasts
- focal interstitial fibrosis
- honeycombing;
- Bronchial mucosa with preserved structure:
- ectatic lumen;
- Bronchial mucosa with altered structure:
- squamous metaplasia and dysplasia

■ *Special stains:* PAS, collagenous stains, Giemsa.

Hallmark of Diagnosis: Macroscopic findings, secondary chronic-destructive inflammation.

Differential diagnosis: Infantile lobar emphysema, congenital pulmonary lymphangiectasis, adenomatoid cystic malformation of a lobe.

Sequoiosis

Definition: Alteration of the lung parenchyma associated with inhalation of fungi of the genera *Graphium* or *Pullularia*.

Incidence/Epidemiology: Rare disorder seen in lumbermen in sequoia forests.

Etiology/Pathophysiology: Allergic extrinsic alveolitis due to inhalation of moldy wood dust contaminated with fungus.

Clinical Presentation: An acute or a chronic form may occur.

Prognosis: Usually good and without serious sequelae.

Radiology: Chest radiographs are normal or show diffuse, soft, interstitial infiltrates or fine granular densities.

Pathology:

Gross: The lungs are normal in color and consistency, or may display small, firm, reddish-gray nodules.

Histology: The characteristic findings include nonnecrotizing epithelioid granulomas near the terminal bronchioles, desquamation, hypertrophy and hyperplasia of cells of the alveolar lining, marked eosinophilic inflammatory infiltrates, bronchiolitis obliterans, and focal acute vasculitis. For details, see Allergic (Extrinsic) Alveolitis.

➤ *Descriptors:* Lung parenchyma with altered structure:
- noncaseous epithelioid granulomas
- eosinophils
- multinucleated giant cells
- intrabronchiolar fibrinoid material and histiocytes
- ulceration of bronchiolar mucosa;
- Lung parenchyma with preserved structure:
- macrophages
- desquamation, hypertrophy, hyperplasia and dysplasia of pneumocytes
- mononuclear inflammatory infiltrates
- intraalveolar serous fluid

■ *Special stains:* PAS, collagenous stains, Giemsa. For details, see Allergic (Extrinsic) Alveolitis.

Hallmark of Diagnosis: Clinical history, nonnecrotizing epithelioid granulomas, morphologic findings related to desquamative interstitial pneumonia, lymphocytic interstitial pneumonia, bronchiolitis obliterans.

Differential diagnosis: Infectious and noninfectious granulomatous diseases such as sarcoidosis, fungal infections, or berylliosis. For details, see Allergic (Extrinsic) Alveolitis.

Sericite Fibers

Definition: Alteration of the lung parenchyma associated with inhalation of sericite fibers.

Incidence/Epidemiology: A few cases of sericite fibers in the peripheral lung parenchyma have been reported.

Etiology/Pathophysiology: Sericite fibers do not induce fibrosis or other lung disorders such as carcinoma.

Clinical Presentation: Patients are asymptomatic.

Prognosis: Usually good and without serious sequelae.

Radiology: Chest radiographs are normal.

Pathology:

Gross: No specific findings have been reported.

Histology: The fibers are located in the bronchioles and alveolar ducts. The lung parenchyma is of normal appearance.

➤ *Descriptors:* Lung parenchyma with preserved structure:
- dust (birefringent fibers)

■ *Special stains:* Scanning electron microscopy, X-ray diffraction techniques, or related physical methods.

Hallmark of Diagnosis: Normal lung parenchyma. Identification of sericite fibers.

Differential diagnosis: Other asbestos and nonasbestos mineral fibers.

Sericulturist's Lung

Definition: Allergic extrinsic alveolitis related to silk larvae.

Incidence/Epidemiology: Infrequently seen in sericulturists or persons involved in silk production. Ripe silk larvae excrete urine and feces which may induce allergic pulmonary reaction.

Etiology/Pathophysiology: Usually immune complex formation (type III immune reaction of the lung) in combination with cell-mediated hypersensitivity (type IV).

Clinical Presentation: Acute and chronic courses have been described. Patients present with dyspnea, cough, slight fever, and sputum production several hours after exposure to silk larvae or silk cocoons.

Prognosis: Usually good and without serious sequelae.

Radiology: Diffuse, soft infiltrates or fine micronodular densities.

Pathology:

Gross: Firm, rubbery, reddish-gray lungs in chronic cases, while acute cases may still show normal lungs.

Histology: Prominent, patchy interstitial infiltrate with close relation to the terminal bronchioles. It is composed of histiocytes, lymphocytes, plasma cells, and occasional multinucleated giant cells and eosinophilic granulocytes. Noncaseating granulomatous formation and bronchiolitis obliterans occur.

➤ *Descriptors:* Lung parenchyma with altered structure:
- noncaseous epithelioid granulomas

- eosinophils
- multinucleated giant cells
- intrabronchiolar fibrinoid material and histiocytes
- ulceration of bronchiolar mucosa;
- Lung parenchyma with preserved structure:
- macrophages
- desquamation, hypertrophy, hyperplasia and dysplasia of pneumocytes
- mononuclear inflammatory infiltrates
- intraalveolar serous fluid

■ *Special stains:* PAS, collagenous stains, endogenous lectins.

Hallmark of Diagnosis: Noncaseating granulomas with moderate dysplasia of pneumocytes, focal bronchiolitis obliterans, clinical history, findings of chest radiographs.

Differential diagnosis: Sarcoidosis, tuberculosis, fungal infections, berylliosis.

Serrapeptase

Definition: Alteration of the lung parenchyma associated with intake of serrapeptase, see Drug Toxicity.

Serratia

Definition: Infection of the lung by *Serratia marcescens.*

Incidence/Epidemiology: The gram negative bacterium *S. marcescens* has been used in aerosol experiments and was assumed to be a nonpathogenic bacterium. Endemic outbreaks of *Serratia* pneumonia have been reported from various hospitals.

Etiology/Pathophysiology: *Serratia* is usually transmitted by contaminated aerosol fluids or by direct contact with contaminated persons. It has been demonstrated in wound infections, sputum of patients with bacterial pneumonia, cerebral fluid of patients with meningitis, and septic arthritis.

Clinical Presentation: Symptoms are those of acute necrotizing bronchopneumonia.

Prognosis: Fair, the prognosis varies with the age and associated circumstances such as alcoholism, malnutrition, or immunodeficiency.

Radiology: Chest radiographs show the findings of bronchopneumonia.

Pathology:

Gross: The lungs are edematous and rubbery in consistency and may show small and somewhat larger necrotic areas.

Histology: The histomorphologic findings include exudation of proteinaceous fluid, neutrophilic leucocytes, lymphocytes, plasma cells, erythrocytes, and macrophages within the distant airways, necrosis and microabscess formation in the lung parenchyma, and organizing bronchopneumonia which may be associated with bronchiolitis obliterans in later stages.

➤ *Descriptors:* Lung parenchyma with altered structure:

- necrosis and hemorrhage
- mixed inflammatory infiltrates
- intrabronchiolar fibrinoid material and histiocytes
- ulceration of bronchiolar mucosa
- focal interstitial fibrosis

■ *Special stains:* PAS, collagenous stains, Giemsa, Gram's, Wharthin-Starry stain, immunofluorescence.

Hallmark of Diagnosis: Necrotizing bronchopneumonia, identification of the bacteria.

Differential diagnosis: Bronchopneumonia caused by other organisms.

Sezary Syndrome

Definition: Pruritic skin infiltrations seen in leukemic diseases, see Mycosis Fungoides.

Shaver's Lung

Definition: Alteration of the lung parenchyma associated with inhalation of bauxite, see Bauxite Lung.

Shock lung

Definition: Alteration of the lung parenchyma associated with serious extrapulmonary trauma, shock, or sepsis.

Incidence/Epidemiology: Most of the cases have been reported in war casualities. It can be seen in victims of traffic accidents or in patients with hemorrhagic, septic, neurogenic, and cardiogenic disorders.

Etiology/Pathophysiology: A number of factors are involved in the development of shock lung. Vasoactive peptides released by necrotic tissue may induce alteration of vascular permeability in the lung and favor microthromboembolism in the capillaries followed by metabolic acidosis and local hypotension. Alteration of oncotic pressure or iatrogenic factors such as overhydration or oxygen therapy can also be involved.

Clinical Presentation: Symptoms are related to respiratory failure and include progressive dyspnea, cyanosis, and severe hypoxemia with high mortality.

Prognosis: Poor, as death will occur in about 40–60% of patients.

Radiology: Chest radiographs show findings related to acute edema on the first day. Later stages reveal diffuse, patchy densities or ground-glass appearance of the lung.

Pathology:

Gross: The lungs are heavy, wet, and pale-red.

Histology: The microscopic findings are related to diffuse alveolar damage (DAD) and show interstitial edema followed by formation of hyaline membranes, desquamation of cells of the alveolar lining, microthrombi in the capillaries, marked hyperplasia of cells of the alveolar lining, intraalveolar deposits of fibrin intermingled with macrophages and fibroblasts, intraalveolar hemorrhage, and interstitial fibroblast proliferation.

➤ *Descriptors:* Lung parenchyma with preserved structure:
- interstitial edema
- mixed inflammatory infiltrates
- desquamation, hypertrophy, hyperplasia and dysplasia of pneumocytes
- hyaline membranes
- hemorrhage;
- Pulmonary vessels with preserved structure:
- microthrombosis (intracapillary);
- Lung parenchyma with altered structure:
- mononuclear inflammatory infiltrates
- proliferating fibroblasts
- diffuse interstitial fibrosis
- honeycombing

■ *Special stains:* PAS, collagenous stains, Giemsa.

Hallmark of Diagnosis: Clinical history, histomorphologic findings of adult respiratory distress syndrome (diffuse alveolar damage), usual interstitial pneumonia, hyaline membranes, diffuse interstitial mononuclear inflammatory infiltrates.

Differential diagnosis: Usual interstitial pneumonia, diffuse alveolar damage due to other agents.

Siderosilicosis

Definition: Alteration of the lung parenchyma associated with inhalation of iron sesquioxide (hematite), see Hematite Miner's Lung.

Silicon Carbide

Definition: Alteration of the lung parenchyma associated with inhalation of silicon carbide, see Carborundum Pneumoconiosis.

Silicosis

Definition: Alteration of the lung parenchyma associated with inhalation of crystalline silica.

Incidence/Epidemiology: Crystalline silica is a constituent of quartz, coesite, cristobalite, tridymite, and stishovite. Persons working in mining (copper, coal, graphite, gold, etc.), sandblasting, potteries, ceramics manufacture, fire-brick manufacture, stone masonry, quarries, molding, and grinding may be exposed to silica and, therefore, develop silicosis. The prevalence of silicosis naturally depends upon the amount of inhaled silica, i.e., the technical standard of the factories and the protection of the workers. However, it may reach 20–30% of exposed persons in nonmetallic mineral manufacture even today. Persons working in the pottery industry, in steel foundries, and in certain mines such as tin or gold (Cornish tin miners, South African gold miners) are particularly at risk.

Etiology/Pathophysiology: Crystalline silica is fibrogenic. Exposed persons usually need 20–40 years of exposure in an occupation in order to develop a clinically relevant silicosis. The changes of the lung parenchyma can be classified into four forms:

(a) simple silicosis,

(b) complicated silicosis,

(c) acute silicosis,
(d) mixed-dust fibrosis.

Simple or nodular silicosis develops after 20–40 years of exposure. A minority of heavily exposed persons may develop nodular silicosis after heavier exposure of 5–15 years (accelerated form). In these forms fibrosis occurs only if the amount of quartz exceeds 15–20% of the total dust content in the lung. Most fibrogenic quartz particles measure 1–2 μm in length. Longer or shorter ones are considered to be less effective in their fibrogenic potency.

The theories of pathogenesis of fibrosis due to silica comprise:

(a) mechanical irritation including piezoelectric effects (this theory could not be satisfactorily confirmed),
(b) silica solubility (this theory could not be confirmed by experimental data; however, it led to experiments in which the fibrogenic potency of particles could be diminished either by coating their surface with ferric oxide or by adding metallic aluminum. Canadian gold miners are protected against silicosis by inhalation of metallic aluminum after exposure to quartz dust),
(c) a membrane effect, especially on macrophages (the toxic effect of silica is thought to be associated with hydrogen donation by polymeric silicic acid. The absorption of the hydrogens by polyvinylpyridine-*N*-oxide (PNO) is assumed to be the underlying cause of the protective potential of PNO against fibrosis. Crystals phagocytized by macrophages can be released again, and in addition, acid hydrolases such as cytoplasmic lactate hydrolase may reach the extracellular matrix),
(d) macrophage fibrogenic factor (MFF, which appears to be a relatively nonspecific stimulant for protein synthesis. It is located on a 20 000 *g* supernatant of rat peritoneal macrophages, and can augment collagen synthesis in granuloma slices),
(e) immunologic component (formation of silicotic nodules may be modified by immunologic components; however, these components probably play no part in the initiation of fibrogenesis).

Simple silicosis is characterized by "onion"-shaped fibrotic nodules of various sizes. Complicated silicosis comprises clusters of fused silicotic nodules, progressive massive fibrosis, bacterial superinfection (tuberculosis), association with rheumatoid disorders (Caplan's syndrome), or development of scleroderma. Acute silicosis is a form of alveolar proteinosis due to heavy exposure to silica, and mixed-dust silicosis occurs when a mixture of quartz particles and other dusts are inhaled simultaneously.

Clinical Presentation: Symptoms of silicosis have an insidious onset and include cough, shortness of breath during exercise, and progressive dyspnea.

Prognosis: Fair, as most patients show slow progressive respiratory failure.

Radiology: Chest radiographs show dense, circumscribed nodules without cavitation, larger confluent masses, or patchy infiltrates.

Pathology:

Gross: The lungs contain several firm nodules measuring a few millimeters to a few centimeters in maximum diameter. They are white, grayish or black depending on the amount of exposed coal dust.

Histology: The nodules are composed of concentric bands of collagen (onion-shaped) which are well-demarcated from the surrounding, usually normal lung parenchyma. Birefringent particles are clustered at the boundaries of the lesions and may also be observed in dust-laden macrophages within the adjacent distant airways. The central and hilar lymph nodes usually show similar alterations. Central necrosis with cholesterol clefts may occur in larger nodules. Formation of epithelioid cell granulomas or multinucleated giant cells are not a feature of simple silicosis and suggest superinfection with tuberculosis. Acute silicosis displays all the features of alveolar proteinosis, i.e., alveoli filled with granular eosinophilic material, missing or weak inflammatory response of the host tissue, preserved texture of the distant airways. Complicated silicosis has the features of simple silicosis in addition to the features of tuberculosis, rheumatoid disorder, scleroderma, or large fibrotic masses with still preserved shadows of the original silicotic nodules.

➤ *Descriptors:* Lung parenchyma with altered structure:

- dust (birefringent fibers)
- focal interstitial fibrosis (onion-shaped)
- enlarged distant air spaces;
- Lung parenchyma with preserved structure:
- intraalveolar serous fluid

- hyaline material;
- Lymphatic tissue with altered structure:
- dust (birefringent fibers)
- focal interstitial fibrosis

■ *Special stains:* PAS, collagenous stains, Giemsa, polarization, X-ray diffraction method or related physical techniques, scanning electron microscopy.

Hallmark of Diagnosis: Clinical history, silicotic nodules, alveolar proteinosis, massive fibrosis.

Differential diagnosis: Pneumoconiosis related to other agents, tuberculosis.

Sillimanite

Definition: Alteration of the lung parenchyma associated with inhalation of sillimanite fibers.

Incidence/Epidemiology: Sillimanite fibers have rarely been reported to be found in human lung parenchyma.

Etiology/Pathophysiology: Sillimanite fibers are considered to be nonfibrogenic and noncarcinogenic.

Clinical Presentation: No specific symptoms have been reported.

Prognosis: Usually good and without serious sequelae.

Radiology: Chest radiographs are usually normal.

Pathology:

Gross: Findings are normal or related to nonfibrous pneumoconiotic lesions.

Histology: The fibers can be found in the distant airways and partly ingested by macrophages. They are birefringent under polarized light.

➤ *Descriptors:* Lung parenchyma with preserved structure:

- dust (birefringent fibers)

■ *Special stains:* Collagenous stains, Prussian blue, scanning electron microscopy, X-ray diffraction or related physical techniques, polarization.

Hallmark of Diagnosis: Clinical history, identification of sillimanite fibers.

Differential diagnosis: Deposits of asbestos fibers and other nonasbestos fibers.

Silo Filler's Lung

Definition: Alteration of the lung parenchyma seen in silo fillers.

Incidence/Epidemiology: Unusual disorder seen in silo fillers or in persons exposed to nitrogen dioxide (NO_2) or nitrous dioxide (N_2O_4). The chemical agent is usually inhaled by persons exposed to chemical accidents (burns).

Etiology/Pathophysiology: Nitrogen dioxide causes acute damage of the lung parenchyma by formation of nitric acid. The chemical pneumonitis is characterized by diffuse alveolar damage with prominent hemorrhage.

Clinical Presentation: Symptoms include dyspnea, chest pain, cough, and hemoptysis.

Prognosis: Fair, as patients usually show slow progressive respiratory failure.

Radiology: Chest radiographs show diffuse interstitial densities.

Pathology:

Gross: The findings are related to diffuse alveolar damage (DAD).

Histology: The findings of diffuse alveolar damage include desquamation of cells of the alveolar lining, formation of hyaline membranes, intraalveolar hemorrhage, bronchiolitis obliterans, and generalized lymphocytic interstitial inflammation. Late stages may show organizing pneumonia, interstitial fibrosis, and honeycombing.

➤ *Descriptors:* Lung parenchyma with altered structure:

- noncaseous epithelioid granulomas
- eosinophilis
- multinucleated giant cells
- intrabronchiolar fibrinoid material and histiocytes
- ulceration of bronchiolar mucosa
- honeycombing;
- Lung parenchyma with preserved structure:
- macrophages
- desquamation, hypertrophy, hyperplasia and dysplasia of pneumocytes
- mononuclear inflammatory infiltrates
- intraalveolar serous fluid

■ *Special stains:* PAS, collagenous stains, endogenous lectins, immunohistochemistry for immunoglobulins and lymphocytic subpopulations.

Hallmark of Diagnosis: Clinical history, diffuse alveolar damage, usual interstitial pneumonia.

Differential diagnosis: Diffuse alveolar damage due to other agents, organizing bacterial pneumonia, lymphocytic interstitial pneumonia, usual interstitial pneumonia due to other agents.

Silver Polisher's Lung

Definition: Alteration of the lung parenchyma seen in silver polishers.

Incidence/Epidemiology: Unusual disorder seen in persons working in silverware factories, who are exposed to dust of abrasive material.

Etiology/Pathophysiology: The abrasive material is composed of a mixture of iron dioxide and silver particles. The inhalation of the abrasive dust is considered to be nonfibrogenic, although cases with severe interstitial lung fibrosis have been reported.

Clinical Presentation: Patients may be asymptomatic or may present with cough, dyspnea and progressive shortness of breath.

Prognosis: Usually good; however, some patients may show slow progressive respiratory failure.

Radiology: Chest radiographs may be normal or may show findings of massive fibrosis.

Pathology:

Gross: The lungs may be normal or may show various degrees of fibrosis, including honeycombing.

Histology: The mixture of inhaled dust is separated by physiologic defence mechanisms into deposits of iron dioxide and deposits of silver. The iron particles are usually found within the interstitial perivascular tissue. These deposits do not stain with Prussian blue. The silver deposits are found within the distant airways and within the alveolar walls. They have a black color with HE stains.

➤ *Descriptors:* Lung parenchyma with preserved structure:
- dust (birefringent fibers, silver particles, crystals, iron);
- Lung parenchyma with altered structure:
- focal interstitial fibrosis
- enlarged distant air spaces

■ *Special stains:* PAS, collagenous stains, Prussian blue, X-ray diffraction or related physical techniques, endogenous lectins.

Hallmark of Diagnosis: Clinical history, identification of iron dioxide and silver deposits.

Differential diagnosis: Other pneumoconioses, interstitial fibrosis due to other agents.

Sinusitis

Definition: Alteration of the lung parenchyma associated with sinusitis (bronchiectasis), see Cartagener's Syndrome.

Sjögren's Syndrome

Definition: Alteration of the lung parenchyma associated with Sjögren's syndrome.

Incidence/Epidemiology: The lung is involved in about 10–20% of patients with Sjögren's syndrome. Lung involvement is usually not related to specific findings; however, an increased percentage of pulmonary function abnormalities associated with biliary liver cirrhosis has been found. The majority of patients are middle-aged women, often with insufficiency of the ovaries.

Etiology/Pathophysiology: Sjögren's syndrome is a rheumatoid disorder involving the major salivary glands and other glandular structures and is often associated with rheumatoid arthritis.

Clinical Presentation: Patients complain about cough, dyspnea, recurrent pneumonia, chest pain, and pleural effusions. The time between the onset of Sjögren's disease and the onset of pulmonary symptoms ranges from several months to several years.

Prognosis: Usually fair, as slow progressive respiratory dysfunction is the common course.

Radiology: Chest radiographs may be normal or show diffuse interstitial infiltrates, diffuse alveolar densities, or findings related to pleural effusions.

Pathology:

Gross: The lungs may be normal or may show macroscopic findings related to the various histomorphologic findings.

Histology: The histomorphologic findings vary to a large extent and are related to involvement of the tracheobronchial glands and diminished pulmonary defence mechanisms. The findings comprise fibrosis of the bronchial submucosa associated with scarred glands, organizing pneumonia, bronchiolitis obliterans, amyloidosis, pseudolymphoma, granulomatous lesions, usual interstitial pneumonia, mononuclear vasculitis and interstitial fibrosis with focal honeycombing.

➤ *Descriptors:* Lung parenchyma with preserved structure:

- intraalveolar fibrinoid material
- macrophages
- mononuclear inflammatory infiltrates;
- Lung parenchyma with altered structure:
- intrabronchiolar fibrinoid material and histiocytes
- ulceration of bronchiolar mucosa
- diffuse interstitial fibrosis
- noncaseous epithelioid granulomas
- mononuclear inflammatory infiltrates
- interstitial hyaline material (amyloidosis)
- focal interstitial fibrosis (scarring)
- enlarged distant air spaces
- honeycombing;
- Pulmonary vessels with preserved structure:
- mononuclear inflammatory infiltrates;
- Bronchial mucosa with altered structure:
- destruction of submucosal glands
- fibrosis

■ *Special stains:* PAS, collagenous stains, Congo, endogenous lectins, immunohistochemistry for immunoglobulins and lymphocytic subpopulations.

Hallmark of Diagnosis: Clinical history, lymphocytic inflammation and atrophy of the tracheobronchial mucus glands.

Differential diagnosis: Due to the histomorphological changes, i.e., tracheobronchitis, bacterial pneumonia, usual interstitial pneumonia, or lymphocytic interstitial pneumonia.

Small Cell Carcinoma

Definition: Malignant tumor of the lung with characteristic histomorphological appearance and biological behavior.

Incidence/Epidemiology: The tumor type accounts for 20% of all malignant lung tumors. Its occurrence is related to the risk factors of other lung carcinoma cell types, especially to smoking and exposure to asbestos. The incidence is similar in men and women.

Etiology/Pathophysiology: Small cell carcinoma is thought to derive from the neuroendocrine system of the lung (APUD cells) or from the endodermally derived bronchial epithelium base. Small cell anaplastic carcinomas frequently express antigens to neuroendocrine markers such as bombesin (gastrin-releasing peptide), neuron-specific enolase, synaptophysin (in about 60% of cases), chromogranin (in about 30% of cases). They may produce hormones such as calcitonin or ACTH or may have receptors for estrogen or progesterone. They have an extremely high proliferation rate and a high capacity to metastasize into various organs, especially into the liver, bone marrow, brain, adrenal glands, and kidneys. They give a good response to cytostatic therapy (patients show a complete or partial remission in about 60–80% of cases) which lasts about 6 months. However, recurrence and drug resistance are the usual outcome after 4–8 months.

Clinical Presentation: Patients with small cell carcinoma have a poor prognosis and usually die within 6 months if not treated by cytostatic therapy and radiation. The majority of small cell carcinomas are located within the proximal bronchi, and symptoms include cough, malaise, dyspnea, and loss of weight or are related to metastases already developed.

Prognosis: Very poor, about 50% of patients die within 1 year after clinical manifestation, and only 10% survive for 2 years or longer.

Radiology: Chest radiographs show a central, large tumor mass with obstruction of the corresponding bronchi. Only 5–10% of all small cell carcinoma are located peripherally.

Pathology:

Gross: The tumors consist of a soft, yellowish-white mass with focal hemorrhagic necroses. Fibrosis may be present if the patient has been treated by cytostatic therapy. The tumors tend to grow beneath the mucosa presenting a mass with continuous involvement of the adjacent lymph nodes.

Histology: The tumors grow without texture in solid bundles. Pseudoglandular patterns may be present. Characteristic features are large areas of hemorrhagic necrosis without inflammatory infiltrations. Fibrosis may be present within such areas. The tumor cells themselves are of small size with scanty cytoplasm. The nuclei measure 4–6 µm in diameter (lymphocytes 3–5 µm) and have a fairly uniform appearance with finely dispersed chromatin and inconspicuous nucleoli. Mitotic figures are frequent. Inflammatory cells are rarely seen at the boundary of small cell carcinomas in contrast to epidermoid carcinomas. The tumor cell nuclei tend to show so-called molding which is a mosaic-like layer under light microscopic magnification. Three different cellular subtypes are distinguished by the classification of the WHO: (a) the oat-cell type with fusiform nuclei of lymphocytic cellular appearance, (b) the intermediate cell type with larger nuclei and more clearly defined cytoplasm, these tumor cells often resemble undifferentiated epidermoid carcinoma cells, (c) the combined cell type which is characterized by two or more histomorphologically different cell types comprising (a) small cell carcinoma and (b) non-small cell carcinoma such as adenocarcinoma, epidermoid carcinoma, or large cell anaplastic carcinoma. There is no difference in staining behavior within these three tumor subtypes in respect of immunohistochemistry or endogenous lectins. (It may be noted that there is evidence that small cell anaplastic carcinoma can change to epidermoid carcinoma and large cell anaplastic carcinoma and vice versa in tissue cultures and in vivo).

➤ *Descriptors:* Newly formed textures with metastasis potential:
- epithelial growth pattern
- solid textures
- small cells
- finely distributed nuclear chromatin
- inhomogeneous nuclear and cellular size
- frequent mitoses
- molding
- necrosis and hemorrhage
- absent or weak inflammatory infiltrations

■ *Special stains:* PAS (small cell anaplastic carcinoma cells are usually PAS-negative), immunohistochemistry (neuroendocrine markers, keratin, vimentin, lymphocytic markers, CEA, EMA, S-100 protein), endogenous lectins (small cell anaplastic carcinomas usually do not express sugar receptors at a glycohistochemically detectable level), DNA analysis.

Hallmark of Diagnosis: Small PAS-negative cells, molding, fine granular chromatin, large areas of necrosis, absent inflammatory cells.

Differential diagnosis: Poorly differentiated adenocarcinoma, epidermoid carcinoma, lymphoma, Ewing's sarcoma, blastoma, carcinoid.

Smoking

Definition: Alteration of the lung parenchyma associated with smoking.

Incidence/Epidemiology: Approximately 15–30% of all adult persons are moderate to heavy smokers. The incidence of smokers is decreasing slightly, especially in men, and increasing slightly in women. Smoking is somewhat related to social status and difficult to treat. It induces increased risk of lung cancer, obstructive bronchitis in large and small bronchi, and emphysema. Mesotheliomas are not associated with smoking.

Etiology/Pathophysiology: Cigarette smoke contains a mixture of chemical components which are alkylated polynuclear aromatic hydrocarbons (PAH, carcinogenic), methyl alcohol, phenol, hydrocyanic acid, anthracenes, pyrenes, arsenic, lead, cadmium, radioactive plutonium, benzanthracenes, benzofluoranthracenes, dibenzopyrenes, chrysenes, nicotine, and carbon monoxide. The inhaled agents reach the distant airways in the form of gases, droplets, and small particles. The particles usually remain close to the bronchioles. All inhaled agents are ingested by macrophages. Cigarette smoke is usually not fibrogenic, although fibrotic changes in relation to dust deposits may occur in heavy smokers.

Clinical Presentation: Heavy smoking induces chronic bronchitis and related symptoms (chronic obstructive lung disease). Sleep apnea syndrome in overweight persons or histiocytosis X are usually associated with heavy smoking.

Prognosis: Heavy smokers have a decreased life expectancy which is about 5–15 years less than that of a nonsmoking population.

Radiology: Chest radiographs usually show normal lungs or morphologic changes associated with emphysema.

Pathology:

Gross: The lungs are red-brown with randomly distributed, small (a few millimeters in maximum diameter), black densities. The bronchial mucosa is thickened, and emphysematous cysts are present with surrounding fibrosis.

Radiology: Agglutinations of dust particles can be seen near and within the bronchioles and in the BALT. The dust-laden macrophages are clustered in the alveoli. Fibrotic changes are rare. The bronchial mucosa is usually hyperplastic and may show squamous metaplasia and dysplasia. The submucosa contains an increased number of mucus glands and shows a thicker basal membrane.

➤ *Descriptors:* Lung parenchyma with preserved structure:

- macrophages (dust-laden)
- dust;
- Bronchial mucosa with altered structure:
- increased number of goblet cells
- squamous metaplasia and dysplasia
- mononuclear inflammatory infiltrates

■ *Special stains:* PAS, collagenous stains, Prussian blue.

Hallmark of Diagnosis: Clinical history, agglutination of dust-laden macrophages, and dust deposits in the distant airways.

Differential diagnosis: Pneumoconiosis, especially coal worker's lung.

Sodium Diatrizoate

Definition: Alteration of the lung parenchyma associated with intake of diatrizoate sodium, see Drug Toxicity.

Sparganosis

Definition: Infection of the lung by sparganum, i.e., second stage larva of pseudophyllidean cestodes (*Spirometra mansonoides*).

Incidence/Epidemiology: The tapeworms have a worldwide distribution. Most human infections have been reported from southeast Asia, China, and Japan.

Etiology/Pathophysiology: The adult parasites live in the intestines of dogs and cats. The eggs reach fresh water with the feces and develop into coracidia which are eaten by cyclops (ubiquitous zooplanktonic organism). Within the cyclops the coracidia develop into procercoid larvae. The first stage larvae develop into the second stage larvae (plerocercoid larvae, sparganum) when the cyclops is eaten by a second intermediate host (fish, snake, amphibian). When the definite host eats the second intermediate host, the sparganum remains in its gut and develops into the adult worm. Humans become infected by eating raw or insufficiently cooked snakes, frogs, fish, or copecods or by drinking contaminated water.

Clinical Presentation: The parasites may involve any organ. Most patients present with tender, slowly growing, subcutaneous nodules. The pulmonary symptoms are usually caused by parasites involving the pleura and the pulmonary arteries, and include chest pain, pleural effusions and dyspnea. Eosinophilia and leucocytosis are common.

Prognosis: Usually good and without serious sequelae, but serious for immunocompromised patients.

Radiology: Chest radiographs show pleural effusions or a mediastinal mass displacing the heart to one side.

Pathology:

Gross: The parasites are white, flat, ribbonlike worms measuring a few millimeters to several centimeters in length and show a slow undulating movement if alive.

Histology: The parasites are usually seen in tissue sections with a provoked inflammatory reaction or in different-sized arterial and venous vessels. The inflammatory infiltrate includes lymphocytes, plasma cells, histiocytes, neutrophilic granulocytes, and various amounts of eosinophilic granulocytes. In immunocompromised patients a different species, the aberrant sparganum, has been reported, which has lost its organization and the symmetry of its histologic body components, which usually causes ulcerating cutaneous and subcutaneous lesions, and which involves the regional lymph nodes, blood vessels, and the parenchyma of any organ.

➤ *Descriptors:* Lung parenchyma with altered structure:

- mixed inflammatory infiltrates (perivascular)
- eosinophils

- noncaseous epithelioid granulomas (poorly defined)
- parasites (intragranulomatous, degenerated);
- Pulmonary vessels with altered structure:
- parasites (arteries, veins)
- noncaseous epithelioid granulomas
- eosinophils

■ *Special stains:* PAS, Movat, collagenous stains, Giemsa.

Hallmark of Diagnosis: Clinical history, perivascular inflammatory infiltrates including neutrophilic and eosinophilic granulocytes, noncaseous epithelioid granulomas, eosinophils, identification of the parasites.

Differential diagnosis: Infection by other parasites, especially *Taenia solium* or *multiceps*.

Spirochetes

Definition: Infection of the lung by spirochetes.

Incidence/Epidemiology: Spirochetes have been described to be present in lung abscesses in earlier times. However, we have seen no such recent reports.

Etiology/Pathophysiology: Zoonotic spirochetes infect many mammalian and some avian species. Man becomes infected by contact with infected animals, contaminated water, or mud. Skin lesions or mucus membranes are the preferred entrances of spirochetes into the body. Congenital infection occurs as well.

Clinical Presentation: Symptoms are abrupt after an incubation period lasting 4–19 days and include headache, fever, myalgia, nausea, vomiting, and "fever of unknown origin".

Prognosis: Congenital pulmonary involvement of spirochetes may cause death due to severe pulmonary hemorrhage.

Radiology: Chest radiographs may be normal or may show abscess formation with cavitation.

Pathology:

Gross: Depending upon the severity of the liver infection the lungs show different intensities of yellowish color (jaundice) and may display circumscribed abscess formation.

Histology: Although the liver, voluntary muscles, and kidneys are the preferred organs of infection by spirochetes, the lungs may be affected and show hemorrhagic abscess formation. The spirochetes have been described as appearing in the growing rims of necrosis.

➤ *Descriptors:* Lung parenchyma with altered structure:

- necrosis and hemorrhage
- mixed inflammatory infiltrates
- infectious organisms (spirochetes, boundary of necrotic areas)

■ *Special stains:* PAS, collagenous stains, Warthin-Starry.

Hallmark of Diagnosis: Clinical history, demonstration of spirochetes in the liver, kidneys, or lung abscess.

Differential diagnosis: Lung abscess due to other agents (aspiration, anaerobic bacteria), toxic injury to the liver and lung (carbon tetrachloride, phosphorus), acute viral hepatitis, drug-induced cholestasis.

Splendore-Hoeppli Reaction

Definition: Radiating, eosinophilic, hyaline, peripheral clubs surrounding colonies of infectious organisms (bacteria), see Actinomycosis, Aspergillosis, Botryomycosis, Coccidioidomycosis, Sporotrichosis.

Spondylitis, Ankylosing

Definition: Alteration of the lung parenchyma associated with ankylosing spondylitis.

Incidence/Epidemiology: Only 1–5% of all patients suffering from ankylosing spondylitis show involvement of the lung.

Etiology/Pathophysiology: Patients with ankylosing spondylitis often have a family history and may show alterations of the lung parenchyma associated with ankylosis of the costovertebral junctions. The etiology of the involvement of the interstitial lung parenchyma is not known.

Clinical Presentation: The majority of patients with involvement of the lung parenchyma do not show related symptoms. Some, however, may complain about dyspnea and shortness of breath during exercise.

Prognosis: Pulmonary involvement does not affect the prognosis which is usually characterized by slow progression of the ankylosis.

Radiology: Chest radiographs usually show bilateral, apical, fibro-bullous changes of the lung parenchyma.

Pathology:

Gross: The apices of both lungs show emphysematous changes with fibrous alterations of pleura and adjacent lung parenchyma.

Histology: Bullous emphysema of both apical lung areas is surrounded by fibrous lung parenchyma and fibrotic pleura. Additional findings include the usual interstitial pneumonia (UIP), organizing pneumonitis, changes similar to LIP, bronchiolitis obliterans, and superinfection of the altered lung areas by *Aspergillus*, (atypical) tuberculosis, or development of lung carcinoma.

➤ *Descriptors:* Lung parenchyma with altered structure:
- enlarged distant air spaces (apical)
- focal interstitial fibrosis
- intrabronchiolar fibrinoid material and histiocytes
- ulceration of bronchiolar mucosa
- mononuclear inflammatory infiltrates;
- Lung parenchyma with preserved structure:
- macrophages
- intraalveolar fibrinoid material;
- Pleura with altered structure:
- acellular collagen
- fibrosis
- mononuclear inflammatory infiltrates

■ *Special stains:* PAS, collagenous stains, Gram, Ziehl-Neelsen.

Hallmark of Diagnosis: Clinical history, radiologic findings, fibrobullous disease of the apices of both lungs.

Differential diagnosis: Chronic obstructive lung disease, congenital emphysema, usual interstitial pneumonia, lymphocytic interstitial pneumonia.

Sporotrichosis

Definition: Infection of the lung by *Sporothrix schenckii*.

Incidence/Epidemiology: *S. schenckii* is found worldwide as a saprophyte of soil, plants, trees, timber, and Sphagnum moss. The majority of infected patients have been reported from the USA, Mexico, South Africa, and South America. The infection is considered to be an occupational disease occurring most frequently in forestry workers, gardeners, farmers, and florists. Primary lung infection usually occurs in patients with chronic obstructive lung disease or in alcoholics.

Etiology/Pathophysiology: Man becomes infected either by cutaneous lesions or rarely by inhalation of the infectious conidia. The organisms may disseminate into various organs such as the bones, joints, lungs, meninges or may just cause lymphocutaneous manifestation (skin ulcerations).

Clinical Presentation: Symptoms are rather variable and include fever, chills, chest pain, hemoptysis, dyspnea, loss of weight, cough, and malaise.

Prognosis: Usually good, if adequate treatment is performed.

Radiology: Chest radiographs show solid circumscribed masses in one or both lungs resembling tuberculosis or histoplasmosis. Calcification does not occur.

Pathology:

Gross: The lesions measure a few millimeters to a few centimeters in maximum diameter and are yellowish-white and soft in consistency. Cavitation may be present.

Histology: The granulomatous lesions are formed by a mixed suppurative and histiocytic-lymphocytic inflammatory reaction with central caseation or cavitation. The organisms do not stain with HE, but can be detected with GMS stain. They form spherical or oval, cigar-shaped buds, often attached to each other. A Splendore-Hoeppli phenomenon may be seen as well as asteroid bodies.

➤ *Descriptors:* Lung parenchyma with altered structure:
- caseous epithelioid granulomas
- mixed inflammatory infiltrates
- necrosis and hemorrhage (cavitation)
- sulfur granules (Splendore-Hoeppli phenomenon)

■ *Special stains:* PAS, collagenous stains, GMS, methenamine silver stain, immunofluorescence, latex agglutination test.

Hallmark of Diagnosis: Clinical history, necrotizing pneumonia, cavitation, identification of *S. schenckii*.

Differential diagnosis: Tuberculosis, histoplasmosis, infection of the lung by other fungi such as *Torulopsis* or *Candida*.

Squamous Cell Carcinoma

Definition: Malignant epithelial neoplasm of the lower respiratory tract, see Epidermoid Carcinoma.

Stannosis

Definition: Alteration of the lung parenchyma associated with exposure to tin.

Incidence/Epidemiology: Tin is mined as tin oxide (cassiterite) and is now produced in Africa, South America, southeast Asia, and China. Tin miners often develop silicosis due to the admixture of quartz-containing rock. The incidence of stannosis was quite high in the past and has now decreased remarkably due to the introduction of wet drilling techniques. Tin miners have an increased risk of lung carcinoma.

Etiology/Pathophysiology: Tin is a nonfibrogenic metal, and stannosis is considered to be a benign pneumoconiosis. Tin is widely ingested by macrophages, and tin deposits are usually located close to the distant airways (peribronchiolar).

Clinical Presentation: Patients are usually asymptomatic.

Prognosis: Usually good and without serious sequelae.

Radiology: Chest radiographs show dense well-circumscribed nodules due to the high atomic number of tin (Z=50).

Pathology:

Gross: The lungs show several, randomly distributed, small, black to dark gray nodules soft in consistency.

Histology: The tin crystals are birefringent and can be seen in macrophages and in small clusters close to the perivascular and peribronchiolar regions. Fibrosis and emphysema are not a characteristic finding in stannosis.

➤ *Descriptors:* Lung parenchyma with preserved structure:

- dust (birefringent fibers, crystals)
- macrophages (birefringent crystals)

■ *Special stains:* Collagenous stains, Prussian blue, X-ray diffraction and related physical techniques, endogenous lectins.

Hallmark of Diagnosis: Clinical history, deposits of birefringent dust particles without associated fibrosis, identification of tin by X-ray diffraction technique.

Differential diagnosis: Pneumoconiosis due to other metallic deposits.

Staphylococcus

Definition: Infection of the lung by *Staphylococcus aureus* or *epidermidis*.

Incidence/Epidemiology: Staphylococcal pneumonia is usually a community-acquired pneumonia following a preceding viral pneumonia or due to sepsis. It may, in addition, occur in infants (nursery pneumonia).

Etiology/Pathophysiology: Staphylococcal pneumonia may occur either in an acute fulminant form, a subacute (abscess-forming) stage, or in a chronic pneumonia syndrome (botryomycosis). *Staphylococcus* colonizes the nose, throat, and the skin of 10–30% of healthy adults.

Clinical Presentation: The onset of symptoms may be acute or insidious. Symptoms include fever, cough, chest pain, chills, and dyspnea. Pyopneumothorax and pneumatocele are often seen in infants and young children.

Prognosis: Despite the usual successful treatment with antibiotics, some patients continue to die with staphylococcal pneumonia, especially elderly and immunocompromised patients. Abscess formation and pleural involvement induce prolonged courses and possibly necessitate surgical treatment.

Radiology: Chest radiographs show a wide range of findings including areas of consolidation, small rounded densities, diffuse infiltrates, bilateral or unilateral foci of abscess formation, and air trapping.

Pathology:

Gross: The lungs show areas of hemorrhage and necrosis as well as consolidated nodules.

Histology: The texture of the lung parenchyma is destroyed and replaced by a purulent hemorrhagic infiltrate. Abscess formation occurs in prolonged stages and may be surrounded by fibrotic material. Sulfur granules are present in the chronic pulmonary syndrome (botryomyces). The walls of the small bronchi and vessels and the bronchioles are dissolved by dense granulocytic infiltrates. Septic emboli may be seen in the arteries and veins. The bacteria are gram-positive, measure 1 μm in maximum diameter, and may be seen in clusters, in pairs, or as single organisms.

➤ *Descriptors:* Lung parenchyma with altered structure:

- necrosis and hemorrhage (abscess formation)
- mixed inflammatory infiltrates
- bacteria (gram-positive)
- sulfur granules
- proliferating fibroblasts
- focal interstitial fibrosis (circumferential);
- Pulmonary vessels with preserved structure:
- emboli (septic)

■ *Special stains:* PAS, collagenous stains, Gram's.

Hallmark of Diagnosis: Clinical history, abscess formation with gram-positive bacteria or sulfur granules, identification of the bacteria.

Differential diagnosis: *Actinomyces*, fungal infections, bacterial pneumonia due to other organisms such as *Streptococcus, Legionella, Pneumococcus, Klebsiella.*

Storage Diseases

Definition: Alteration of the lung parenchyma associated with storage disorders.

Incidence/Epidemiology: The lung may become involved in various storage disorders such as Niemann-Pick disease, adult Niemann-Pick-like lipoidosis, Gaucher's disease, Fabry's disease, glycogen storage disorders, and Hermansky-Pudlak syndrome. The percentage of involvement of the lung amounts to 10–80% depending upon the nature of the disorder.

Etiology/Pathophysiology: Storage disorders often affect reticulo-histiocytic cells in various organs such as reticuloendothelial cells of the liver or interstitial and alveolar macrophages of the lung. The cells accumulate large amounts of corresponding substances due to missing or insufficient enzymatic activity.

Clinical Presentation: Symptoms include cough, dyspnea, and sometimes severe abnormalities of lung function.

Prognosis: Usually fair, with slow progressive pulmonary involvement.

Radiology: Chest radiographs usually show diffuse patchy densities.

Pathology:

Gross: The lungs are heavy and spongy or rubbery in consistency and may have small, granulomatous, grayish-yellow nodules.

Histology: The texture of the lung parenchyma is usually preserved. The distant airways are filled with dense agglutinations of foamy macrophages. The cytoplasm may be filled with vacuoles (Niemann-Pick disease). Lymphocytic infiltrates may surround the macrophages. The details are discussed under the particular headings.

➤ *Descriptors:* Lung parenchyma with preserved structure:

- macrophages (foamy)
- mononuclear inflammatory infiltrates
- desquamation, hypertrophy, hyperplasia and dysplasia of pneumocytes

■ *Special stains:* PAS, Fontana, Prussian blue, oil red O stain.

Hallmark of Diagnosis: Clinical history, agglutination of foamy macrophages in the distant airways, preserved lung texture.

Differential diagnosis: Desquamative interstitial pneumonia, giant cell interstitial pneumonia, Whipple's disease, malakoplakia.

Streptococcus Infection

Definition: Infection of the lung by β-hemolytic streptococci.

Incidence/Epidemiology: Streptococcal pneumonia is a community-acquired infection. Historically, it was described in many soldiers during World War I. It is now rare, although serious infection still occurs, especially in diseased or immunocompromised persons.

Etiology/Pathophysiology: Streptococcal infection may have an acute or subacute course. The majority of patients have a history of preceding viral infection or laryngitis/pharyngitis. The bacteria can multiply very fast, inducing large areas of necrosis and empyema.

Clinical Presentation: Symptoms include abrupt onset of cough, high fever, chills and dyspnea. The subacute course is more like bronchopneumonia, lasting for 7 days or more.

Prognosis: Usually good and without serious sequelae, if adequate antibiotic therapy is performed.

Radiology: Chest radiographs show dense, patchy infiltrates and areas of consolidation. Cavitation may occur in late stages.

Pathology:

Gross: The lungs are heavy and edematous and may show, in addition, large areas of dry consolidation and hemorrhagic necrosis. Empyema is common in severe cases.

Histology: The interalveolar septula are necrotic. The distant airways are filled with neutrophilic granulocytes, lymphocytes, plasma cells, fibrin, and numerous gram-positive bacteria. The cocci are usually clustered in pairs and measure 1 μm in maximum diameter. Organizing pneumonia and fibrotic changes are findings in late stages.

➤ *Descriptors:* Lung parenchyma with preserved structure:

- intraalveolar fibrinoid material
- mixed inflammatory infiltrates
- bacteria;
- Lung parenchyma with altered structure:
- necrosis and hemorrhage
- mixed inflammatory infiltrates
- bacteria (gram-positive)
- macrophages
- proliferating fibroblasts
- enlarged distant air spaces
- focal interstitial fibrosis

■ *Special stains:* PAS, collagenous stains, Gram.

Hallmark of Diagnosis: Necrotizing bacterial pneumonia with identification of the bacteria.

Differential diagnosis: Bacterial pneumonia due to other organisms such as *Staphylococcus, Hemophilus, Legionella*.

Streptomycin

Definition: Alteration of the lung parenchyma associated with intake of streptomycin, see Drug Toxicity.

Strongyloidiasis

Definition: Infection of the lung by *Strongyloides stercoralis*.

Incidence/Epidemiology: It has been estimated that about 35 million people are infected with the nematode *S. stercoralis*. The highest incidence has been reported from Brazil, where about 85% of the population may be infected. It is most frequent in tropical climates; however, epidemics have also been reported in temperate climates. A high risk of infection exists in patients with mental diseases, immunocompromised persons, or those with burns or malnutrition.

Etiology/Pathophysiology: Three different life cycles of the parasite are known, (a) the direct development cycle, the rhabditiform larvae reach the soil in feces where they develop into filariform larvae which infect man by penetrating his skin. (b) the indirect development cycle, the rhabditiform larvae passed in feces molt several times in the soil and mature to free-living adults. These larvae remain noninfective for several cycles, and may change into filariform infective larvae which again penetrate the skin of man. (c) the autoinfection cycle, the rhabditiform larvae already within the intestines change into infective filariform larvae which invade the skin of the host directly. After penetrating the skin, the larvae enter the venous vessels and are carried into the lungs where they invade the distant air spaces. The larvae develop into adult worms within the alveoli and move into the major bronchi. They are swallowed and mature to adult female worms in the small intestines.

Clinical Presentation: The worms are well-adapted to man and seldom cause symptoms in healthy persons. Three clinical phases can be distinguished, (a) the cutaneous phase characterized by focal erythema, edema, itching, urticaria, and petechiae a few hours after the larvae have entered the skin; (b) the pulmonary phase, which occurs 1 week later and is characterized by cough, irritation of the throat, or in severe infections by hemoptysis, dyspnea and respiratory distress; (c) the intestinal phase, which starts 3 weeks after infection and is characterized by diarrhea, cramps, nausea, and vomiting. All the clinical symptoms are closely related to the burden of parasites. In immunocompromised patients thousands of worms may penetrate into the lungs.

Prognosis: Usually good; however, in severe cases with hyperinfection or in immunocompromised patients it is poor.

Radiology: Chest radiographs are usually normal or may show mild diffuse interstitial infiltrates.

Pathology:
Gross: The worms measure 1 mm in length and 50–75 μm in width. The lungs are usually of normal appearance or may be altered by small foci of necrosis and hemorrhage.
Histology: The parasites are usually embedded in inflammatory infiltrates with various amounts of eosinophilic granulocytes. Adult worms may be seen in the bronchial lumen. Rhabditiform larvae may be found in the sputum. Formation of granulomas with centrally localized degenerating parasites is an additional finding in the lung parenchyma.

➤ *Descriptors:* Lung parenchyma with altered structure:
- necrosis
- mixed inflammatory infiltrates
- eosinophils
- parasites (larvae and eggs)

■ *Special stains:* PAS, collagenous stains, Movat.
Hallmark of Diagnosis: Clinical history, eosinophilic bronchitis with adult worms, identification of the parasites.
Differential diagnosis: Infection by other nematodes, bacterial pneumonia, granulomatous lung diseases.

Suberosis

Definition: Alteration of the lung parenchyma associated with inhalation of *Thermoactinomyces viridis*.
Incidence/Epidemiology: Unusual disorder seen in persons exposed to cork-dust mold.
Etiology/Pathophysiology: Hypersensitivity pneumonitis due to inhalation of *T. viridis*.
Clinical Presentation: An acute or subacute onset may occur. Symptoms include cough, dyspnea, and asthmatic complaints.
Prognosis: Usually good and without serious sequelae.
Radiology: Chest radiographs show diffuse, patchy densities in both lungs, which may change in size and location within a few days.
Pathology:
Gross: The lungs are wet, heavy, and grayish-red.
Histology: The cells of the alveolar lining are hyperplastic and hypertrophic. Noncaseating granulomas may be seen as well as aggregates of histiocytes with scattered lymphocytes. Desquamation of the cells of the alveolar lining and clusters of intraalveolar macrophages are common. For details, see Allergic (Extrinsic) Alveolitis.

➤ *Descriptors:* Lung parenchyma with altered structure:
- noncaseous epithelioid granulomas
- eosinophils
- multinucleated giant cells
- intrabronchiolar fibrinoid material and histiocytes
- ulceration of bronchiolar mucosa;
- Lung parenchyma with preserved structure:
- macrophages
- desquamation, hypertrophy, hyperplasia and dysplasia of pneumocytes
- mononuclear inflammatory infiltrates
- intraalveolar serous fluid

■ *Special stains:* PAS, collagenous stains, Giemsa, immunohistochemistry for immunoglobulins and lymphocytic subpopulations, endogenous lectins.
Hallmark of Diagnosis: Clinical history, histomorphological features consistent with allergic extrinsic alveolitis.
Differential diagnosis: Usual interstitial pneumonia, desquamative interstitial pneumonia, sarcoidosis, tuberculosis, berylliosis, lymphocytic interstitial pneumonia, Wegener's granulomatosis, fungal infection.

Succinylcholine

Definition: Alteration of the lung parenchyma associated with intake of succinylcholine, see Drug Toxicity.

Sudden Infant Death Syndrome

Definition: Acute death of virtually healthy infants due to acute respiratory distress.
Incidence/Epidemiology: Sudden infant death is not infrequently seen in immature infants or in those with undetected disorders such as respiratory infections, cardial abnormalities, or in those exposed to silent toxicologic agents.
Etiology/Pathophysiology: The infants die during sleep (crib death). The underlying causes are respiratory infections (especially respiratory syncytial virus) or a "reflex death"

due to an immature central nervous system with increased duration of apnea episodes.

Clinical Presentation: The acute death of the infants occurs during the night (sleep) without any preceding symptoms and is usually not noted until the next morning.

Prognosis: Acute death without preceding symptoms.

Radiology: Chest radiographs are usually normal.

Pathology:

Gross: The lungs are edematous and heavy due to acute cardio-respiratory death.

Histology: Interalveolar and interstitial edema may be present. No specific histomorphologic findings are known.

➤ *Descriptors:* Lung parenchyma with preserved structure:

- intraalveolar serous fluid
- interstitial edema

■ *Special stains:* None.

Hallmark of Diagnosis: Clinical history, normal appearance of the lung.

Differential diagnosis: Criminal smothering.

Sugar Tumor

Definition: Benign tumor of the lung with specific histomorphologic appearance, see Benign Clear Cell Tumor of the Lung.

Sulfachrysceidine

Definition: Alteration of the lung parenchyma associated with intake of sulfachrysceidine, see Drug Toxicity.

Sulfadimethoxine

Definition: Alteration of the lung parenchyma associated with intake of sulfadimethoxine, see Drug Toxicity.

Sulfanilamide

Definition: Alteration of the lung parenchyma associated with intake of sulfanilamide, see Drug Toxicity.

Sulfasalazine

Definition: Alteration of the lung parenchyma associated with intake of sulfasalazine, see Drug Toxicity.

Sulfonamides

Definition: Alteration of the lung parenchyma associated with intake of sulfonamides, see Drug Toxicity.

Sulfur Dioxide

Definition: Alteration of the lung parenchyma associated with inhalation of sulfur dioxide.

Incidence/Epidemiology: Sulfur dioxide is a major component of industrial processes producing air pollution. It is released into the air when oil or coal are burned as well as in paper manufacture, fruit preservation, or oil refining. High concentrations of sulfur dioxide in the air have been measured in concentrated smog (smog alarm levels).

Etiology/Pathophysiology: Chronic inhalation of air with high concentrations of sulfur dioxide induces functional and histomorphologic changes in the lower respiratory tract such as chronic bronchitis and bronchiolitis, alveolitis, increase of mucus production in monkeys and probably in man. Its fibrogenic potential is considered to be rather weak.

Clinical Presentation: Symptoms include chronic cough, expectoration, and shortness of breath during exercise.

Prognosis: Usually good in acute stages; however, little is known about long-term exposure to small concentrations.

Radiology: Chest radiographs are usually normal.

Pathology:

Gross: The bronchial mucosa is edematous, swollen, covered with mucus, and reddish.

Histology: The findings include hyperplasia of goblet cells and of basal cells in the bronchial mucosa. The submucosa is invaded by mononuclear inflammatory infiltrates. The cells of the alveolar lining are hyperplastic and hypertrophic.

➤ *Descriptors:* Bronchial mucosa with preserved structure:
- increased number of goblet cells
- mononuclear inflammatory infiltrates
- hyaline basal membrane

■ *Special stains:* PAS, collagenous stains, Giemsa.

Hallmark of Diagnosis: Clinical history, findings of chronic bronchitis and bronchiolitis.

Differential diagnosis: Mild bacterial or viral infection.

Sulfur Granules

Definition: Characteristic yellowish amorphous material (sulfur granules) seen in necrotic lung parenchyma, see Actinomycosis, Botryomycosis.

Summer Pneumonitis

Definition: Allergic extrinsic pneumonitis caused by inhalation of *Trichosporon cutaneum.*

Incidence/Epidemiology: Unusual disorder reported in Japan during the summertime. Aged persons living in old wooden houses situated in wet areas are at increased risk.

Etiology/Pathophysiology: Inhalation of the fungus causes an allergic response of the lung parenchyma. For details, see under Allergic (Extrinsic) Alveolitis.

Clinical Presentation: Acute and subacute forms of this allergic pneumonitis have been described.

Prognosis: Usually good and without serious sequelae.

Radiology: Chest radiographs are normal or show diffuse, soft, interstitial infiltrates or fine granular densities.

Pathology:

Gross: The lungs are of normal color and consistency or may display small, firm, reddish-gray nodules.

Histology: The characteristic findings include nonnecrotizing epithelioid granulomas near the terminal bronchioles, desquamation, hypertrophy and hyperplasia of cells of the alveolar lining, marked eosinophilic inflammatory infiltrates, bronchiolitis obliterans, and focal acute vasculitis. For details, see under Allergic (Extrinsic) Alveolitis.

➤ *Descriptors:* Lung parenchyma with altered structure:
- noncaseous epithelioid granulomas
- eosinophils
- multinucleated giant cells
- intrabronchiolar fibrinoid material and histiocytes
- ulceration of bronchiolar mucosa;
- Lung parenchyma with preserved structure:
- macrophages
- desquamation, hypertrophy, hyperplasia and dysplasia of pneumocytes
- mononuclear inflammatory infiltrates
- intraalveolar serous fluid

■ *Special stains:* PAS, collagenous stains, Giemsa. For details, see under Allergic (Extrinsic) Alveolitis.

Hallmark of Diagnosis: Clinical history, nonnecrotizing epithelioid granulomas, morphologic findings related to desquamative interstitial pneumonia, lymphocytic interstitial pneumonia, bronchiolitis obliterans.

Differential diagnosis: Infectious and noninfectious granulomatous diseases such as sarcoidosis, fungal infections or berylliosis. For details, see under Allergic (Extrinsic) Alveolitis.

Swyer-James Syndrome

Definition: Unilateral hyperlucent lung (synonym MacLeod syndrome).

Incidence/Epidemiology: Specific radiologic findings are related to partial obstruction of a larger conducting airway with air trapping. It is not an infrequent finding in older patients with centrally localized tumors or in younger patients with endobronchial tumors.

Etiology/Pathophysiology: Air trapping causes hyperinflation of the lung and can also be induced by bronchiolitis obliterans with small foci of obstructive pneumonia or atelectasis. Unilateral hypoplasia of a pulmonal artery may also induce hyperlucent lung (Bret's syndrome).

Clinical Presentation: Patients often show asthmatic symptoms with attacks of cough, dyspnea, and chest pain.

Prognosis: Depends upon the underlying disease.

Radiology: Chest radiographs show a hyperlucent lung and a possible shift of the mediastinum to the opposite side.

Pathology:

Gross: The lung is enlarged in size and may collapse after surgical excision or at autopsy. Proximal stenosis is usually present.

Histology: The texture of the peripheral lung parenchyma is preserved. The alveoli are enlarged. The proximal stenosis may be caused by an endobronchial tumor, scarring of the bronchial walls, or collapse of the bronchial walls due to severe inflammation or destroyed cartilage (flapping bronchus). Small foci of atelectasis are usually present.

➤ *Descriptors:* Lung parenchyma with preserved structure:

- enlarged distant air spaces
- macrophages
- mononuclear inflammatory infiltrates

■ *Special stains:* PAS, collagenous stains.

Hallmark of Diagnosis: Radiologic findings, enlarged alveoli, proximal localization of stenosis, or findings of bronchiolitis obliterans.

Differential diagnosis: Artificial ventilation, congenital emphysema.

Syphilis, Congenital

Definition: Infection of the lung by *Treponema pallidum.*

Incidence/Epidemiology: The incidence of congenital syphilis is steadily decreasing and is now estimated to occur in 5/100 000 births in the USA.

Etiology/Pathophysiology: The infection of the fetus may occur at any time during pregnancy. Infection of the lung is common.

Clinical Presentation: The infant usually shows respiratory distress.

Prognosis: In about 60% of infants congenital syphilis remains latent and becomes late congenital syphilis with iritis, dental abnormalities (Hutchinson's teeth), and syphilitic periostitis. Mortality rate of acute congenital syphilis has been estimated at 5–15% of infected infants and is usually caused by pulmonary hemorrhage.

Radiology: Chest radiographs show dense, bilateral infiltrates.

Pathology:

Gross: The lungs are firm in consistency and grayish-white.

Histology: The interalveolar septula are altered by severe fibrosis with a zonal distribution. The corresponding inflammatory infiltrates are low in number and comprise mainly lymphocytes and plasma cells. Spirochetes may be detected within the distant airways. Presence of neutrophilic granulocytes indicates bacterial superinfection.

➤ *Descriptors:* Lung parenchyma with altered structure:

- necrosis and hemorrhage
- mononuclear inflammatory infiltrates
- focal interstitial fibrosis
- infectious organisms (spirochetes)
- honeycombing

■ *Special stains:* PAS, collagenous stains, methenamine silver stains, Giemsa.

Hallmark of Diagnosis: Clinical history, pulmonary hemorrhage and fibrosis, presence of spirochetes in the distant airways.

Differential diagnosis: Pulmonary fibrosis due to other causes.

Tacainide

Definition: Alteration of the lung parenchyma associated with intake of tacainide, see Drug Toxicity.

Taeniasis

Definition: Infection of the lung with the larval stage of *Taenia solium*, see Cysticercosis.

Talc

Definition: Alteration of the lung parenchyma associated with inhalation of talc, see Talcosis, Drug Abuse.

Talcosis

Definition: Alteration of the lung parenchyma associated with inhalation of talc (talc pneumoconiosis).

Incidence/Epidemiology: Occupational exposure may occur in miners or in persons working in the leather, rubber, paper, ceramic, cosmetic, pharmaceutical, soap, and textile industries. Talc consists of hydrated magnesium silicate, i.e., a sandwich consisting of two layers of silica tetrahedra and magnesium hydroxide between. Of practical importance are contaminants with quartz and amphibole asbestos (tremolite, anthophyllite). Talcosis may also be seen in persons who abuse cosmetic talc or who inject intravenously crushed tablets containing talc (drug abuse). Talc miners are at increased risk of lung cancer, which is probably related to contamination with asbestos.

Etiology/Pathophysiology: Contaminated talc is highly fibrogenic, whereas "pure" talc primarily induces a cellular macrophage response with little fibrosis. In drug abusers, however, marked fibrosis may occur, probably associated with the larger size of talc particles as compared with occupational exposure.

Clinical Presentation: Depending upon the number of inhaled particles, patients may be asymptomatic or present with cough, dyspnea, massive fibrosis and pulmonary hypertension (especially drug abusers).

Prognosis: Usually fair, but slow progressive respiratory distress is the common course.

Radiology: Chest radiographs show multiple, fine, granular densities and diffuse interstitial infiltrates.

Pathology:

Gross: The lungs show multiple, grayish-white to grayish-black granulomas measuring a few millimeters to a few centimeters in diameter. Massive, diffuse fibrosis with honeycombing may also be present in severe cases.

Histology: The histologic features include agglutinations of macrophages in the distant airways, foreign body granulomas with birefringent, small needles measuring 0.5–10 μm in length, and focal, diffuse, interstitial fibrosis or poorly defined fibrotic nodules. Multinucleated giant cells are usually numerous in the granulomas which may resemble sarcoidosis. Drug abusers may develop granulomas localized within the vessels and in the distant airways.

➤ *Descriptors:* Lung parenchyma with altered structure:

- macrophages (dust-laden)
- dust (birefringent fibers, crystals)
- noncaseous epithelioid granulomas
- multinucleated giant cells
- mononuclear inflammatory infiltrates
- focal interstitial fibrosis;
- Pulmonary vessels with altered structure:
- noncaseous epithelioid granulomas
- multinucleated giant cells

■ *Special stains:* PAS, collagenous stains, Giemsa, polarization, X-ray diffraction and related physical techniques.

Hallmark of Diagnosis: Clinical history, identification of talc, foreign body granulomas with numerous birefringent needles resembling sarcoidosis.

Differential diagnosis: Sarcoidosis, berylliosis, granulomatous lung lesions with varied etiology.

Tartrazine

Definition: Alteration of the lung parenchyma associated with intake of tartrazine, see Drug Toxicity.

Tea Grower's Lung

Definition: Alteration of the lung parenchyma seen in persons working in tea plantations.

Incidence/Epidemiology: Unusual disorder seen in workers planting, farming, and harvesting tea.

Etiology/Pathophysiology: The changes in the lung parenchyma are induced by an allergic pneumonitis resulting from an unknown antigen.

Clinical Presentation: Acute and subacute onset of the disorder have been noted.

Prognosis: Usually good and without serious sequelae.

Radiology: Chest radiographs are normal or show diffuse, soft, interstitial infiltrates or fine granular densities.

Pathology:

Gross: The lungs are of normal color and consistency, or may display small, firm, reddish-gray nodules.

Histology: The characteristic findings include nonnecrotizing epithelioid granulomas near the terminal bronchioles, desquamation, hypertrophy and hyperplasia of cells of the alveolar lining, marked eosinophilic inflammatory infiltrates, bronchiolitis obliterans, and focal acute vasculitis. For details, see under Allergic (Extrinsic) Alveolitis.

➤ *Descriptors:* Lung parenchyma with altered structure:
- noncaseous epithelioid granulomas
- eosinophils
- multinucleated giant cells
- intrabronchiolar fibrinoid material and histiocytes
- ulceration of bronchiolar mucosa;
- Lung parenchyma with preserved structure:
- macrophages
- desquamation, hypertrophy, hyperplasia and dysplasia of pneumocytes
- mononuclear inflammatory infiltrates
- intraalveolar serous fluid

■ *Special stains:* PAS, collagenous stains, Giemsa. For details, see under Allergic (Extrinsic) Alveolitis.

Hallmark of Diagnosis: Clinical history, nonnecrotizing epithelioid granulomas, morphologic findings related to desquamative interstitial pneumonia, lymphocytic interstitial pneumonia, bronchiolitis obliterans.

Differential diagnosis: Infectious and noninfectious granulomatous diseases such as sarcoidosis, fungal infections or berylliosis. For details, see under Allergic (Extrinsic) Alveolitis.

Teratocarcinoma

Definition: Extremely rare malignant tumor presenting all three germ layers, see Teratoma.

Teratoma

Definition: Predominantly benign and rarely malignant tumor of the lung or mediastinum involving all three germ cell layers (only about 10 cases with metastizing teratoma have ever been reported).

Incidence/Epidemiology: Primary teratomas of the lung are infrequent lesions, and only about 30–40 cases have been reported. Teratomas of the mediastinum are about 30-fold more frequent. The tumors may be detected in any age group, including infants.

Etiology/Pathophysiology: Teratomas are thought to derive from thymic nests which may be left in the lung after the outpouching of the lung buds.

Clinical Presentation: Patients may be asymptomatic or present with cough, chest pain, hemoptysis, and dyspnea.

Prognosis: Usually good and without serious sequelae.

Radiology: Chest radiographs show solid tumors with either calcification or hyperlucent areas.

Pathology:

Gross: The tumors resemble epidermoid cysts of the ovary and may contain large cysts filled with brown granular masses. They may contain sebum, bone, fat, and epidermoid layers.

Histology: The tumors are well-demarcated from the surrounding lung parenchyma and contain all three germ cell layers. Epidermoid layers, sebum, fat, and fragments of thymic or pancreatic tissue are frequently seen as well as skeletal and smooth muscle and cartilage. Inflammatory response of host tissue is weak or missing. Immature epithelial and stromal cells are often noted in some areas, suggesting a malignant variety of these tumors. Malignant behavior, however, was not observed in the majority of these tumors.

➤ *Descriptors:* Newly formed textures without metastasis potential:
- epithelial growth pattern
- mesenchymal growth pattern
- adenoid textures
- fibromatous textures
- chondromatous textures
- osteoid textures
- cysts
- large tumor cells
- homogeneous nuclear and cellular size
- absent or infrequent mitoses
- smooth muscle cells
- keratin production
- mucus production
- mononuclear inflammatory infiltrates

■ *Special stains:* PAS, collagenous stains, Giemsa, immunohistochemistry for keratin, vimentin, neuroendocrine markers, desmin, desmoplakin, endogenous lectins, DNA analysis.

Hallmark of Diagnosis: Identification of all three germ cell layers within these tumors.

Differential diagnosis: Coelom cyst, hamartoma.

Tetracycline

Definition: Alteration of the lung parenchyma associated with intake of tetracycline, see Drug Toxicity.

Thatched Roof Lung

Definition: Alteration of the lung parenchyma associated with inhalation of substances released by dead grasses and leaves.

Incidence/Epidemiology: Unusual disorder seen in rural areas with high humidity and warm climate.

Etiology/Pathophysiology: Hypersensitivity reaction of the lung parenchyma due to an unknown antigen.

Clinical Presentation: Acute and subacute onsets have been reported.

Prognosis: Usually good and without serious sequelae.

Radiology: Chest radiographs are normal or show diffuse, soft, interstitial infiltrates or fine granular densities.

Pathology:

Gross: The lungs are of normal color and consistency or may display small, firm, reddish-gray nodules.

Histology: The characteristic findings include nonnecrotizing epithelioid granulomas near the terminal bronchioles, desquamation, hypertrophy and hyperplasia of cells of the alveolar lining, marked eosinophilic inflammatory infiltrates, bronchiolitis obliterans, and focal acute vasculitis. For details, see under Allergic (Extrinsic) Alveolitis.

➤ *Descriptors:* Lung parenchyma with altered structure:

- noncaseous epithelioid granulomas
- eosinophils
- multinucleated giant cells
- intrabronchiolar fibrinoid material and histiocytes
- ulceration of bronchiolar mucosa;
- Lung parenchyma with preserved structure:
- macrophages
- desquamation, hypertrophy, hyperplasia and dysplasia of pneumocytes
- mononuclear inflammatory infiltrates
- intraalveolar serous fluid

■ *Special stains:* PAS, collagenous stains, Giemsa. For details, see under Allergic (Extrinsic) Alveolitis.

Hallmark of Diagnosis: Clinical history, nonnecrotizing epithelioid granulomas, morphologic findings related to desquamative interstitial pneumonia, lymphocytic interstitial pneumonia, bronchiolitis obliterans.

Differential diagnosis: Infectious and noninfectious granulomatous diseases such as sarcoidosis, fungal infections, or berylliosis. For details, see under Allergic (Extrinsic) Alveolitis.

Thiozides

Definition: Alteration of the lung parenchyma associated with intake of thiozides, see Drug Toxicity.

Thoracoblastoma

Definition: Malignant blastoma of the thoracopulmonary region (extrapulmonary blastoma).

Incidence/Epidemiology: Very rare tumor, sometimes seen in children and young adults.

Etiology/Pathophysiology: Pulmonary blastomatous histogenesis with extrapulmonary location.

Clinical Presentation: Patients present with large, pleural-based masses with pleural effusions, chest pain, and dyspnea.

Prognosis: Usually poor as median survial is under 2 years.

Radiology: Chest radiographs show circumscribed masses within the pleural cavity.

Pathology:

Gross: Soft, pink masses with hemorrhage and necrosis, extrapulmonary location, and connection to the pleura.

Histology: The morphology of the tumor cells is related to primitive mesenchymal cells with large variation in nuclear size and numerous mitoses. Islands of primitive cartilage, tumor cells resembling rhabdomyoblasts, and primitive stromal cells or primitive tubules are usually present.

➤ *Descriptors:* Newly formed textures with metastasis potential:
- mesenchymal growth pattern
- lymphomatoid textures
- adenoid textures (primitive tubules)
- chondromatous textures (primitive cartilage)
- small tumor cells
- inhomogeneous nuclear and cellular size
- frequent mitoses
- necrosis and hemorrhage

■ *Special stains:* PAS, Giemsa, immunohistochemistry for vimentin, keratin, desmin, neurofilaments, α_1-antitrypsin, desmoplakin, NSE, DNA analysis.

Hallmark of Diagnosis: Blastomatous histomorphology with extrapulmonary location.

Differential diagnosis: Askin tumor, rhabdomyosarcoma, carcinosarcoma.

Tin

Definition: Alteration of the lung parenchyma associated with exposure to tin, see Stannosis.

Titanium

Definition: Alteration of the lung parenchyma associated with exposure to titanium.

Incidence/Epidemiology: Exposed persons may be seen in the dye industry (titanium dioxide) or in the hard metal industry (titanium carbide). Titanium dioxide associated with silica is called rutile which may affect miners.

Etiology/Pathophysiology: Titanium dioxide and titanium carbide are considered to be inert substances and not fibrogenic. Increased risk of bronchial carcinoma associated with exposure to titanium has not been noted.

Clinical Presentation: Patients are usually asymptomatic.

Prognosis: Usually good and without serious sequelae.

Radiology: Chest radiographs are usually normal or may show perihilar densities.

Pathology:

Gross: The lungs may have a grayish-white appearance with a greenish hue.

Histology: Dust-laden macrophages can be seen in the distant airways with perivascular and peribronchiolar distribution. The titanium fibers are birefringent and may also be seen in enlarged hilar lymph nodes. Fibrosis is usually absent.

➤ *Descriptors:* Lung parenchyma with preserved structure:
- dust
- macrophages (dust-laden)
- mononuclear inflammatory infiltrates (weak)

■ *Special stains:* PAS, collagenous stains, Giemsa, Prussian blue, X-ray diffraction or related physical techniques.

Hallmark of Diagnosis: Clinical history, identification of titanium particles.

Differential diagnosis: Inhaled particles of other inert metals such as iron, tin, zirconium, antimony, barium, cerium.

Tobacco

Definition: Alteration of the lung parenchyma associated with inhalation of tobacco smoke, see Smoking.

Tobacco Grower's Lung

Definition: Alteration of the lung parenchyma associated with inhalation of antigens related to tobacco plants.

Incidence/Epidemiology: Unusual disorder seen in tobacco growers and persons working with tobacco plants, especially in humid and warm areas.

Etiology/Pathophysiology: Hypersensitivity pneumonitis due to extrinsic antigens. The antigens are not known.

Clinical Presentation: Acute and subacute courses have been observed.

Prognosis: Usually good and without serious sequelae.

Radiology: Chest radiographs are normal or show diffuse, soft, interstitial infiltrates or fine granular densities.

Pathology:

Gross: The lungs are of normal color and consistency, or may display small, firm, reddish-gray nodules.

Histology: The characteristic findings include nonnecrotizing epithelioid granulomas near the terminal bronchioles, desquamation, hypertrophy and hyperplasia of cells of the alveolar lining, marked eosinophilic inflammatory infiltrates, bronchiolitis obliterans, and focal acute vasculitis. For details, see under Allergic (Extrinsic) Alveolitis.

➤ *Descriptors:* Lung parenchyma with altered structure:
- noncaseous epithelioid granulomas
- eosinophils
- multinucleated giant cells
- intrabronchiolar fibrinoid material and histiocytes
- ulceration of bronchiolar mucosa;
- Lung parenchyma with preserved structure:
- macrophages
- desquamation, hypertrophy, hyperplasia and dysplasia of pneumocytes
- mononuclear inflammatory infiltrates
- intraalveolar serous fluid

■ *Special stains:* PAS, collagenous stains, Giemsa. For details, see under Allergic (Extrinsic) Alveolitis.

Hallmark of Diagnosis: Clinical history, nonnecrotizing epithelioid granulomas, morphologic findings related to desquamative interstitial pneumonia, lymphocytic interstitial pneumonia, bronchiolitis obliterans.

Differential diagnosis: Infectious and noninfectious granulomatous diseases such as sarcoidosis, fungal infections, or berylliosis. For details, see under Allergic (Extrinsic) Alveolitis.

Tolazamide

Definition: Alteration of the lung parenchyma associated with intake of tolazamide, see Drug Toxicity.

Tolbutamide

Definition: Alteration of the lung parenchyma associated with intake of tolbutamide, see Drug Toxicity.

Torulopsosis

Definition: Infection of the lung with *Torulopsis glabrata* (fungus of the family *Cryptococcaceae*).

Incidence/Epidemiology: The fungus has a very low virulence and is considered to be an opportunistic organism. It has a worldwide distribution.

Etiology/Pathophysiology: The organisms usually infect immunocompromised patients and may cause fungemia, pyelonephritis, pneumonia, osteomyelitis, endocarditis, meningoencephalitis, etc. Fungemia is usually induced by a contaminated catheter, injection needles, or intravenous tubes.

Clinical Presentation: Infection is self-healing and limiting in about 50% of cases. The remainder may show high fever, chills, dyspnea, and cardiac failure.

Prognosis: Usually good, self-healing occurs in more than 50% of patients; however, a few fatal cases have been reported.

Radiology: Chest radiographs show patchy or nodular, bilateral densities in severe infections.

Pathology:
Gross: The lungs may show necrotic areas of various sizes and organizing pneumonia.

Histology: The organisms are small round yeasts measuring 2–5 μm in maximum diameter. They have single buds. Mononuclear and histiocytic inflammatory cells are usually present at the boundary. The fungal cells resemble *Histoplasma capsulatum* and can be distinguished from *Histoplasma* by their larger size, increased pleomorphism, and the lack of granulomatous reaction of the host tissue usually present in *Histoplasma* infections.

➤ *Descriptors:* Lung parenchyma with preserved structure:
- intraalveolar fibrinoid material
- fungus (yeast and spores)
- mixed inflammatory infiltrates

■ *Special stains:* PAS, GMS, Giemsa, immunofluorescence.

Hallmark of Diagnosis: Clinical history, organizing pneumonia, identification of the fungus.

Differential diagnosis: Histoplasmosis, cryptococcosis, candidiasis.

Toxic Injury

Definition: Reaction of the lung parenchyma induced by toxic agents.

Incidence/Epidemiology: A great number of toxic agents are known to induce functional and morphologic changes in the lung parenchyma. These include various drugs, inhalants, and radiation.

Etiology/Pathophysiology: The pattern of reaction of the lung parenchyma due to toxic agents is limited. The damage usually starts by disturbance of the air-blood barrier and consequent extravasation of proteinaceous fluid and blood substances. Cellular damage may be seen simultaneously in the epithelial and endothelial cells of the distant airways. Formation of granulomas, invasion of eosinophilic granulocytes, stenosis of lymphatic or venous drainage, and fibrosis may follow. The mechanisms of toxic injury include oxidant lung damage or direct toxicity, hypersensitivity phenomena, and individual susceptibility. Toxic agents may be drugs, parasites (*Ascaris lumbricoides*), inhalation of irritant gases or metal fumes, or exposure to radiation.

Clinical Presentation: The clinical onset may be acute, subacute or chronic according to the degree and form of toxic exposure.

Prognosis: Usually fair, as most patients with acute toxic injury survive but develop chronic lung damage. Those with a history of chronic toxic injury often present with slow progressive respiratory failure.

Radiology: Chest radiographs usually show diffuse, unilateral or bilateral densities which may undergo consolidation.

Pathology:

Gross: The lungs are heavy and edematous in acute stages. They show consolidated or fibrotic areas in later stages.

Histology: The histomorphological changes are as follows: diffuse alveolar damage (edema, congestion, hemorrhage, formation of hyaline membranes, desquamation of pneumocytes, microatelectasis), usual interstitial pneumonia (mononuclear interstitial infiltrates, desquamation of pneumocytes, organizing pneumonia with various degrees of fibrosis, fibroblast proliferation, loss of normal lung texture, cellular atypias), eosinophilic pneumonia (eosinophilic infiltrates, small histiocytic granulomas), alveolar proteinosis, lymphocytic interstitial pneumonia, pleural and cardiac serositis (lupus-like syndrome), desquamative interstitial pneumonia, lipoid pneumonia, angiitis, fibrinoid necrosis, and microthrombi of the capillaries (radiation pneumonitis).

➤ *Descriptors:* Lung parenchyma with preserved structure:

- intraalveolar serous fluid
- hemorrhage
- hyaline membranes
- desquamation, hypertrophy, hyperplasia and dysplasia of pneumocytes
- mononuclear inflammatory infiltrates
- macrophages;
- Lung parenchyma with altered structure:
- necrosis
- noncaseous epithelioid granulomas
- multinucleated giant cells
- eosinophils
- enlarged distant air spaces
- proliferating fibroblasts
- focal interstitial fibrosis
- honeycombing

■ *Special stains:* PAS, collagenous stains, Giemsa, Prussian blue, immunohistochemistry for immunoglobulins and lymphocytic subpopulations, endogenous lectins.

Hallmark of Diagnosis: Clinical history, lung function tests, chest radiographic findings, histomorphology.

Differential diagnosis: Bacterial infections, collagenous disorders, bronchial carcinoma.

Toxocariasis

Definition: Infection of the lung by *Toxocara*, see Larva migrans.

Toxoplasmosis

Definition: Infection of the lung by *Toxoplasma gondii*.

Incidence/Epidemiology: Involvement of the lung in persons who are infected with toxoplasma occurs only in immunocompromised patients. Patients with AIDS or patients receiving immunosuppressive therapy are especially at risk.

Etiology/Pathophysiology: Infection is seen in about 50% of healthy persons without any major symptoms. In the majority of these patients lymphadenopathy is found. Infection of immunocompromised patients induces a disseminated form with pulmonary involvement in about two-thirds of patients, whereas lymphadenopathy is not seen. The organisms are sporozoa which alternate sexual generation with asexual multiplication. They multiply in histiocytes. The definite hosts are cats in whose intestines the organisms develop oocysts. The oocysts pass with the feces and become infective by sporulation. The infective sporozoites stay alive in soil for about 1 year. Man becomes infected by eating poorly cooked meat from chronically infected animals or by ingesting oocysts from soil or contaminated objects.
Clinical Presentation: The symptoms include tachypnea and dyspnea with or without fever, usually with acute onset.

Prognosis: Acquired toxoplasmosis has a good prognosis. Congenital toxoplasmosis seldom causes death but may heal with sequelae.

Radiology: Chest radiographs show diffuse, bilateral, interstitial or intraalveolar infiltrates.

Pathology:
Gross: The lungs are heavy, edematous and congested and may show zones of necrosis and fibrinous exudate.

Histology: The distant airways are filled with macrophages and histiocytes which contain numerous organisms (tachyzoites). The interalveolar septula are edematously widened and are filled with lymphocytes, plasma cells, and neutrophilic granulocytes. Areas of hemorrhage and necrosis are frequently seen. The organisms stain well with HE, PAS, or Giemsa and can be demonstrated in pseudocysts or in histiocytes.

➤ *Descriptors:* Lung parenchyma with altered structure:
- necrosis and hemorrhage
- infectious organisms (tachyzoites)
- macrophages (tachyzoites)
- mixed inflammatory infiltrates

■ *Special stains:* PAS, Giemsa, GMS, immunofluorescence.

Hallmark of Diagnosis: Clinical history, necrotizing pneumonia, identification of the infectious organisms.

Differential diagnosis: Leishmaniasis, histoplasmosis, trichomoniasis, *Pneumocystis carinii* infection.

Tracheobronchiomegaly

Definition: Diffuse or circumscribed enlargement of the trachea and bronchi of unknown etiology (Mounier-Kuhn syndrome).
Incidence/Epidemiology: Rare disorder seen in children and in young to middle-aged adults (30–40 years old).
Etiology/Pathophysiology: Familial occurrence has been reported suggesting an autosomal recessive type of inheritance.
Clinical Presentation: Patients show symptoms related to asthmatic complaints and bronchiectasis.
Prognosis: Fair, as slow progressive obstructive lung damage is often seen.
Radiology: Chest radiographs show a diffuse or circumscribed outpouching of the trachea or major bronchi.
Pathology:
Gross: The trachea shows circumscribed enlargement and diverticula of the lumen between the tracheal cartilage rings.
Histology: The mucosa and the submucosa are affected by chronic inflammation and may be atrophic. The submucosal glands are destroyed, and the smooth muscle fibers are replaced by connective tissue. The cartilage is preserved.

➤ *Descriptors:* Bronchial mucosa with altered structure:
- atrophic mucosa
- mononuclear inflammatory infiltrates
- fibrosis

■ *Special stains:* PAS, collagenous stains.
Hallmark of Diagnosis: Clinical history, macroscopic findings, increase of collagenous tissue and atrophic muscular tissue in the submucosa.
Differential diagnosis: Tracheomalacia, traumatic lesion.

Tracheobronchitis

Definition: Acute or chronic inflammation of the trachea and bronchi, see Bronchitis.

Tracheobronchomalacia

Definition: Degeneration and atrophy of tracheal or bronchial cartilage, see Bronchomalacia.

Tracheobronchopathia Osteoplastica

Definition: Increase of irregularly shaped cartilage in the trachea and bronchi.

Incidence/Epidemiology: Rare disorder. It is usually an incidental finding in autopsies or surgical specimens. It is more common in men than in women and most frequently seen in elderly persons.

Etiology/Pathophysiology: The morphological findings resemble ecchondrosis. The etiology is not known. Its association with tracheobronchial amyloid has been discussed; however, there is evidence that tracheobronchopathia osteoplastica develops without simultaneous or preceding amyloidosis.

Clinical Presentation: Patients may be asymptomatic or present with cough, wheezing, expectoration and dyspnea.

Prognosis: Usually good; however, slow progressive lung damage has been reported.

Radiology: Chest radiographs may be normal or show a dilated trachea and bronchi.

Pathology:

Gross: The trachea or the major bronchi show a rubbery surface with multiple, circumscribed, ossified nodules. The lower parts of the trachea are usually involved. Ulceration and granulation may be present.

Histology: The nodules are formed from mature bone and cartilage including bone marrow. The epithelial cells are atrophic and may undergo squamous metaplasia. The ossified nodules are randomly distributed in the submucosa and extend into the mucosa. Amyloidosis and chronic inflammation may be seen in addition.

➤ *Descriptors:* Bronchial mucosa with altered structure:

- ossification (ossified nodules, multiple)
- ulceration
- histiocytes
- mononuclear inflammatory infiltrates

■ *Special stains:* PAS, collagenous stains, Congo, Giemsa.

Hallmark of Diagnosis: Macroscopic findings, increased deposits of irregularly shaped bone and cartilage in the submucosa of the trachea or bronchi.

Differential diagnosis: Tracheal amyloidosis, tracheobronchiomegaly, tracheobronchomalacia.

Tracheoesophageal Fistula

Definition: Congenital or acquired abnormal connection between the trachea and esophagus.

Incidence/Epidemiology: Unusual disorder seen in adults with esophageal carcinoma or with malignant bronchial/tracheal tumor. Infants with congenital esophageal atresia will show a tracheoesophageal fistula in 80–90% of cases.

Etiology/Pathophysiology: Tracheoesophageal fistula in adults is usually a consequence of chronic inflammation or of destructive malignant growth. In infants, congenital tracheoesophageal fistula usually connects the lower part of the trachea with the corresponding segment of the esophagus. Maternal polyhydramnios is usually present. Additional malformations are common and include pulmonary hypoplasia, hydrocephalus, micrognathia, renal malposition, malrotation and atresia of the intestines, ventricular septal defect, and other cardiovascular abnormalities.

Clinical Presentation: Patients present with dysphagia, dyspnea, cough, cyanosis, and choking during feeding or intake of meals.

Prognosis: Depends upon the underlying disease, but usually poor.

Radiology: Chest radiographs usually show a mediastinal mass due to malignant growth or inflammation and dense, localized, pulmonary infiltrates due to aspiration.

Pathology:

Gross: Abnormal connection between the esophagus and trachea of varied size embedded in tumorous or necrotic tissue in adults; in infants usually blind fistula associated with esophageal atresia.

Histology: In adults necrosis and ulceration of the mucosa and submucosa, in infants only mild inflammatory changes and possible squamous metaplasia of the tracheal mucosa.

➤ *Descriptors:* Bronchial mucosa with altered structure:
- necrosis
- ulceration
- mixed inflammatory infiltrates
- squamous metaplasia and dysplasia

■ *Special stains:* PAS, collagenous stains, Giemsa.

Hallmark of Diagnosis: Clinical history, macroscopic findings, necrotizing inflammation.

Differential diagnosis: Due to the underlying cause.

Transplantation

Definition: Alteration of the lung parenchyma associated with organ transplants.

Incidence/Epidemiology: Although still rare, organ transplantations are of increasing importance. The majority are kidney followed by liver and bone marrow transplantations. Other transplants include heart, single lung and heart-lung. All patients receive immunosuppressive therapy and are vulnerable to all kinds of opportunistic infections.

Etiology/Pathophysiology: Immunosuppressive therapy alters the cellular defence mechanisms. The patients show different susceptibilities to infectious organisms depending upon the transplanted organ: Bone marrow transplant patients have an increased risk of cytomegalovirus infections (50%) in contrast to renal transplant patiens (less than 20%). Single lung transplant patients suffer from serious bacterial infections, whereas heart transplant recipients often present with fungal infections. *Pneumocystis carinii* infection is most frequently seen in patients with AIDS.

Clinical Presentation: The patients present with fever, cough, dyspnea, and chest pain.

Prognosis: Fair, about 10–40% of the patients may die from pneumonias depending upon the infectious agent and the transplanted organ.

Radiology: Chest radiographs show dense, patchy infiltrates in both lungs, often with involvement of a complete lobe. Cavitation may be present.

Pathology:

Gross: The lungs are heavy and reddish-yellowish and show multiple consolidated areas. Necrosis and cavitation may be noted.

Histology: The histomorphological findings are consistent with those of severe necrotizing pneumonia. Viral inclusion bodies or fungal yeast may be seen. Graft versus host reaction in lung transplants presents with microthomboses in the septular capillaries, fibrinoid debris in the distant airways, and necrosis of the cells of the alveolar lining.

➤ *Descriptors:* Lung parenchyma with preserved structure:
- intraalveolar fibrinoid material
- degeneration of pneumocytes
- mixed inflammatory infiltrates
- intraalveolar serous fluid
- enlarged distant air spaces;
- Lung parenchyma with altered structure:
- necrosis and hemorrhage
- infectious organisms (bacteria, virus, fungus, protozoans)
- mixed inflammatory infiltrates
- macrophages
- proliferating fibroblasts
- focal interstitial fibrosis;
- Pulmonary vessels with preserved structure:
- microthrombosis

■ *Special stains:* PAS, collagenous stains, methenamine silver stain, immunohistochemistry, endogenous lectins.

Hallmark of Diagnosis: Clinical history, necrotizing pneumonia, microthrombosis.

Differential diagnosis: Pneumonia due to the underlying infectious organism, adult respiratory distress syndrome.

Tranylcypromine

Definition: Alteration of the lung parenchyma associated with intake of tranylcypromine, see Drug Toxicity.

Trematodes

Definition: Infection of the lung by trematodes.

Incidence/Epidemiology: Infection by trematodes is a frequent parasitic disorder in man; however, pulmonary involvement is less frequent. Most human infections have been reported from Asian and African countries. Of specific importance is infection by *Schistosoma* (see schistosomiasis).

Etiology/Pathophysiology: The trematodes infective to man include *Alaria, Clinostomum, Clonorchis, Fasciola, Fasciolopsis, Opisthorchis, Paragonimus* and *Schistosoma.* The life cycle is described under the particular headings. It usually comprises one or two intermediate hosts (snails, fish, crab). Infection of man occurs either by eating poorly cooked meat (*Paragonimus, Clonorchis, Opisthorchis, Alaria, Clinostomum*), by eating contaminated water plants (*Fasciola, Faciolopsis*), or by active penetration of the parasite through the skin of man (*Schistosoma*). The parasites usually reach the lung via the pulmonary arteries and settle down in the peripheral lung parenchyma.
Clinical Presentation: Patients may be asymptomatic or present with cough, dyspnea, hemoptysis, and pulmonary hypertension.

Prognosis: Usually good, depending upon the species of parasite; infection with *Schistosoma japonicum* is serious and fatal, if not treated early.

Radiology: Chest radiographs may be normal or may show diffuse interstitial infiltrates.

Pathology:
Gross: The parasites usually induce circumscribed, grayish-white, granulomatous nodules measuring a few millimeters in maximum diameter.

Histology: The histomorphologic findings are described under the particular headings. They usually comprise granulomas with central necrosis containing the worms or their eggs.

➤ *Descriptors:* Lung parenchyma with altered structure:
- caseous epithelioid granulomas
- parasites (intragranulomatous, larvae and eggs)
- mixed inflammatory infiltrates
- eosinophils

■ *Special stains:* PAS, collagenous stains, Giemsa, Movat.

Hallmark of Diagnosis: Clinical history, necrotizing histiocytic granulomas, identification of the parasites.

Differential diagnosis: Depends on the underlying parasite, lentil pneumonia (Liesegang phenomenon).

Tremolite

Definition: Alteration of the lung parenchyma associated with inhalation of tremolite fibers, see Asbestos-Associated Diseases.

Trichinosis

Definition: Infection of the lung by *Trichinella spiralis.*
Incidence/Epidemiology: *Trichinella* is a nematode with worldwide distribution. Trichinosis is most common in areas with high consumption of pork, especially in eastern and central Europe, North America, Central and South America.
Etiology/Pathophysiology: Infection in man occurs upon eating raw or poorly cooked pork containing encysted larvae. The adult male and female parasites live in the intestines of man, pigs, bears, and other mammals. The infected animals serve as intermediate and also as definite hosts. The worms produce infective larvae which migrate through most organs and invade and encyst in the skeletal muscle. Encysted larvae stay infective for several years.
Clinical Presentation: The lungs are rarely infected. Patients with pulmonary infection may present with cough, dyspnea, and hemoptysis in addition to the more common features such as eosinophilia, slight edema of the face and eyelids, myalgia of the neck, transient diarrhea followed by encephalitis, meningitis, and nephritis after 4–6 weeks.
Prognosis: Usually good even for patients with cerebromeningeal infections. The overall mortality rate is less than 5%.
Radiology: Chest radiographs are usually normal or may show diffuse, patchy, intraalveolar infiltrates.
Pathology:
Gross: The female worms measure 3–4 mm in length (males 1–2 mm) and 40–70 μm in diameter (males 30–50 μm). The larvae measure 100 μm in length and 6 μm in maximum diameter, and encysted larvae 1 mm in length and 40 μm in maximum diameter.
Histology: The encysted larvae are surrounded by a hyaline layer which induces only a weak inflammatory reaction of host tissue. Some cysts may be seen with a granulomatous reac-

tion including multinucleated giant cells. Migrating larvae may induce a mild to moderate mononuclear inflammatory reaction.

➤ *Descriptors:* Lung parenchyma with preserved structure:
- parasites (larvae)
- mononuclear inflammatory infiltrates;
- Lung parenchyma with altered structure:
- caseous epithelioid granulomas (with central cysts)
- cysts
- parasites (intragranulomatous)
- multinucleated giant cells
- eosinophils

■ *Special stains:* PAS, collagenous stains, Giemsa, Movat, complement fixation test.

Hallmark of Diagnosis: Clinical history, necrotizing histiocytic granulomas, identification of the parasites.

Differential diagnosis: Infection by other nematodes.

Trichomoniasis

Definition: Infection of the lung by the protozoan *Trichomonas tenax*.

Incidence/Epidemiology: *T. tenax* has a worldwide distribution. Infections of the oral cavity and subsequent pulmonary involvement have been reported from Europe (USSR), Asia, and America. Infection usually occurs in persons with preexisting lung disorders or with an inefficient immune system.

Etiology/Pathophysiology: The flagellates are transmitted by direct contact and are usually present in persons with poor oral hygiene. Infections of the buccal cavity and of the lower respiratory tract occur simultaneously in only 30–40% of the cases. It is considered to be an opportunistic organism.

Clinical Presentation: Patients may be asymptomatic or show progressive fever, dyspnea, cough, empyema, and pleural effusions.

Prognosis: Usually good and without serious sequelae.

Radiology: Chest radiographs are either normal or may show patchy densities with cavitation and pleural effusion.

Pathology:

Gross: The lungs show areas of consolidation or necrosis and suppurative inflammation.

Histology: The histomorphological findings are nonspecific and include suppurative necrotic areas, zones of organizing pneumonia, and intraalveolar edema. The organisms may be seen in necrotic tissue appearing as grayish-reddish cells which measure 5 μm in maximum diameter. The cytoplasm contains multiple, reddish and bluish granules. The organisms are best demonstrated in Papanicolaou-stained or fresh cytological specimens.

➤ *Descriptors:* Lung parenchyma with preserved structure:
- intraalveolar serous fluid
- intraalveolar fibrinoid material
- mixed inflammatory infiltrates;
- Lung parenchyma with altered structure:
- necrosis
- infectious organisms (flagellates)
- proliferating histiocytes
- mixed inflammatory infiltrates

■ *Special stains:* PAS, Giemsa, Papanicolaou.

Hallmark of Diagnosis: Progressive opportunistic pulmonary infection, identification of the organisms.

Differential diagnosis: Infection with other protozoan or bacterial organisms.

Trichosporosis

Definition: Infection of the lung by *Trichosporon species*.

Incidence/Epidemiology: The yeastlike fungi *T. beigelii* and *capitatum* are considered to be superficial infective organisms causing white piedra (*T. beigelii*). They are, however, opportunistic organisms and may cause disseminated infections in immunocompromised patients.

Etiology/Pathophysiology: The organisms usually infect the hair shafts and cause a superficial mycosis. Fungemia with dissemination into several organs has been reported in patients receiving cytostatic drugs or immunosuppressive therapy.

Clinical Presentation: Symptoms include high fever, cough, dyspnea, expectoration, and symptoms related to fungemia and sepsis.

Prognosis: Usually poor, the mortality rate is 50–70%.

Radiology: Chest radiographs show dense, patchy, usually bilateral infiltrates.

Pathology:

Gross: The lungs show multiple, randomly distributed, reddish-yellowish, hemorrhagic-necrotic areas.

Histology: The necrotic areas contain densely packed fungal organisms appearing as pleomorphic yeast cells with septated hyphae. The hyphae are segmentated and fragmentated. Inflammatory response of host tissue is weak and granulomas are usually not present. Often an arthoconidia formation of the yeastlike cells can be seen. The trichosporon organisms are more pleomorphic than those of *Candida* or *Aspergillus*.

➤ *Descriptors:* Lung parenchyma with altered structure:
- necrosis and hemorrhage
- fungus (yeast)
- mixed inflammatory infiltrates
- proliferating fibroblasts

■ *Special stains:* PAS, Giemsa, methenamine silver stain.

Hallmark of Diagnosis: Clinical history, necrotizing pneumonia, identification of the fungus.

Differential diagnosis: Infection by other fungal organisms, especially *Candida*, *Aspergillus*.

Trimethadione

Definition: Alteration of the lung parenchyma associated with intake of trimethadione, see Drug Toxicity.

Tripelennamine

Definition: Alteration of the lung parenchyma associated with intake of tripelennamine, see Drug Toxicity.

Triphenamines

Definition: Alteration of the lung parenchyma associated with intake of triphenamines, see Drug Toxicity.

Tropical Eosinophilic Pneumonia

Definition: Infection of the lung by *Wuchereria bancrofti* or *Brugia malayi* (Weingarten's syndrome), see Filariasis.

Trypsin

Definition: Alteration of the lung parenchyma associated with exposure to trypsin, see Drug Toxicity.

Tuberculosis

Definition: Infection of the lung by *Mycobacterium tuberculosis*.

Incidence/Epidemiology: The incidence of tuberculosis has decreased remarkably in the developed countries since tuberculostatic drugs have become available. It is, however, still a common disorder in persons with partial or complete immunodeficiency and in alcoholics, aged people, or persons suffering from malnutrition. A broad prevalence is still seen in Third World countries.

Etiology/Pathophysiology: Tuberculosis infects the lung primarily, and is an airborne infection in 80–90% of cases. Primary infection of the gut by contaminated milk (*M. bovis*) has almost completely disappeared due to adequate sterilization of the milk and extensive control of cattle.

Pulmonary infection affects the host in different ways depending on the immune status of patients:

(a) Infection of a nonsensitized, immune-competent host represents a "localized pneumonia" and may be induced by as little as three bacteria. So-called primary tuberculosis starts with a focal suppurative infection which becomes "organized" and develops into a "caseous" necrosis surrounded by multinucleated giant cells and epithelioid cells with increasing immune response of the host tissue. The bacteria usually spread into the regional lymph nodes which also develop caseous granulomas. So-called primary tuberculosis is usually a self-healing disorder. The morphological manifestation is the so-called primary complex (Ghon focus) which can be seen as a small, calcified nodule

in the middle zones of the lung and, in addition, calcified lymph nodes localized within the lymphatic drainage of the Ghon focus (Ghon complex).
(b) Infection of a nonsensitized, immune-incompetent host may develop into a progressive primary complex usually occurring in infants or children below the age of 3 years. The morphologic and physiologic equivalent is a progressive destructive pneumonia with cavity formation and transbronchial dissemination. It tends to progress into the lower lobes, induce liquefaction of the draining lymph nodes, and may cause bronchoesophageal fistulae. It usually does not spread in the "subapical localization" which is the predominant topography of "reactivated tuberculosis".
(c) Infection of a nonsensitized, immunocompromised patient with complete or nearly complete immune deficiency induces either a hematogenous dissemination (sepsis) or an extensive aerogen dissemination (consumption). Hematogenous spread into extrapulmonary organs may be clinically unsuspicious and self-healing.
(d) Reinfection of a sensitized patient may occur either by late hematogenous reinfection of the lung, or "reactivation" of the encapsulated organisms, or by repeated inhalation of the bacilli. Depending upon immune competence, the following manifestations may be observed: (a) with competent immune system, infection of the upper lobe with granulomatous reaction and organization (Simon's focus); (b) with lost immune memory with a nearly immunocompetent system, chronic or adult tuberculosis usually seen in the elderly with slowly progressive disorder; (c) in immunodeficiency, miliary tuberculosis, usually seen in alcoholics or persons with high individual susceptibility.

Clinical Presentation: Symptoms include loss of weight, mild fever, cough, dyspnea or progressive dyspnea, and signs of sepsis.

Prognosis: It has been estimated that about 90–95% of infected patients can be treated successfully; however, the mortality rate is still above 5%. The recuperation is often limited by accompanying diseases.

Radiology: Chest radiographs show various findings depending upon the status of the disease: (a) a small calcified nodule in the middle zone (Ghon focus); (b) circumscribed densities in one or both upper lobes (Simon's focus); (c) cavitation and dense infiltrations (reactivation); (d) small miliary nodules (miliary tuberculosis); (e) diffuse densities occupying one lobe or lung with inhomogeneous necrotic areas (galloping consumption).

Pathology:
Gross: The lungs contain caseous or calcified, yellowish nodules which are localized within the middle zones, apical zones, or randomly distributed throughout the lungs. Necrotic cavitations usually have a connection to the bronchi, are located in the upper zones, and measure several centimeters in diameter.

Histology: The characteristic histomorphological finding is the so-called caseous necrosis which has a central "homogeneous necrotic area with ghosts of former vascular and bronchial walls", surrounding epithelioid cells, scattered multinucleated giant cells, and numerous lymphocytes and plasma cells. Formation of well-defined, epithelioid granulomatous infiltrates is usually not seen in immunocompromised patients. Depending upon the potency of the immune system, only weak or even no granulomas may be present. Nonactive, "old" tuberculous lesions have calcified central areas surrounded by a ring of collagenous tissue without epithelioid cells or multinucleated giant cells and by only a few scattered mononuclear inflammatory cells.

➤ *Descriptors:* Lung parenchyma with altered structure:

- caseous epithelioid granulomas
- bacteria (intragranulomatous)
- multinucleated giant cells
- calcification
- mononuclear inflammatory infiltrates
- necrosis (cavitation)
- proliferating fibroblasts
- enlarged distant air spaces
- focal interstitial fibrosis
- honeycombing;
- Bronchial mucosa with altered structure:
- caseous epithelioid granulomas
- bacteria (intragranulomatous)
- multinucleated giant cells
- mononuclear inflammatory infiltrates
- necrosis (cavitation);
- Lymphatic tissue with altered structure:
- caseous epithelioid granulomas
- bacteria (intragranulomatous)

- multinucleated giant cells
- mononuclear inflammatory infiltrates
- necrosis

■ *Special stains:* PAS, collagenous stains, Giemsa, Ziehl-Neelsen, auramine, methenamine silver stain, Brown-Hopps, Brown-Brenn.

Hallmark of Diagnosis: Clinical history, caseating epithelioid granulomas, identification of the bacilli (which may be difficult due to their small number).

Differential diagnosis: Sarcoidosis, epithelioid granulomas due to other infective organisms (fungus), noninfective granulomatous disorders such as Wegener's disease, Churg-Strauss syndrome, berylliosis.

Tuberous Sclerosis

Definition: Alteration of the lung parenchyma associated with tuberous sclerosis.

Incidence/Epidemiology: Tuberous sclerosis is a progressive neuro-cutaneous syndrome with multiple, calcified nodules in the brain and ventricles and multiple sebaceous adenomas. It is seen in both men and women and is of familial occurrence with an autosomal dominant inheritance. Pulmonary involvement is seen in less than 1% of patients.

Etiology/Pathophysiology: The etiology is not known. Although it is thought to be a disorder of dominant inheritance, the sporadic cases outnumber the familial ones. In addition to the sclerosing lesions of the skin and nervous system, association with renal tumors and cardiac rhabdomyomas has been reported.

Clinical Presentation: Patients show mental retardation, epileptic seizures, and progressive dyspnea. Pneumothorax may develop.

Prognosis: Usually poor, most patients die before the age of 30 years.

Radiology: Chest radiographs show small, dense, miliary nodules with random distribution in the lungs.

Pathology:

Gross: The lungs show small cystic spaces measuring about 1–2 cm in maximum diameter surrounded by dense, grayish-white tissue (focal honeycombing).

Histology: The nodules and cystic spaces resemble those seen in lymphangioleiomyomatosis. Proliferating smooth-muscle fibers intermingled with collagenous fibers may be seen in one nodule, whereas in another the emphysematous changes may be predominant. Engorged capillaries and adenomatous foci of metaplastic pneumocytes may be present. The alterations of the lung parenchyma are usually diffuse and tend to spread from interstitial tissue to the distant air spaces.

➤ *Descriptors:* Lung parenchyma with altered structure:

- enlarged distant air spaces
- cysts
- mononuclear inflammatory infiltrates
- proliferating smooth muscle cells
- focal interstitial fibrosis
- squamous metaplasia and dysplasia of pneumocytes;
- Pulmonary vessels with preserved structure:
- tortuous vessels

■ *Special stains:* PAS, collagenous stains, Giemsa, endogenous lectins, immunohistochemistry for vimentin, desmin, desmoplakin, keratin, endothelial cells.

Hallmark of Diagnosis: Clinical history, miliary nodules consisting of smooth muscle fibers and collagen.

Differential diagnosis: Lymphangioleiomyomatosis, leiomyosarcoma, benign metastasizing leiomyoma, diffuse leiomyomatosis of the lung.

Tularemia

Definition: Infection of the lung by the gram-negative bacterium *Francisella tularensis*.

Incidence/Epidemiology: Human infection with *F. tularensis* usually occurs upon contact with infected or contaminated rodents or insects.

Etiology/Pathophysiology: Tularemia is usually a serious infection which may show five different forms: (a) ulceroglandular infection with a papulomatous ulcer of the skin and regional lymphadenitis; (b) oculoglandular infection (Parinaud's conjunctivitis) with small, yellowish nodules in the conjunctiva and cervical lymphadenitis; (c) glandular infection without detectable localization of the infection; (d) septicemic infection with involvement of the lungs, liver, kidneys, central nervous system, and meninges; (e) glandular-pharyngeal infection with involvement of the oral cavity and pharynx.

Clinical Presentation: Symptoms include high fever after an incubation period of 1–3 days, malaise, chills, dyspnea, and cough.

Prognosis: Usually good and without serious sequelae; about 5% of untreated patients will die.

Radiology: Chest radiographs show multiple, patchy densities with a lobar pattern of consolidation.

Pathology:

Gross: The lungs show several areas of pink color with increased density, fibrin deposits, and hemorrhagic necrosis.

Histology: The distant airways are filled with debris, fibrin, dense neutrophilic granulocytes, erythrocytes, lymphocytes, and plasma cells. Fresh thromboses may be present in the small arteries and veins which are usually located in the center of the necrotic areas. A granulomatous reaction of the lung parenchyma may be present, but multinucleated giant cells are usually absent.

➤ *Descriptors:* Lung parenchyma with altered structure:

- necrosis and hemorrhage
- mixed inflammatory infiltrates
- caseous epithelioid granulomas (ill-defined);
- Pulmonary vessels with preserved structure:
- thrombosis (in small arteries)

■ *Special stains:* PAS, collagenous stains, Giemsa, Warthin-Starry stain, methenamine silver stain, GMS.

Hallmark of Diagnosis: Clinical history, necrotizing bacterial pneumonia with vasculitis and thrombosis, immunofluorescence.

Differential diagnosis: Other bacterial infections, especially anthrax, plague.

Tumorlet

Definition: Small neoplastic proliferation with infiltrative microscopic appearance mimicking carcinoids.

Incidence/Epidemiology: The incidence of tumorlets depends upon the accuracy of analysis of the lung parenchyma due to their small size. The rate of tumorlets has been suggested to range between 10–20% of all autopsied persons. They have been observed more frequently in women. They usually occur in middle-aged to elderly persons.

Etiology/Pathophysiology: Tumorlets are considered to be foci of hyperplastic neuroepithelial cells (APUD-like cells) associated with the epithelium of small bronchi or bronchioles. A relationship between tumorlets and other types of bronchial carcinoma has not been observed so far.

Clinical Presentation: The tumors do not cause clinical symptoms.

Prognosis: Accidental findings, no influence on prognosis or mortality.

Radiology: The tumors are not detectable on chest radiographs.

Pathology:

Gross: The tumors measure 1–4 mm in maximum diameter and may be visible on lung examination as small, grayish nodules.

Histology: The tumors are composed of small tumor cells with a moderate amount of eosinophilic cytoplasm and fairly uniform, round nuclei. The nuclei have finely dispersed chromatin, and mitoses are usually not detectable. Inflammatory response of host tissue is absent as well as necrotic areas or hemorrhage. They usually grow within the distant air spaces and may show a central fibrosis. The cell type and growth pattern of the tumors resemble those of carcinoids.

➤ *Descriptors:* Newly formed textures without metastasis potential:

- epithelial growth pattern
- solid textures
- endocrine textures
- small tumor cells
- homogeneous nuclear and cellular size
- absent or infrequent mitoses
- finely distributed nuclear chromatin
- absent inflammatory infiltrates

■ *Special stains:* PAS, Giemsa, immunohistochemistry for neuroendocrine markers, endogenous lectins, DNA analysis.

Hallmark of Diagnosis: Tumors of small size with neuroendocrine (carcinoid) appearance and staining characteristics.

Differential diagnosis: Carcinoid, hyperplasia of basal cells or Kulchitsky's cells, pulmonary chemodectoma.

Tungsten Carbide

Definition: Alteration of the lung parenchyma associated with exposure to tungsten carbide.

Incidence/Epidemiology: Tungsten carbide, a metal of extreme hardness and heat resistance, is widely used in the machine tool industry especially for dental and other drills. Additional metals in the tungsten carbide matrix include titanium, tantalum, and vanadium. "Hard metal disease" is seen in dental technicians and persons employed in the machine tool industry. Persons suffering from hard metal lung are at increased risk of lung cancer.

Etiology/Pathophysiology: The tungsten carbide crystals measure 1–2 μm in length and are usually deposited in the distant airways. Tungsten carbide itself is considered to have no or only weak fibrogenic potency. The fibrotic changes in the lung parenchyma seen in persons exposed to tungsten carbide are assumed to be induced by the admixture of cobalt.

Clinical Presentation: Symptoms include progressive shortness of breath during exercise, cough, and dyspnea.

Prognosis: Fair, as slow progressive respiratory failure is often seen.

Radiology: Chest radiographs show diffuse or patchy, bilateral densities.

Pathology:

Gross: The lungs show diffuse fibrosis of mild to moderate degree with focal honeycombing.

Histology: The distant airways are filled with dust-laden macrophages. The predominant histomorphological image is related to desquamative interstitial pneumonia (DIP) or giant cell interstitial pneumonia (GIP). The interalveolar septula are widened and contain a moderate number of mononuclear inflammatory cells and a moderate amount of collagen. Hyperplasia and hypertrophy of the cells of the alveolar lining may be seen as well as cuboidal metaplasia. Epithelioid granulomas as seen in sarcoidosis are not a feature of tungsten-carbide-related changes.

➤ *Descriptors:* Lung parenchyma with preserved structure:

- macrophages (dust laden)
- multinucleated giant cells
- desquamation, hypertrophy, hyperplasia and dysplasia of pneumocytes;
- Lung parenchyma with altered structure:
- diffuse interstitial fibrosis (mild)

■ *Special stains:* PAS, collagenous stains, Giemsa, X-ray diffraction or related physical techniques, endogenous lectins.

Hallmark of Diagnosis: Clinical history, identification of tungsten carbide and cobalt in the lung.

Differential diagnosis: Desquamative interstitial pneumonia due to other agents.

Tween

Definition: Alteration of the lung parenchyma associated with intake of tween, see Drug Toxicity.

Typhoid Fever

Definition: Alteration of the lung parenchyma associated with infection by *Salmonella*.

Incidence/Epidemiology: Involvement of the lung parenchyma associated with typhoid fever is an unusual disorder. However, development of a lung abscess caused by *S. typhi* or *paratyphi* may occur even years after the initial infection.

Etiology/Pathophysiology: The organisms may induce either acute pulmonary infection (pneumonia) and abscess formation or may reinfect the lung many years after the initial outbreak of the disease. The late recurrence may be due to reactivation of dormant organisms or to a second exposure to *Salmonella*.

Clinical Presentation: Symptoms include suppurative expectoration, cough, dyspnea, chest pain, and malaise.

Prognosis: Usually good. The mortality rate is 2–4%; death occurs most frequently in infants or patients with severe underlying diseases such as malnutrition or decreased immune defence.

Radiology: Chest radiographs show either circumscribed, necrotizing nodules or diffuse intraalveolar and interstitial densities.

Pathology:

Gross: The lungs are heavy, edematous, and reddish-grayish and may show hemorrhagic necrotic areas of various sizes.

Histology: The lung parenchyma is destroyed and invaded by granulocytes, lymphocytes, and plasma cells. Extravasation of erythrocytes and suppurative detritus is present. In addition, mononuclear angiitis and suppurative bronchitis may be seen.

➤ *Descriptors:* Lung parenchyma with altered structure:

- necrosis and hemorrhage
- mixed inflammatory infiltrates;
- Bronchial mucosa with preserved structure:
- mixed inflammatory infiltrates
- fibrinoid material;
- Pulmonary vessels with preserved structure:
- mononuclear inflammatory infiltrates

■ *Special stains:* PAS, collagenous stains, Giemsa.

Hallmark of Diagnosis: Clinical history, histomorphologic findings of bacterial abscessing pneumonia and bronchopneumonia.

Differential diagnosis: Abscess formation and bacterial pneumonia due to other organisms.

Uranium

Definition: Alteration of the lung parenchyma associated with exposure to uranium.

Incidence/Epidemiology: Uranium miners (Schneeberg, Erzgebirge) have been found to have an increased risk of lung cancer and development of radiation pneumonitis. Similar observations have been reported in miners working in Joachimsthal and in miners exposed to other radioactive metals such as plutonium.

Etiology/Pathophysiology: The toxicity of uranium is related to its long decay chain with the emission of several radioactive particles including α, β, and γ emission. All types of malignant tumours can be induced by exposure to radioactive substances, especially adenocarcinoma (but also bronchioloalveolar carcinoma, epidermoid carcinoma, small cell anaplastic carcinoma, hemangiosarcoma and lymphosarcoma).

Clinical Presentation: Symptoms include cough, dyspnea, chest pain, loss of weight, and malaise.

Prognosis: Fair; exposed persons usually show slow progression of respiratory failure. The risk of developing bronchial carcinoma is 10–20 times the risk for a nonsmoker population.

Radiology: Chest radiographs show diffuse interstitial infiltrates or circumscribed densities.

Pathology:

Gross: The lungs have an increased consistency and may show honeycombing or a circumscribed tumor mass.

Histology: The fibrotic changes are described under the heading Radiation. They include hyperplasia and hypertrophy of cells of the alveolar lining, mononuclear interstitial infiltrates, diffuse fibrosis, desquamative interstitial pneumonia, and exudation of fibrinoid substances. The specific tumour cell types are described under the particular headings.

➤ *Descriptors:* Lung parenchyma with preserved structure:

- desquamation, hypertrophy, hyperplasia and dysplasia of pneumocytes
- mononuclear inflammatory infiltrates
- macrophages
- intraalveolar fibrinoid material;
- Lung parenchyma with altered structure:
- proliferating fibroblasts
- diffuse interstitial fibrosis
- enlarged distant air spaces
- honeycombing

■ *Special stains:* PAS, collagenous stains, Giemsa, immunohistochemistry for the different tumor cell types, endogenous lectins, DNA analysis, X-ray diffraction or related physical techniques.

Hallmark of Diagnosis: Clinical history, measurement of the radioactivity of the lung, identification of uranium.

Differential diagnosis: Desquamative interstitial pneumonia, usual interstitial pneumonia, organizing pneumonia, interstitial fibrosis or lung cancer associated with other agents.

Urbach-Wiethe Syndrome

Definition: Alteration of the lung parenchyma associated with hyalinosis (and lipoidosis) cutis et mucosae.

Incidence/Epidemiology: Unusual disorder with autosomal recessive inheritance.

Etiology/Pathophysiology: The disorder is characterized by deposits of lipoproteins in the submucosa of the esophagus, upper respiratory tract, and skin. So-called lipid proteinosis may also involve the trachea and major bronchi.

Clinical Presentation: Symptoms include hoarseness, cough, and asthmatic complaints.

Skin papules, dental abnormalities, and symmetric calcifications in the region of the sella turcica are observed..

Prognosis: Usually good; the disease is compatible with long life.

Radiology: Chest radiographs are usually normal.

Pathology:

Gross: The walls of the trachea, larynx, and major bronchi are thickened, and the lumen may be obliterated.

Histology: The mucosa of the trachea and major bronchi may undergo squamous metaplasia with atypias. The submucosa shows deposits of hyaline substances with intermingled foamy macrophages replacing the submucosal glands and smooth muscle fibers.

➤ *Descriptors:* Bronchial mucosa with altered structure:

- hyaline material (submucosa)
- macrophages (foamy)
- squamous metaplasia and dysplasia

■ *Special stains:* PAS, Giemsa, Congo, oil red O.

Hallmark of Diagnosis: Clinical history, deposits of lipoprotein in the submucosa of the major conducting airways.

Differential diagnosis: Amyloidosis, bronchial gland adenoma, hyalinosis.

Uremic Lung

Definition: Alteration of the lung parenchyma associated with renal failure.

Incidence/Epidemiology: The changes of the lung parenchyma seen in patients with renal failure are also seen in patients with left ventricular failure from essential hypertension or in patients with acute rheumatic fever. Alteration of the lung parenchyma associated with these disorders is not infrequent.

Etiology/Pathophysiology: The changes are now recognized as a specific form of pulmonary edema (chronic pulmonary edema) which is induced by disturbance of the colloid-osmotic pressure or of the physical pressure in the arteries. Deficient fibrinolysis or other (toxic) factors may also be involved.

Clinical Presentation: Symptoms include progressive dyspnea, cough, chest pain, and renal and cardiac insufficiency. Increased agitation and restlessness usually precede sudden paroxysmal dyspnea.

Prognosis: Fair; patients usually show slow progressive respiratory failure.

Radiology: Chest radiographs show bilateral, perihilar, "butterfly" or "batwing"-like interstitial densities.

Pathology:

Gross: The lungs are heavy, rubbery in consistency, and bluish-red.

Histology: The alveoli are filled with fibrinoid deposits intermingled with macrophages and histiocytes. Formation of hyaline membranes and interstitial edema are present as well as intraalveolar, hemosiderin-laden macrophages. The early stages are characterized by a proteinaceous fluid within the distant airways, which is reabsorbed or organized in the later stages. Fibrosis and honeycombing may be the end-stage.

➤ *Descriptors:* Lung parenchyma with preserved structure:

- intraalveolar serous fluid
- interstitial edema
- intraalveolar fibrinoid material
- macrophages (hemosiderin-laden)
- hyaline membranes
- mononuclear inflammatory infiltrates;
- Lung parenchyma with altered structure:
- focal interstitial fibrosis
- enlarged distant air spaces
- honeycombing

■ *Special stains:* PAS, collagenous stains, Giemsa, Prussian blue.

Hallmark of Diagnosis: Clinical history, chronic pulmonary edema.

Differential diagnosis: Usual interstitial pneumonia, pulmonary congestion, bacterial pneumonia, congenital edema, adult respiratory distress syndrome, hyaline membrane syndrome.

Usual Interstitial Pneumonia

Definition: Chronic interstitial pneumonia with characteristic histomorphologic findings (synonyms, cryptogenic fibrosing alveolitis, idiopathic pulmonary fibrosis, Hamman-Rich syndrome, organizing interstitial pneumonia, chronic interstitial pneumonia, acute diffuse interstitial pulmonary fibrosis, bronchiolar emphysema, and muscular cirrhosis of the lung), see also Idiopathic Interstitial Fibrosis.

Incidence/Epidemiology: Usual interstitial pneumonia (UIP) is the most common histomorphological type of the chronic interstitial pneumonias. It occurs most frequently in middle-aged to elderly patients with equal sex distribution.

Etiology/Pathophysiology: The etiology is not known. The pathogenesis includes various stages of acute lung damage and repair mechanisms. Humoral factors, rheumatoid factors, nuclear-specific antibodies, cryoglobulins, chemotactic factors, and alterations in cell-mediated immune response mechanisms are probably involved.

Clinical Presentation: Symptoms include insidious onset of cough, dyspnea, hyperpnea, loss of weight, pleuritic chest pain, and progressive shortness of breath during exercise. Additionally, episodes of pneumonia are frequent.

Prognosis: Usually poor, most patients evolve honeycombing within weeks or a period of years, and seldom survive longer than 5 years.

Radiology: Chest radiographs show bilateral, diffuse or reticulonodular densities with accentuation at the basal lung zones. A patchy, ground-glass pattern may be present. Late stages may suggest honeycombing.

Pathology:

Gross: Both lungs show dense fibrotic zones with enlarged cystic areas intermingled with normal-appearing lung parenchyma. Emphysematous changes may predominate. Some lungs may show large areas of fibrosis and fibrotic nodules.

Histology: The distant airways contain clusters of fibrinoid material which is intermingled with histiocytes and surrounded by macrophages or hyperplastic cells of the alveolar lining. The differentiation between the former air spaces and the former interstitial tissue is not possible. Young and old collagen fibers mark the older lesions which may, in addition, coalesce to larger zones. Lymphocytes and plasma cells are localized within the still recognizable interalveolar septula. The noninvolved lung zones are completely normal and display neither hyperplasia and hypertrophy of pneumocytes nor recognizable interstitial changes. The end-stage is honeycombing.

➤ *Descriptors:* Lung parenchyma with preserved structure:

- intraalveolar serous fluid
- desquamation, hypertrophy, hyperplasia and dysplasia of pneumocytes
- hyaline membranes
- mononuclear inflammatory infiltrates;
- Lung parenchyma with altered structure:
- proliferating fibroblasts
- mononuclear inflammatory infiltrates
- focal interstitial fibrosis
- enlarged distant air spaces
- honeycombing

■ *Special stains:* PAS, collagenous stains, Giemsa, endogenous lectins.

Hallmark of Diagnosis: Clinical history, histomorphologic changes with organizing pneumonia, fibrosis, emphysema, normal lung zones, and interstitial mononuclear infiltrates.

Differential diagnosis: Bacterial pneumonia, desquamative interstitial pneumonia, viral pneumonia, bronchioloalveolar carcinoma, adult respiratory distress syndrome.

Vanadium Lung

Definition: Alteration of the lung parenchyma associated with exposure to vanadium.

Incidence/Epidemiology: Persons exposed to vanadium work in vanadium mines, which are mainly located in South Africa, USSR, USA, and Peru, or work close to oil-fired boilers, heat exchangers or gas turbines. Vanadium pentoxide is also used as a catalyst for producing sulfuric acid. The majority of steel material contain admixtures of vanadium.

Etiology/Pathophysiology: Vanadium is considered to have a nonfibrogenic potency. Vanadium fumes do not usually induce long-lasting pulmonary effects. An increased risk of lung cancer has not been found.

Clinical Presentation: Symptoms include cough, wheezing, and chest pain.

Prognosis: Usually good and without serious sequelae.

Radiology: Chest radiographs are normal.

Pathology:

Gross: The trachea and the major bronchi are reddish and may contain increased amounts of mucus. No other changes have been reported.

Histology: The histomorphologic findings are consistent with acute bronchitis and acute pneumonitis, usually with a desquamative component. The changes are completely reversible.

➤ *Descriptors:* Lung parenchyma with preserved structure:
- intraalveolar serous fluid
- mononuclear inflammatory infiltrates
- macrophages;
- Bronchial mucosa with preserved structure:
- viscous mucus
- increased number of goblet cells
- mononuclear inflammatory infiltrates

■ *Special stains:* PAS, Giemsa, X-ray diffraction or related physical techniques.

Hallmark of Diagnosis: Clinical history, acute bronchitis, identification of vanadium in the peripheral lung zones.

Differential diagnosis: Acute bronchitis and bronchopneumonia due to other agents.

Vanishing Lung

Definition: Term synonymous with panacinar emphysema, see Emphysema, Panacinar.

Varicella Zoster

Definition: Infection of the lung parenchyma by herpes virus V-Z, see Chickenpox.

Vasculitis

Definition: Inflammation of intrapulmonary vessels associated with infectious or inflammatory disorders of the lung.

Incidence/Epidemiology: The pulmonary vessels may be involved in association with various pulmonary disorders. Vasculitis is seen in Rocky Mountain spotted fever, drug abuse, polyarteritis nodosa, radiation pneumonitis, pulmonary hypertension, scleroderma, or lupus erythematosus, in about 20–50% of cases with pulmonary tuberculosis, pulmonary histoplasmosis, fungal and mycobacterial pneumonias, and *Pseudomonas* pneumonia. Vasculitis is of diagnostic significance in other disorders, especially Wegener's disease, Churg-Strauss syndrome, lymphomatoid granulomatosis, and necrotizing sarcoid-like granulomatosis.

Etiology/Pathophysiology: The inflammatory vascular infiltrates may be induced by intravascular thrombi contaminated with infectious organisms, by antigenic properties of the vascular walls, especially of the basal membranes or endothelial cells, or by extensive surrounding inflammation. These various pathways can be differentiated to some degree by analyzing the appearance of vessels inside, at the boundary of, and outside the center of the specific lesion.

Clinical Presentation: Symptoms are usually related to the changes in the pulmonary parenchyma and not to the involvement of the vessels.

Prognosis: Usually good, depending upon the underlying disease.

Radiology: Chest radiographs are usually not related to the presence or absence of vasculitis.

Pathology:

Gross: The gross alterations of the lung parenchyma are related to the general morphologic changes of the lung.

Histology: The walls of small and medium-sized arteries show an invasion of mononuclear inflammatory infiltrates which destroy the lamina elastica interna and externa and degrade the regular order of collagen fibers. Granulocytic inflammatory infiltrates and infarctlike necrosis of the vascular walls indicate bacterial infection or superinfection. Granulomatous vasculitis indicates a delayed immunoresponse. Thrombotic lesions are usually secondary to the primary inflammation.

➤ *Descriptors:* Pulmonary vessels with altered structure:
- mononuclear inflammatory infiltrates
- mixed inflammatory infiltrates
- caseous epithelioid granulomas
- noncaseous epithelioid granulomas
- fragmentation of elastic fibers
- thrombosis;
- Lung parenchyma with altered structure:
- necrosis and hemorrhage
- mononuclear inflammatory infiltrates
- palisading histiocytes
- proliferating fibroblasts
- focal interstitial fibrosis
- enlarged distant air spaces
- honeycombing

- *Special stains:* PAS, collagenous stains, Giemsa.

Hallmark of Diagnosis: Clinical history, inflammation of the vascular walls.

Differential diagnosis: Depends on the underlying disorder.

VATER

Definition: Congenital malformations (vertebral, anal, tracheo-esophageal, renal), see Congenital Abnormalities.

Vegetable Dust Lung

Definition: Alteration of the lung parenchyma associated with exposure to vegetable dust.

Incidence/Epidemiology: Persons exposed to the following vegetable dusts may develop pulmonary symptoms: hay, grain, silage, sugar cane, mushroom, cork, barley, wood, maple, cheese, oak, cedar, mahogany, paprika, coffee, tea, tobacco, and other plants. The risk of pulmonary abnormalities increases with increasing temperature and humidity of the environment.

Etiology/Pathophysiology: Most of the reported changes of the lung parenchyma are induced by fungal contaminations and subsequent hypersensitivity reaction of the lung as described under the heading Allergic (Extrinsic) Alveolitis.

Clinical Presentation: Symptoms are either acute or may show an insidious onset and a chronic stage.

Prognosis: Usually good and without serious sequelae.

Radiology: Chest radiographs usually show diffuse, bilateral interstitial infiltrates or fine granular densities.

Pathology:

Gross: The lungs are heavy, rubbery in consistency, and edematous.

Histology: The histomorphologic features cover a broad spectrum and include mononuclear interstitial inflammatory infiltrates, pleural fibrosis, usual interstitial pneumonia, noncaseating granulomas, eosinophilic infiltration, bronchiolitis obliterans, interstitial edema, desquamative interstitial pneumonia, giant cell interstitial pneumonia, and angiitis.

➤ *Descriptors:* Lung parenchyma with altered structure:
- noncaseous epithelioid granulomas
- eosinophils
- multinucleated giant cells
- intrabronchiolar fibrinoid material and histiocytes
- ulceration of bronchiolar mucosa;
- Lung parenchyma with preserved structure:
- macrophages
- desquamation, hypertrophy, hyperplasia and dysplasia of pneumocytes
- mononuclear inflammatory infiltrates
- intraalveolar serous fluid

- *Special stains:* PAS, collagenous stains, Giemsa, immunohistochemistry for immunoglobulins and lymphocytic subpopulations, endogenous lectins.

Hallmark of Diagnosis: Clinical history, histomorphologic findings consistent with allergic extrinsic pneumonitis.

Differential diagnosis: According to the predominant histomorphologic features.

Veno-occlusive Disease

Definition: Occlusive changes of the small and medium-sized venous vessels due to different causes and associated with pulmonary hypertension.

Incidence/Epidemiology: Children and young adults (below the age of 16 years) are the most frequent victims of venous occlusive disease. Men are more often affected than women. The overall incidence is difficult to estimate, because a broad variety of agents can induce venous occlusive disease.

Etiology/Pathophysiology: Hypertrophy of the media and intimal fibrosis are induced by several agents including viral infection, chemotherapy, and toxic substances. The primary morphologic changes are probably thrombotic lesions which are followed by intimal fibrosis and hypertrophy of the muscular wall.

Clinical Presentation: Patients suffer from progressive dyspnea usually with preceding flu-like infections, cough, and syncope.

Prognosis: Fair, slow progressive pulmonary hypertension can cause death after a few years, although some exceptional cases with complete or partial reversibility have been reported.

Radiology: Chest radiographs show enlarged pulmonary arteries, Kerley's A and B lines, and possible pleural effusions.

Pathology:

Gross: The medium-sized pulmonary veins and the small arteries are occluded by old, organized thrombotic lesions and show surrounding fibrosis. The interlobar septa are thickened and fibrotic.

Histology: The small and medium-sized veins contain old, organized thrombi with complete occlusion of the lumen. Additional concentric and excentric intimal fibrosis and usually mild hypertrophy of the media are present. The distant air spaces contain hemosiderin-laden macrophages clustering around the occluded veins. The small arteries exhibit various degrees of medial hypertrophy. Angiitic lesions are not associated with veno-occlusive disease. The interalveolar septula may show a foreign-body reaction with inclusion of multinucleated giant cells, encrusted deposits of iron-containing proteins, and fibrosis.

➤ *Descriptors:* Pulmonary vessels with preserved structure:
- thrombosis (in small and medium sized veins)
- recanalization (partial)
- intimal fibrosis;
- Lung parenchyma with preserved structure:
- macrophages (hemosiderin-laden)

■ *Special stains:* PAS, collagenous stains, Giemsa, Prussian blue, endogenous lectins.

Hallmark of Diagnosis: Clinical history (pulmonary hypertension), chronic occlusion of small and medium-sized veins, associated changes in small arteries.

Differential diagnosis: Idiopathic pulmonary hemosiderosis, primary pulmonary hypertension, occlusion of major pulmonary veins, thromboembolic disorders.

Vermiculite

Definition: Alteration of the lung parenchyma associated with inhalation of vermiculite fibers, see Nonasbestos Mineral Fibers.

Vinblastine

Definition: Alteration of the lung parenchyma associated with intake of vinblastine, see Drug Toxicity.

Viral Infection

Definition: Infection of the lung by virus.

Incidence/Epidemiology: Viral infections of the lung are a frequent disorder, although pulmonary viral infections seen by pathologists are usually rare and limited to newborns, infants, children, aged persons, and immunocompromised patients. Viral pneumonias in newborns are often caused by enterovirus, echovirus, coxsackievirus, or adenovirus.

Etiology/Pathophysiology: Viruses may infect the lung directly via the conducting airways or may be transferred to the lung by viremia. Some viruses such as herpes or measles enter the body via the terminal air spaces but seldom induce infections of the lung. A considerable number of viral agents infect the lower respiratory tract, including adenovirus, Epstein-Barr virus, influenza A and B viruses, cytomegalovirus, parainfluenzavirus, and rhinovirus.

Clinical Presentation: Symptoms are usually abrupt and include high fever, headache, malaise, cough, and dyspnea.

Prognosis: Usually good and self-limited; however, infections of immunocompromised patients may be life-threatening.

Radiology: Chest radiographs show patchy or diffuse interstitial densities with patterns that indicate alveolar involvement.

Pathology:

Gross: The lungs are heavy, reddish, and of increased consistency resembling segmental bacterial pneumonia.

Histology: The histomorphologic findings vary widely. Depending upon the particular virus, any of the following changes may be seen: adenovirus, influenza, parainfluenza, rhinovirus, herpes, measles, and respiratory syncytial virus cause bronchiolitis, hemorrhagic mononuclear pneumonitis, and necrotizing pneumonitis. Chronic interstitial pneumonitis with diffuse alveolar damage may also be seen in pulmonary viral infections which can be induced by cytomegalovirus. Nuclear inclusion bodies are most characteristic in cytomegaloviral infections and less intensive in influenzavirus infections. Other histomorphologic findings include bronchiolitis obliterans, eosinophilic inflammatory infiltrates, thrombotic occlusions and intimal fibrosis of small veins, alveolar hemorrhage, hyaline membrane formation, and organizing pneumonia.

➤ *Descriptors:* Lung parenchyma with preserved structure:
- desquamation, hypertrophy, hyperplasia and dysplasia of pneumocytes (inclusion bodies)
- intraalveolar serous fluid
- hyaline membranes
- mononuclear inflammatory infiltrates;
- Lung parenchyma with altered structure:
- necrosis and hemorrhage
- eosinophils
- intrabronchiolar fibrinoid material and histiocytes
- ulceration of bronchiolar mucosa

■ *Special stains:* PAS, Giemsa, immunofluorescence, in situ hybridization.

Hallmark of Diagnosis: Clinical history, identification of the virus by virologic diagnosis, and corresponding histomorphologic findings.

Differential diagnosis: Toxic reaction of the lung parenchyma, bronchioloalveolar carcinoma, usual interstitial pneumonia, desquamative interstitial pneumonia, idiopathic hemosiderosis, bacterial pneumonia.

Visciodol

Definition: Alteration of the lung parenchyma associated with intake of visciodol, see Drug Toxicity.

Vitamin D

Definition: Alteration of the lung parenchyma associated with intake of vitamin D, see Drug Toxicity.

Volcanic Ash Lung

Definition: Alteration of the lung parenchyma associated with inhalation of volcanic ash.

Incidence/Epidemiology: Eruption of volcanic mountains such as Mount St. Helens in 1980 or Mount Pinatubo in 1991 may expose a large population to ash consisting of amorphous silicates, iron oxide, aluminum oxide, quartz, and related components. The eruption of a volcano may distribute the dust particles over hundreds of miles.

Etiology/Pathophysiology: The toxic effects of volcanic ash depend upon their concentration in the air and are considered to be negligible if they do not exceed 10 mg of dust/m^3 of air. Higher concentrations have a fibrogenic potential as shown in animal experiments. The fibrogenic potential is usually directly related to the concentration of quartz.

Clinical Presentation: Symptoms are related to the dust concentration in the inhaled air and include dyspnea, cough, and acute respiratory distress. In addition, death has been reported due to blockage of the conducting airways by dust-laden mucus.

Prognosis: Usually good; depending upon the amount of inhaled ash, slow progressive respiratory failure may develop.

Radiology: Chest radiographs show diffuse or patchy, intraalveolar densities.

Pathology:

Gross: The lungs are heavy, edematous, and dark-grayish.

Histology: The alveoli are filled with dust-laden macrophages. The major bronchi contain dark, viscous mucus. Acute inflammatory infiltrations are present in the bronchial walls and in the interstitial tissue.

➤ *Descriptors:* Lung parenchyma with preserved structure:
- dust
- macrophages (dust-laden)
- mononuclear inflammatory infiltrates;
- Bronchial mucosa with preserved structure:
- viscous mucus (dark color)
- mixed inflammatory infiltrates

■ *Special stains:* PAS, Giemsa, Prussian blue, polarization, X-ray diffraction or related physical techniques.

Hallmark of Diagnosis: Clinical history, acute inflammation of conducting airways, and acute pneumonitis with abnormal dust concentration.

Differential diagnosis: Acute bronchitis and pneumonitis due to other agents.

Waldenström's, Macroglobulinemia

Definition: Alteration of the lung parenchyma associated with Waldenström's macroglobulinemia, see Macroglobulinemia of Waldenström.

Weber-Christian Disease

Definition: Panniculitis nodularis (relapsing panniculitis). The disease has been associated with lymphocytic angiitis and granulomatosis, see Lymphocytic Angiitis and Granulomatosis, Benign.

Wegener's Granulomatosis

Definition: Pulmonary lesions characterized by necrotizing granulomatous inflammation combined with severe vasculitis.

Incidence/Epidemiology: Unusual disorder seen in children older than 10 years and in adults of any age. The majority of patients are over 50 years old, and the sex ratio shows a slight predominance of women.

Etiology/Pathophysiology: The etiology is still not known. The presence of vasculitis and granulomatosis suggests the involvement of the cell-mediated immune system, especially the presence of autoimmune antibodies against neutrophils. Wegener's granulomatosis is a multisystemic disorder involving the upper respiratory tract (nose, paranasal sinus), the kidneys (glomerulitis), and the lung. Other organs that may be involved include the eyes, ears, skin, and central and peripheral nervous systems.

Clinical Presentation: Symptoms include ulceration of the nose, cough, hemoptysis, chest pain, fever, or renal failure.

Prognosis: Fair, as modern immunosuppressive treatment has been very effective in controlling the disease; however, recurrences are frequent, and death may occur due to the cytotoxic drugs.

Radiology: Chest radiographs show multiple, often bilateral, dense nodules of various sizes which are frequently cavitated. The sizes range from a few millimeters to some centimeters in maximum diameter.

Pathology:

Gross: The lungs show multiple irregularly shaped, necrotic areas with hemorrhage. The surrounding "healthy" lung parenchyma is usually pink and of increased consistency.

Histology: The lesions consist of two characteristic histomorphological features, (a) irregularly shaped infarctlike necrosis which still shows the "ruins" of the arterial walls in the center. The boundary is composed of polymorphous inflammatory cells with intermingled multinucleated giant cells and palisading histiocytes. (b) Transmural inflammation of the arterial walls of small and medium-sized vessels localized in the periphery and outside the major foci. The inflammatory cells comprise neutrophilic granulocytes, lymphocytes, plasma cells, histiocytes, and rarely multinucleated giant cells. Additional findings include pulmonary hemorrhage, chronic bronchiolitis with occasional multinucleated giant cells, obstructive pneumonitis, and moderate interstitial fibrosis close to the necrotic areas.

➤ *Descriptors:* Lung parenchyma with altered structure:

- necrosis and hemorrhage
- palisading histiocytes
- multinucleated giant cells
- mixed inflammatory infiltrates
- proliferating fibroblasts
- focal interstitial fibrosis;
- Pulmonary vessels with altered structure:
- mixed inflammatory infiltrates
- multinucleated giant cells;
- Bronchial mucosa with preserved structure:
- mononuclear inflammatory infiltrates (small bronchi)

■ *Special stains:* PAS, collagenous stains, Giemsa, immunohistochemistry for immunoglobulins and lymphocytic subpopulations, endogenous lectins.

Hallmark of Diagnosis: Clinical history, necrotizing vasculitis and granulomatosis.

Differential diagnosis: Infectious granulomatous disorders such as those of fungus or parasites, other forms of pulmonary angiitis and granulomatosis (allergic angiitis and granulomatosis, necrotizing sarcoid-like granulomatosis, lymphomatoid granulomatosis, bronchocentric granulomatosis).

Wegener's Limited Granulomatosis

Definition: Wegener's granulomatosis without involvement of the upper respiratory tract and clinical glomerulitis.

Incidence/Epidemiology: It has been estimated that about 40–50% of all patients with Wegener's granulomatosis can be classified as belonging to the "limited group".

Etiology/Pathophysiology: Similar to that suggested for Wegener's granulomatosis.

Clinical Presentation: Symptoms are related to the pulmonary involvement, possibly to lesions of the skin and of the gastrointestinal tract.

Prognosis: The prognosis of patients with limited Wegener's granulomatosis is more favorable than that of patients with Wegener's granulomatosis.

Radiology: Chest radiographs show findings of Wegener's granulomatosis.

Pathology:

Gross: The findings correspond to those of Wegener's granulomatosis.

Histology: The findings correspond to those of Wegener's granulomatosis.

➤ *Descriptors:* Lung parenchyma with altered structure:

- necrosis and hemorrhage
- palisading histiocytes
- multinucleated giant cells
- mixed inflammatory infiltrates
- proliferating fibroblasts
- focal interstitial fibrosis;
- Pulmonary vessels with altered structure:
- mixed inflammatory infiltrates
- multinucleated giant cells;
- Bronchial mucosa with preserved structure:
- mononuclear inflammatory infiltrates (small bronchi)

■ *Special stains:* PAS, collagenous stains, Giemsa, immunohistochemistry for immunoglobulins and lymphocytic subpopulations, endogenous lectins.

Hallmark of Diagnosis: Clinical history, necrotizing vasculitis and granulomatosis.

Differential diagnosis: Infectious granulomatous disorders such as those of fungus or parasites; other forms of pulmonary angiitis and granulomatosis (allergic angiitis and granulomatosis, necrotizing sarcoid-like granulomatosis, lymphomatoid granulomatosis, bronchocentric granulomatosis, Wegener's granulomatosis).

Welder's Pneumoconiosis

Definition: Alteration of the lung parenchyma seen in arc welders, see Arc Welder's Lung.

Weingarten's Syndrome

Definition: Infection of the lung with *Wuchereria bancrofti*, see Eosinophilia, Tropical Pulmonary.

Whipple's Disease

Definition: Alteration of the lung parenchyma associated with Whipple's disease.

Incidence/Epidemiology: Whipple's disease or so-called intestinal lipodystrophy may involve in addition to the small intestines other organs such as lymph nodes, serosa, and the lung parenchyma. It is most frequently seen in young to middle-aged adults.

Etiology/Pathophysiology: Whipple's disease is probably induced by bacteria (α-hemolytic streptococci?), although the final proof is still missing.

Clinical Presentation: Patients present with diarrhea, abdominal pain, loss of weight, arthralgia, polyserositis, pleurocarditis and progressive cough, which may precede the abdominal symptoms.

Prognosis: Usually good and without serious sequelae if adequate therapy is performed.

Radiology: Chest radiographs may be normal or show bilateral, peribronchiolar infiltrates, predominantly in the basal parts of the lung. An interstitial pattern may also be present.

Pathology:

Gross: The pleura has a "sunken" surface and may be covered with fibrin. The bronchial walls are thickened and stiff.

Histology: Granulomatous inflammation with characteristic macrophages are present in the walls of small bronchi and arteries, in the pleura, and in the adjacent lung parenchyma. Lymphocytes and plasma cells are seen in the periphery of the granulomas. Fibrosis, necrosis, and giant cells are not present.

➤*Descriptors:* Lung parenchyma with altered structure:

- noncaseous epithelioid granulomas
- mononuclear inflammatory infiltrates
- macrophages (large cytoplasmic granules);
- Bronchial mucosa with altered structure:
- noncaseous epithelioid granulomas
- mononuclear inflammatory infiltrates;
- Pulmonary vessels with altered structure:
- noncaseous epithelioid granulomas
- mononuclear inflammatory infiltrates;
- Pleura with altered structure:
- noncaseous epithelioid granulomas
- fibrinoid material
- mononuclear inflammatory infiltrates

■ *Special stains:* PAS, Giemsa, oil red O stain.

Hallmark of Diagnosis: Clinical history, noncaseating granulomas with characteristic "Whipple cells" which contain PAS-positive bodies in the cytoplasm.

Differential diagnosis: Malacoplakia, *Pneumocystis carinii* infection, endogenous lipid pneumonia, and storage disorders such as Niemann-Pick, Gaucher, and atypical tuberculosis (*Mycobacterium avium-intracellulare*).

Williams-Campbell Syndrome

Definition: Congenital disorder characterized by absence of cartilage in the major bronchi.

Incidence/Epidemiology: Rare congenital disorder with a few reported cases.

Etiology/Pathophysiology: The absence of bronchial cartilage (fourth to the eighth generation) induces instability of the conducting airways and consequent chronic infection with bronchiectasis, obliterative bronchiolitis, and focal emphysema. A true congenital defect in the development of the bronchial cartilage is assumed.

Clinical Presentation: Patients present with asthmatic complaints accompanied by attacks of dyspnea, cough, and chest pain.

Prognosis: Usually good, if the correct diagnosis and the adequate therapy avoid secondary infectious damage of the lung parenchyma. Spread of chronic infection into other parts of the lung may occur.

Radiology: Chest radiographs show destructive bronchitis and bronchiolitis. Poststenotic atelectasis may be the most impressive finding.

Pathology:

Gross: The involved portions of the bronchi are soft, floppy, inflamed, and ectatic and may show collapsed lumens.

Histology: Number and size of cartilaginous rings are decreased as well as the number of submucosal glands. The bronchial walls are invaded by chronic inflammatory cells. The smooth muscle cells are attenuated.

➤*Descriptors:* Bronchial mucosa with altered structure:

- absent cartilage
- decreased number of submucosal glands
- mixed inflammatory infiltrates

■ *Special stains:* PAS, collagenous stains, Giemsa.

Hallmark of Diagnosis: Clinical history, missing bronchial cartilage, bronchiectasis.

Differential diagnosis: Congenital bronchomalacia, Kartegener's syndrome, chronic obstructive bronchitis, bronchiectases due to other causes such as cystic fibrosis, impairment of the pulmonary defence mechanisms.

Wilms's Tumor

Definition: Metastasis of Wilms's tumor into the lung, see Metastases into the Lung.

Wollastonite

Definition: Alteration of the lung parenchyma associated with inhalation of wollastonite fibers, see Nonasbestos Mineral Fibers.

Woodworker's Lung

Definition: Alteration of the lung parenchyma associated with exposure to wood dust.

Incidence/Epidemiology: Acute and chronic interstitial pneumonitis has been reported in persons exposed to oak, cedar, or mahogany dust and to pine and spruce pulp.

Etiology/Pathophysiology: The alterations of the lung parenchyma associated with wood dust are thought to be induced by an allergic extrinsic alveolitis. Wood dust usually induces desquamative interstitial pneumonia (DIP).

Clinical Presentation: Symptoms include acute or insidious onset of chest pain, dyspnea, and dry cough.

Prognosis: Usually good and without serious sequelae.

Radiology: Chest radiographs show diffuse or patchy, bilateral densities.

Pathology:

Gross: The lungs are edematous and pink-reddish.

Histology: The histomorphologic findings usually show a desquamative interstitial pneumonia. However, all alterations of the lung parenchyma associated with allergic extrinsic pneumonitis may be seen such as noncaseating granulomas, lymphocytic interstitial pneumonia, usual interstitial pneumonia, eosinophilic lung and organizing pneumonia or bronchiolitis obliterans.

➤ *Descriptors:* Lung parenchyma with altered structure:

- noncaseous epithelioid granulomas
- eosinophils
- multinucleated giant cells
- intrabronchiolar fibrinoid material and histiocytes
- ulceration of bronchiolar mucosa;
- Lung parenchyma with preserved structure:
- macrophages
- desquamation, hypertrophy, hyperplasia and dysplasia of pneumocytes
- mononuclear inflammatory infiltrates
- intraalveolar serous fluid

■ *Special stains:* PAS, collagenous stains, Giemsa, immunohistochemistry for immunoglobulins and lymphocytic subpopulations, endogenous lectins.

Hallmark of Diagnosis: Clinical history, histomorphologic findings consistent with allergic extrinsic pneumonitis.

Differential diagnosis: Infectious and noninfectious granulomatous diseases, for details, see Allergic (Extrinsic) Pneumonitis.

Woolsorter's Lung

Definition: Infection of the lung by *Bacillus anthracis*, see Anthrax Pneumonia.

Zeolite Fibers

Definition: Alteration of the lung parenchyma associated with inhalation of zeolite fibers, see Nonasbestos Mineral Fibers.

Zirconium Lung

Definition: Alteration of the lung parenchyma associated with exposure to zirconium.

Incidence/Epidemiology: Zirconium is broadly used in the ceramic industry in the form of zircon (ZrO_2SiO_2), and workers may be exposed to zircon dust.

Etiology/Pathophysiology: Whereas little is known about the fibrogenic potency of zirconium in man, zircon induces noncaseating granulomas and chronic desquamative interstitial pneumonia in various species of animals. In man, application of deodorants containing zircon can induce cutaneous granulomas.

Clinical Presentation: Symptoms may include shortness of breath during exercise, dyspnea, and cough.

Prognosis: Usually good; however, details about long-term exposure are lacking.

Radiology: Chest radiographs may show diffuse, bilateral densities or fine reticulogranular nodules.

Pathology:

Gross: The lungs are of increased consistency and have a rubbery surface.

Histology: The histomorphologic changes include diffuse interstitial, mononuclear inflammatory infiltrates and noncaseating granulomas with scattered multinucleated giant cells similar to those seen in berylliosis.

➤ *Descriptors:* Lung parenchyma with altered structure:

- noncaseous epithelioid granulomas
- multinucleated giant cells
- mononuclear inflammatory infiltrates
- macrophages

■ *Special stains:* PAS, collagenous stains, Giemsa, X-ray diffraction or related physical techniques.

Hallmark of Diagnosis: Clinical history, identification of zirconium by X-ray diffraction or related physical techniques.

Differential diagnosis: Disorders inducing noncaseating granulomas or diffuse (desquamative) interstitial pneumonia.

Zygomycosis

Definition: Infection of the lung by a fungus of the order *Mucorales*, see Mucormycosis.

References

Textbooks:

Anacker H (1991) Teschendorf, Radiologische Differentialdiagnostik Lunge, Pleura, Mediastinum. Thieme, Stuttgart

Antman K, Aisner J (1987) Asbestos related malignancy. Grune & Stratton, Orlando, New York

Ash LR, Orihel TC (1984) Atlas of human parasitology. American Society of Clinical Pathologists Press, Chicago

Becker HD, Kayser K, Schulz V, Tuengerthal S, Vollhaber HH (1989) Atlas der Brocnhoskopie. Schattauer, Stuttgart

Binford CH, Connor DH (1976) Pathology of tropical and extraordinary diseases. Armed Forces Institute of Pathology, Washington DC

Carter D, Eggleston (1979) Tumors of the lower respiratory tract. Armed Forces Institute of Pathology, Washington

Clemmesen J (1977) Statistical studies in malignant neoplasms I,II,III,IV,V, Munksgaard, Kopenhagen

Colby TV, Lombard C, Yousem SA, Kitaichi M (1990) Atlas of pulmonary surgical pathology. WB Saunders, Philadelphia

Dail DH, Hammar SP (1987) Pulmonary pathology. Springer, New York, Berlin

Doerr W, Seifert G (1983) Pathologie der Lunge I und II. Springer, Berlin Heidelberg

Dunnill MS (1987) Pulmonary Pathology. Churchill Livingstone, Edinburgh, London

Edington, GM, Gilles, HM (1968) Pathology in the Tropics.Edward Arnold, London

Enzinger FM, Weiss SW (1988) Soft tissue tumors. CV Mosby, St.Louis

Fabel H (1989) Pneumologie. Urban & Schwarzenberg, München

Farnell PM, Taussig LM (1986) Bronchopulmonary dysplasia and related chronic disorders. Columbus, Ross Laboratories

Fraser RG, Pare IAP, Pare PD, Fraser RS, Genereux GP (1991) Diagnoses of diseases of the chest, Vol I, II, III, IV. WB Saunders, Philadelphia

Gabius H-J, Gabius S (1991) Lectins and cancer. Springer, Berlin Heidelberg

Gabius H-J, Nagel G (1988) Lectins and glycoconjugates in oncology. Springer, Berlin Heidelberg

Goodman LS, Gilman A (1990) The pharmacological basis of therapeutics, Pergamon, Oxford

Howard JK, Tyrer FH (1987) Textbook of occupational medicine. Churchill Livingstone, Edingburgh

Jones JSP (1987) Pathology of the mesothelium. Springer, London Berlin

Katzenstein AL, Askin FB (1990) Surgical pathology of non-neoplastic lung disease. Philadelphia, London

Kayser K (1987) Height and weight in human beings. Verlag für angewandte Wissenschaften, München

Kittle GF (1987) Mesothelioma: Diagnosis and management. Year Book Medical Publishers, Chicago, Longon

Kjeldsberg CR, Knight JA (1986) Body fluids. American Society of Clinical Pathologists Press, Chicago

Konietzko J, Dupuis H (1990) Handbuch der Arbeitsmedizin. Ecomed, Landsberg

Laraya-Cuasay LR, Hughes WT (1988) Interstitial lung diseases in children Vol I, II. CRC Press, Boca Raton

Liebow A, Smith D (1969) The lung. Williams & Wilkens, Baltimore

McKay B, Lukeman JM, Ordonez NG (1990) Tumors of the lung. Major problems in pathology, Vol 24, WB Saunders, Philadelphia

Nakhosteen JA, Niederle N, Zavala DC (1989) Atlas und Lehrbuch der Bronchoskopie. Springer, Berlin

Remington JS, Klein JO (1983) Infectious diseases of the fetus and newborn infant. WB Saunders, Philadelphia

Rippon WJ (1988) Medical Mycology, The pathogenic fungi and the pathogenic actinomyces. WB Saunders, Philadelphia

Schwarz MI, King TE (1988) Interstitial lung disease. BC Becker, Toronto

Spencer H (1985) Pathology of the lung. Pergamon, Oxford

Speissl B, Beahrs OH, Hermanek P, Hutter RVP, Scheibe O, Sobin LH, Wagner G (1990) TNM-Atlas, illustrierter Leitfaden zur TNM/pTNM Klassifikation maligner Tumoren. Springer, Berlin Heidelberg

Thurlbeck WM (1988) Pathology of the Lung. Thieme, Stuttgart, New York

Voegeli E (1990) Praktische Thoraxradiologie. Huber, Bern

Webster J (1980) Introduction to fungi. Cambridge University Press, Cambridge

Weill H, Turner-Warwick M (1981) Occupational lung diseases. Marcel Decker, New York

Wilson JD, Braunwald E, Isselbacher KJ, Petersdorf RG, Martin JB, Fauci AS, Root RK (1991) Harrison's principles of internal medicine. McGraw-Hill, New York

Selected articles

Abbondanzo SL, English CK, Kagan E, McPherson (1989) Fatal adenovirus pneumonia in a newborn identified by electron microscopy and in situ hybridisation. Arch Pathol Lab Med 113:1349-1353

Adamson JYR, Letourneau HL, Bowden DH (1991) Comparison of alveolar and interstitial macrophages in fibroblast stimulation after silica and long and short asbestos. Lab Invest 64:339-344

Adamson JYR, Young L, Bowden DH (1988) Relationship of alveolar epithelial injury and repair to the induction of pulmonary fibrosis. Am J Pathol 130:377-383

Aigner K, Schindl R (1989) Fibrosierender Lungenprozess durch TEL-Mineralwolle. Z Erkr Atmungsorgane 173:247-249

Akslen LA, Myking AO, Morkve O, Gulsvik A, Raithel HJ, Schaller KH (1990) Increased content of chromium and nickel in lung tissues from patients with bronchial carcinoma. Path Res Pract 186:717-722

Albright SG, Katz VL (1989) α-fetoprotein findings in a case of cystic adenomatoid malformation of the lung. Clin Genet 35:75-76

Alvarez-Fernandez E, Carretero-Albinana L (1990) Lectin histochemistry of normal bronchopulmonary tissues and common forms of bronchogenic carcinoma. Arch Pathol Lab Med 114:475-481

Alvarez-Fernandez E, Carretero-Albinana L, Menarguez-Palanca J (1989) Sclerosing hemangioma of the lung – an immunohistochemical study of intermediate filaments and endothelial markers. Arch Pathol Lab Med 113:121-124

Baker JW, Fistel SJ, Jones RV, Weiss RB (1990) Interstitial pneumonitis associated with ifosfamide therapy. Cancer 65:2217-2221

Balis JU, Paterson JF, Lundh JM, Haller EM, Shelley SA, Montgomery MR (1991) Ozone stress initiates acute perturbations of secreted surfactant membranes. Am J Pathol 138:847-857

Bellis D, Andrion A, Delsedime L, Mollo F (1989) Minimal pathologic changes of the lung and asbestos exposure. Hum Pathol 20:102-106

Beluffi G, Brokensha C, Kozlowski K, Lucaya J, Masel J, Morris L, Rosso R, Stronati M, Thomson R (1989) Congenital cystic adenomatoid malformation of the lung. Presentation of 16 cases. Rofo 150:523-530

Benjamin DR (1989) Herpes simplex tracheobronchitis and pneumonitis. Pediatr Pathol 9:773-777

Berger U, Khagani A, Pomerance A, Yacoub M, Coombes RC (1990) Pulmonary lymphangioleiomyomatosis and steroid receptors. Am J Clin Pathol 93:609-614

Burnett JW (1990) Berylliosis. Cutis 45:151-154

Cagle PT, Truong LD, Holland VA, Lawrence EC, Rogers BB, Schwartz MR, Kolda T, Buffone GJ, Noon GP, Greenberg SD (1989) Factors contributing to mortality in lung transplant recipients: an autopsy study. Mod Pathol 2:85-89

Cartier A, Molo JL (1990) Occupational asthma due to tea dust. Thorax 45:203-206

Chandraratnam EA, Henderson DW, Meredith DJ, Jain S (1987) Regenerative atypical squamous metaplasia in fibreoptic bronchial biopsy sites —- a lesion liable to misinterpretion as carcinoma on rebiopsy: report of 5 cases. J Pathol 19:419-424

Chiba T, Ohi R, Hayashi Y, Uchida T (1989) Bronchopulmonary foregut malformation in 3 infants – with special reference to cases in childhood. Z Kinderchir 44:105-108

Churg A, Wright JL, DePaoli L, Wiggs B (1989) Mineralogic correlates of fibrosis in chrysotile miners and millers. Am Rev Respir Dis 139:891-896

Colby T, Bilbao JE, Battifora H, Krishnan U (1989) Primary osteosarcoma of the lung – a reappraisal following immunohistochemical study. Arch Pathol Lab Med 113:1147-1150

Dillman RO, Berry C, Ryan KP, Green MR, Seagren SL (1991) Recent outcomes for patients with carcinoma of the lung. Cancer Invest 9:9-17

Drlicek M, Grisold W, Lorber J, Hackl H, Wuketich S, Jellinger K (1991) Pulmonary meningioma – immonuhistochemical and ultrastructural features. Am J Surg Pathol 15:455-459

Duarte MI, da Matta VL, Corbett CE, Laurenti MD, Chebabo R, Goto H (1989) Interstitial pneumonitis in human visceral leishmaniasis. Trans R Soc Trop Med Hyg 83:73-76

Dunnill MS (1990) Pulmonary fibrosis. Histopathology 16:321-329

Egen MJ, Crocker J (1990) Evaluation of nuclear organizer region in pulmonary pathology. Thorax 45:225-232

Elsasser S, Dalquen P, Soler M, Perruchoud AP (1989) Methotrexate-induced pneumonitis: appearance four weeks after discontinuitation of treatment. Am Rev Respir Dis 140:1089-1092

Fauci AS, Schnittmann SM, Poli G, Koenig S, Pantaleo G (1991) Immunopathogenic mechanisms in human immunodeficiency virus (HIV) infection. Ann Int Med 114:678-693

Fend F, Prior C, Margreiter R, Mikuz G (1990) Cytomegalovirus pneumonitis in heart-lung transplant recipients: histopathology and clinicopathologic considerations. Hum Pathol 21:918-926

Feng YE, Huang S-W, Dong H-J (1990) Histiocytosis X – S-100 protein, peanut agglutinin, and transmission electron microscopy study. Am J Clin Pathol 94:627-631

Frieman J, Müller KM, Pott F (1990) Mesothelial proliferation due to asbestos and man-made fibres – experimental studies on rat omentum. Path Res Pract 186:117-123

Fujimoto T, Matsumoto T, Shoji S (1989) Disorganizing-fibrosing processes in alveolar walls of interstitial pneumonia, "alveolopneumonitis": a morphopathological study. Tohoku J Exp Med 158:237-251

Fukuda Y, Masuda Y, Ishizaki M, Masugi Y, Ferrans V (1989) Morphogenesis of abnormal elastic fibers in lungs of patients with panacinar and centriacinar emphysema. Hum Pathol 20:652-659

Gabius H-J (1988) Tumor lectinology: at the intersection of carbohydrate chemistry, biochemistry, cell biology, and oncology. Angew Chem Int Ed Engl 27:1267-1276

Gabius H-J, Kayser K (1989) Elucidation of similarities of sugar receptor (lectin) expression of human lung metastases from histogenetically different types of primary tumors. Anticancer Res 9:1599-1604

Gatzinsky P, Olling S (1989) A case of carcinoma in intralobular pulmonary sequestration. Thorac Cardiovasc Surg 36:290-291

Genner J, Settnes OP (1990) Pathological charateristics for the diagnosis of *Pneumocystis carinii* pneumonia – a restrospcetive autopsy study. APMIS 98:1098-1104

Golden IL, Sherwin RP (1989) Desquamative interstitial pneumonia in an infant. Mimicry of sudden infant death syndrome. Am J Forensic Med Pathol 10:344-348

Gosney J, Heath D, Smith P, Harris P, Yacoub M (1989) Pulmonary endocrine cells in pulmonary arterial disease. Arch Pathol Lab Med 113:337-341

Graeme-Cook F, Mark E (1991) Pulmonary mucinous cystic tumors of borderline malignancy. Hum Pathol 22:185-190

Green DM, Finklestein JZ, Tefft ME, Norkool P (1989) Diffuse interstitial pneumonitis after pulmonary irradiation for metastatic Wilms's tumor. A report from the National Wilms' Tumor Study. Cancer 63:450-453

Griffin M, Pushpanathan C, Andrews W (1990) *Chlamydia trachomatis* pneumonitis: a case study and literature review. Pediatr Pathol 10:843-852

Hillerdal G (1990) Pleural and parenchymal fibrosis mainly affecting the upper lung lobes in persons exposed to asbestos. Respir Med 84:129-134

Horcher E, Helmer F (1987) Scimitar syndrome and associated pulmonary sequestration: report of a successfully corrected case. Prog Pediatr Surg 21:107-111

Hornig D, Kühn H (1984) Beitrag zur "limitierten" Wegenerschen Granulomatose beim Kind mit primärem Befall der Lunge. Pathologe 5:134-142

Hu SN, Vallyathan V, Green FH, Weber KC, Laqueur W (1990) Pulmonary arteriolar muscularization in coal worker's pneumoconiosis and its correlation with right ventricular hypertrophy. Arch Pathol Lab Med 114:1063-1070

Itai S, Nishikata J, Takahashi N, Tanaka O, Matsubara Y, Hasegawa S, Yanai N, Takaoka K, Arii S, Tobe T, Kannagi R (1990) Differentiation-dependent expression of I and sialyl I antigens in the developing lung of human embryos and in lung cancers. Cancer Res 50:7603-7611

Karpel JP, Aldrich TK, Mitsudo S, Norin AJ (1989) Lung lymphocytes in bleomycin-induced pulmonary disease. Lung 167:163-172

Kawai T, Greenberg SD, Truong LD, Mattioli CA, Klima M, Titus JL (1988) Differences in lectin binding of malignant pleural mesothelioma and adenocarcinoma of the lung. Am J Pathol 130:401-410

Kayser K (1988) Metastasis into the lung – the pathologists's point of view. Contr Oncol 30:1-16

Kayser K, Bach S, Bülzebruck H, Vogt-Moykopf I, Probst G (1990) Site, size, and tumour involvement of resected extrapulmonary lymph nodes in lung cancer. J Surg Oncol 43:45-49

Kayser K, Bülzebruck H, Probst G, Vogt-Moykopf I (1987) Retrospective and prospective tumor staging evaluating prognostic factors in operated bronchus carcinoma patients. Cancer 59:355-361

Kayser K, Ernst M, Bubenzer J (1991) Expression of transferrin- and interleukin-2-receptors, and HLA-DR in human lung carcinomas. Exp Pathol 41:37-43

Kayser K, Gabius H-J, Carl S, Bubenzer J (1990) Alterations of human lung parenchyma after cytostatic therapy. APMIS 99:121-128

Kayser K, Gabius H-J, Köhler A, Runtsch T (1990) Binding of neuroendocrine markers and biotinylated sex hormones and the survival in human lung cancer. Lung Cancer 6:171-183

Kayser K, Heil M, Gabius H-J (1989) Is the profile of binding of a panel of neoglycoproteins useful as a diagnostic marker in human lung cancer? Path Res Pract 184:621-629

Kayser K, Probst F, Gabius H-J, Müller KM (1990) Are there characteristic alterations of lung tissue associated with Crohn's disease? Path Res Pract 186:485-490

Kayser K, Schönberg M, Tuengerthal S, Vogt-Moykopf I (1986) Chronic progredient diffuse alveolar damage probably related to exposure to herbicides. Klin Wschr 64:44-48

Kayser K, Stute H (1989) DNA content and minimum spanning tree in primary and metastatic adenocarcinoma of the lung. Acta Stereol 8:117-121

Kayser K, Stute H (1989) Minimum spanning tree, Voronoi's tesselation and Johnson-Mehl diagrams in human lung cancer. Path Res Pract 729-734

Kayser K, Stute H, Bubenzer J, Paul J (1990) Combined morphometrical and syntactic structure analysis as tools for histomorphological insight into human lung carcinoma growth. Anacel 2:167-178

Kayser K, Stute H, Tuengerthal S (1987) Diffuse pulmonary ossification associated with metastatic melanoma of the lung. Respiration 22:221-227

Kayser K, Stute H, Tuengerthal S, Burkhardt H-U, Bubenzer J (1990) Pathoanatomische und klinische Befunde beim malignen kleinzelligen Tumor der

Thorakopulmonal-Region. Tumordiagn Ther 11:68-73

Kayser K, Weisse G, Gabius H-J, Bubenzer J, v.Eberstein M, Hintze T (1990) Differentiation-related expression of epidermal growth factor receptors in human lung carcinoma demonstrated histochemically by biotinylated epidermal growth factor. Mod Pathol 3:327-311

Kayser K, Weisse G, Gabius H-J, Hintze T (1990) Biotinylated epidermal growth factor: a useful tool for the histochemical analysis of specific binding sites. Histochem J 22:426-432

King TE (1989) Bronchiolitis obliterans. Lung 167:69-93

Kinoshita M, Nakamura Y, Nakano R, Morimatsu M, Fukuda S, Nishimi Y, Hashimoto T (1989) Thirty-one autopsy cases of trisomy 18; clinical features and pathological findings. Pediatr Pathol 9:445-457

Kish JK, Ro JY, Ayala AG, McMurtrey MJ (1989) Primary mucinous adenocarcinoma of the lung with signet-ring cells: a histochemical comparison with signet-ring cell carcinomas of other sites. Hum Pathol 20:1097-1102

Koss LG, Czerniak B, Herz F, Wersto R (1989) Flow cytometric measurements of DNA and other cell components in human tumors: a critical appraisal. Hum Pathol 20:528-548

Lakhanpal S, Duffy J, Engel AG (1988) Eosinophilia associated with perimyositis and pneumonitis. Mayo Clin Proc 63:37-41

Lang L (1990) Bronchiolitis obliterans organizing pneumonia (clinical conference) Del Med J 62:1101-1108

Larivee P, Cantin A, Dufresne A, Begin R (1990) Enzyme activities of lung lavage in silicosis. Lung 168:151-158

Lauque D, Dongay G, Levade T, Caratero C, Carles P (1990) Bronchoalveolar lavage in liquid paraffin pneumonitis. Chest 98:1149-1155

Lee JS, Ro JY, Sahin AA, Hong WK, Brown BW, Mountian CF, Hittelman WN (1991) Expression of blood-group antigen A – a favorable pronostic factor in non-small cell lung cancer. N Engl J Med 324:1084-1090

Lee MM, Schinella RA (1991) Pulmonary calcification caused by *Pneumocystis carinii pneumonia,* a clinicopathological study of 13 cases in acquired immune deficiency syndrome patients. Am J Surg Pathol 15:376-380

Levine B, Chaisson E (1991) *Mycobacterium kansasii*: a cause of treatable pulmonary disease associated with advanced human immunodeficiency virus (HIV) infection. Ann Int Med 114:861-868

Lin RY, Gruber PJ, Saunders R, Perla EN (1988) Lymphocytic interstitial pneumonitis in adult HIV infection. N Y State J Med 88:273-276

Liu YC, Tomashefski JF, Tomford W, Green H (1989) Necrotizing *Pneumocystis carinii* vasculitis associated with lung necrosis and cavitation in a patient with acquired immunodeficiency syndrome. Arch Pathol Lab Med 113:494-497

Lombard CM, Colby TV, Elliott CG (1989) Surgical pathology of the lung in anti-basement membrane antibody-associated Goodpasture's syndrome. Hum Pathol 20:445-451

Mady C, Abensur H, Jatene F, Pereira-Barreto AC, Bellotti G, Pileggi F (1987) Sequestro intra-lobar pulmonar. Relato de caso e revisao da literatura. Arq Bra Cardiol 49:101-104

Meyrick B, Christman B, Jesmok G (1991) Effects of recombinant tumor necrosis factor-α on cultured pulmonary artery and lung microvascular endothelial monolayers. Am J Pathol 138:93-101

Miller R (1990) Bronchioloalveolar cell adenomas. Am J Surg Pathol 14:904-912

Miskovits G, Appel J, Varnai Z (1989) Pneumothorax durch histiozytäre Pneumonitis. Pneumologie 43:669-672

Morin C, Filiatrault D, Russo P (1989) Pulmonary sequestration with histologic changes of cystic adenomatoid malformation. Pediatr Radiol 19:130-132

Nagata N, Sueishi K, Tanaka K (1991) Anatomic pathway of pulmonary fluid leakage in endotoxemia induced in rats. Am J Pathol 138:183-193

Nakazawa T, Umegae Y (1990) Sericulturist's lung disease: hypersensitivity pneumonitis related to silk production. Thorax 45:233-234

Newman LS, Kreiss K, King TE Jr, Seay S, Campbell PA (1989) Pathologic and immunologic alterations in early stages of beryllium disease. Re-examination of disease definition and natural history. Am Rev Respir Dis 139:1479-1486

Nielsen H, Frederiksen J, Sherson D, Milman N (1990) Comparison of alveolar macrophage and blood monocyte oxidative burst response in pulmonary sarcoidosis. APMIS 98:401-406

Nyberg P, Klockkars M (1990) Quartz-induced production of reactive oxygen metabolites by activated human monocyte-derived macrophages. APMIS 98:823-827

Ofek I, Sharon N (1990) Adhesions as lectins: specificity and role in infection. Curr Top Microbiol Immunol 151:91-113

Ohori NP, Sciurba FC, Owens GR, Hodgson MJ, Yousem SA (1989) Giant-cell interstitial pneumonia and hard-metal pneumoconiosis. A clinicopathologic study of four cases and review of the literature. Am J Surg Pathol 13:581-587

Ohshima S (1990) Studies on pulmonary anthracosis. With special reference to the mineral constitution of intrapulmonary particulate pollutants in the human lung. Acta Pathol Jpn 40:41-49

Ortiz J, Val-Bernal JF, Gonzalez-Rodilla I, Miranda C, Mazorra F (1989) Hallazgos morfologicos en amebiasis sistemica. A proposito de un caso. Rev Esp Enferm Apar Dig 75:717-719

Oulton M, Moores HK, Scott JE, Janigan DT, Hajela R (1991) Effects of smoke inhalation on surfactant phospholipids and phospholipase A_2 activity in the mouse lung. Am J Pathol 138:195-202

Pauli BU, Augustin-Voss HG, El-Sabban ME, Johnson RC, Hammer DA (1990) Organ-preference of metastasis. The role of endothelial cell adhesion molecules. Cancer Metastais Rev 9:175-189

Pennza PT (1989) Aspiration pneumonia, necrotizing pneumonia, and lung abscess. Emerg Med Clin North Am 7:279-307

Perez-Arellano JL, Sanchez-Sanchez R, Pastor-Encinas I, Losa-Garcia JE, Garcia-Martin MJ, Gonzalez-Villaron L (1989) Pathogenesis of hypersensitivity pneumonitis. Allergol Immunopathol 17:225-232

Perlman EJ, Moore W, Hutchins GM (1989) The pulmonary vasculature in meconium aspiration. Hum Pathol 20:701-706

Peyrol S, Cordier JF, Grimaud JA (1990) Intra-alveolar fibrosis of idiopathic bronchiolitis obliterans-organizing pneumonia. Cell-matrix patterns. Am J Pathol 137:155-170

Piguet PF, Grau GE, Collart MA, Vassalli P, Kapanci Y (1989) Pneumopathies of the graft-versus-host reaction. Alveolitis associated with an increased level of tumor necrosis factor mRNA and chronic interstitial pneumonitis. Lab Invest 61:37-45

Pollard RB (1988) Cytomegalovirus infections in renal, heart, heart-lung and liver transplantation. Pediatr Infect Dis J 7:S97-S102

Radenbach D, Morgenroth K, Staud RD, Magnussen H (1990) Pulmonale Risiken durch Glasfaserstaubexposition. Pneumologie 44 Suppl 1:250-251

Rau B, Paul K, Branscheid D, Krysa S, Vogt-Moykpf I (1990) Das lobäre Emphysem – Symptome, Diagnostik, Therapie. Z Herz Thorax Gefäßchir 4:125-129

Reynolds HY (1988) Hypersensitivity pneumonitis: correlation of cellular and immunologic changes with clinical phases of disease. Lung 166:189-208

Risher WH, Crocker EF Jr, Beckman EN, Blalock JB, Ochsner JL (1989) Pulmonary dirofilariasis. The largest single-institution experience. J Thorac Cardiovasc 97:303-308

Ro JY, Tsakalakis PJ, White VA, Luna MA, Chang-Tung EG, Green L, Cribbett L, Ayala AG (1989) Pulmonary dirofilarisasis: the great imitator of primary or metastatic lung tumor. Hum Pathol 20:69-76

Rödelsperger K, Woitowitz H-J, Patrich R, Brückel B (1990) Asbestfasern und ferruginous bodies in der menschlichen Lunge. Staub 50:73-80

Salazar-Flores M, Rodriguez-Esparza J, Laufer-Dorotinski B, Sosa-Trejo F (1987) Paragonimiasis pulmonar. Informe de un caso. Salud Publica Mex 29:470-473

Samuels T, Morava-Protzner I, Youngson B, Huang SN (1989) Calcification in bronchopulmonary sequestration. Can Assoc Radiol J 40:106-107

Schuh D, Kemmer C (1988) Die Strahlenpneumonitis. Morphologisches Bild und Pathogenese. Zentralbl Allg Pathol 134:611-626

Schürmann D, Ruf B, Fehrenbach FJ, Jautzke G, Pohle HD (1988) Fatal legionnaire's pneumonia: frequency of legionellosis in autopsied patients with pneumonia from 1969 to 1985. J Pathol 155:35-39

Schwartz GF, Anderson ST (1990) Methotrexate induced pneumonitis in a young woman with psoriasis and rheumatoid arthritis (letter). J Rheumatol 17:980

Shintaku M, Mase K, Ohtsuki H, Yasumizu R, Yasunaga K, Ikehara S (1989) Generalized sarcoidlike granulomas with systemic angiitis, crescentic glomerulonephritis, and pulmonary hemorrhage. Arch Pathol Lab Med 113:1295-1298

Shiue ST, Scherzer HH, DeGraff AC Jr, Cole SR (1990) Hypersensitivity pneumonitis associated with the use of ultrasonic humidifiers. N Y State J Med 90:263-265

Siegel C, Johnston S, Adair S (1990) Isolation of measles virus in primary rhesus monkey cells from a child with acute interstitial pneumonia who cytologically had giant-cell pneumonia without a rash. Am J Clin Pathol 94:464-469

Sison RF, Hruban RH, Moore GW, Kuhlman JE, Wheeler PS, Hutchins GM (1989) Pulmonary disease associated with pleural "asbestos" plaques. Chest 95:831-835

Skeens JL, Fuhrman CR, Yousem SA (1989) Bronchiolitis obliterans in heart-lung transplantation patients: radiologic findings in 11 patients. AM J Roentgenol 153:253-256

Smith DB, Janmey PA, Lind SE (1988) Circulating actin-gelsolin complexes following oleic acid-induced lung injury. Am J Pathol 130:261-267

Spagnolo DV, Whitaker D, Carello S, Radosevich J, Rosen S, Gould V (1991) The use of monoclonal antibody 44-3A6 in cell blocks in the diagnosis of lung carcinoma, carcinomas metastatic to lung and pleura, and pleural malignant mesothelioma. Am J Clin Pathol 95:322-329

Stevens JH, Raffin TA, Baldwin JC (1989) The status of the transplantation of the human lung. Surg Gynecol Obstet 169:179-185

Sugano K, Ohkura H, Matsudo A, Mita S, Sakai T, Hatakawa Y, Ushioda T, Hoshikawa N (1990) Bronchogenic lung cyst with elevated serum type I chain related carbohydrate antigens, CA19-9, CA50 and FH-7. Jpn J Clin Oncol 20:182-187

Sullivan L (1989) Primary choriocarcinoma of the lung in a man. Arch Pathol Lab Med 113:82-83

Takemura T, Matsui Y, Oritsu M, Akiyama O, Hiraga Y, Omichi M, Hirasawa M, Saiki S, Tamura S, Mochizuki I, Mikami R (1991) Pulmonary vascular involvement in sarcoidosis: granulomatous angiitis and microangiopathy in transbronchial lung biopsies. Virchows Arch (A) 418:361-368

Tarroch X, Rovirosa M, Toran N, Lozano C (1989) Hipoplasia e hipertension pulmonar en un sindrome de Down: valoracion pronostica mediante la biopsia pulmonar. Rev Esp Cardiol 42:348-350

Tazelaar HD, Viggiano RW, Pickersgill J, Colby TV (1990) Interstitial lung disease in polymyositis and dermatomyositis. Clinical features and prognosis as correlated with histologic findings. Am Rev Respir Dis 141:727-733

Tomashefski, JF Jr, Konstan MW, Bruce MC, Abramowsky CR (1989) The pathologic characteristics of interstitial pneumonia cystic fibrosis. Am J Clin Pathol 91:522-530

Torikata C, Kijimoto C, Koto M (1991) Ultrastructure of respiratory cilia of WIC-Hyd male rats. An animal model for human immotile cilia syndrome. Am J Pathol 138:341-347

Travis WD, Colby TV, Lombard C, Carpenter HA (1990) A clinicopathologic study of 34 cases of diffuse pulmonary hemorrhage with lung biopsy confirmation. Am J Surg Pathol 14:1112-1125

Travis WD, Hoffman GS, Leavitt RY, Pass HI, Fauci AS (1991) Surgical pathology of the lung in Wegener's granulomatosis. Review of 87 open lung biopsies from 67 patients. Am J Surg Pathol 15:315-333

Travis WD, Pittaluga S, Lipschik GY, Ognibene FP, Suffredini AF, Masur H, Feuerstein I, Kovacs J, Pass HI, KS Condron, JH Shelhamer (1990) Atypical pathologic manifestation of *Pneumocystis carinii* pneumonia in the acquired immune deficiency syndrome. Am J Pathol Surg 14:615-625

Tsutsumi Y (1989) Immunohistochemical analysis of calcitonin and calcitonin gene-related peptide in human lung. Hum Pathol 20:896-902

Tuna IC, Jamieson SW (1989) Human heart and lung transplantation. Adv Surg 22:251-276

Verbeken EK, Demedts M, Vanwing J, Deneffe G, Lauweryns JM (1989) Pulmonary phospholipid accumulation distal to an obstructed bronchus. Arch Pathol Lab Med 113:886-890

Wagner U, Meerbach W, Fischer W, Otto J, Jahn R, Schneider WD (1990) Kasuistischer Beitrag zur Schweisserlunge. Z Erkr Atmungsorgane 174:149-154

Wallaert B, Lassalle P, Fortin F, Aerts C, Bart F, Fournier E, Voisin C (1990) Superoxide anion generation by alveolar inflammatory cells in simple pneumoconiosis and in progressive massive fibrosis of nonsmoking coal workers. Am Rev Respir Dis 141:129-133

Walz R, Koch HK (1990) Malignant pleural mesothelioma: some aspects of epidemiology, differential daignosis and prognosis. Histological and immunohistochemical evaluation and follow-up of mesotheliomas diagnosed from 1964 to January 1985. Path Res Pract 186:124-134

Weiss LM, Mohaved BS, Berry GJ, Billingham ME (1990) In situ hybridization studies for viral nucleic acids in heart and lung allograft biopsies. Am J Clin Pathol 93:675-679

Wick MR, Mills SE, Swanson PE (1990) Expression of "myelomonocytic" antigens in mesotheliomas and adenocarcinomas involving the serosal surfaces. Am J Clin Pathol 94:18-26

Wied GL, Bartels PH, Bibbo M, Dytch HE (1988) Image analysis and quantitative cyto- and histopathology. Technical Report 2, International Academy of Cytology, Chicago

Wilkinson JL (1989) Heart and heart/lung transplantation in children. Aust Paediatr J 25:117-118

Wilson L, Tomita T, Braniecki M (1991) Fatal pulmonary hypertension in identical twins with systemic lupus erythematosus. Hum Pathol 22:295-297

Woodward Sc (1989) Elastin breakdown and regeneration in emphysema. Hum Pathol 20:613-614

Wreghitt T (1989) Cytomegalovirus infections in heart and heart-lung transplant recipients. J Antimicrob Chemother 23, Suppl E:49-60

Appendix

Figures of Lung Diseases

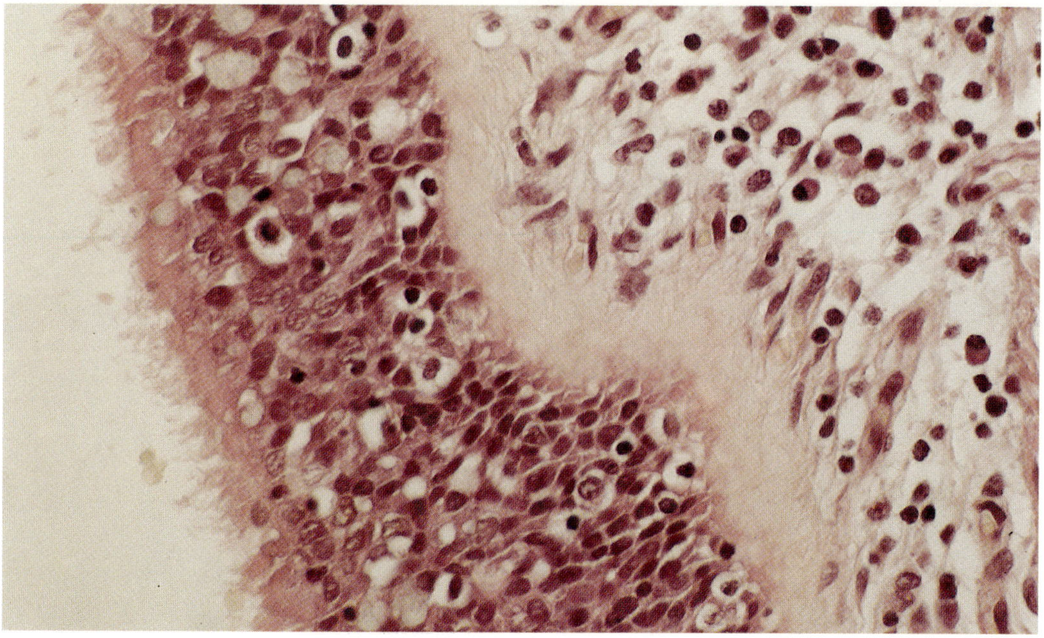

Descriptors: Bronchial mucosa with preserved structure:
- desquamation, hypertrophy, hyperplasia and dysplasia of epithelial cells
- mononuclear inflammatory infiltrates
- hyaline basal membrane

Diagnosis: Chronic asthmoid bronchitis. (HE, ×400)

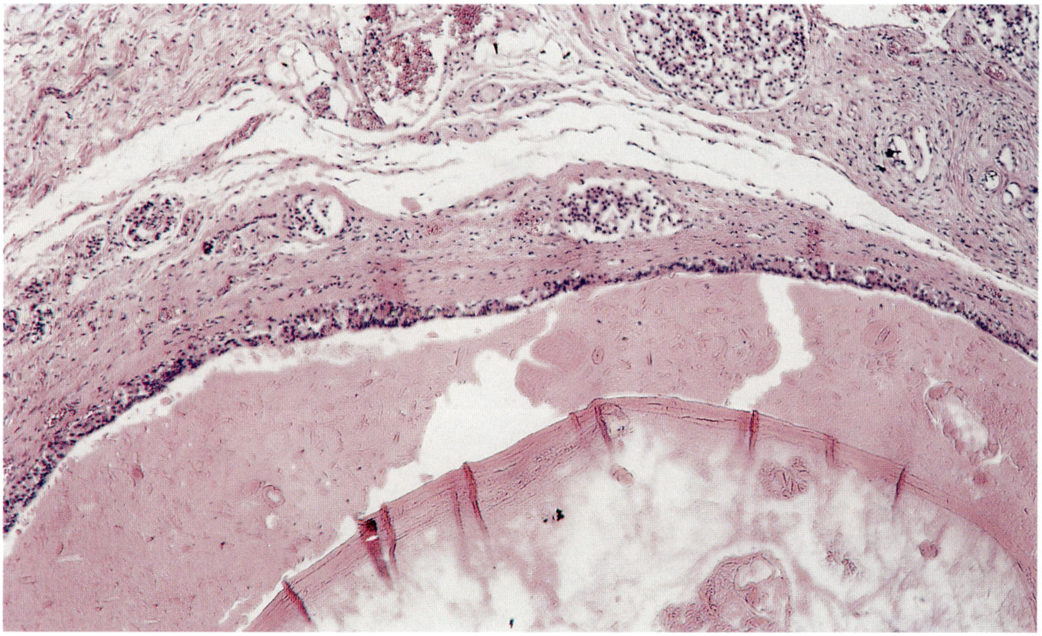

Descriptors: Bronchial mucosa with preserved structure:
- atrophy
- ectatic lumen
- viscous mucus
- mononuclear inflammatory infiltrates

Diagnosis: Cystic fibrosis. (HE, ×120)

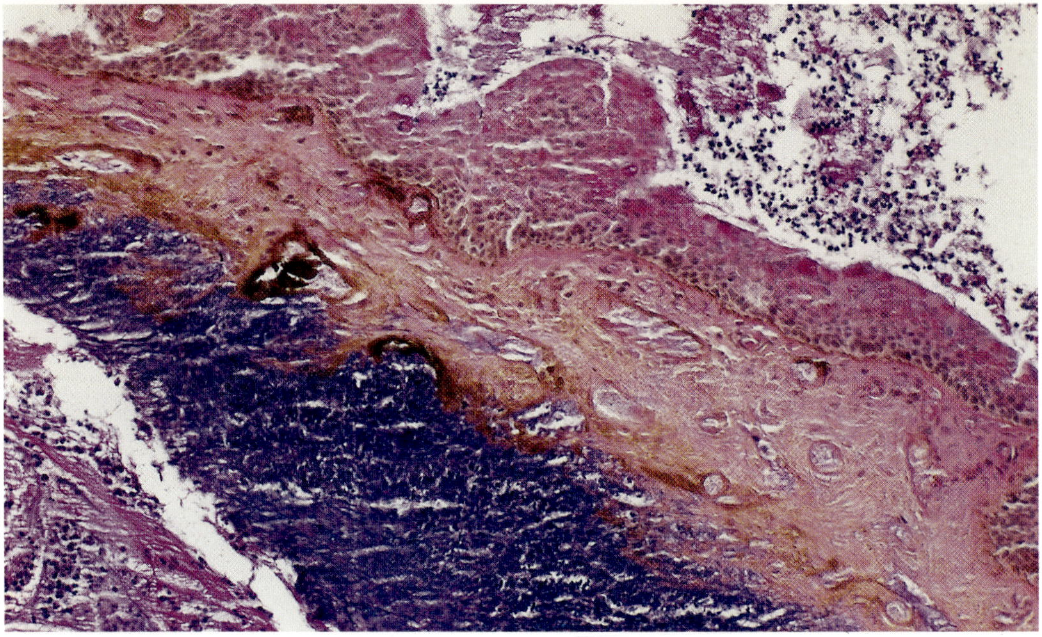

Descriptors: Bronchial mucosa with altered structure:
- ulceration
- fibrinoid material
- mixed inflammatory infiltrates
- squamous metaplasia and dysplasia
- necrosis

Diagnosis: Chemical burn. (PAS, ×120)

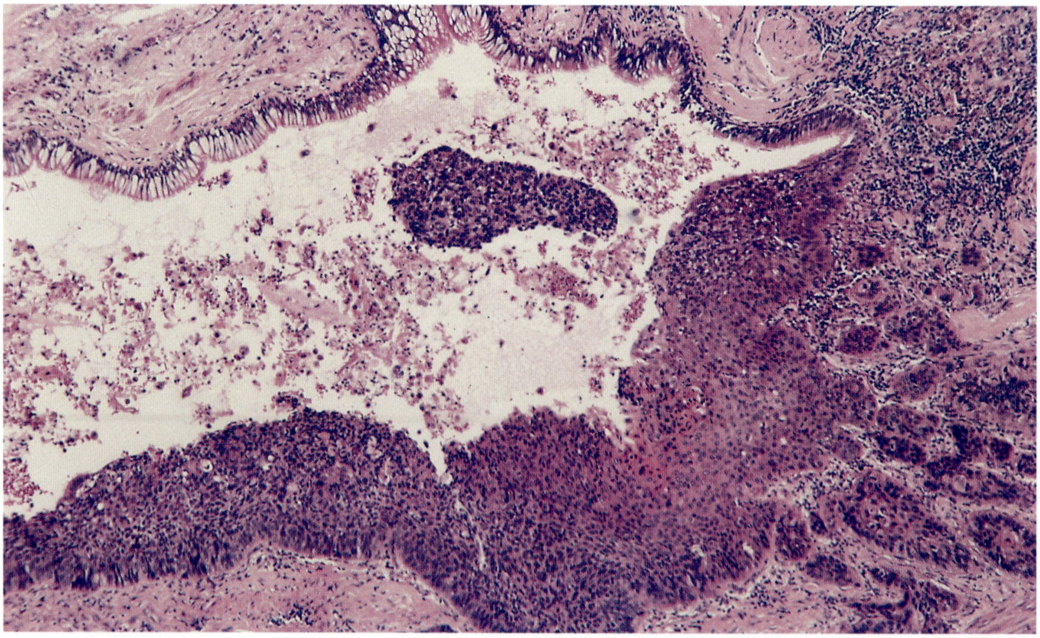

Descriptors: Bronchial mucosa with preserved structure:
- ectatic lumen
- hyaline basal membrane
- increased number of goblet cells
- mononuclear inflammatory infiltrates;

Newly formed textures with metastasis potential:
- epithelial growth pattern
- epidermoid textures
- inhomogeneous nuclear and cellular size

Diagnosis: Carcinoma in situ (epidermoid carcinoma). (HE, ×120)

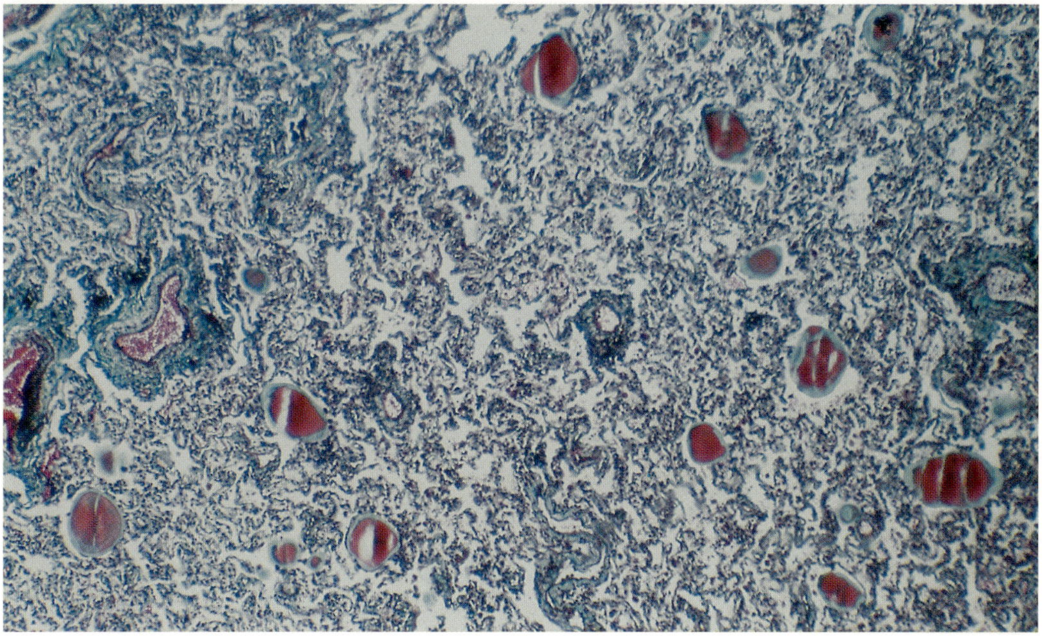

Descriptors: Lung parenchyma with preserved structure:
- absent hyaline membranes
- mononuclear inflammatory infiltrates (mild)
- calcium deposits
- unsuspicious pneumocytes

Diagnosis: Alveolar microlithiasis. (Masson's trichrome, ×120)

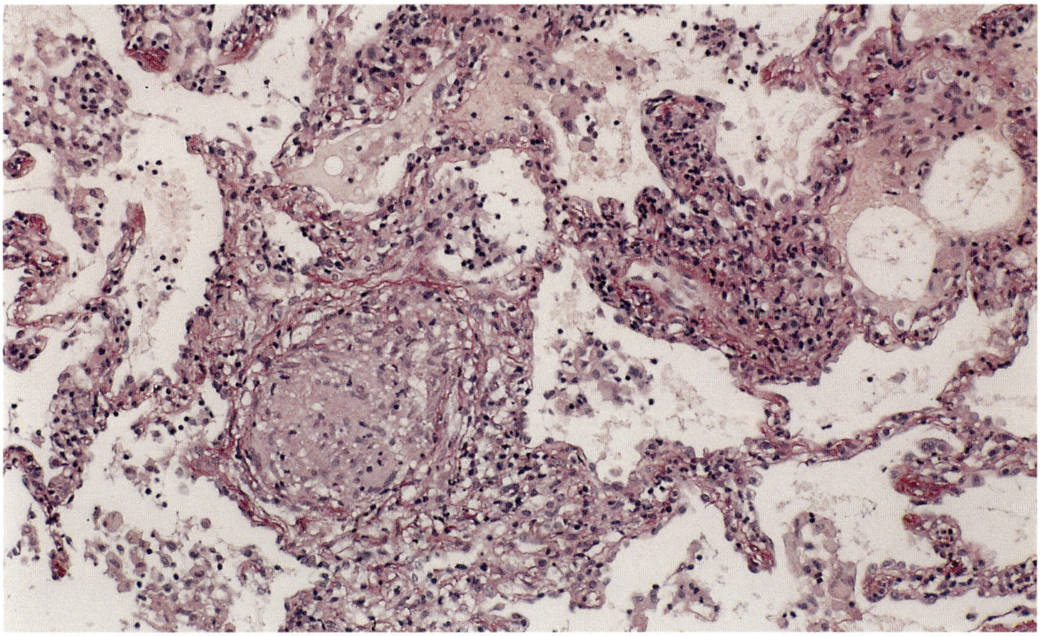

Descriptors: Lung parenchyma with preserved structure:
- desquamation, hypertrophy, hyperplasia and dysplasia of pneumocytes
- mixed inflammatory infiltrates
- intraalveolar serous fluid

Diagnosis: Psittacosis. (HE, ×180)

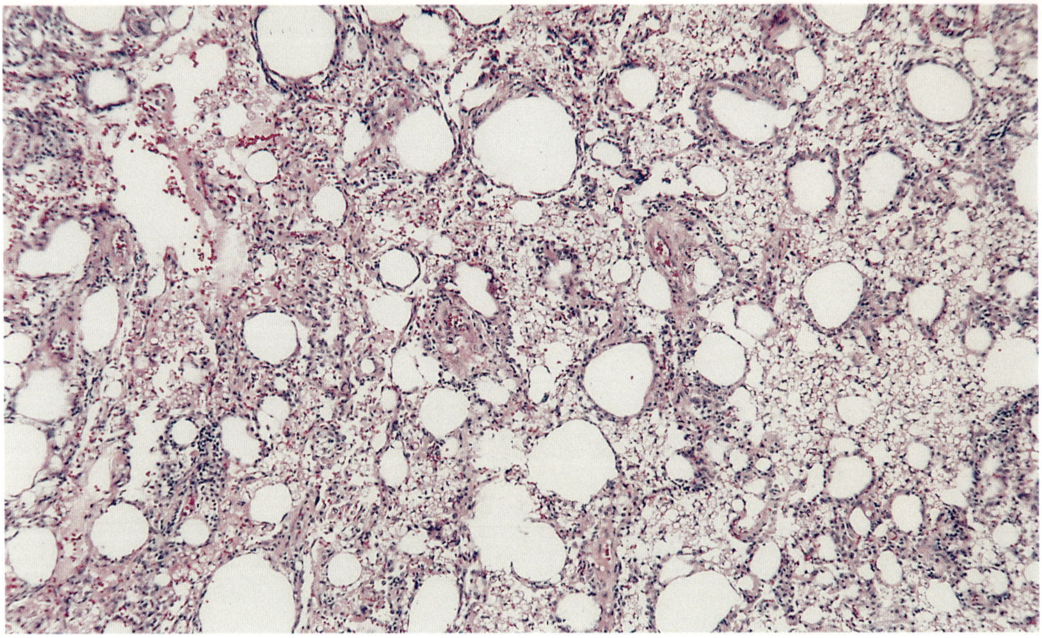

Descriptors: Lung parenchyma with preserved structure:
- lipoid material (intraalveolar droplets)
- macrophages (foamy)
- mononuclear inflammatory infiltrates (mild);

Lung parenchyma with altered structure:
- diffuse interstitial fibrosis (mild)

Diagnosis: Lipoid pneumonia. (HE, ×120)

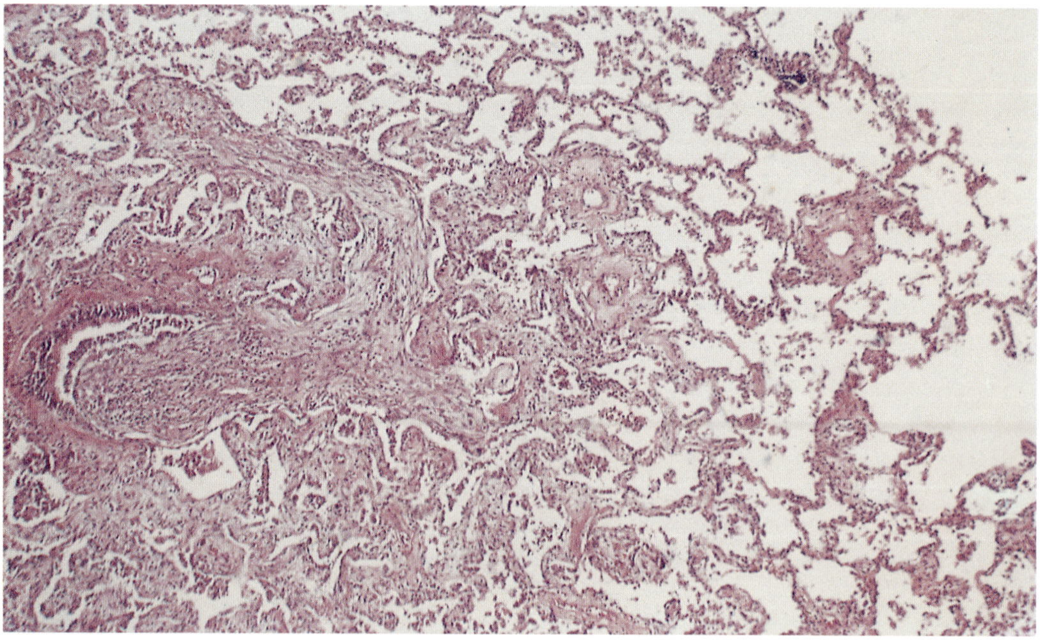

Descriptors: Lung parenchyma with altered structure:
- ulceration of bronchiolar mucosa
- intrabronchiolar fibrinoid material and histiocytes

Diagnosis: Bronchiolitis obliterans (associated with cytostatic drug regimes). (HE, ×120)

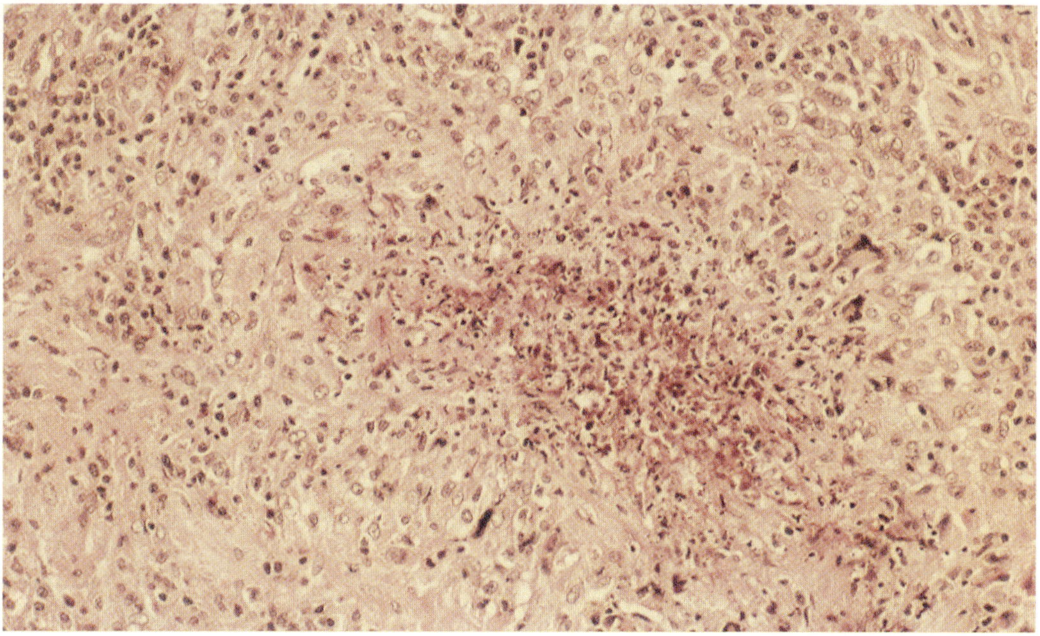

Descriptors: Lung parenchyma with altered structure:
- necrosis and hemorrhage
- palisading histiocytes
- multinucleated giant cells
- mixed inflammatory infiltrates
- proliferating fibroblasts

Diagnosis: Wegener's granulomatosis. (HE, ×340)

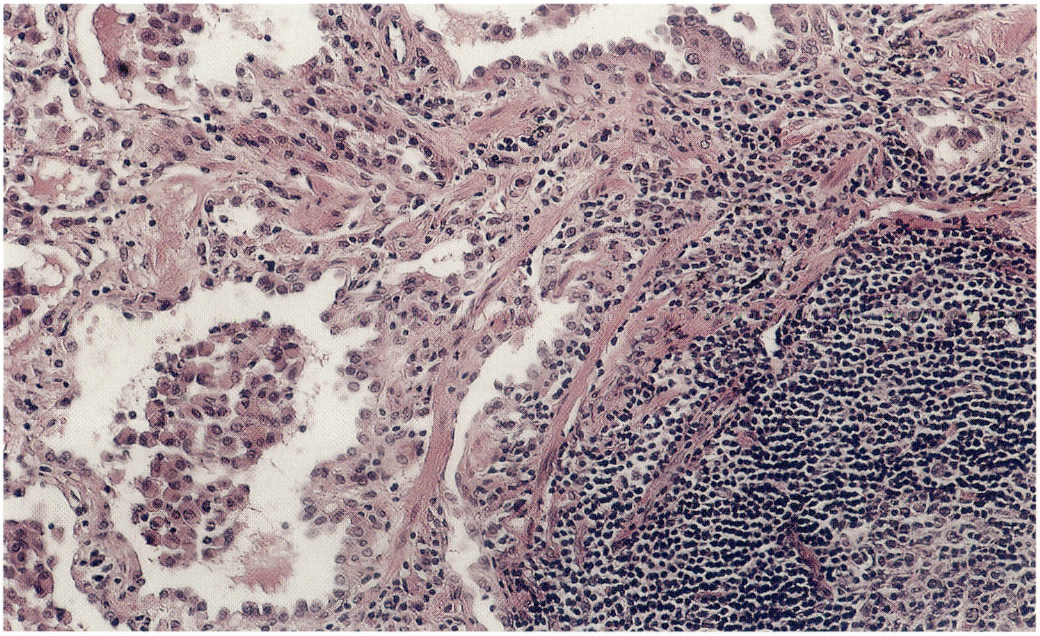

Descriptors: Lung parenchyma with preserved structure:
- intraalveolar fibrinoid material
- mononuclear inflammatory infiltrates
- desquamation, hypertrophy, hyperplasia and dysplasia of pneumocytes;

Lung parenchyma with altered structure:
- lymphomatoid granulomas

Diagnosis: Rheumatoid disease, acute stage. (HE, ×340)

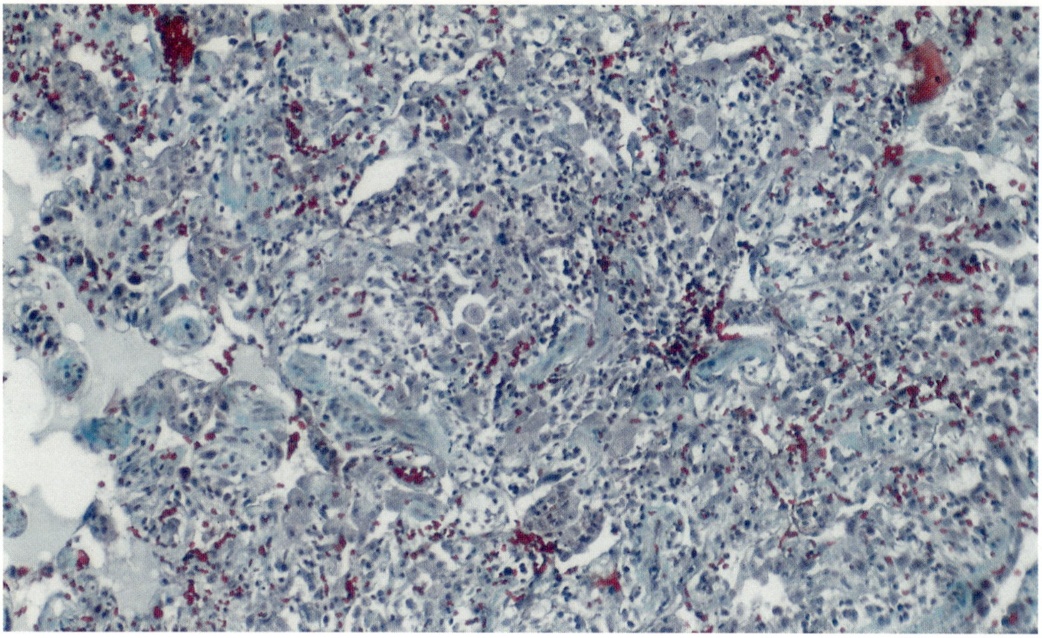

Descriptors: Lung parenchyma with preserved structure:
- intraalveolar serous fluid
- hyaline membranes
- desquamation, hypertrophy, hyperplasia and dysplasia of pneumocytes
- mixed inflammatory infiltrates;

Lung parenchyma with altered structure:
- proliferating fibroblasts

Diagnosis: Radiation pneumonitis, acute stage. (Masson's trichrome, ×340)

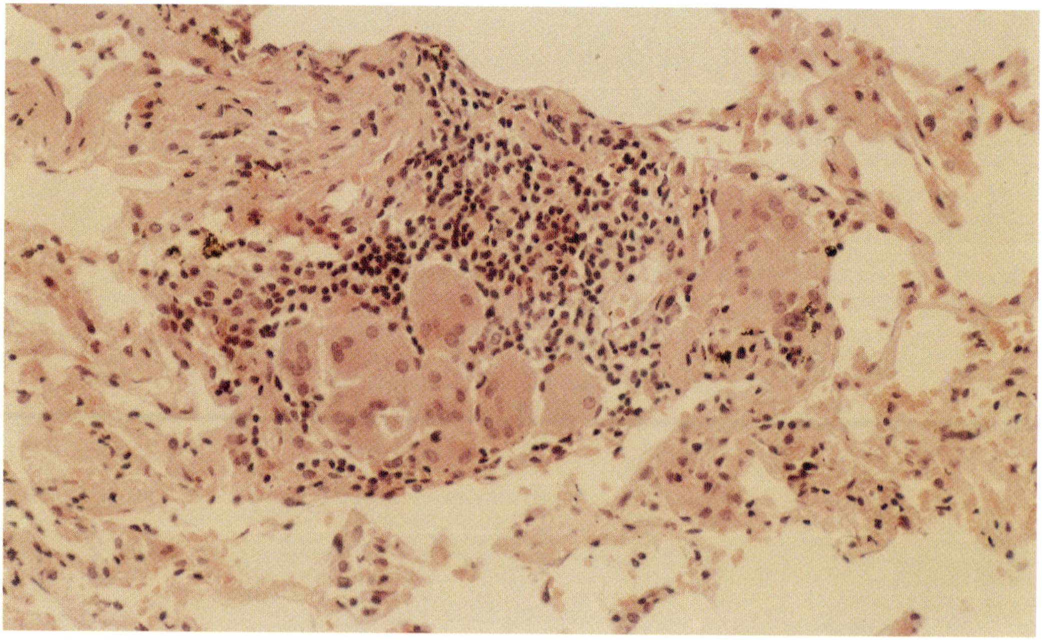

Descriptors: Lung parenchyma with altered structure:
- noncaseous epitheloid granulomas
- mononuclear inflammatory infiltrates
- multinucleated giant cells;

Lung parenchyma with preserved structure:
- unsuspicious pneumocytes

Diagnosis: Sarcoidosis, early lesion. (HE, ×340)

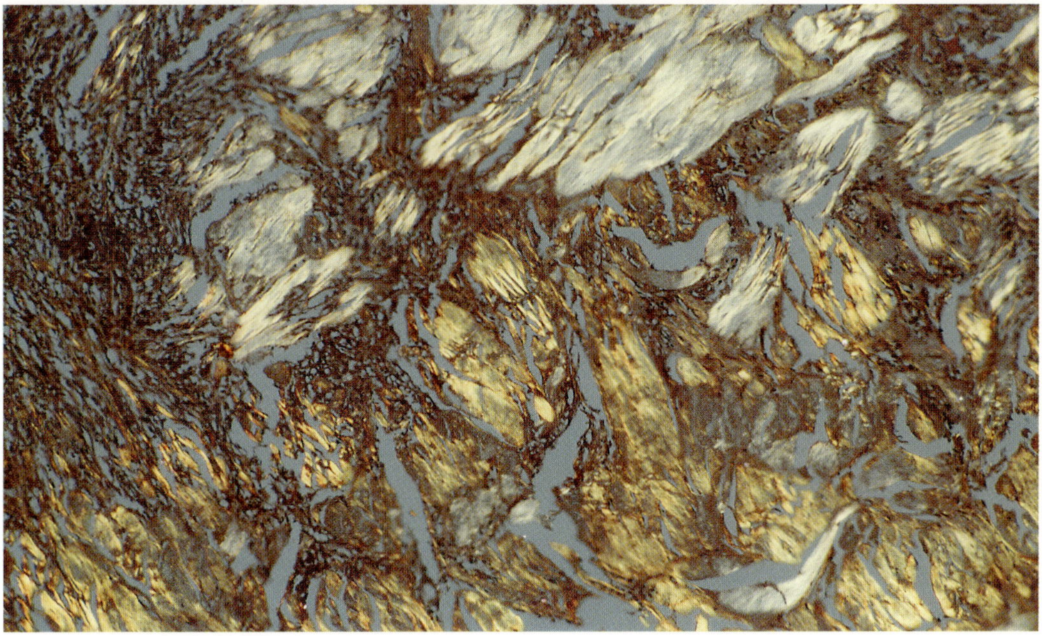

Descriptors: Lung parenchyma with altered structure:
- interstitial hyaline material
- mononuclear inflammatory infiltrates

Diagnosis: Amyloidosis. (Modified Congo, ×320)

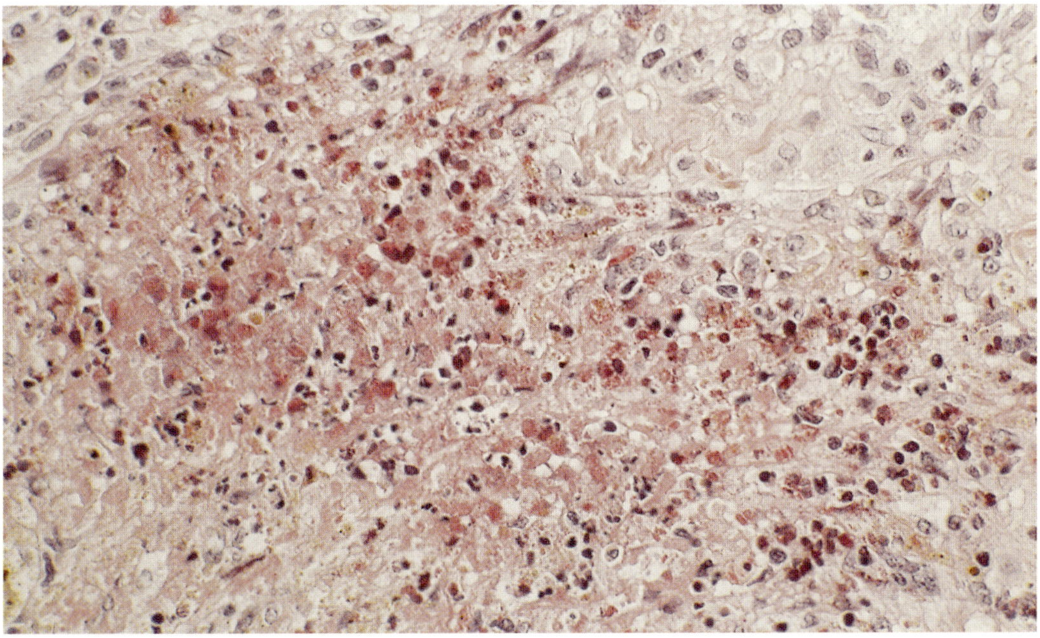

Descriptors: Lung parenchyma with altered structure:
- necrosis and hemorrhage
- palisading histiocytes
- eosinophils
- multinucleated giant cells

Diagnosis: Allergic angiitis and granulomatosis (Churg-Strauss Syndrome). (HE, ×340)

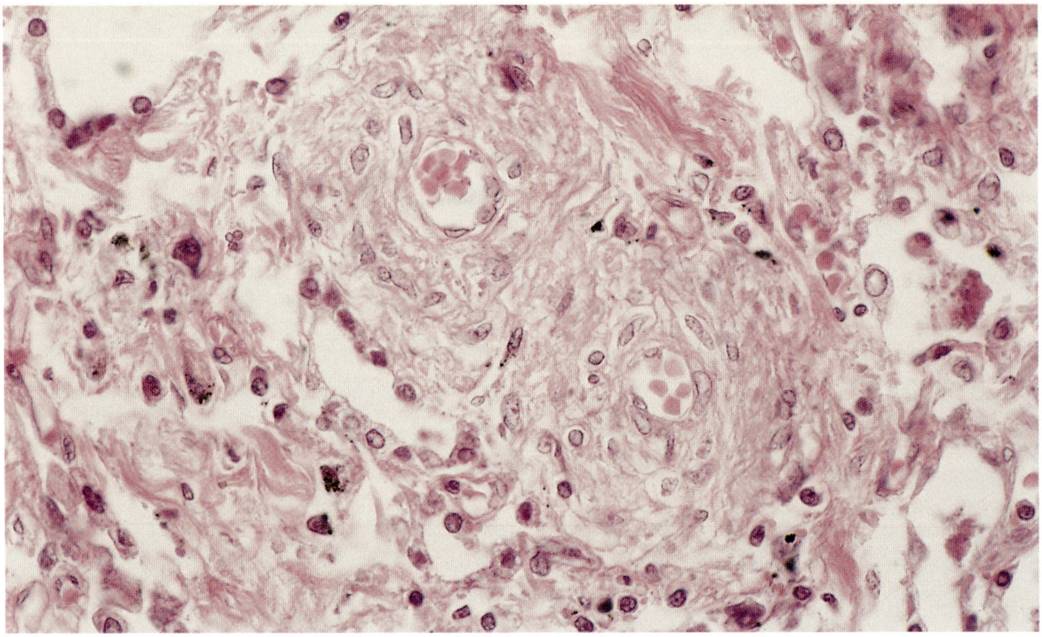

Descriptors: Lung parenchyma with preserved structure:

- intraalveolar fibrinoid material
- macrophages
- hyaline membranes;

Lung parenchyma with altered structure:

- proliferating fibroblasts;
- Pulmonary vessels with altered structure:
- proliferating smooth muscle cells

Diagnosis: Scleroderma lung. (HE, ×400)

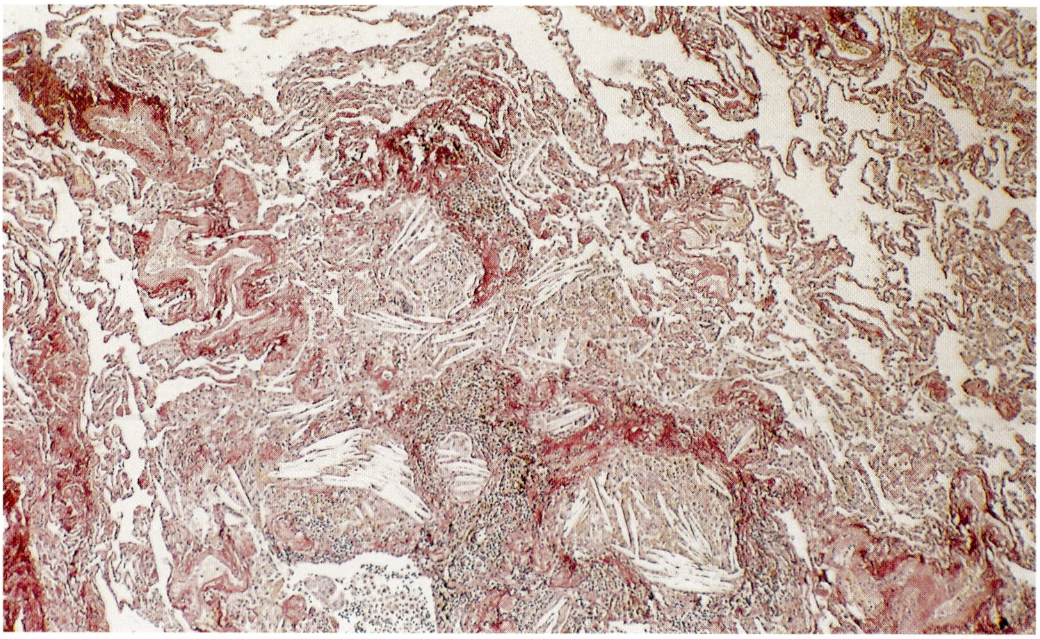

Descriptors: Lung parenchyma with altered structure:

- lipoid material (cholesterin crystals)
- mononuclear inflammatory infiltrates
- focal insterstitial fibrosis
- unsuspicious pneumocytes

Diagnosis: Lipoid pneumonia associated with hypercholesterinemia. (Sirius, ×120)

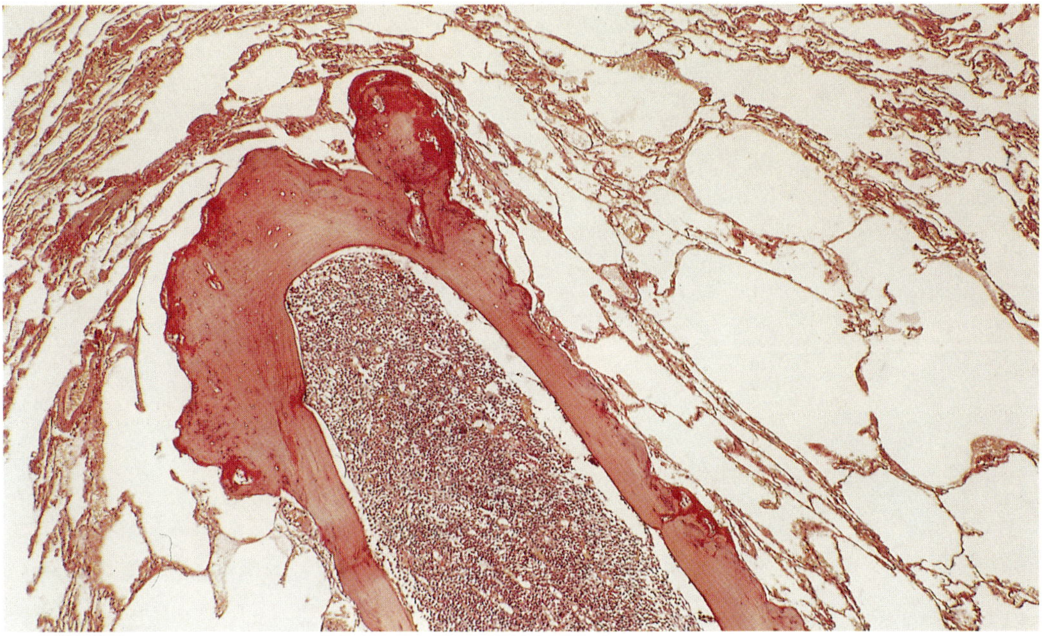

Descriptors: Lung parenchyma with altered structure:
- bony nodules (intraalveolar, mature)
- unsuspicious pneumocytes
- mononuclear inflammatory infiltrates (weak)

Diagnosis: Ossification, pulmonary. (HE, ×120)

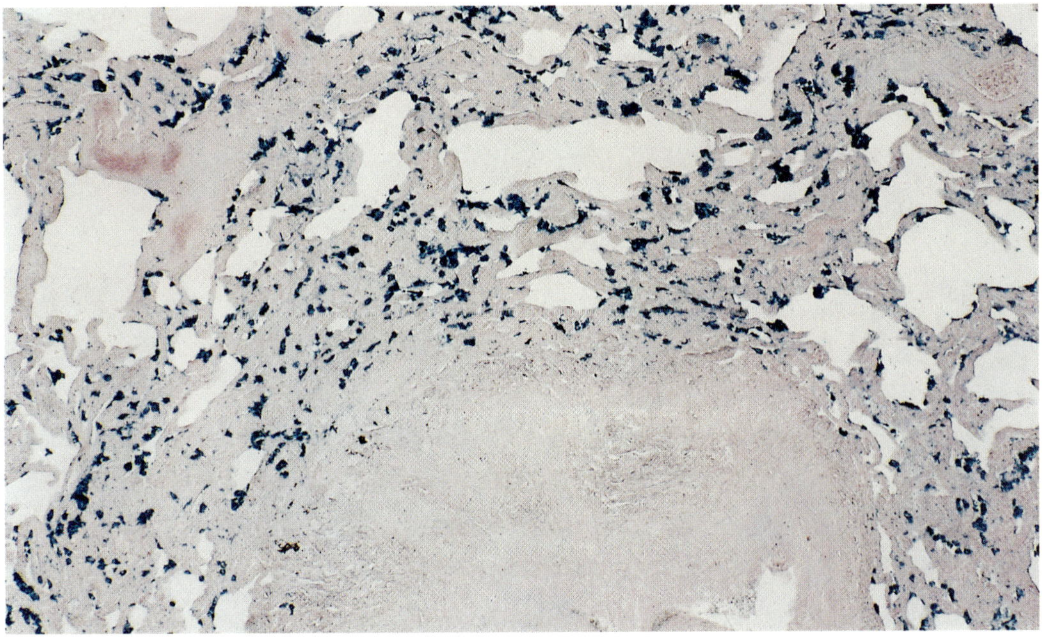

Descriptors: Lung parenchyma with altered structure:
- macrophages (hemosiderin-laden)
- mononuclear inflammatory infiltrates
- foreign body material (iron)
- focal interstitial fibrosis
- honeycombing

Diagnosis: Severe hemosiderosis (Welder's lung). (Prussian blue, ×120)

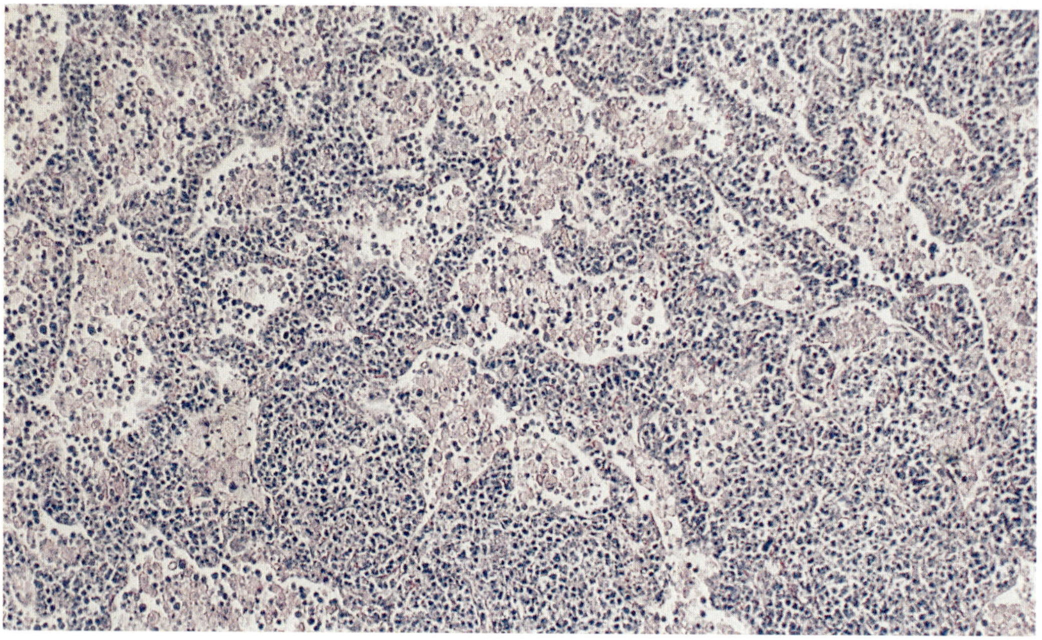

Descriptors: Lung parenchyma with preserved structure:
- mononuclear inflammatory infiltrates
- atypical lymphoid cells
- unsuspicious pneumocytes

Diagnosis: Lymphocytic interstitial pneumonia resembling lymphocytic lymphoma. (HE, ×180)

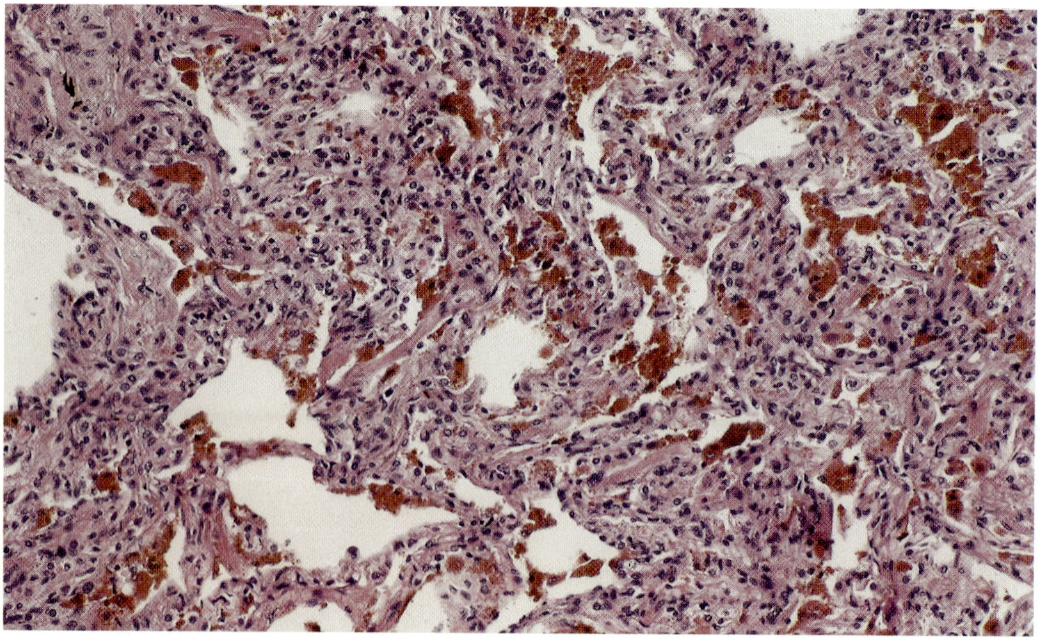

Descriptors: Lung parenchyma with preserved structure:
- mononuclear inflammatory infiltrates
- macrophages (hemosiderin-laden)
- desquamation, hypertrophy, hyperplasia and dysplasia of pneumocytes
- hyaline material

Diagnosis: Idiopathic hemosiderosis. (HE, ×180)

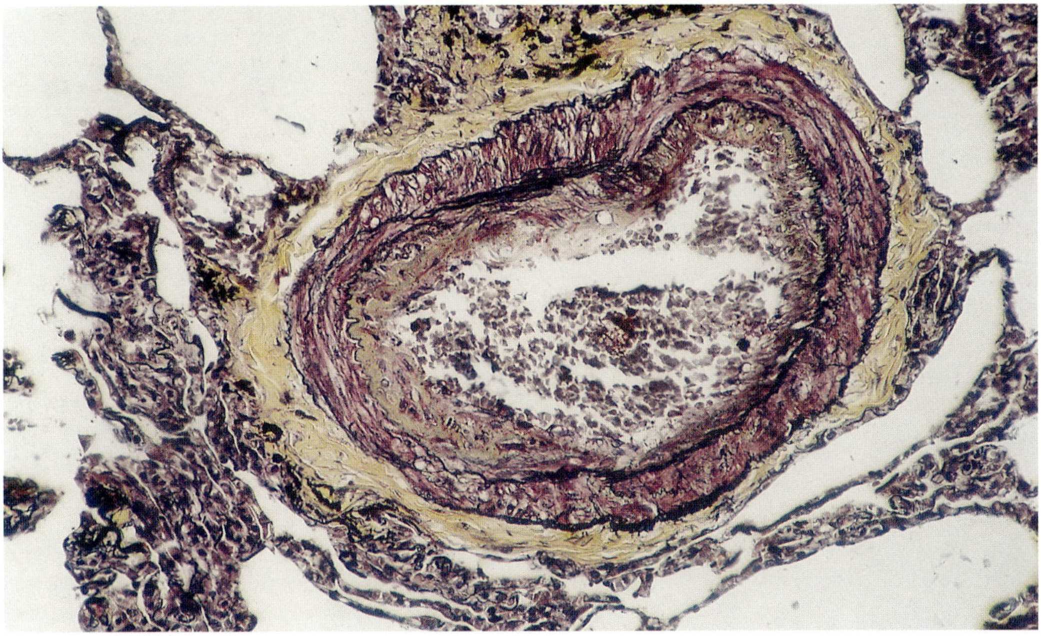

Descriptors: Pulmonary vessels with altered structure:

- fibrosis (intimal, patchy eccentric)
- proliferating smooth muscle cells
- stenosis

Diagnosis: Pulmonary hypertension (idiopathic). (Reticulin, ×340)

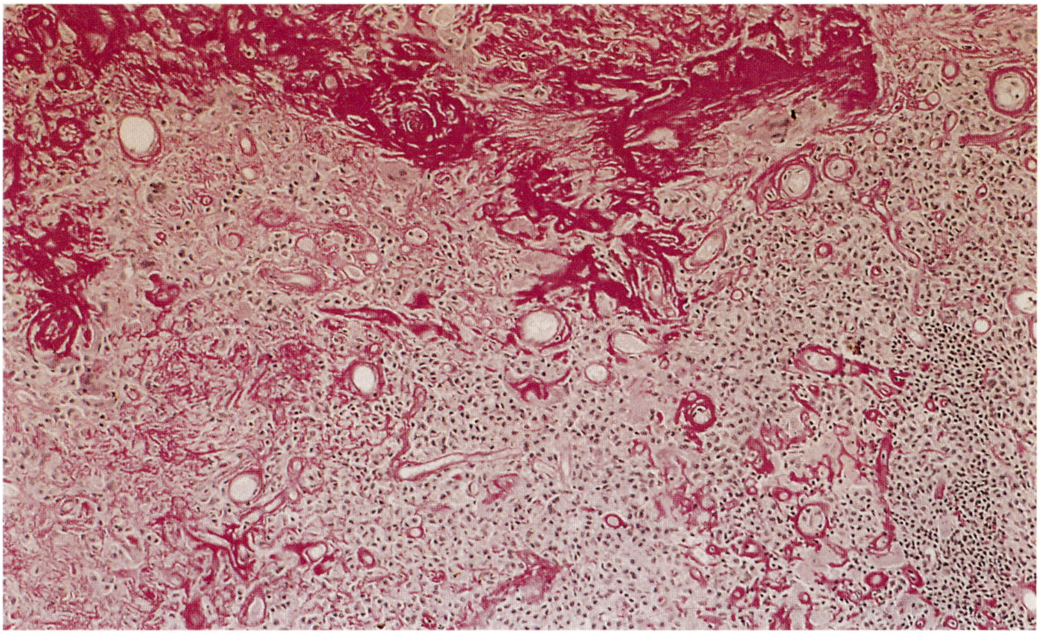

Descriptors: Newly formed textures without metastasis potential:

- mesenchymal growth pattern
- lymphomatoid textures
- mononuclear inflammatory cells (lymphocytes and plasma cells, mature)
- fibroblasts and myofibroblasts
- homogeneous nuclear and cellular size
- multinucleated giant cells
- hyaline deposits (perivascular)

Diagnosis: Pseudotumor, inflammatory. (PAS, ×240)

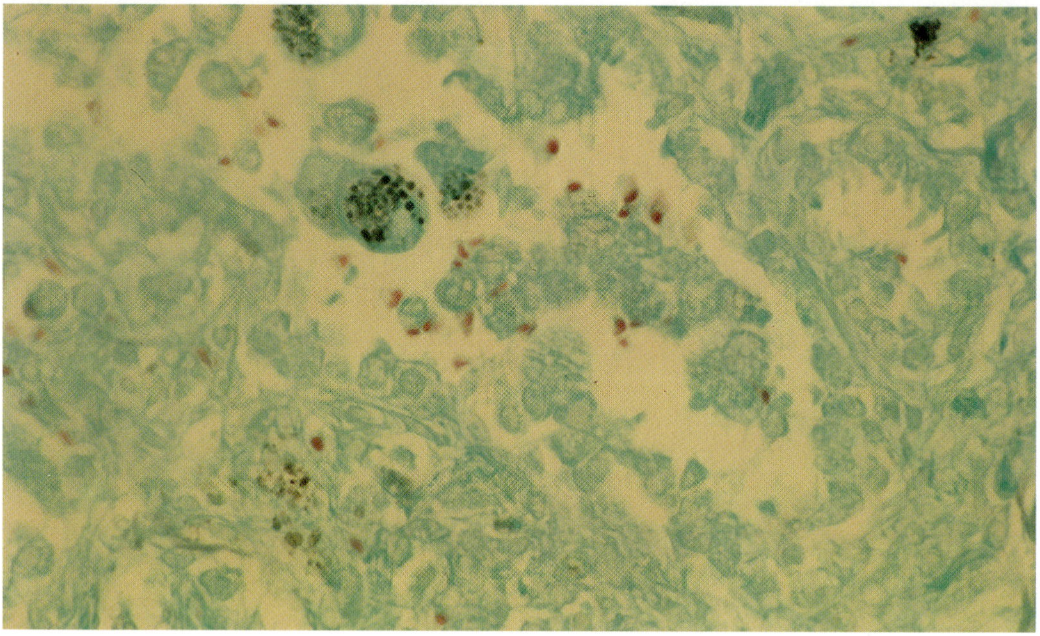

Descriptors: Lung parenchyma with preserved structure:
- intraalveolar serous fluid
- mononuclear inflammatory infiltrates
- macrophages (precysts)
- infectious organisms (cysts and precysts)

Diagnosis: Pneumocystis carinii pneumonia. (Grocott's stain, ×400)

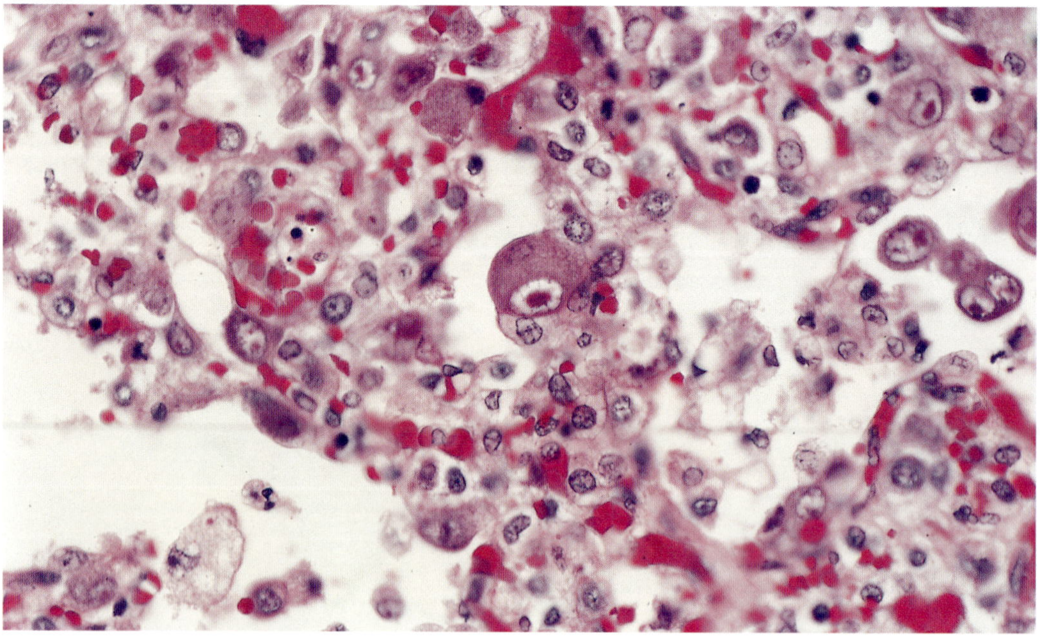

Descriptors: Lung parenchyma with preserved structure:
- intraalveolar fibrinoid material
- mononuclear inflammatory infiltrates
- desquamation, hypertrophy, hyperplasia and dysplasia of pneumocytes
- inclusion bodies

Diagnosis: Cytomegalovirus pneumonia. (PAS, ×600)

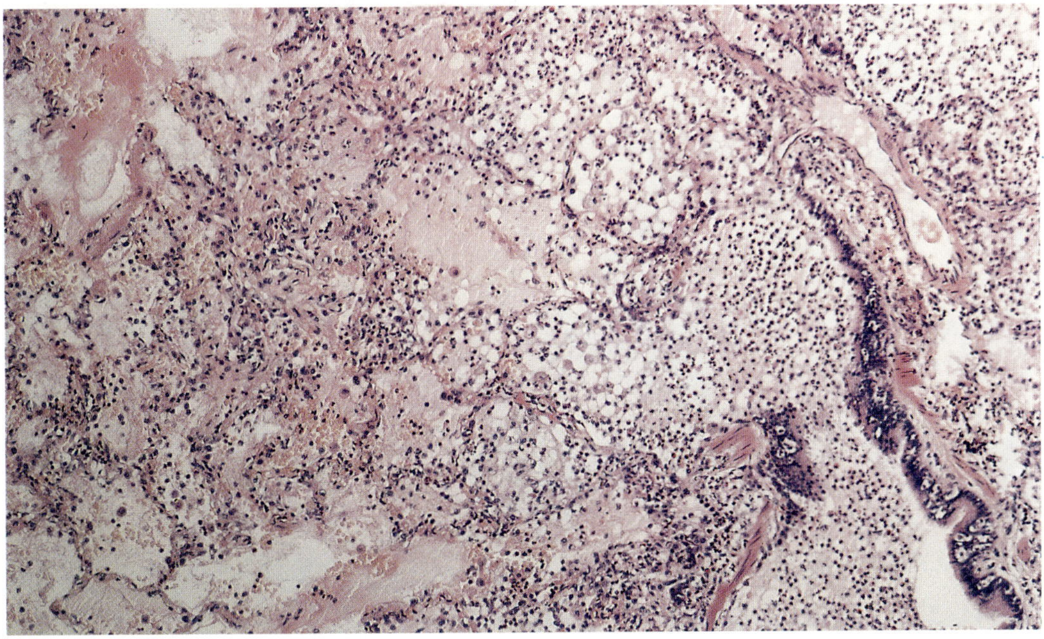

Descriptors: Lung parenchyma with preserved structure:
- bacteria
- mixed inflammatory infiltrates
- intraalveolar serous fluid
- hemorrhage

Diagnosis: Bacterial pneumonia, early stage. (HE, ×240)

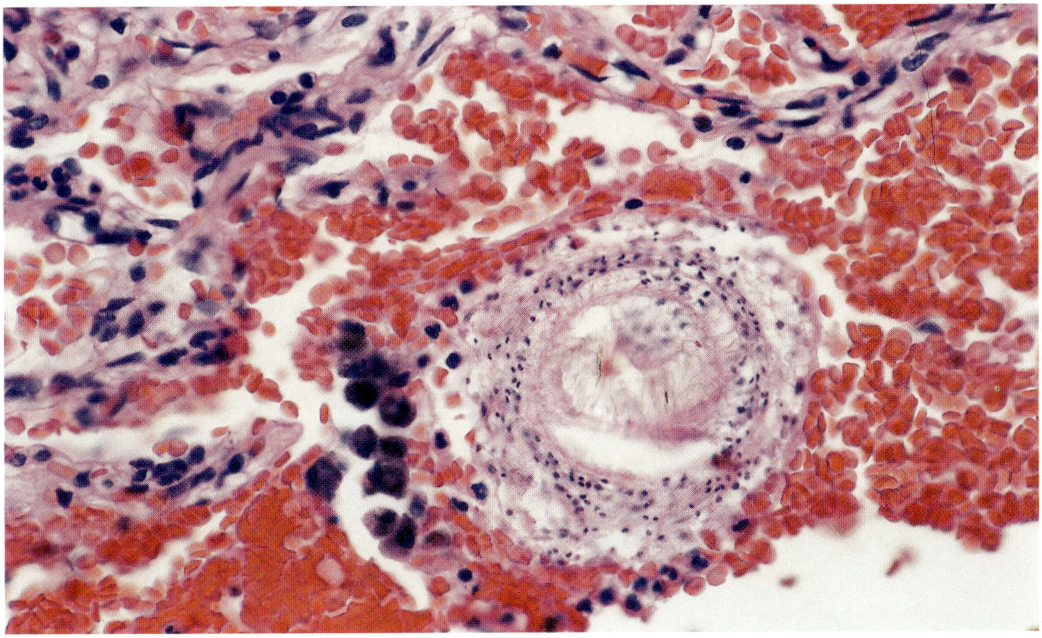

Descriptors: Lung parenchyma with altered structure:
- parasites
- necrosis
- mixed inflammatory infiltrates
- eosinophils

Diagnosis: Echinococcosis. (HE, ×400)

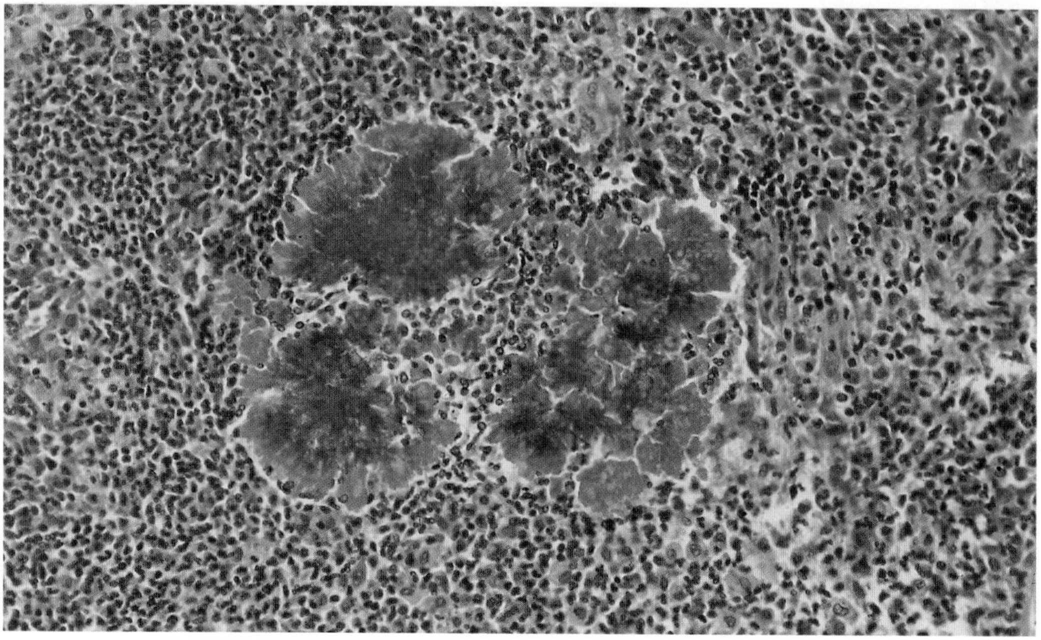

Descriptors: Lung parenchyma with altered structure:
- necrosis and hemorrhage
- mixed inflammatory infiltrates
- bacteria
- sulfur granules

Diagnosis: Actinomycosis. (PAS, ×340)

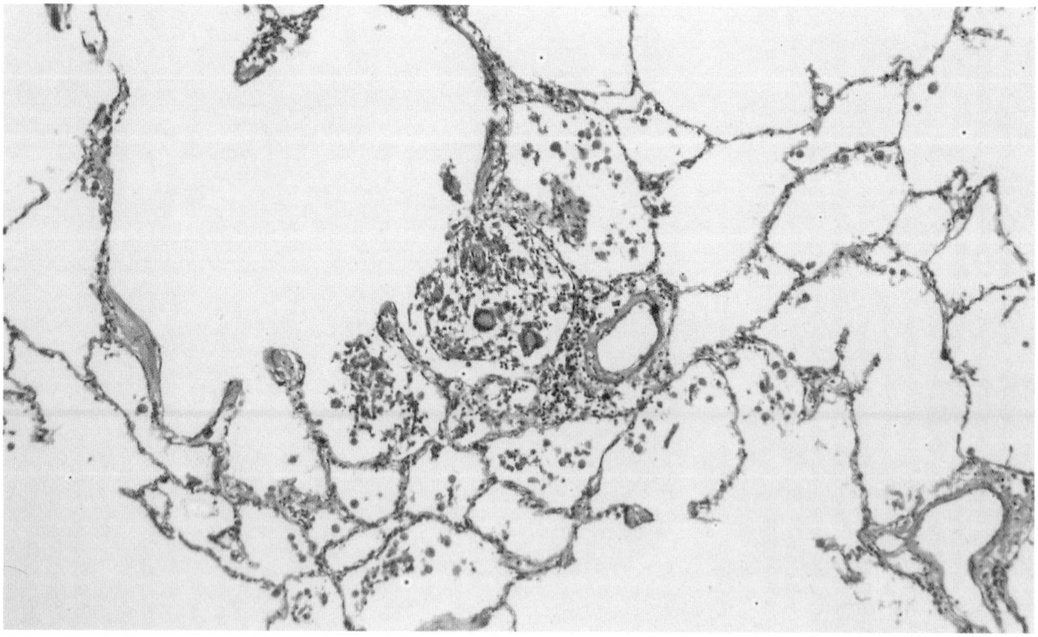

Descriptors: Lung parenchyma with altered structure:
- caseous epitheloid granulomas (early)
- multinucleated giant cells
- mononuclear inflammatory infiltrates

Diagnosis: Early tuberculosis. (HE, ×180)

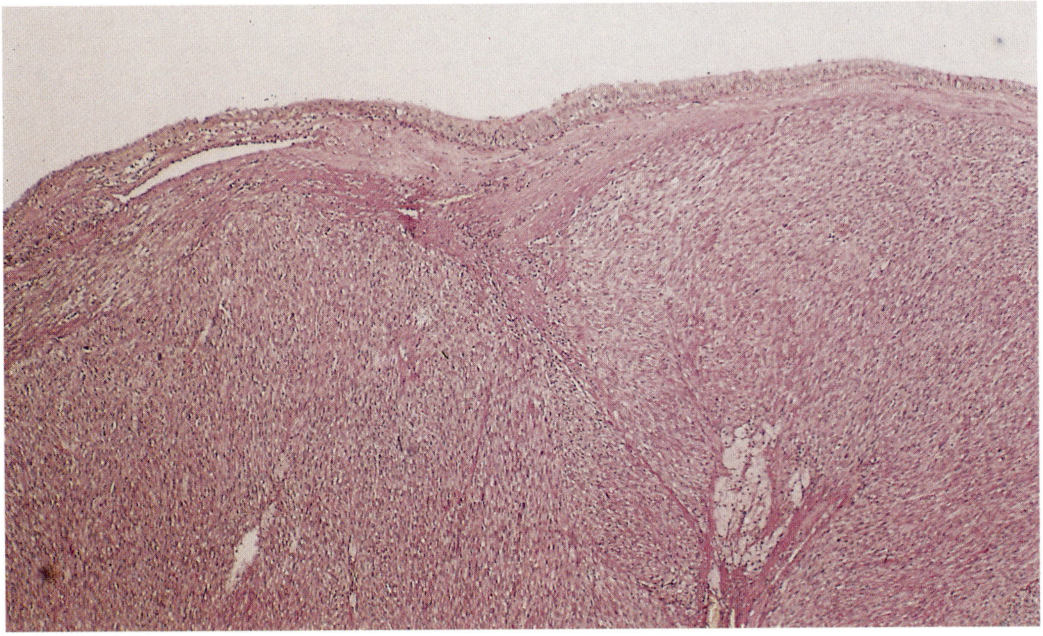

Descriptors: Newly formed textures without metastasis potential:

- mesenchymal growth pattern
- fibromatous textures
- plump spindle cells
- homogeneous nuclear and cellular size
- absent or infrequent mitoses

Diagnosis: Bronchial leiomyoma. (HE, ×180)

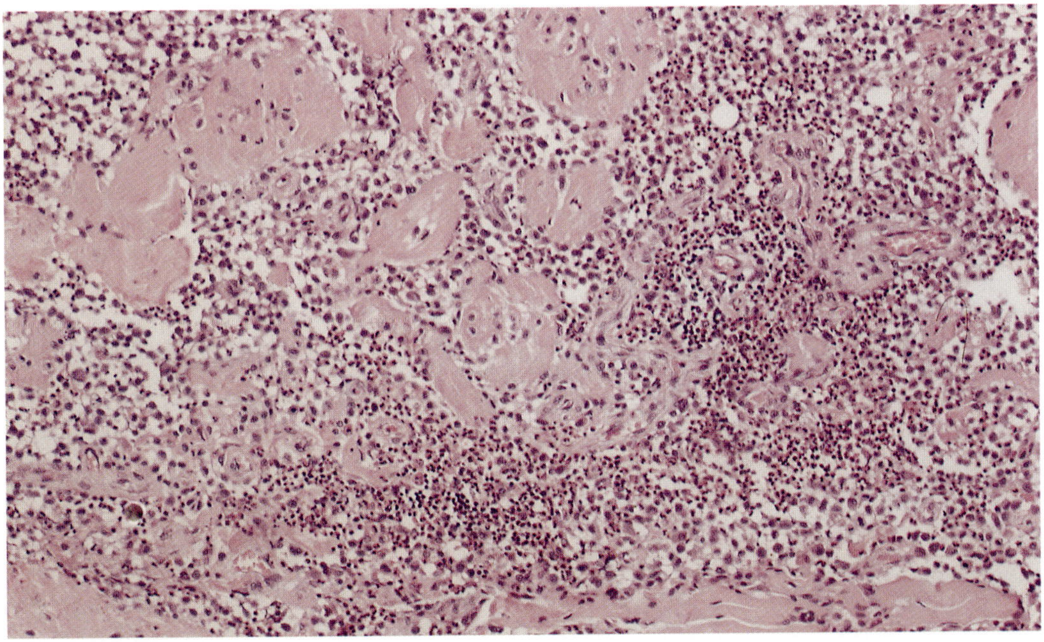

Descriptors: Lung parenchyma with altered structure

- atypical cells (spindle shaped, histiocytosis X)
- eosinophils
- macrophages
- focal interstitial fibrosis

Diagnosis: Histiocytosis X. (HE, ×240)

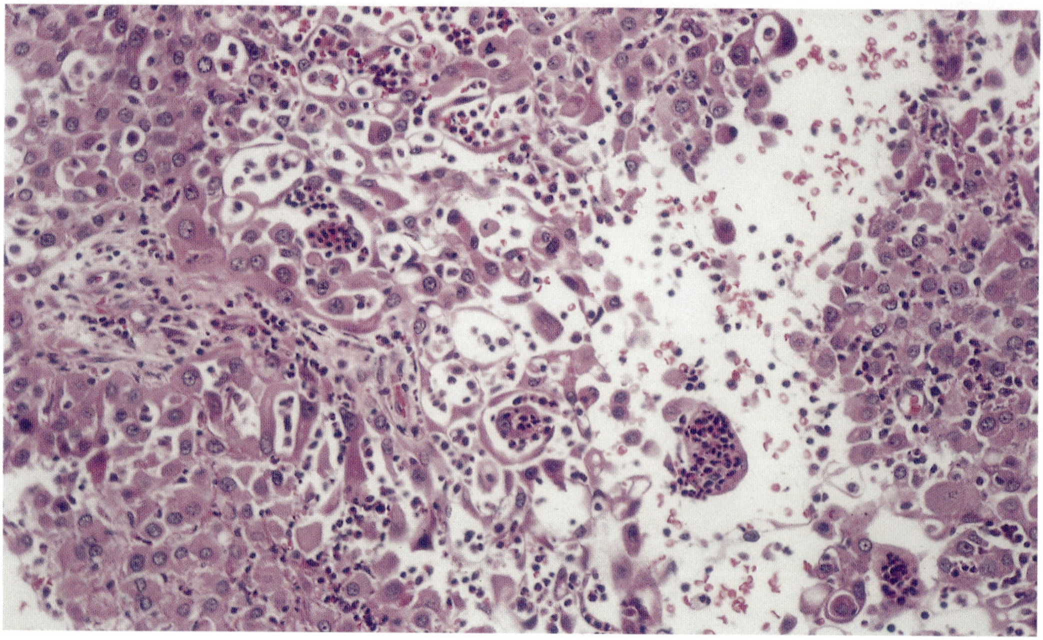

Descriptors: Newly formed textures with metastasis potential:

- epithelial growth pattern
- adenoid textures
- solid textures
- large tumor cells
- homogeneous nuclear and cellular size
- prominent nucleoli
- infrequent mitoses
- necrosis (small areas)

Diagnosis: Epithelial mesothelioma. (HE, ×340)

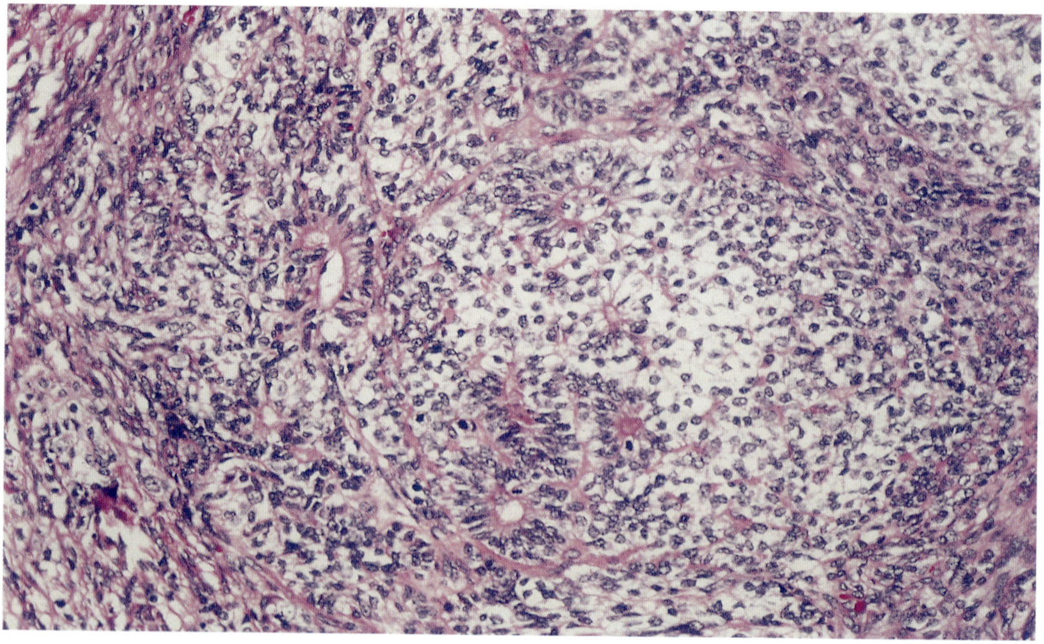

Descriptors: Newly formed textures with metastasis potential:

- mesenchymal growth pattern
- vascular texture (antler-like spaces)
- plump spindle cells
- inhomogeneous nuclear and cellular size
- frequent mitoses

Diagnosis: Hemangiopericytoma (high grade). (PAS, ×240)

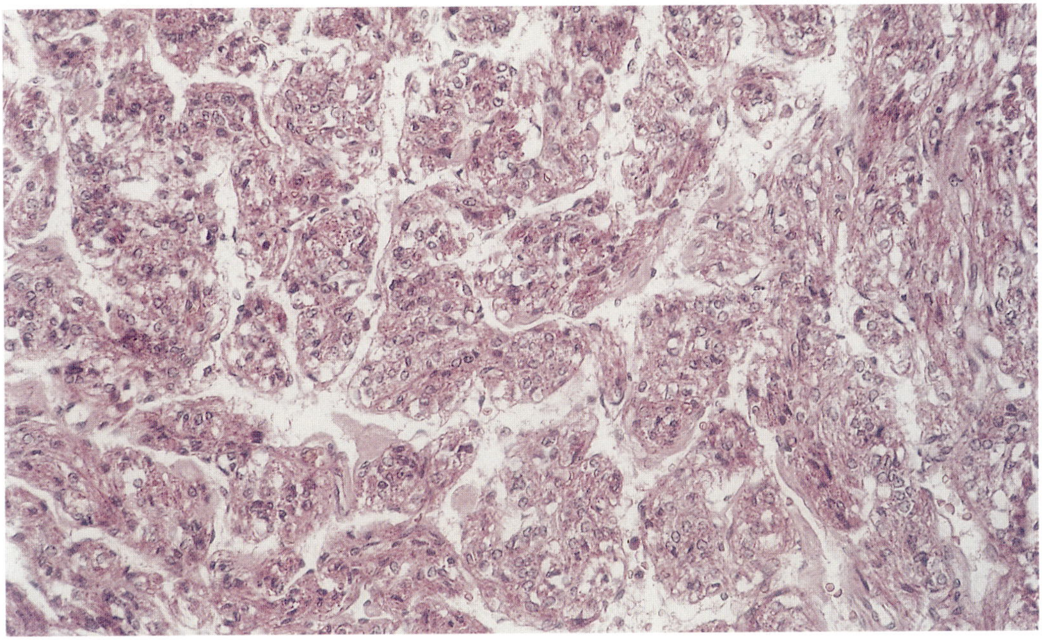

Descriptors: Newly formed textures with metastasis potential:

- mesenchymal growth pattern
- lymphomatoid textures
- small tumor cells (lymphoplasmacytoid)
- homogeneous nuclear and cellular size
- infrequent mitoses

Diagnosis: Macroglobulinemia of Waldenström. (PAS, ×240)

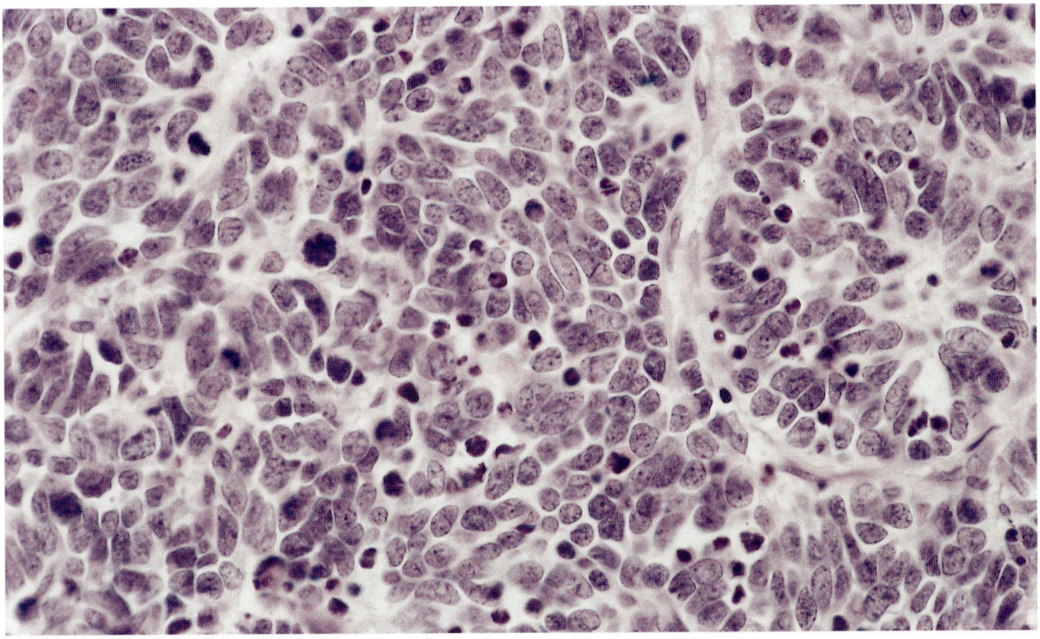

Descriptors: Newly formed textures with metastasis potential:

- epithelial growth pattern
- solid textures
- small cells
- finely distributed nuclear chromatin
- inhomogeneous nuclear and cellular size
- frequent mitoses
- molding

Diagnosis: Small cell carcinoma (oat cell type). (HE, ×800)

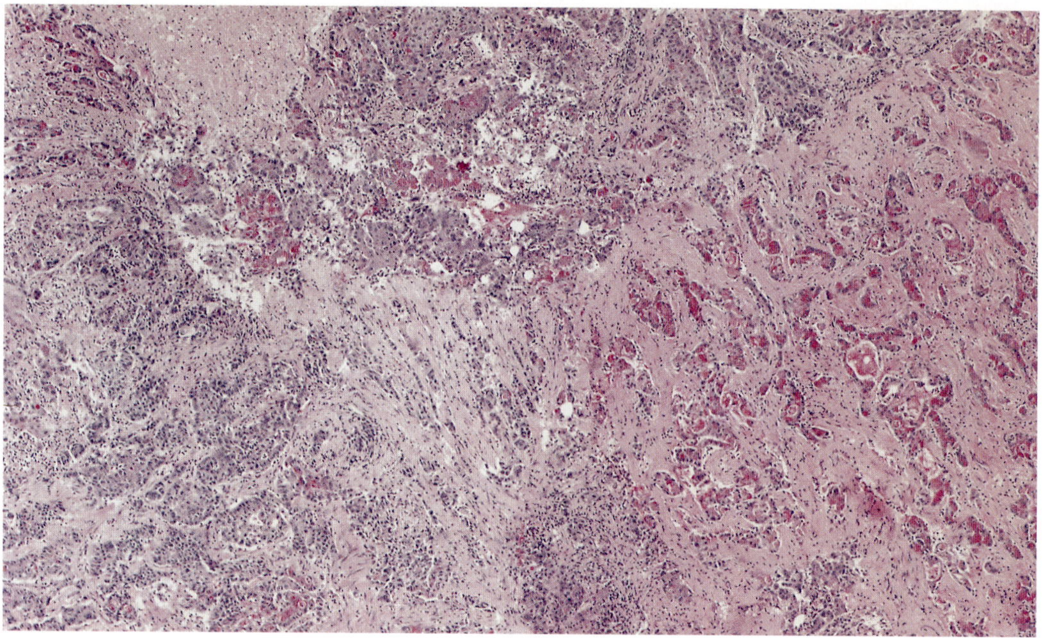

Descriptors: Newly formed textures with metastasis potential:

- epithelial growth pattern
- adenoid textures
- epidermoid textures
- mucus production
- inhomogenous nuclear and cellular size
- prominent nucleoli
- necrosis
- absent or weak inflammatory infiltrates

Diagnosis: Adeno-squamous carcinoma. (PAS, ×180)

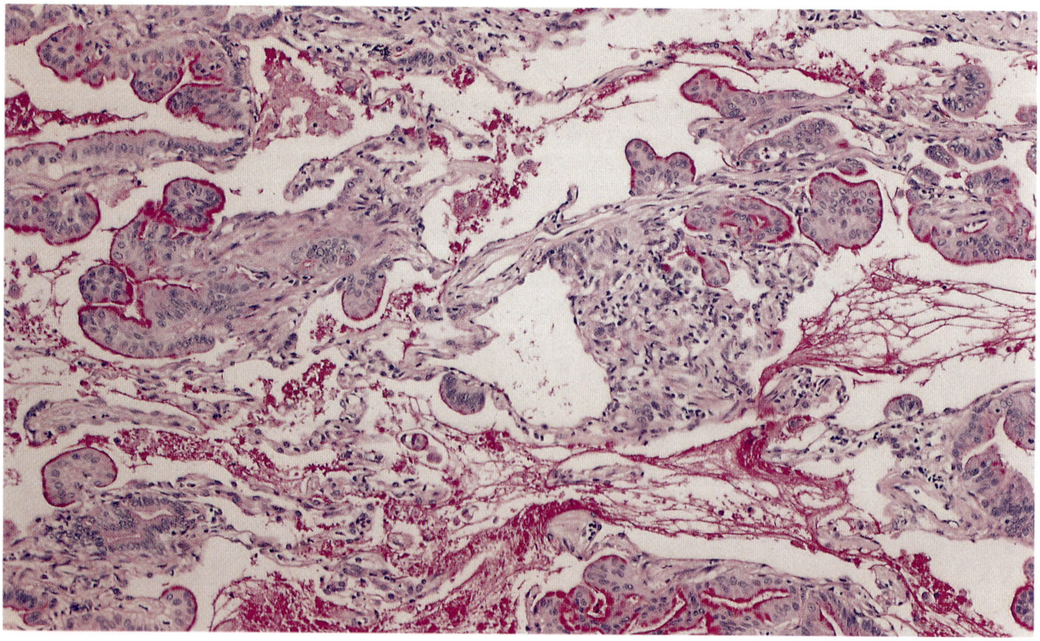

Descriptors: Newly formed textures with metastasis potential:

- epithelial growth pattern
- adenoid textures
- lining of tumor cells
- island of tumor cells
- mucus production
- homogeneous nuclear and cellular size
- infrequent mitoses
- absent or weak inflammatory infiltrates

Diagnosis: Bronchioloalveolar carcinoma (diffuse). (PAS, ×240)

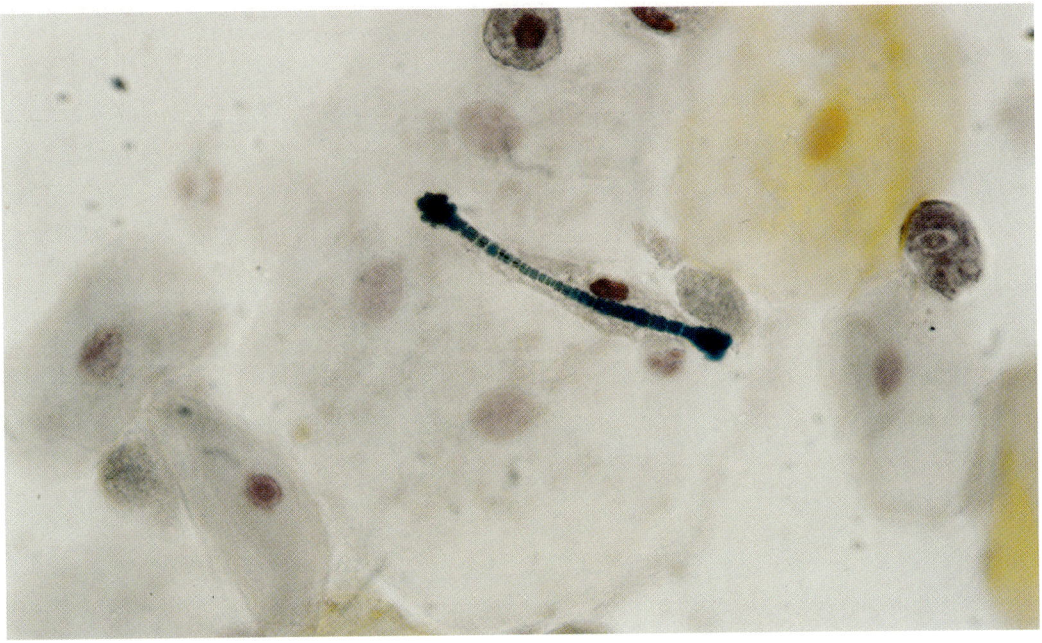

Descriptors: Lung parenchyma with altered structure:

- asbestos bodies (intraalveolar)
- macrophages

Diagnosis: Asbestos body. (Prussian blue, ×800)

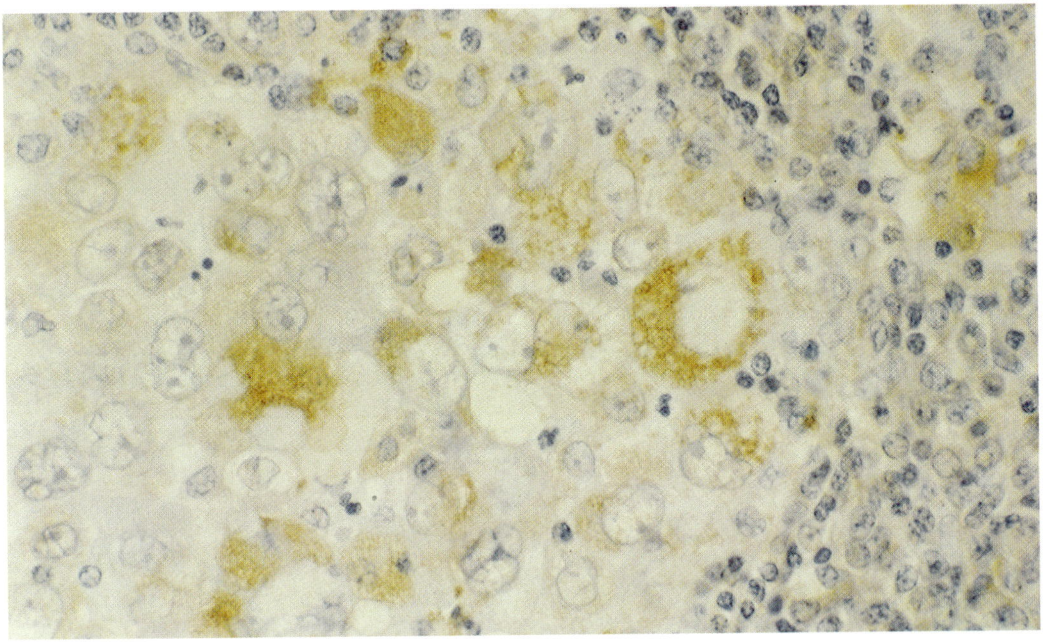

Descriptors: Newly formed textures with metastasis potential:

- epithelial growth pattern
- solid textures
- large tumor cells
- prominent nucleoli
- inhomogeneous nuclear and cellular size
- dense inflammatory infiltrates
- hormone receptors

Diagnosis: Large cell anaplastic carcinoma with positive staining to biotinylated testosteron. (ABC, ×600)

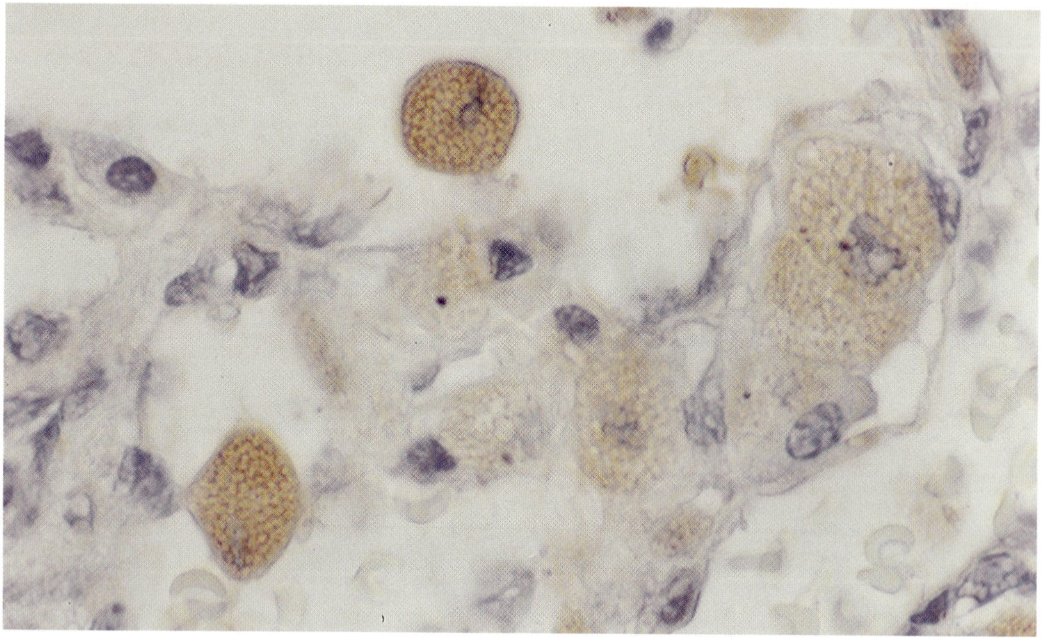

Descriptors: Lung parenchyma with altered structure:

- desquamation, hypertrophy, hyperplaisa and dysplasia of pneumocytes
- mononuclear inflammatory infiltrates

Diagnosis: Crohn's disease, altered endogenous lectins of macrophages and pneumocytes (N-acetyl-D-galactosamine-receptors). (ABC, ×800)

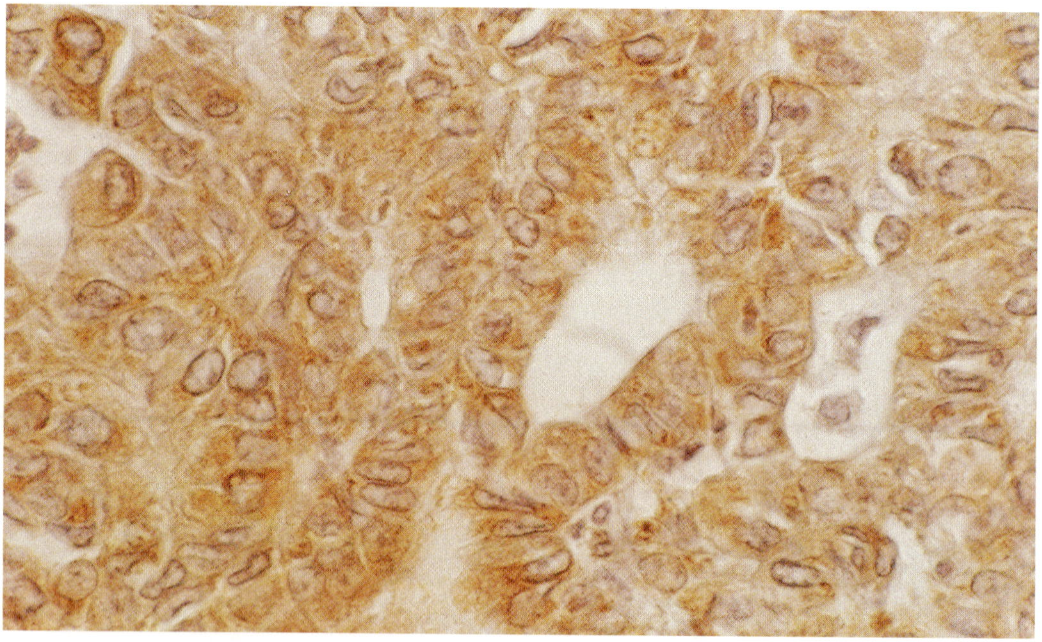

Descriptors: Newly formed textures with metastasis potential:

- epithelial growth pattern
- adenoid textures
- inhomogeneous nuclear and cellular size
- moderate number of mitoses
- prominent nucleoli
- absent or weak inflammatory infiltrates
- growth factor receptors (epidermal growth factor)

Diagnosis: Intrapulmonary metastasis of colon carcinoma, positive staining to biotinylated epidermal growth factor. (ABC, ×600)